Textbook of Veterinary Medicine

Textbook of Veterinary Medicine

Edited by **Mel Roth**

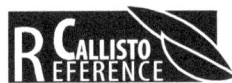

R CALLISTO REFERENCE

New York

Published by Callisto Reference,
106 Park Avenue, Suite 200,
New York, NY 10016, USA
www.callistoreference.com

Textbook of Veterinary Medicine
Edited by Mel Roth

International Standard Book Number: 978-1-63239-676-1 (Hardback)

Contents

Preface

This book explores all the important aspects of veterinary medicine in the present day scenario as well as its future prospects. It aims to shed light on some of the unexplored areas and recent researches of this discipline. Veterinary medicine primarily deals with prevention, diagnosis and treatment of diseases in animals. It also helps to prevent the spread of diseases from animals to human beings. Different approaches, evaluations, methodologies, and advanced studies have been included in this book. It will prove to be immensely beneficial to veterinary doctors, paraveterinary workers, students and researchers in this field.

This book is a comprehensive compilation of works of different researchers from varied parts of the world. It includes valuable experiences of the researchers with the sole objective of providing the readers (learners) with a proper knowledge of the concerned field. This book will be beneficial in evoking inspiration and enhancing the knowledge of the interested readers.

In the end, I would like to extend my heartiest thanks to the authors who worked with great determination on their chapters. I also appreciate the publisher's support in the course of the book. I would also like to deeply acknowledge my family who stood by me as a source of inspiration during the project.

Editor

Clinical and Breed Characteristics of Idiopathic Head Tremor Syndrome in 291 Dogs: A Retrospective Study

Linda G. Shell,[1] John Berezowski,[2,3] Mark Rishniw,[4] Belle M. Nibblett,[1] and Patrick Kelly[1]

[1]Department of Clinical Sciences, Ross University School of Veterinary Medicine (RUSVM),
 P.O. Box 334, Basseterre, Saint Kitts and Nevis
[2]Department of Biomedical Sciences, Ross University School of Veterinary Medicine (RUSVM),
 P.O. Box 334, Basseterre, Saint Kitts and Nevis
[3]Veterinary Public Health Institute, Swiss Veterinary Faculty, University of Bern, Hochschulstrasse 4, 3012 Bern, Switzerland
[4]Department of Clinical Studies, Cornell University, 602 Tower Road, Ithaca, NY 14853, USA

Correspondence should be addressed to Linda G. Shell; lshell@rossvet.edu.kn

Academic Editor: Pedro J. Ginel

Objective. To establish signalment and phenomenology of canine idiopathic head tremor syndrome (IHTS), an episodic head movement disorder of undetermined pathogenesis. *Design.* Retrospective case series. *Animals.* 291 dogs with IHTS diagnosed between 1999 and 2013. *Procedures.* Clinical information was obtained from an online community of veterinary information aggregation and exchange (Veterinary Information Network, 777 W Covell Boulevard, Davis, CA 95616) and conducted with their approval. Information on breed, sex, age of onset, tremor description, mentation during the event, effect of distractions and drugs, diagnostics, presence of other problems, and outcome was analyzed. *Results.* IHTS was found in 24 pure breeds. Bulldogs, Labrador Retrievers, Boxers, and Doberman Pinschers comprised 69%; mixed breeds comprised 17%. Average onset age was 29 months (range: 3 months to 12 years). First episode occurred before 48 months of age in 88%. Vertical (35%), horizontal (50%), and rotational (15%) movements were documented. Possible trigger events were found in 21%. Mentation was normal in 93%. Distractions abated the tremor in 87%. Most dogs did not respond to antiepileptic drugs. *Conclusions and Clinical Relevance.* This retrospective study documents IHTS in many breeds including Labrador Retrievers, Boxers, and mixed breeds.

1. Introduction

Canine idiopathic head tremor syndrome (IHTS), also sometimes referred to as episodic rapid repetitive myoclonus, is generally regarded as a benign condition manifesting as episodic uncontrolled head tremors that start and stop spontaneously. These head tremors have been reported to occur in "vertical" ("yes") or "horizontal" ("no") directions. Affected dogs appear alert during the tremors [1]. The diagnosis has been based on signalment, history, and characteristic head tremors as described above. Recent reports in the literature have characterized IHTS phenomenology in Doberman Pinschers [2] and English Bulldogs [3]. Although the cause of IHTS is unknown, affected Doberman Pinschers were traced to a common sire suggesting the condition may be inherited [1].

The veterinary literature, including neurology textbooks, does not contain significant information about IHTS for the practicing veterinarian. Affected dogs may initially be considered to have seizure activity, since this is the closest condition that might explain the signs. Thus, treatment with antiepileptic drugs (AEDs) may be attempted. Noting numerous cases of IHTS described by members of an online veterinary database (Veterinary Information Network, 777 W Covell Boulevard, Davis, CA 95616; this study was conducted with approval from Veterinary Information Network and its members), we sought to gain more information about IHTS by analyzing data from these cases. Specifically, we sought to document affected breeds, detail the character (duration and frequency) and direction of the head movement, investigate effects of stressful events and treatments on IHTS episodes, and determine whether or not the life span of affected dogs was affected.

2. Materials and Methods

Data on IHTS cases was obtained in two surveys.

2.1. Survey 1. Clinical information was reviewed from veterinarians who participate in an online community of veterinary information aggregation and exchange (Veterinary Information Network, 777 W Covell Boulevard, Davis, CA 95616: this study was conducted with approval from Veterinary Information Network and its members). Archived cases were searched for by key words: head tremor syndrome, head bob, head bobble, head bobbing, head bobbers, bobble head, bobble doll, shakes head yes, and shakes head no; these are all descriptors that investigators (LGS and MR) had observed veterinarians use to describe clinical signs of IHTS. Cases with at least one key word were evaluated by two investigators (LGS and BMN or PK) to confirm that the following inclusion criteria were met: characteristic description of head tremors associated with IHTS (up and down motions or side to side motions), absence of limb or truncal tremors and other signs of cerebellar origin, short duration (seconds to minutes) of head tremors, intermittent occurrence of head tremors, and lack of other neurological signs. Inclusion was further supported by the opinion of one or more veterinary neurologists who agreed that the description of signs suggested a diagnosis of IHTS.

From the written data and from the available videos of cases, we created a database containing details of age, breed, sex, age of onset, tremor description and direction, duration (in seconds/minutes), frequency and timing of events, mentation during the event, effect of distraction and types of distractors, and diagnostics performed.

2.2. Survey 2. An online survey of veterinarians identified additional cases of IHTS from which data was collected and reviewed (LGS and MR). In the survey, veterinarians were given a written description of IHTS, viewed a video of IHTS in a dog, and were asked to provide information (age of onset of tremor, breed, sex, tremor description including frequency, direction, etc.) from their medical charts if they had managed a case that clinically fit the description of IHTS. In addition to the information collected in survey one, additional information was obtained on body position during tremors (standing, sternal, and lateral), presence of behavioral problems, other diseases and seizures, history of littermates with signs, drugs administered prior to or during the tremor, and outcome.

2.3. Statistical Analysis. Wilcoxon Rank Sum Tests, Fischer's Exact Tests, and Chi Squared tests were used to compare groups. All analyses were performed using standard statistical software (R: a language and environment for statistical computing: Version i386.3.1.0. R Core Team (2014); R Foundation for Statistical Computing, Vienna, Austria; URL http://www.R-project.org/). A value of $P < 0.05$ was considered significant.

TABLE 1: Breed distribution of 291 dogs with IHTS.

Breed	Percentage (number)
Bulldog	37% (107)
Mixed	16% (48)
Boxer	13% (37)
Labrador Retriever	11% (33)
Doberman Pinscher	8% (24)
Staffordshire Terrier	3% (9)
Basset Hound	1% (3)
Boston Terrier	1% (3)
Golden Retriever	1% (3)
Greyhound	1% (3)
Parson Russell Terrier	1% (3)
Beagle	0.6% (2)
Great Dane	0.6% (2)
Miniature Schnauzer	0.6% (2)
Vizsla	0.6% (2)
Australian Shepherd	0.3% (1)
Border Collie	0.3% (1)
English Springer Spaniel	0.3% (1)
German Shorthaired Pointer	0.3% (1)
Papillon	0.3% (1)
Pembroke Welsh Corgi	0.3% (1)
Redbone Coonhound	0.3% (1)
Rhodesian Ridgeback	0.3% (1)
Shetland Sheepdog	0.3% (1)
Standard Poodle	0.3% (1)
Total	100% (291)

3. Results

3.1. Study Population. Of 197 potential cases of IHTS reported in the online database between January 1999 and April 2013, descriptive information and data were sufficient to meet the inclusion criteria for 137 cases and of these, 50 had accompanying videos which were reviewed and confirmed to be representative of IHTS. Of the 174 responses from the online survey, 154 responses also met the inclusion criteria and were included in the study. Data obtained in the two surveys were very similar and hence were combined for the analyses reported below (291 cases).

3.2. Breed Data. Table 1 presents the breed data. Most dogs with IHTS were purebreds (84%; 243/291) with Bulldogs being the most commonly reported (37%, 107/291) followed by mixed breeds (16%, 48/291), Boxers (13%, 37/291), Labrador Retrievers (11%, 33/291), and Doberman Pinschers (8%, 24/291). Videos 1, 2, and 3 show the head tremors in a miniature Schnauzer, a Labrador Retriever, and a Boxer, respectively.

3.3. Age of Onset. Age of onset was available for 280 cases and varied from 3 to 144 months. Mean and median ages were 29 and 25 months, respectively. The majority (88%) of dogs had

TABLE 2: Direction of head tremor based on breeds affected.

Breed	Horizontal	Vertical	Rotary	Total
Bulldog	41% (32)	42% (33)	17% (13)	78
Boxer	59% (17)	34% (10)	7% (2)	29
Labrador Retriever	44% (11)	44% (11)	12% (3)	25
Doberman Pinscher	48% (10)	33% (7)	19% (4)	21
Other pure breeds	49% (16)	33% (11)	18% (6)	33
Mixed	67% (29)	19% (8)	14% (6)	43
Total	50% (115)	35% (80)	15% (34)	229

TABLE 3: Duration of head tremors.

Time	Percent (number)	Cumulative %
0 to 0.5 min	21% (52)	21
0.5 to 1.0 min	20% (48)	41
1-2 min	18% (43)	58
2–5 min	24% (59)	82
5–60 min	15% (37)	98
1-2 hr	1% (3)	99
>2 hr	1% (3)	100
Total	100% (245)	

TABLE 4: Frequency of occurrence of head tremors.

Frequency category	Percent (number)
Continuously over 12–24 hours	1% (3)
Multiple times/day	26% (65)
Once a day	9% (21)
Every few days	25% (61)
Weekly	7% (18)
Monthly	9% (23)
Quarterly	4% (9)
Less frequently than every 3-4 months	10% (24)
Sporadically	9% (22)
Total	100% (246)

their first episode of IHTS before 48 months of age. Bulldogs had a statistically significantly earlier age of onset (average 24 months) compared to the averages for the other breeds (32 months) ($P = 0.017$).

3.4. Sex. Overall, fewer females (41%; 115/279) were documented with IHTS than males (59%; 164/279). The percent of females varied by breed from a low of 27% females among Doberman Pinschers to a high of 51% in Bulldogs ($P = 0.158$).

3.5. Description of Head Tremor

3.5.1. Direction of Head Tremor. Horizontal head motions ("no") occurred in half the dogs (115/229). Rotational motions were the least common, found only in 15% of the dogs (Table 2). There were no significant differences in the horizontal and vertical directions between the five most commonly affected breeds: Bulldogs, mixed breeds, Boxers, Labradors, and Dobermans ($P = 0.306$). Video 1 shows more of a rotational type of tremor in a miniature Schnauzer See Video 1 in Supplementary Materials available online at http://dx.doi.org/10.1155/2015/165463. Video 2 shows vertical head tremors in a Boxer and video 3 shows horizontal tremors in a Labrador Retriever.

3.5.2. Mentation. Ninety-three percent (246/264) of cases were considered to be alert or responsive during the episode. Only a few veterinarians described their patients' mentation as confused or disoriented (12), anxious (3), or lethargic (3).

3.5.3. Duration of Tremor. In the majority of affected dogs (82%; 202/245) the tremors lasted less than 5 minutes (Table 3) with only 15% (37/245) lasting between 5 minutes and 1 hour. Three dogs were reported to have tremors occurring continuously over 12–48 hours.

3.5.4. Frequency of Occurrence. Frequency data is presented in Table 4. The most commonly reported occurrences were multiple times/day (26%; 65/246) and every few days (25%; 61/246). However 22% (55/246) of the cases occurred infrequently based on combined results for the categories of "sporadically", "quarterly," and "less frequently than 3-4 months."

3.5.5. Body Position and Relationship to Rest. Affected dogs could be found in standing (41 cases), sitting (34 cases), or sternal (40 cases) positions at the onset of the tremor. Tremors did occur in lateral recumbency (5) but less commonly. Additional unprompted information indicated that head tremors were observed while the dog was resting, sleeping or waking from sleep in 66 cases.

3.5.6. Effect of Distractions. In 87% (142/163) of dogs, distractions caused the tremor to disappear for an undisclosed time. Distractors included voluntary turning of the head to one side or the other, calling the dog by its name, offering it food, making a sound so that the dog turned its head, and asking the dog to perform a task. More than one distractor was frequently reported as being helpful.

3.5.7. Time of Day That Tremor Was Observed. Most veterinarians (76%) did not have information about the time of day the tremors occurred (220/291 cases). For 71 dogs, a time of day was known: 58% (41/71) had tremors occurring in the evening/night hours, 34% (24/71) in the daytime hours, and 8% (6/71) during both day and night hours.

3.6. Predisposing Factors

3.6.1. Concurrent Medications. Forty-four percent (67/154) of affected dogs were receiving medications at the time of onset of IHTS. For the majority (85%; 57/67), these medications were heartworm and flea control products; the rest of medications were prednisolone, diphenhydramine, tramadol, antibiotics, fludrocortisone, oral cyclosporine, and various eye medications.

3.6.2. Concurrent Illness, Trauma, or Disease. Concurrent illness, trauma, or stressful events were noted in 21% of patients (33/154). Traumatic events (hit by car, dog fight), surgeries (castration, skin tumor removal, and cherry eye repair), and medical conditions (allergies; upper or lower respiratory infection; gastrointestinal, skin, or urinary tract infection; heart failure; demodicosis; heartworm disease; bee sting; papilloma; and immune mediated hemolytic anemia) had been diagnosed within a week (18 cases) or a month (6 cases) of the IHTS onset. Nine cases experienced a stressful event such as moving or a change in household members, travel, kennel confinement, or shock collar use. Specific triggers (gastrointestinal upset, shock collar training, and thunderstorm phobia) for repeated IHTS signs were identified in 3 cases.

3.6.3. Concurrent Behavioral Issues. History of behavioral problems was positive in 13% (20/153) of cases either prior to (10 cases), concurrently with (3 cases), or after (7 cases) the onset of IHTS. Behavioral problems included fear or aggression (8), thunderstorm phobia (4), separation anxiety (3), and unspecified problems (5).

3.6.4. Family History. Familial history was unknown for 89% (137/154) of cases, reported positive for IHTS in 4/154 (2.6%), and reported negative for IHTS in 13. Of the 4 cases with familial information, the known affected dog had littermates (2) or unspecified family members (2) with IHTS.

3.7. Outcome

3.7.1. Treatment. Treatment was documented for 43/254 (17%) dogs. A variety of medications were used including bromide (5), phenobarbital (20), diazepam (12), and calcium carbonate (3). Less commonly used treatments included various antibiotics, corticosteroids, supplements (fish oil, antioxidants), clonazepam, and diphenhydramine. Veterinarians reported possible positive responses for oral maintenance phenobarbital (5/20), diazepam (3/12), calcium carbonate (1/3), and fish oil (1/1).

3.7.2. Neurological Diagnostics. Results of cerebrospinal fluid analysis and advanced brain imaging were normal in 8 of 15 cases evaluated and unknown for 7 cases.

3.7.3. Development of Other Neurological Disorders. Other neurological disorders did not develop in the majority (95%; 146/154) of dogs after the onset of IHTS. The neurological signs or disorders that developed in 8 dogs (5%) were diverse and were comprised of seizures (3) and one case of each of the following metronidazole-induced ataxia that resolved when medication was discontinued, degenerative myelopathy, idiopathic Horner's syndrome, cervical spondylopathy, and episodic collapse. Of the 3 cases that developed seizure activity, one developed it 9 years after IHTS was recognized; brain neoplasia was suspected but not proven. Another case developed seizures 2 months after onset of IHTS and

subsequent results of spinal fluid analysis and brain magnetic resonance imaging studies were normal.

3.7.4. Long Term Outcome. Of the 135 dogs for which long term data was available, 91% were still alive; the remaining 9% had died or been euthanized for reasons unrelated to IHTS. All or most of the clinical signs of IHTS had resolved in 67% (90/135) while 24% (33/135) continued to have intermittent clinical signs.

4. Discussion

Currently the diagnosis of IHTS is a clinical one based on signalment (breed disposition), history (no exposure to toxins, intermittent nature of signs, etc.), lack of concurrent neurological and physical signs that might explain the tremors, and presence of characteristic head tremors occurring sporadically and of short duration. No diagnostic tests have been identified to date that allow a more specific diagnosis of IHTS. Likewise, no other diseases have been described to produce the same signs as IHTS. Only a few IHTS cases have been documented to have advanced diagnostics (spinal fluid analysis, brain scans) and in those no abnormalities were reported [2, 3]. Therefore, the diagnosis of IHTS in this study was based on inclusion criteria that fit with IHTS as has been defined in other published studies [2, 3]. The authors acknowledge the inherent weakness of relying upon case descriptions and survey data but the clinical signs and historical data were sufficiently characteristic enough to hypothesize a diagnosis of IHTS and to eliminate cases that were not IHTS.

While previous studies centered on Bulldogs [2] and Doberman Pinschers [3], with an anecdotal report that Bulldog and Boxer breeds were commonly affected [1], we found IHTS in 24 pure breeds and in a substantial number of mixed breed dogs (17%). Although there are no data on relative breed prevalence in the US, it did seem that certain breeds appeared overrepresented, mainly, Bulldogs (37%), Boxers (13%), Labrador Retrievers (11%), and Doberman Pinschers (8%). Our scant familial information and the propensity for certain breeds to be affected suggest a possible hereditary basis to the condition which is consistent with the report that affected Doberman Pinschers could be traced to a common sire [1].

Most dogs in our study had onset of signs at a mature age with 88% occurring before 4 years of age. This onset agrees with prior reports that suggested onset age was usually between 6 months and 3 years [1–3]. However it is important to note that age of onset varied from as early as 3 months of age to as old as 12 years.

The previously described phenomenology of IHTS in Bulldogs [3] and Doberman Pinschers [2] is generally similar to our findings across 24 breeds and mixed breed dogs. Generally, IHTS presents as head tremors in a vertical, horizontal, or rotary direction, usually in mature dogs under 4 years of age. Episodes are spontaneous in onset and sporadic in number and occurrence. Duration is variable from seconds to several hours but most episodes do not last longer than

5 minutes. Tremors can occur while the dog is standing, resting, or sleeping. Most dogs are alert during an episode but some are anxious or lethargic. No drug therapy was identified that influenced the condition.

A number of new phenomenological findings emerged in our study. First, we documented the presence of a rotational head tremor in 15% of cases. This might be similar to the 9.2% of affected Dobermans that Wolf et al. [2] described with motions in both vertical and horizontal directions, which could be construed as rotational [2]. The significance of direction of head tremors is unknown. Second, getting the dog's attention so that it moved its head seemed to make the tremor disappear or cease momentarily in 87% of our cases. Most of the distractors reported in this study as well as those in Wolf et al.'s [2] study would result in mental stimulation or a change in neck position. Why the head tremor would cease with a change in neck position is unknown but warrants further investigation into one proposed theory that IHTS involves the stretch reflex mechanism [4]. Finally, although the data were limited, there was more of a trend toward evening or nighttime occurrence. However, this could be explained by the time of day that most owners are home and interacting with or observing their pet.

The relationship of the head tremor with body/neck posture, rest, the sleep/wake cycle, and neck movement needs further investigation. In the Bulldog study, IHTS episodes occurred predominately at rest [3]. Likewise, many of the Doberman Pinschers were reported to be reclining or dozing when the IHTS started [2]. Dogs in our study were reported to manifest IHTS while resting or being in stationary positions (sitting, standing, or being in sternal or lateral recumbency). The condition did not appear to be initiated by movement.

This study confirmed that the majority of cases do not have any other neurological or behavioral problems. However, stressful events or concurrent illness or trauma, occurring predominantly within a week of the tremor onset, was noted in about one-fifth of our cases. In prior studies, stressful events were associated with IHTS in 46.7% of Dobermans and in 7% of Bulldogs [2, 3]. Thus underlying diseases and environmental stressors should be investigated in any dog presenting with signs of IHTS.

Outcome obtained from 135 cases indicated that the majority of affected dogs were still alive (91%) and that none had died or been euthanized because of IHTS. Thus IHTS is not a life-threatening disease. Furthermore the intermittent head tremors eventually disappeared in the majority of affected dogs (67%) although the survey did not gather data on the time it took for signs to resolve. One might assume that if underlying diseases and environmental stressors are addressed, clinical signs may resolve. Intermittent signs were reported, however, to occur in some dogs.

Focal seizure activity has been mentioned as a possible cause of IHTS [2] but currently there is little to no data to support that possibility. Other authors [4] have noted that AEDs do not appear effective in treating this disorder; that appeared to be the case for the few dogs that were medicated with maintenance AEDs in our study. We acknowledge, however, that, given the sporadic nature and short duration of clinical signs, it would be difficult to access AED efficacy;

likewise, for the same reasons, it would be difficult to justify using AEDs in these patients unless more obvious generalized seizure activity was documented.

Unfortunately, tremors have many possible causes. In humans, tremors are the most common type of movement disorders [5–7] but tremors can also occur with stereotypies, tics, and psychogenic disorders [8, 9]. Tremors can also be a part of other movement disorders such as essential tremor syndrome, cervical dystonia [10], and paroxysmal dyskinesias [11]. However, tremors associated with these movement disorders are not paroxysmal, nor is the head a commonly affected area. Thus at the present time, IHTS does not appear to be similar to known movement disorders in humans.

In summary, our study shows that IHTS can be found in a wide range of dog breeds. The data we collected more clearly defines the clinical presentation and signs. IHTS is a benign condition that frequently resolves spontaneously and is nonresponsive to treatment with a wide range of conventional drugs. The condition is of concern to dog owners, however, and further studies appear warranted to establish its pathogenesis.

Disclosure

This paper is presented partially in abstract form at the 26th Annual ESVN-ECVN Symposium, Paris, France, September 2013.

Conflict of Interests

The authors declare that there is no conflict of interests regarding the publication of this paper.

Acknowledgments

The authors thank Veterinary Information Network and the many veterinarian members for their contributions to this study and RUSVM veterinary medicine students who assisted in verifying data. It is supported in part by RUSVM, Center for Integrative Mammalian Research.

References

[1] A. De Lahunta, E. N. Glass, and M. Kent, "Classifying involuntary muscle contractions," *Compendium on Continuing Education for the Practicing Veterinarian*, vol. 28, no. 7, pp. 516–529, 2006.

[2] M. Wolf, A. Bruehschwein, C. Sauter-Louis, A. C. Sewell, and A. Fischer, "An inherited episodic head tremor syndrome in Doberman pinscher dogs," *Movement Disorders*, vol. 26, no. 13, pp. 2381–2386, 2011.

[3] J. Guevar, S. DeDecker, L. M. L. Van Ham, A. Fischer, and H. A. Volk, "Idiopathic head tremor in English bulldogs," *Movement Disorders*, vol. 29, no. 2, pp. 191–194, 2014.

[4] A. Delahunta and E. Glass, "Upper motor neuron," in *Veterinary Neuroanatomy and Clinical Neurology*, pp. 192–220, Saunders, St. Louis, Mo, USA, 3rd edition, 2009.

[5] G. Grimaldi and M. Manto, "Definition of tremor," in *Mechanisms and Emerging Therapies in Tremor Disorders*, G. Grimaldi and M. Manto, Eds., pp. 3–10, 2012.

[6] P. Crawford and E. E. Zimmerman, "Differentiation and diagnosis of tremor," *American Family Physician*, vol. 83, no. 6, pp. 697–702, 2011.

[7] S. Smaga, "Tremor," *American Family Physician*, vol. 68, no. 8, pp. 1545–1553, 2003.

[8] E. F. Augustine and J. W. Mink, "Tic disorders and stereotypies," in *Oxford Textbook of Movement Disorders*, D. Burn, Ed., pp. 247–254, 2013.

[9] S. G. Reich, "Psychogenic movement disorders," *Seminars in Neurology*, vol. 26, no. 3, pp. 289–296, 2006.

[10] C. Godeiro-Junior, A. C. Felicio, P. C. Aguiar, V. Borges, S. M. A. Silva, and H. B. Ferraz, "Head tremor in patients with cervical dystonia: different outcome?" *Arquivos de Neuro-Psiquiatria*, vol. 66, no. 4, pp. 805–808, 2008.

[11] K. P. Bhatia, "Familial (idiopathic) paroxysmal dyskinesias: an update," *Seminars in Neurology*, vol. 21, no. 1, pp. 69–74, 2001.

Serological Survey of Foot-and-Mouth Disease Virus in Buffaloes (*Syncerus caffer*) in Zambia

T. K. W. Sikombe,[1,2] A. S. Mweene,[1] John Muma,[1] C. Kasanga,[3] Y. Sinkala,[1,4] F. Banda,[2] M. Mulumba,[5] E. M. Fana,[6] C. Mundia,[7] and M. Simuunza[1]

[1]*Department of Disease Control, School of Veterinary Medicine, University of Zambia, P.O. Box 32379, Lusaka, Zambia*
[2]*Central Veterinary Research Institute, P.O. Box 33980, Lusaka, Zambia*
[3]*Faculty of Veterinary Medicine, Sokoine University of Agriculture, P.O. Box 3021, Morogoro, Tanzania*
[4]*National Livestock Epidemiology and Information Centre, P.O. Box 30041, Lusaka, Zambia*
[5]*Southern African Development Community Secretariat, SADC House, Plot No. 54385, Central Business District, Private Bag 0095, Gaborone, Botswana*
[6]*Botswana Vaccine Institute, Private Bag 0031, Gaborone, Botswana*
[7]*Department of Veterinary Services, Southern African Development Community, Trans-Boundary Animal Disease Section, Ministry of Agriculture and Livestock, P.O. Box 50060, Lusaka, Zambia*

Correspondence should be addressed to T. K. W. Sikombe; tingiyasikombe@yahoo.com

Academic Editor: Timm C. Harder

A study was conducted to determine the serotypes of foot-and-mouth disease viruses (FMDV) circulating in African buffaloes (*Syncerus caffer*) from selected areas in Zambia. Sera and probang samples were collected between 2011 and 2012 and analysed for presence of antibodies against FMDV while probang samples were used to isolate the FMDV by observing cytopathic effect (CPE). Samples with CPE were further analysed using antigen ELISA. High FMD seroprevalence was observed and antibodies to all the three Southern African Territories (SAT) serotypes were detected in four study areas represented as follows: SAT2 was 72.7 percent; SAT1 was 62.6 percent; and SAT3 was 26.2 percent. Mixed infections accounted for 68.6 percent of those that were tested positive. For probang samples, CPE were observed in three of the samples, while the antigen ELISA results showed positivity and for SAT1 ($n = 1$) and SAT2 ($n = 2$). It is concluded that FMDV is highly prevalent in Zambian buffaloes which could play an important role in the epidemiology of the disease. Therefore livestock reared at interface with the game parks should be included in all routine FMDV vaccination programmes.

1. Introduction

Foot-and-mouth disease (FMD) is a highly infectious viral disease of domestic and wild cloven hoofed animals [1–3]. The disease is caused by the foot-and-mouth disease virus (FMDV) of the genus *Aphthovirus* belonging to the family Picornaviridae. The first report of FMD in Zambia dated from 1933 in Barotseland (now Western Province). Typing of the virus from Zambian FMD outbreaks began in 1948 when the Southern African Territories (SAT) immunological types of FMD virus were recognised [4]. Currently, FMD is endemic in some parts of Northern and Muchinga Provinces along areas bordering Tanzania and in southern border areas between Zambia and Zimbabwe, Botswana and Namibia and along the Kafue and Zambezi flood plains which are also bordered by parts of Kafue National Park. These areas are densely populated with domestic and game animals which are usually in contact for most part of the year. The FMD scenario in Zambia is complicated by the presence of a stable wildlife reservoir, the African buffaloes "*Syncerus caffer*," and traditional practice of transhumant grazing, where cattle farmers trek their animals to wildlife sanctuaries in search of water and pasture [5–7] and where there are several viruses with high sequence diversity due to the nature of

FMDV [8, 9]. African buffaloes are known to be carriers of FMDV and as such contact exposes cattle to the risk of being infected. It has also been reported that FMD may circulate undetected in vaccinated cattle herds and in some indigenous breeds reared in areas where FMD is endemic [10].

Zambia has continued to experience isolated outbreaks of FMD such as those that occurred in Namwala in 2005 [11] and in 2008 [12]; Itezhi-Tezhi in 2006 [13] and in 2008 [12]; and Monze and Mazabuka in 2007 [14] and in 2008 [12]. These outbreaks were considered as reoccurrences of the 2004 SAT1 outbreak (Yona Sinkala, personal communications, 2012). In December 2007, SAT2 FMDV outbreaks occurred in Sesheke district in Western Province and Kazungula district of Southern Province [12]. The disease spilled over in 2008 and spread to Senanga, Mongu, Shang'ombo, and Kalabo districts of Western Province [12]. In 2009, there was an outbreak in Mbala, Northern Province, where SAT1 was isolated [15]. In 2010, there was another outbreak in Mbala district, which spread to Chinsali district, and serotype O was isolated [16]. In 2012, Mbala district and Kazungula/Livingstone experienced further outbreaks, where SAT2 and SAT1 were isolated, respectively [17, 18].

FMD is endemic in Zambia and continues to impact negatively on the livestock industry development. Little understanding of the epidemiology of FMDV has led to the continuous occurrences of the disease in Zambia. Cattle movement and trade restrictions resulting from occurrence of this disease have led to severe negative impacts for pastoral and agropastoral families who are most reliant on livestock products for food and economic security [19]. In addition trade restrictions imposed by other countries mean that the country is not able to participate fully in trade of livestock and its byproducts regionally and internationally.

FMD vaccination campaigns are conducted biannually in most parts of Zambia, where the disease is endemic. Although vaccination offers a potential solution, there are questions surrounding the efficacy of the vaccines used since there are many different serotypes (SAT1, SAT2, and SAT3, type O and type A) of FMD viruses reported to be circulating in Zambia [4, 20]. Due to this the vaccines used may not sufficiently match the field strains circulating that often even their homologous potency is unknown and the cold chain crucial for the success of any FMD vaccination is difficult to maintain. Trivalent vaccines (SAT1, SAT2, and SAT3) were used annually in Southern, Central, and Western Provinces of Zambia before 2006. After 2006, bivalent vaccines (SAT1 and SAT2) were used in Southern, Central, and Western Provinces of Zambia where our study was based, while bivalent vaccines (SAT1 and SAT2 or SAT1 and type A or SAT1 and type O) have been used in Northern and Muchinga Provinces of Zambia, bordering Tanzania; unfortunately this area was not covered by our study. This study therefore was conducted to determine the infection status and FMD virus (FMDV) serotypes circulating in buffaloes in Zambia. Thus the epidemiological situation of FMDV will be discussed.

2. Material and Methods

2.1. Study Area. The study was carried out in areas located in National Parks (NP) and Game Management Areas

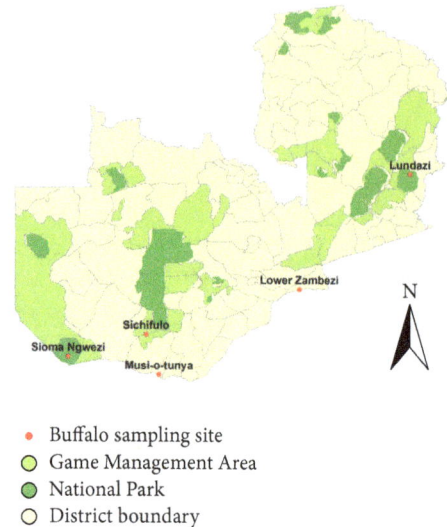

FIGURE 1: Map of Zambia with sampling sites in Game Management Areas (GMA) and National Parks (NP).

(GMA) in Zambia (Figure 1). Five locations were selected for this study which included Mosi-oa-tunya (S: 17°52.370′; E: 025°50053′), Sichifulo (S: 16°49.470′; E: 025°29.482′), Lower Zambezi (S: 15°38.384′; E: 029°36.756′), Lundazi (S: 12°17.157′; E: 033°10.836′), and Sioma (S: 17°08.8900′; E: 23°65.3367′). These areas were purposively selected because of the presence of interactions between cattle and wildlife resulting from the transhumant cattle husbandry practice where traditional cattle farmers bring their livestock for grazing into wildlife habitats in search of greener pastures and water. These areas are among the major ecosystems of buffaloes in Zambia. Luangwa National Park has the highest density of buffaloes in Zambia (Chuma Simukonda, personal communications, 2011). However, cattle-wildlife interactions are more pronounced in the Kafue flats where FMD outbreaks occur frequently [5].

2.2. Study Design. This was a cross-sectional survey carried out from 2011 to 2012 under a special research licence provided by the Zambia Wildlife Authority (ZAWA). It was part of a wider survey undertaken by the Southern African Development Community Transboundary Animal Diseases (SADC TADs) disease surveillance programme. The licence approved sampling of 25 buffaloes from each of the five study areas (Mosi-oa-tunya, Sichifulo, Lower Zambezi, Lundazi, and Sioma) (DVLD/3/22/1: National Parks, Game Reserves and Wildlife). Therefore, we targeted to sample 125 animals.

2.3. Sample Collection. Targeted animals were buffaloes aged between six months and six years. This was done to exclude young animals that still had maternal antibodies and those older animals that were no longer prone to infection. The age range of the buffalo was determined by the protrusions of the horns based on aerial view first and before sampling the age range was determined by checking the horns and dentition [21]. Animals were first immobilised through remotely injecting chemical anaesthetic agent, etorphine hydrochloride (M99, Immobilon; Novartis, South Africa).

From the immobilised animals, about 8 mL of blood was collected from all the 99 buffaloes through the jugular vein puncture using a sterile vacutainer needle into plain vacutainer tubes. The blood was left to clot overnight at room temperature and then centrifuged at 2500 rpm for 5 minutes to separate the serum. Sera were stored at −20°C until needed for laboratory analysis.

Probang samples were collected from 49 buffaloes using probang cups as recommended in the OIE Terrestrial Manual [22]. The collected probang samples were mixed with FMDV transport media (composed of 0.08 M phosphate buffer containing 0.01% bovine serum albumin, 0.002% phenol red, 1000 units/mL penicillin, 100 units/mL mycostatin, 100 units neomycin, and 50 units/mL polymyxin and adjusted to pH 7.2) [22] in the ratio of 1 : 3 in a conical tube after which the mixture was transferred into a cryotube. The cryotube containing probang sample was then put into a liquid nitrogen tank. Probang cups were disinfected using citric acid (0.2%, wt/vol) and rinsed three times in water and then in PBS between samplings. Probang samples were stored in liquid nitrogen or in the freezer at −70°C in the laboratory awaiting treating and passaging. Furthermore, information on age and sex was recorded and latitude and longitude coordinates were collected with a handheld GPS device (nüvi 205 series; Garmin, USA).

After sampling, the immobilised buffaloes were revived by injection with diprenorphine (M5050, Revivon; Novartis, South Africa). All the samples were collected and processed following World Reference Laboratory (WRL) and World Organisation for Animal Health (Office International des Epizooties (OIE)) guidelines [10].

2.4. Sample Analysis. Detection of antibodies against FMDV in sera was done at Central Veterinary Research Institute (CVRI) in Lusaka and Botswana Vaccine Institute (BVI) using the liquid phase blocking ELISA (Institute for Animal Health, Pirbright Laboratory, UK) technique for the detection of antibodies against FMDV in sera as described by [23] and the PrioCHECK FMDV-NS test (Prionics Lelystad B.V., Netherlands), a blocking ELISA that can measure antibody level to 3ABC nonstructural proteins [24].

The probang samples were treated and passaged in RM monolayer cell cultures and then examined for cytopathic effect (CPE). If no CPE was detected after 48 hours, the cells were frozen and thawed, used to inoculate fresh cell cultures, and examined for CPE for another 48 hours. Some field viruses may require several passages before they become adapted [22]. In antigen ELISA (Institute for Animal Health, Pirbright Laboratory, UK) we tested the supernatants of CPE positive cell cultures inoculated with probang samples in order to confirm the specificity of the CPE and to serotype the isolate. The antigen ELISA kit was based on a standard indirect sandwich ELISA technique to determine the presence of FMDV antigens in samples as described by [22].

2.5. Data Analysis. Data was stored in basic Excel format for easy handling and storage. The data was transferred to SPSS 16.0 for statistical analysis. Proportion of positive

sera, with the 95% confidence intervals (CI) on both LPBE and PrioCHECK FMDV-NS test, were estimated. The associations between categorical variables and the ELISA tests results were evaluated using Fisher's exact test, while Kappa test was used to evaluate the agreement between the LPBE and PrioCHECK FMDV-NS test cross-tabulation results. p values <0.05 were considered statistically significant. Spatial mapping of the distribution of FMD in the study areas was done using ArcView_GIS (Environmental Systems Resource Institute, 1992–1999 ArcView 3.2, Redlands, CA).

3. Results

3.1. Serology Results

3.1.1. LPBE Test. A total of 99 serum samples were tested and the results are shown in Table 1. The overall FMD prevalence based on LPBE SAT serotype results was 92.9 percent (95% CI = 87.8–98.0). The SAT1 prevalence was highest in Lower Zambezi and Lundazi (88.0%, 95% CI = 68.8–97.4), while no animals tested positive to SAT1 serotypes in Sioma National Park. There was a significant difference in SAT1 prevalence among the sampling sites ($p = 0.001$). SAT2 prevalence was highest in Lundazi where all animals tested positive (100%, 95% CI = 83.3–100), with no animals testing positive in Sioma. There was a significant difference in prevalence among the sampling sites ($p = 0.001$). SAT3 prevalence was highest in Sichifulo (50%, 95% CI = 27.2–72.8), with no animals testing positive in Sioma. There was a significant difference in SAT3 prevalence among the sampling sites ($p = 0.001$). All the buffaloes sampled (100%, 95% CI = 83.3–100) from Lower Zambezi and Lundazi were positive to antibodies against FMDV on the LPBE test and all those from Lundazi were positive to at least (100%, 95% CI = 83.3–100) two serotypes.

The few calves (age ranging from six months to eight months) that were sampled were all from Sioma and were all negative for FMDV SAT antibodies. The highest prevalence according to age range was in the 1-2-year category of which all were positive for antibodies against FMDV. In the 3-4-year age category, 93.1% were positive for antibodies against FMDV, while, in the 5-6-year age category, all the samples were positive for FMDV antibodies. There was no significant difference in SAT serotypes prevalence between the different age groups ($p > 0.05$). Similarly, there was no significant difference in the prevalence of SAT serotypes between male and female buffaloes ($p > 0.05$).

3.1.2. PrioCHECK FMDV-NS Test. A total of 99 serum samples were tested on the assay. FMD overall prevalence, based on the PrioCHECK FMDV-NS ELISA test which detects antibodies to nonstructural viral proteins, was high, 84.8% (95% CI = 77.2–91.5). The prevalence according to area of sampling was as follows: Lower Zambezi ($n = 25$), 96% (95% CI = 88.3–103.7); Lundazi ($n = 25$), 100% (95% CI = 100–100); Mosi-oa-tunya ($n = 25$), 80% (95% CI = 64.3–95.7); and Sichifulo ($n = 20$), 75% (95% CI = 56.0–94.0). The few calves (age ranging from six months to eight months) that were sampled were all from Sioma and were all negative

TABLE 1: Seroprevalence of FMDV by LPBE SAT.

Study area NP/GMA	Number tested	SAT serotype			Overall prevalence %	Mixed infection %
		SAT1 %	SAT2 %	SAT3 %		
Lower Zambezi	25	88.0 (68.8–97.4)	84.0 (63.9–95.5)	8.0 (0.98–26)	100.0 (83.3–100)	84.0 (63.9–95.5)
Lundazi	25	88.0 (68.8–97.4)	100.0 (83.3–100)	12.0 (2.5–31.2)	100.0 (83.3–100)	100.0 (83.3–100)
Mosi-oa-tunya	25	32.0 (14.9–53.5)	76.0 (59.3–92.7)	44.0 (24.4–65.1)	92.0 (74.0–99.9)	60.0 (38.7–78.9)
Sichifulo	20	45.0 (23.1–68.3)	35.0 (15.4–59.2)	50.0 (27.2–72.8)	95.0 (75.1–99.9)	35.0 (15.4–59.2)
Sioma	4	0	0	0	0	0

TABLE 2: Prevalence of LPBE results, mixed infection, and PrioCHECK FMDV-NS test results in relation to age.

Age category	n	Prevalence (95% CI)—LPBE	Mixed infection	Prevalence (95% CI)—PrioCHECK FMDV-NS
Less than 1 year	4	0	0	0
1-2 years	37	100 (100-100)	64.9 (57.6–72.2)	100 (100-100)
3-4 years	49	93.9 (87.2–100)	87.7 (78.1–97.4)	85.7 (75.9–95.5)
5-6 years	9	100 (100-100)	88.9 (87.1–90.7)	100 (100-100)
p value		0.413	0.497	0.451

TABLE 3: Prevalence of LPBE results, mixed infection, and PrioCHECK FMDV-NS results in buffalo according to sex category.

Sex	n	Prevalence (95% CI)—LPBE			Mixed infection	Prevalence (95% CI)—PrioCHECK FMDV-NS
		SAT1	SAT2	SAT3		
Female	61	59 (46.7–71.0)	75 (64.1–85.9)	24.5 (13.7–35.2)	76.5 (64.5–88.5)	86.9 (78.4–95.4)
Male	38	63.2 (47.9–78.5)	71.1 (56.7–65.5)	28.9 (14.5–43.3)	62.4 (54.9–69.9)	81.6 (69.3–93.9)
p value		0.861	0.278	0.778	0.533	0.567

for FMDV antibodies on PrioCHECK FMDV-NS test. There was a significant difference in prevalence among the different sampling sites ($p < 0.05$) and this was statistically significant (p value = 0.001). Of the 84 buffaloes that tested positive for FMDV NPS antibodies, 69 were strong positives (>70) and 15 were weak positives (>50 and <70). The prevalence according to age categories was also not statistically different (p value = 0.413) (Table 2). The overall prevalence of females ($n = 61$) and males ($n = 38$) on PrioCHECK FMDV-NS test was 86.9% (95% CI = 78.4–95.4) and 81.6% (95% CI = 69.3–93.9), respectively. Further, there was no significant difference in the prevalence of antibodies against SAT serotypes tested in LBPE and against nonstructural proteins (PrioCHECK FMDV-NS test) in relation to age and sex (Table 3).

The cross-tabulation of combined test results for the LPBE SAT serotype ELISA and the PrioCHECK FMDV-NS ELISA among the buffaloes sampled in GMA and NP is shown in Table 4. The results showed a fair agreement between results obtained on PrioCHECK FMDV-NS and LPBE SAT serotypes (kappa = 0.296 at 0.001; McNemar = 0.057).

3.1.3. Virus Isolation and Serotyping by Antigen ELISA in Probang Samples. A total of 49 probang samples (Lundazi, $n = 24$, and Lower Zambezi, $n = 25$) were collected, treated,

TABLE 4: LPBE test and PrioCHECK FMDV-NS test cross-tabulation.

	PrioCHECK FMDV-NS test		
	Negative	Positive	Total
LPBE test			
Negative	4	3	7
Positive	11	81	92
Total	15	84	99

and passaged. Overall cytopathic effects (CPE) suggestive of FMDV replication in primary RM cell cultures were observed in three samples from Lundazi ($n = 2$) and Lower Zambezi ($n = 1$). The CPE was characterised by the fast destruction of the cell monolayer from which infected cells were round and seen singly. Complete destruction of the cell sheet was mostly seen within 48 hours of inoculation of the 1st passage or 2nd passage. Samples with CPE were analysed using the antigen ELISA to identify the serotypes. The antigen ELISA analysis showed that two samples from Lundazi were of SAT2 serotypes, and one sample from Lower Zambezi was of the SAT1 serotype.

4. Discussion

The aim of this study was to determine the seroprevalence of the FMD in buffaloes and identify circulating FMDV serotypes in buffalo populations in Zambia. A high prevalence of antibodies against FMDV in buffaloes was observed in all the study areas except in Sioma where only few animals (all calves) were tested. Further, major FMDV SAT types observed to be circulating in buffaloes in Zambia based on the results from LPBE were SAT1, SAT2, and SAT3, while only SAT1 and SAT2 were isolated from probang samples. Our study reveals that FMD could be a problem in study areas. These results corroborate the findings of previous studies which demonstrated high FMDV seroprevalence in buffalo populations in Southern Africa [25, 26]. In our study SAT2 was the most predominant serotype, followed by SAT1 and then SAT3. Overall, all the Game Parks/Game Management Areas had high prevalence of mixed infections, which supports the earlier observation that individual buffaloes may be persistently infected with more than one type of FMDV in the pharyngeal region [27–29]. The LPBE was chosen as it has been used successfully for numerous animal species before, including the African buffalo. While the test shows an almost perfect sensitivity, the specificity in cattle usually is about 95% and similar values were assumed for the African buffalo. However, in cattle up to 18% [30, 31] false positive reactions have been reported. LPBE detects immunoglobulins directed against the capsid or structural proteins of the virus and therefore cannot distinguish antibodies induced by vaccinations using inactivated vaccines from those elicited by infection with live virus [32]. PrioCHECK FMDV-NS detects antibodies against the nonstructural 3ABC protein of FMDV but cannot distinguish between serotypes. However, antibodies to the 3ABC protein are considered to be the most reliable indicators of infection/exposure to FMDV [33, 34]. The specificity of the PrioCHECK FMDV-NS for bovine sera was given as 98.1 percent by [35] while the sensitivity in nonvaccinated, experimentally infected bovines also approached 100 percent. Bronsvoort et al. [36] published sensitivity and specificity estimates of 87.7 percent and 87.3 percent, respectively, for the African buffalo using Bayesian statistics, but their data would be consistent with values closer to those recorded for cattle, in particular if factors like antibody kinetics and sample quality are taken into account.

The study has also revealed that buffaloes within the age of one to two years are most likely to be infected by FMDV as all the buffaloes were positive to FMDV infection at this age. This is in agreement with the findings of previous studies which indicated that, after maternal antibodies wane, the young buffaloes were prone to FMDV infection from the carrier buffaloes [37]. Buffaloes in the age category of 5-6 years were positive for antibodies against FMDV and had mixed infection slightly higher compared to the other categories; this could have been due to the risk that the older the buffaloes are, the more the time they are likely to get infected by different FMDV serotypes is. African buffaloes are efficient maintenance hosts of the SAT type viruses, with an individual animal maintaining the virus up to five years and

isolated herds for up to 24 years, although persistence in an individual buffalo is probably not lifelong [37].

Probang samples were collected with the view of isolating FMDV and identifying serotypes in circulation [29, 37, 38]. However, only a small proportion of samples yielded positive results as two, SAT2, and one, SAT1, virus isolates were obtained. This is in line with the report that the excretion of virus by carriers is intermittent [1] and the findings by [10] that reported that the quantity of virus present in the pharynx of carrier animals can vary considerably over time. As part of future studies, it is recommended to obtain more probang samples for virus isolation and also generate nucleotide sequences of these isolates so that the FMDV circulating in these buffaloes can be differentiated to topotypes level to understand their diversity. In addition, the availability of more local FMDV isolates enables the calculation of r^1 values required to check and possibly adapt preventive and control measures in endemic or epidemic regions where strategic or general vaccination is required with vaccine containing the FMDV subtypes that are active in the area [29].

In this study, based on LPBE, very few SAT3 seropositive buffalo samples were only seropositive for SAT3 ($n = 5$), while slight proportions were SAT1 seropositive only ($n = 9$) or SAT2 seropositive only ($n = 10$). The majority of samples were positive to more than one serotype, and this raises the issue of to what extent the SAT results are cross-reactions [27]. Virus neutralisation assays using local FMDV isolates would be required to further dissect possible cross-reactivities. In addition, the isolation of a SAT3 FMDV from concurrent probang samples would confirm the presence of this serotype in Zambian buffaloes.

The study showed fair agreement between LPBE test and PrioCHECK FMDV-NS test cross-tabulation results. Lack of substantial or perfect agreement could be attributed to the fact that the kinetics and duration of the antibody response to structural and nonstructural viral proteins differ as does the rate of seroconversion [39].

Antibodies to all the three Southern African Territories (SAT) serotypes were detected in buffaloes in the four study areas (Mosi-oa-tunya, Sichifulo, Lower Zambezi, and Lundazi) where age and sex of the buffalo had no effect in FMDV infection/exposure status. This is in agreement with earlier observations in studies conducted in buffaloes in Sub-Saharan Africa [37]. The exception was Sioma where all the four samples collected from buffaloes in age range of six months to eight months were negative for antibodies against FMDV. Therefore no equivocal statement can be made regarding these results as the apparent absence could be attributed to the small sample size and may be that the young buffaloes had not yet been exposed to FMDV.

There is little published on non-SAT serotypes in buffalo in Zambia. From reported outbreaks in Saharan Africa [37], it appears that the majority of outbreaks in the southern regions are due to SAT serotypes with only sporadic introductions of O and A. Zambia being surrounded by other countries which have reported other serotypes cannot be excluded from harbouring other serotypes apart from SAT serotypes due to the reported outbreaks in Kenya (1994 to 2000), Tanzania

(1999 to 2000), and Uganda (1995 to 1999) of SAT1, SAT2, and O (as well as A and C in Kenya) [37]. This needs to be looked at in more detail as recent work on sera has shown consistency in results of antibody screening repeatedly over long storage period. The other interesting studies could be comparison of the prevalence of FMDV in buffalo to that in livestock held in Kazungula/Livingstone during the time period of the buffalo sampling as it could possibly shed light on the role that buffaloes have in transmission of the disease to domestic livestock. This is immanent from the fact that the Department of Veterinary Services in the Ministry of Agriculture and Livestock (MAL) had reported FMDV SAT1 outbreaks which belonged to topotype III (WZ) but were not closely related to other SAT1 viruses [17].

It is known that buffaloes play an important role in maintaining FMD infections and are able to infect other susceptible species in Sub-Saharan Africa [26, 40] and that buffaloes have been shown to be the source of infection for impala and domestic animals in proximity of the Kruger National Park (KNP) and other game parks in Southern Africa [40]. References [41–43] demonstrated natural and experimental transmission from carrier buffalo to cattle. However, it should be noted that even though transmission has been demonstrated, the transmission conditions from carrier buffalo are not well understood and difficult to replicate because many attempts at carrying out transmission from carrier buffalo to naive buffalo or cattle have failed, even under conditions of immunosuppression or coinfection with rinderpest and bovine herpes-1 virus [28, 44–47].

5. Conclusion

In conclusion, our study has demonstrated high FMDV seroprevalence in buffaloes in Zambia and characterised the SAT serotypes circulating in the country. These findings will play a role in the control of FMD in Zambia because knowledge of circulating FMDV is critical in vaccine matching, which is necessary to ensure vaccine efficacy. Most parts of Zambia are endemic to FMD; therefore strategic or general vaccination is required with vaccine containing the FMDV subtypes that are active in the area [29].

There is still need for molecular characterisation of the positive virus samples on antigen ELISA at the same time antigen titrations should also be performed and r^1 values should be determined to enable matching with the FMD.

Conflict of Interests

The authors declare that none of them have financial or personal relationships with individuals or organisations that may have inappropriately influenced them in writing this paper and, therefore, declare that there is no conflict of interests.

Acknowledgments

The authors would like to thank the GRZ, SACIDS (through a grant from the Wellcome Trust (Grant WTO 87546MA)) and SADC TADs program for funding this study. They thank the late Director of Veterinary Services Dr. Joseph Mubanga for his assistance with this work. Many thanks are due to Dr. Paul Fandamu, Ms. Mwauseya, Mr. M. Mukubwali, and Mr. M. Simweemba for the technical support. They thank Ms. L. Seoke of BVI for the assistance with laboratory work. They are grateful to the Quality Control Staff of BVI for the good supply of RM monolayer cells.

References

[1] S. Alexandersen, Z. Zhang, and A. I. Donaldson, "Aspects of the persistence of foot-and-mouth disease virus in animals—the carrier problem," *Microbes and Infection*, vol. 4, no. 10, pp. 1099–1110, 2002.

[2] F. Brown, "The history of research in foot-and-mouth disease," *Virus Research*, vol. 91, no. 1, pp. 3–7, 2003.

[3] N. J. Knowles and A. R. Samuel, "Molecular epidemiology of foot-and-mouth disease virus," *Virus Research*, vol. 91, no. 1, pp. 65–80, 2003.

[4] J. B. Brooksby, "Portraits of viruses: foot-and-mouth disease virus," *Intervirology*, vol. 18, no. 1-2, pp. 1–23, 1982.

[5] P. Chilonda, J. D. Woodford, B. Ahmadu, K. L. Samui, M. Syakalima, and J. E. D. Mlangwa, "Foot and mouth disease in Zambia: a review of the aetiology and epidemiology and recommendations for possible control," *Revue Scientifique et Technique*, vol. 18, no. 3, pp. 585–592, 1999.

[6] E. Overby and G. C. N. Zyambo, "Foot and mouth disease outbreaks in Zambia," *Revue Scientifique et Technique*, vol. 2, no. 1, pp. 189–197, 1999.

[7] M. Munyeme, J. B. Muma, H. M. Munangándu, C. Kankya, E. Skjerve, and M. Tryland, "Cattle owners' awareness of bovine tuberculosis in high and low prevalence settings of the wildlife-livestock interface areas in Zambia," *BMC Veterinary Research*, vol. 6, article 21, 2010.

[8] B. W. J. Mahy, "Foot and mouth disease virus," in *Current Topics in Microbiology and Immunology*, vol. 288, 2005.

[9] M. G. Mateu, "Antibody recognition of picornaviruses and escape from neutralization: a structural view," *Virus Research*, vol. 38, no. 1, pp. 1–24, 1995.

[10] R. P. Kitching, "Clinical variation in foot and mouth disease: cattle," *Revue Scientifique et Technique*, vol. 21, no. 3, pp. 499–504, 2002.

[11] Annonymous, *Annual Reports of the Department of Veterinary and Livestock Development*, Ministry of Agriculture, Livestock and Fisheries, 2005.

[12] *Annual Reports of the Department of Veterinary and Livestock Development*, Ministry of Agriculture, Livestock and Fisheries, 2008.

[13] Annonymous, *Annual Reports of the Department of Veterinary and Livestock Development*, Ministry of Agriculture, Livestock and Fisheries, 2006.

[14] *Annual Reports of the Department of Veterinary and Livestock Development*, Ministry of Agriculture, Livestock and Fisheries, 2007.

[15] *Annual Reports of the Department of Veterinary and Livestock Development*, Ministry of Agriculture, Livestock and Fisheries, 2009.

[16] *Annual Reports of the Department of Veterinary and Livestock Development*, Ministry of Agriculture, Livestock and Fisheries, 2010.

[17] Tech. Rep., OIE/FAO FMD Reference Laboratory Network, 2012.

[18] F. Banda, C. J. Kasanga, R. Sallu et al., "Investigation of foot-and-mouth disease outbreaks in the Mbala and Kazungula districts of Zambia," *Onderstepoort Journal of Veterinary Research*, vol. 81, no. 2, article 721, 2014.

[19] Y. Sinkala, M. Simuunza, D. U. Pfeiffer et al., "Challenges and economic implications in the control of foot and mouth disease in sub-Saharan Africa: Lessons from the Zambian experience," *Veterinary Medicine International*, vol. 2014, Article ID 373921, 12 pages, 2014.

[20] J. S. S. Dillman, "Foot and mouth disease investigations in game animals (lechwe and buffaloes)," Final Report vol.1, Germany Agency for Technical Cooperation, Government Publishers, Lusaka, Zambia, 1976.

[21] H. K. Mwima, "Wildlife research and management in Zambia with special reference to some protected areas where wild and domestic animals co-exist," in *The Effects of Enlargement of Domestic Animal Pasture on the Wildlife in Zambia, Lusaka, Zambia*, pp. 305–308, 1995.

[22] OIE, *Manual of Diagnostic Tests and vaccines for Terrestrial Animals*, Office International des Epizooties, Paris, France, 6th edition, 2010.

[23] C. Hamblin, I. T. R. Barnett, and R. S. Hedger, "A new enzyme-linked immunosorbent assay (ELISA) for the detection of antibodies against foot-and-mouth disease virus I. Development and method of ELISA," *Journal of Immunological Methods*, vol. 93, no. 1, pp. 115–121, 1986.

[24] M. de Diego, E. Brocchi, D. Mackay, and F. de Simone, "The non-structural polyprotein 3ABC of foot-and-mouth disease virus as a diagnostic antigen in ELISA to differentiate infected from vaccinated cattle," *Archives of Virology*, vol. 142, no. 10, pp. 2021–2033, 1997.

[25] J. J. Esterhuysen, G. R. Thomson, J. R. Flammand, and R. G. Bengis, "Buffalo in the northern Natal game parks show no serological evidence of infection with foot-and-mouth disease virus," *Onderstepoort Journal of Veterinary Research*, vol. 52, no. 2, pp. 63–66, 1985.

[26] G. R. Thomson, W. Vosloo, and A. D. S. Bastos, "Foot and mouth disease in wildlife," *Virus Research*, vol. 91, no. 1, pp. 145–161, 2003.

[27] R. S. Hedger, I. T. R. Barnett, D. V. Gradwell, and P. T. Dias, "Serological tests for foot-and-mouth disease in bovine serum samples, problems of interpretation," *Revue Scientifique et Technique*, vol. 1, pp. 387–393, 1992.

[28] E. C. Anderson, W. J. Doughty, J. Anderson, and R. Paling, "The pathogenesis of foot-and-mouth disease in the African buffalo (*Syncerus caffer*) and the role of this species in the epidemiology of the disease in Kenya," *Journal of Comparative Pathology*, vol. 89, no. 4, pp. 541–549, 1979.

[29] P. Sutmoller, S. S. Barteling, R. C. Olascoaga, and K. J. Sumption, "Control and eradication of foot-and-mouth disease," *Virus Research*, vol. 91, no. 1, pp. 101–144, 2003.

[30] A. Clavijo, P. Wright, and P. Kitching, "Developments in diagnostic techniques for differentiating infection from vaccination in foot and mouth disease," *Veterinary Journal*, vol. 167, no. 1, pp. 9–22, 2004.

[31] B. Haas, "Application of the liquid phase blocking sandwich ELISA. Problems encountered in import/export serology and possible solutions," in *Proceedings of the Session of the Research Group of the European Commission for the Control of Foot and Mouth Disease*, pp. 124–127, EuFMD, Vienna, Austria, 1994.

[32] R. M. Armstrong, S. J. Cox, N. Aggarwal et al., "Detection of antibody to the foot-and-mouth disease virus (FMDV) non-structural polyprotein 3ABC in sheep by ELISA," *Journal of Virological Methods*, vol. 125, no. 2, pp. 153–163, 2005.

[33] K. J. Sørensen, K. G. Madsen, E. S. Madsen, J. S. Salt, J. Nqindi, and D. K. J. Mackay, "Differentiation of infection from vaccination in foot-and-mouth disease by the detection of antibodies to the non-structural proteins 3D, 3AB and 3ABC in ELISA using antigens expressed in baculovirus," *Archives of Virology*, vol. 143, no. 8, pp. 1461–1476, 1998.

[34] T. Sun, P. Lu, and X. Wang, "Localization of infection-related epitopes on the non-structural protein 3ABC of foot-and-mouth disease virus and the application of tandem epitopes," *Journal of Virological Methods*, vol. 119, no. 2, pp. 79–86, 2004.

[35] E. Brocchi, I. E. Bergmann, A. Dekker et al., "Comparative evaluation of six ELISAs for the detection of antibodies to the non-structural proteins of foot-and-mouth disease virus," *Vaccine*, vol. 24, no. 47-48, pp. 6966–6979, 2006.

[36] B. M. D. C. Bronsvoort, S. Parida, I. Handel et al., "Serological survey for foot-and-mouth disease virus in wildlife in eastern Africa and estimation of test parameters of a nonstructural protein enzyme-linked immunosorbent assay for buffalo," *Clinical and Vaccine Immunology*, vol. 15, no. 6, pp. 1003–1011, 2008.

[37] W. Vosloo, A. D. S. Bastos, O. Sangare, S. K. Hargreaves, and G. R. Thomson, "Review of the status and control of foot and mouth disease in sub-Saharan Africa," *Scientific and Technical Review*, vol. 21, no. 3, pp. 437–449, 2002.

[38] M. Rémond, C. Kaiser, and F. Lebreton, "Diagnosis and screening of foot-and-mouth disease," *Comparative Immunology, Microbiology and Infectious Diseases*, vol. 25, no. 5-6, pp. 309–320, 2002.

[39] B. M. D. Bronsvoort, N. Toft, I. E. Bergmann et al., "Evaluation of three 3ABC ELISAs for foot-and-mouth disease non-structural antibodies using latent class analysis," *BMC Veterinary Research*, vol. 2, article 30, 2006.

[40] G. R. Thomson and A. D. S. Bastos, "Foot and mouth disease," in *Infectious Diseases of Livestock*, J. A. W. Coetzer and R. C. Tustin, Eds., pp. 1324–1365, Oxford University Press, Cape Town, South Africa, 2nd edition, 2004.

[41] P. S. Dawe, F. O. Flanagan, R. L. Madekurozwa et al., "Natural transmission of foot-and-mouth disease virus from African buffalo (*Syncerus caffer*) to cattle in a wildlife area of Zimbabwe," *Veterinary Record*, vol. 134, no. 10, pp. 230–232, 1994.

[42] P. S. Dawe, K. Sorensen, N. P. Ferris, I. T. Barnett, R. M. Armstrong, and N. J. Knowles, "Experimental transmission of foot-and-mouth disease virus from carrier African buffalo (*Syncerus caffer*) to cattle in Zimbabwe," *Veterinary Record*, vol. 134, no. 9, pp. 211–215, 1994.

[43] A. D. S. Bastos, D. T. Haydon, O. Sangaré, C. I. Boshoff, J. L. Edrich, and G. R. Thomson, "The implications of virus diversity within the SAT2 serotype for control of foot-and-mouth disease in sub-Saharan Africa," *Journal of General Virology*, vol. 84, no. 6, pp. 1595–1606, 2003.

[44] R. G. Bengis, G. R. Thomson, R. S. Hedger, V. De Vos, and A. Pini, "Foot-and-mouth disease and the African buffalo (*Syncerus caffer*). 1. Carriers as a source of infection for cattle," *The Onderstepoort Journal of Veterinary Research*, vol. 53, no. 2, pp. 69–73, 1986.

[45] J. B. Condy and R. S. Hedger, "The survival of foot and mouth disease virus in African buffalo with non transference of infection to domestic cattle," *Research in Veterinary Science*, vol. 16, no. 2, pp. 182–185, 1974.

[46] M. D. Gainaru, G. R. Thomson, R. G. Bengis, J. J. Esterhuysen, W. Bruce, and A. Pini, "Foot-and-mouth disease and the African buffalo (*Syncerus caffer*). II. Virus excretion and transmission during acute infection.," *The Onderstepoort Journal of Veterinary Research*, vol. 53, no. 2, pp. 75–85, 1986.

[47] G. R. Thomson, "The role of carrier animals in the transmission of foot and mouth diseases," OIE Comprehensive Reports on Technical Items Presented to the International Committee or to Regional Commissions, 1996.

3

Platelet-Rich Gel Supernatants Stimulate the Release of Anti-Inflammatory Proteins on Culture Media of Normal Equine Synovial Membrane Explants

Diana L. Ríos, Catalina López, and Jorge U. Carmona

Grupo de Investigación Terapia Regenerativa, Departamento de Salud Animal, Universidad de Caldas, Calle 65 No. 26-10, Manizales, Colombia

Correspondence should be addressed to Jorge U. Carmona; carmona@ucaldas.edu.co

Academic Editor: Philip H. Kass

The aims were as follows: (1) to evaluate the effects at 48 and 96 h of two concentrations (25 and 50%) of leukocyte and platelet-rich gel (L-PRG) and pure PRG (P-PRG) supernatants on the production/degradation in normal equine synovial membrane explants (SME) of platelet derived growth factor isoform BB, transforming growth factor beta-1, tumor necrosis factor alpha, interleukin (IL-) 4 (IL-4), IL-1 receptor antagonist (IL-1ra), and hyaluronan (HA) synthesis and (2) to correlate these molecules with their respective PRG supernatant treatments. SME from 6 horses were cultured for 96 h with L-PRG and P-PRG supernatants at 25 and 50% concentrations, respectively. SME culture media were changed each 48 h and used for determination by ELISA of the molecules, which were also determined in synovial fluid. 25% L-PRG supernatant produced a sustained release over time of IL-1ra and a gradual release of HA, whereas 50% L-PRG supernatant produced a sustained increase over time of IL-4 and HA. 50% P-PRG supernatant produced an increased and sustained production of IL-1ra and IL-4. The cellular composition and the articular concentration (volume) of a platelet-rich plasma preparation could affect the anti-inflammatory and anabolic joint responses in horses with osteoarthritis.

1. Introduction

Osteoarthritis (OA) is a frequent cause of lameness in horses and a potential cause of wastage of valuable animals [1, 2]. This joint disease could appear as a consequence of several predisposing factors, such as repetitive trauma (traumatic arthritis) and synovitis from diverse causes, such as osteochondrosis (OCD) and joint infection [3]. Although OA, in humans is not normally associated with synovitis, this last alteration is a clinical and pathological remark in horses with this pathology [4]. In general, it is well established that synovitis increases the articular cartilage damage by both gene upregulation and production of catabolic cytokines, mainly interleukin-1 (IL-1), tumor necrosis alpha (TNF-α), matrix metalloproteinases (MMPs), and eicosanoids, among others [3, 4].

Although equine OA has routinely been treated with intra-articular injection of corticosteroids and hyaluronan [5], there are currently several emerging regenerative therapies, such as autologous conditioned serum (ACS) [6], autologous protein solution (APS) [7], stem cells [8], and platelet-rich plasma (PRP) [9–11]. Notably, PRP could be considered as one of the most worldwide clinical regenerative therapies used in people [12], horses [10, 11], and dogs with OA [13, 14].

Some reports indicate the beneficial effect of PRP in horses with naturally occurring OA [10, 11] and some *in vitro* studies [15, 16] and *in vivo* research [17] have recently been performed in order to explain how PRP could induce articular tissue anabolism. However, there is little information on the basic mechanisms by which this substance produces pain relief and improvement of the joint function.

Currently, there is no consensus on how to employ the "ideal PRP preparation" for the intraarticular joint treatment in patients with OA [16]. Although some ideas have been proposed in order to classify the plethora of PRP preparations used [18], in general, in the horse, these substances could be classified as leukocyte and platelet-rich plasma (L-PRP) and pure platelet-rich plasma (P-PRP). L-PRP preparations show both increased platelet (PLT) (~3–5-fold or more) and leukocyte (WBC) (3-fold or more) counts with respect to basal cell counts in whole blood. P-PRP products show from low physiological to 2-fold PLT counts and from negligible WBC concentration to 2-fold WBC counts with respect to basal cell counts in whole blood [19]. When these PRP preparations are activated, they are transformed in platelet rich gels (PRGs). Thus, PRG from L-PRP is termed L-PRG and PRG from P-PRP is termed P-PRG [18].

As mentioned, synovitis is a *sine qua* nonclinical and pathological alteration in horses with OA [4]. Bearing in mind this, it is necessary to know how supernatants from L-PRG and P-PPG could affect the inflammatory response and metabolism of the equine synovial membrane. Thus, the aims of this research were (1) to evaluate the temporal effects (at 48 and 96 h) of two concentrations (25 and 50%) of L-PRG and P-PRG supernatants on the production or degradation in normal equine synovial membrane explants (SME) of anabolic growth factors (platelet derived growth factor isoform BB (PDGF-BB) and transforming growth factor beta-1 (TGF-β_1)), the proinflammatory tumor necrosis factor alpha (TNF-α), anti-inflammatory cytokines interleukin- (IL-) 4 (IL-4) and IL-1 receptor antagonist (IL-1ra), and hyaluronan (HA) and (2) to perform a correlation analysis between these molecules and their respective PRG supernatant treatments.

2. Material and Methods

This study was approved by the Ethical Committee for Animal Experimentation of the authors' institution.

2.1. Animals and Samples. Synovial membrane samples from the dorsal metacarpophalangeal joints from 6 horses with a mean age of 9 ($\pm$3.3) years were included. The samples were from horses free from muscle-skeletal disease and euthanized by a pentobarbital intravenous overdose for other medical reasons. All the joints were radiographed and macroscopically evaluated for excluding horses with OA joint associated changes. Further, 2 mL of synovial fluid were obtained from each joint in order to know the actual concentrations of PDGF-BB, TGF-β_1, TNF-α, IL-4, IL-1ra, and HA.

2.2. L-PRP and P-PRP Preparation. Venous blood from 1 adult clinically healthy, 11-year-old mare was used to avoid the great variability in the GF, cytokine, and HA concentrations in the PRGs supernatants used in the experiments. L-PRP and P-PRP were obtained by a manual double centrifugation tube method [20], previously validated and used clinically in horses with OA [10]. Briefly, blood was drawn from jugular venipuncture and deposited in 4.5 mL tubes with sodium citrate solution (BD Vacutainer, Becton Drive, Franklin Lakes, NJ, USA). After centrifugation at 120 g for five minutes, the first 50% of the top supernatant plasma fraction, adjacent to the buffy coat, was collected. This fraction was then centrifuged at 240 g for five minutes and the bottom fourth fraction was collected. This fraction was considered L-PRP. The upper plasma fraction was considered as P-PRP.

Whole blood and both PRP were analyzed for PLT and WBC concentration using an impedance-based hematology device (Celltac-α MEK 6450, Nihon Kohden, Japan).

Both PRP were activated with calcium gluconate (ratio 1 : 10) and remained in incubation at 37°C for 1 h until clot retraction. L-PRG and P-PRG supernatants were always used fresh during each culture media changing at 1 and 49 h. Aliquots of both PRG supernatants obtained at every time point were frozen at −86°C for later quantification of the molecules of interest.

2.3. Culture and Study Design. Synovial membrane samples were obtained aseptically and circular 4 mm diameter explants were obtained using a disposable biopsy punch (KAI Medical, Solingen, Germany). SME were dissected from the joint capsule and washed in phosphate buffered saline. The design of the study included the evaluation of five experimental groups, as follows: 1 SME control group (without addition of any PRG supernatant) and 4 SME groups cultured with L-PRG or P-PRG supernatants at two different concentrations, 25% and 50%.

Synovial membrane explants were stabilized in culture media (DMEM, Lonza Group Ltd., Basel, Switzerland) and supplemented with streptomycin (100 μg/mL) and penicillin (100 μg/mL) without the addition of serum. Cultures were incubated in a 5% CO_2 and water saturated atmosphere for 24 h and then replaced for fresh culture media. After 1 h of incubation L-PRG and P-PRG supernatants were added for obtaining concentrations at 25 and 50%. All SME groups were cultured during 48 h and the culture media were changed and replaced by fresh culture media and fresh PRG supernatants and incubated for other additional 48 h. Culture media obtained at 1, 48, 49, and 96 h were aliquoted and frozen at −86°C for later determination of PDGF-BB, TGF-β_1, TNF-α, IL-4, IL-1ra, and HA.

2.4. ELISA Analysis. L-PRG and P-PRG supernatants, culture media from SME groups obtained at 1, 48, 49, and 96 h, and synovial fluid were analyzed for measuring (by duplicate) the concentrations of the molecules of interest using ELISA kits (R&D Systems, Minneapolis, MN, USA). PDGF-BB (Human PDGF-BB DuoSet, DY220) and TGF-β_1 (Human TGF-β_1 DuoSet, DY240E) were determined using human antibodies, because there is a high homology between these proteins in humans and horses [21, 22]. In addition, these kits have been used for the same purposes in other equine PRP studies [17, 20]. TNF-α (Equine TNF-alpha DuoSet, DY1814), IL-4 (Equine IL-4 DuoSet, DY1809), and IL-1ra (Equine IL-1ra/IL-1F3 DuoSet, DY1814) were assayed with equine specific antibodies and HA (Hyaluronan DuoSet, DY3614) was determined using a multispecies detection ELISA kit. Standards provided for each ELISA kit were used for preparing each standard curve following the manufacturers' instructions. Readings were performed at 450 nm.

2.5. Statistical Analysis. The statistical analysis was performed with the software SPSS 19.0 (IBM, Chicago, IL, USA). A Shapiro-Wilk test was used to assess the fit of data set to

TABLE 1: Mean (mean standard error) of the concentration of the molecules evaluated in both leukocyte and platelet-rich gel (L-PRG) and pure platelet-rich gel (P-PRG) supernatants and synovial fluid.

Variable	Fluid		
	L-PRG	P-PRG	Synovial fluid
TGF-β_1 (pg/mL)	1669.2 ± 313.2	1369.2 ± 21.4	1413.8 ± 4.8
PDGF-BB (pg/mL)	3069. 9 ± 1261.6	383.8 ± 80.9^a	60.5 ± 0.9^a
TNF-α (pg/mL)	60 ± 0.5^{a,b}	59 ± 1.4^a	66.7 ± 3.3^b
IL-4 (pg/mL)	75.7 ± 9.3^a	61.1 ± 1.52^a	101.8 ± 33.7^b
IL-1ra (pg/mL)	160.4 ± 68.0	58.7 ± 3.1^a	77.8 ± 10.7
HA (ng/mL)	6.9 ± 2.9	2.3 ± 1.08	53017.6 ± 12140^a

$^{a-b}$Lowercase letters denote significant differences ($P < 0.01$) between groups in the same column by Tukey test.

a normal distribution (goodness of fit). Both PLT and WBC counts in whole blood and both PRP and PDGF-BB, TGF-β_1, TNF-α, IL-4, IL-1ra, and HA concentrations in all the evaluated groups showed a normal distribution ($P > 0.05$).

Platelet and WBC counts in whole blood, L-PRP, and P-PRP were evaluated by a one-way analysis of variance (ANOVA), followed by a Tukey test. PDGF-BB, TGF-β_1, TNF-α, IL-4, IL-1ra, and HA concentrations from both PRG supernatants, synovial fluid, and blood cells were evaluated in a similar fashion. PDGF-BB, TGF-β_1, TNF-α, IL-4, IL-1ra, and HA concentrations from synovial fluid and culture media obtained at 48 and 96 h from all SME groups were analyzed by a generalized lineal model (GLM) followed when necessary by a Tukey test.

PDGF-BB, TGF-β_1, TNF-α, IL-4, IL-1ra, and HA concentrations in fresh culture media with PRG supernatants at 1 h and 48 h were also compared with the concentrations for these molecules in the culture media from SME groups obtained at 48 h and 96 h using a t-paired test. A correlation analysis was performed to determine the Pearson correlation coefficient (r) between the variables evaluated in the study. A $P < 0.05$ value was accepted as statistically significant for all tests. Data are presented as mean ± standard error (s.e).

3. Results

3.1. Cell and Growth Factor, Cytokine, and HA Concentration in L-PRP/L-PRG, P-PRP/P-PRG, and Synovial Fluid.
Platelet counts were significantly ($P < 0.05_{[Tukey\ test]}$) different between whole blood, L-PRP, and P-PRP, with the lowest concentration for P-PRP (99.4 ± 4.3 PLT/μL (mean ± mean standard error)), followed by whole blood (124.7 ± 3.1 PLT/μL) and L-PRP (311.6 ± 20.4 PLT/μL). WBC counts were also significantly different between the evaluated groups, with a higher concentration for L-PRP (34.2 ± 3.7 WBC/μL), followed by whole blood (8.4 ± 3.6 WBC/μL) and P-PRP (0.13 ± 0.03 WBC/μL).

TGF-β_1 concentration was similar between L-PRG, P-PRG, and synovial fluid. PDGF-BB had a significantly ($P < 0.05_{[Tukey\ test]}$) higher concentration in L-PRG when compared with P-PRG and synovial fluid; however, the concentration for this GF was similar between these two last components. TNF-α concentration was significantly ($P < 0.01_{[Tukey\ test]}$) higher in synovial fluid when compared to P-PRG supernatant. However, there were not significant

differences for this cytokine in supernatants from L-PRG and P-PRG. IL-4 concentration was significantly ($P < 0.05_{[Tukey\ test]}$) higher in synovial fluid when compared to both PRG supernatants; however, the concentration of this cytokine was similar between both PRG supernatants. IL-1ra concentration was similar between L-PRG supernatant and synovial fluid, but the concentration of this cytokine was significantly ($P < 0.01_{[Tukey\ test]}$) lower in P-PRG supernatants. HA concentration was significantly ($P < 0.05_{[Tukey\ test]}$) higher in synovial fluid when compared to both PRG supernatants, but it was similar between both PRG supernatants (Table 1).

3.2. Production/Degradation of Growth Factors, Cytokines, and HA in Culture Media of SME TGF-β_1.
Initial TGF-β_1 concentrations obtained at 1 and 46 h in the culture media were significantly ($P < 0.05_{[t\text{-}paired\ test]}$) lower when compared with every homologous PRG supernatant treatment at 48 and 96 h, respectively (Figures 1(a) and 1(b)). This GF was substantially produced from SME control group and its concentration at 48 h was similar compared to those TGF-β_1 concentrations measured in the culture media from the SME treated with both 25% PRG supernatants. SME group cultured with 50% L-PRG supernatant presented the highest ($P < 0.05_{[Tukey\ test]}$) concentration for this protein when compared with the SME control group and those SME groups treated with both 25% PRG supernatants (Figure 1(a)). At 96 h, a significant ($P < 0.05_{[Tukey\ test]}$) increased TGF-β_1 concentration was observed in SME group cultured with 50% L-PRG supernatant in comparison with SME control group (Figure 1(b)). To note, synovial fluid TGF-β_1 concentration was similar to the culture media from all SME evaluated groups at 48 and 96 h.

3.3. PDGF-BB.
Platelet derived growth factor-BB concentration was significantly ($P < 0.05_{[t\text{-}paired\ test]}$) higher in culture media from all SME groups treated with different PRG supernatant concentrations at 1 and 49 h when compared with those PDGF-BB concentrations measured in the same groups at 48 and 96 h, respectively (Figures 2(a) and 2(b)). At 48 h, a significant diminution of PDGF-BB concentration was noticed for all SME groups treated with all PRG supernatants. At this time point, culture media from SME control group presented PDGF-BB concentration similar to those

(a)

(b)

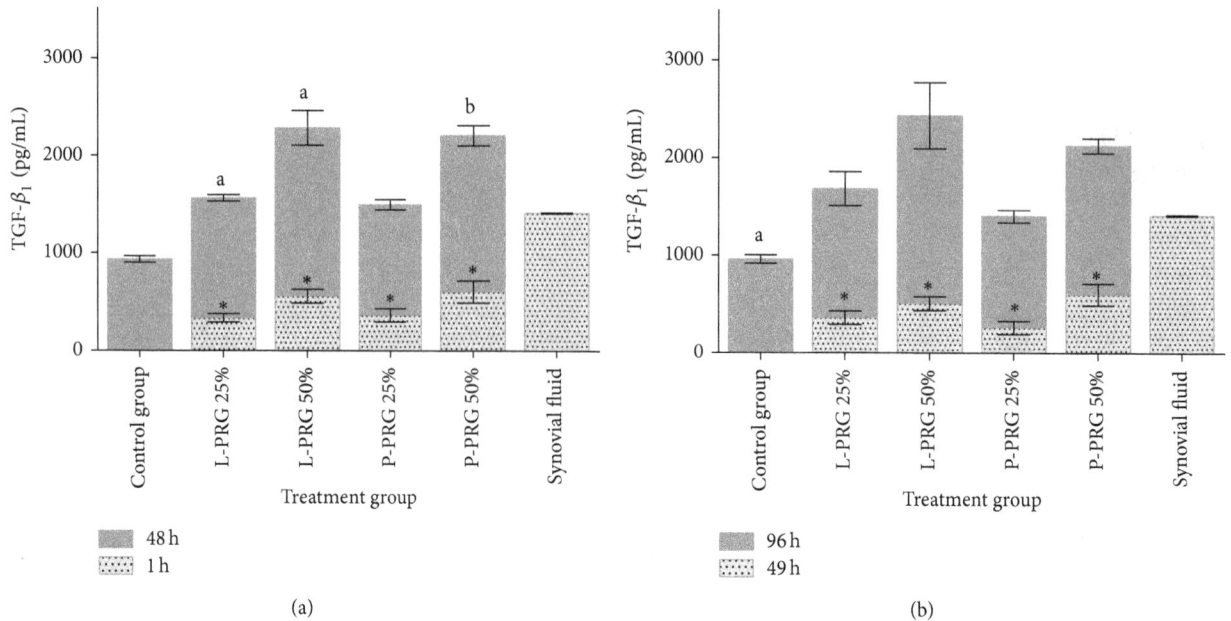

FIGURE 1: (a) [a-b]Lowercase letters denote significant ($P < 0.05$) differences between groups in the same column by Tukey test at 48 h. Significantly different with a: L-PRG 50% and P-PRG 50% and b: L-PRP 50%. (b) [a]Lowercase letters denote significant ($P < 0.05$) differences between groups in the same column by Tukey test at 96 h. Significantly different with a: L-PRG 50%. *Significant differences ($P < 0.01$) between the same variable at 1 h and 48 h and at 49 h and 96 by t-paired test.

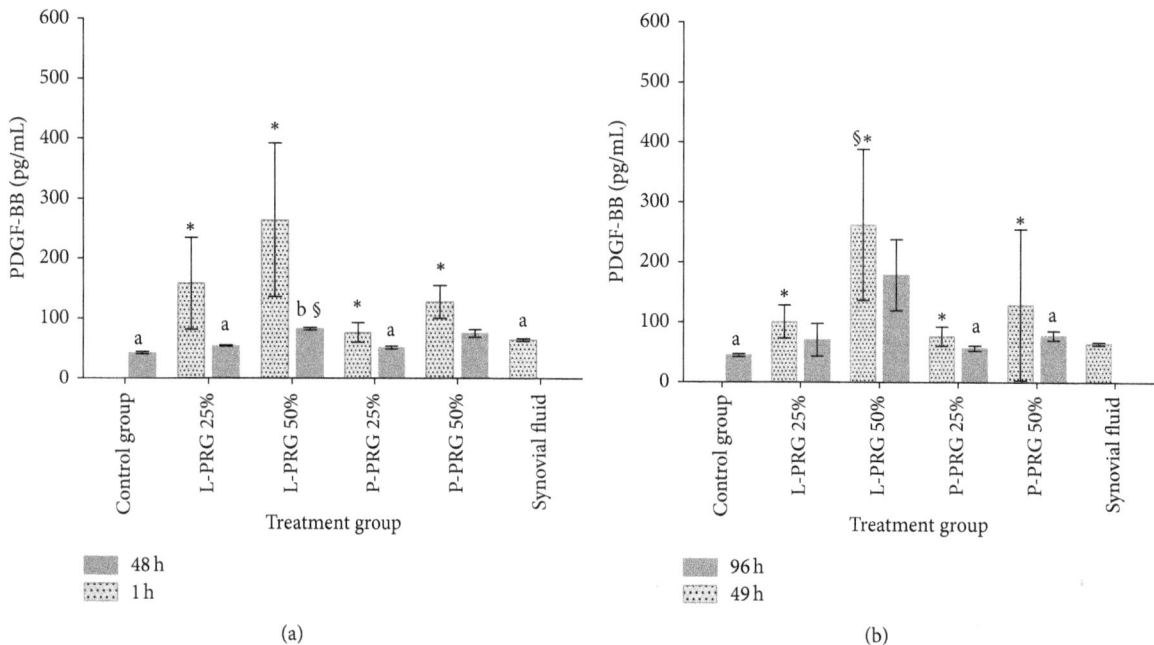

(a)

(b)

FIGURE 2: (a) [a-b]Lowercase letters denote significant ($P < 0.05$) differences between groups in the same column by Tukey test at 48 h. Significantly different with a: L-PRG 50% and P-PRG 50% and b: synovial fluid (SF). (b) [a]Lowercase letters denote significant ($P < 0.05$) differences between groups in the same column by Tukey test at 96 h. Significantly different with a: L-PRG 50%. *Significant differences ($P < 0.01$) between the same variable at 1 h and 48 h and at 49 h and 96 by t-paired test. [§*]Significant differences ($P < 0.05$) between the same variable at 48 and 96 h by Tukey test.

(a)

(b)

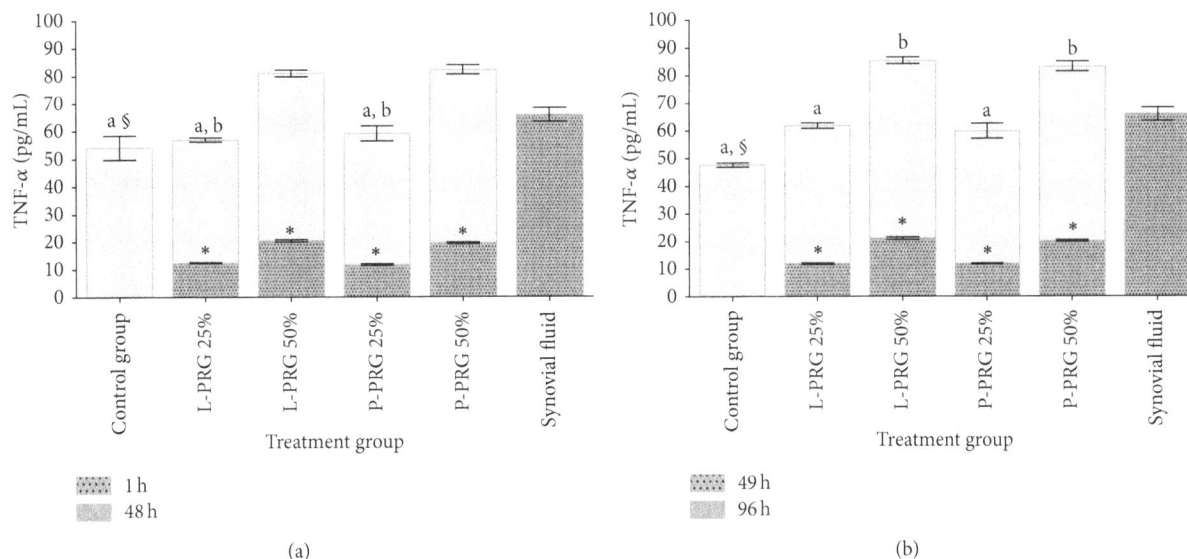

FIGURE 3: (a) [a-b]Lowercase letters denote significant ($P < 0.05$) differences between groups in the same column by Tukey test at 48 h. Significantly different with a: SF and b: L-PRG 50% and P-PRG 50%. (b) [a-b]Lowercase letters denote significant ($P < 0.05$) differences between groups in the same column by Tukey test at 96 h. Significantly different with a: SF and b: control group, L-PRG 25% and P-PRG 25%. *Significant differences ($P < 0.05$) between the same variable at 1 h and 48 h and at 49 h and 96 by t-paired test. §Significant differences ($P < 0.05$) between the same variable at 48 and 96 h by Tukey test.

concentrations obtained in synovial fluid and the SME groups treated with both 25% PRG supernatant concentrations. In addition, culture media from SME treated with 50% L-PRG supernatant displayed a significant ($P < 0.05_{[Tukey\ test]}$) increase of PDGF-BB concentration when compared to the SME control group and SME groups treated with both 25% PRG supernatant concentrations (Figure 2(a)).

At 96 h a similar trend for the concentration of this GF was observed, although PDFG-BB concentration from culture media of the SME treated with 50% of L-PRG supernatant was significantly ($P < 0.05_{[Tukey\ test]}$) higher when compared with the same group at 48 h (Figure 2(b)). Notably, the concentration for this growth factor was maintained in all the evaluated SME groups in a near or similar concentrations to those obtained in synovial fluid, except for the PDFG-BB concentration from the culture medium of the SME treated with 50% of L-PRG at 96 h.

3.4. TNF-α.

Tumor necrosis factor alpha was released to the culture media from all SME groups evaluated. At 48 h, the concentration for this cytokine in the SME control group and the groups treated with both 25% PRG concentrations was significantly different ($P < 0.05_{[Tukey\ test]}$) when compared to synovial fluid. On the other hand, TNF-α concentration was significantly ($P < 0.05_{[Tukey\ test]}$) lower in culture media from SME treated with 25% L-PRG supernatant in comparison with those groups treated with both 50% PRG supernatants (Figure 3(a)). At 96 h, a similar trend in the concentrations for this cytokine in all the evaluated groups was noticed (Figure 3(b)).

3.5. IL-4.

At 48 h, IL-4 concentration was significantly ($P < 0.05_{[Tukey\ test]}$) lower in culture media from the SME control group and those groups treated with both L-PRG supernatant concentrations and the 25% P-PRG concentration in comparison to SME group treated with 50% P-PRG concentration. IL-4 synovial fluid concentration was similar to those obtained in culture media from SME treated with 50% P-PRG supernatant (Figure 4(a)). At 96 h, IL-4 concentration was similar between synovial fluid and culture media from SME groups treated with PRG supernatants. On contrary, the concentration for this cytokine was significantly ($P < 0.05_{[Tukey\ test]}$) lower in culture media from SME control group in comparison to synovial fluid (Figure 4(b)). Furthermore, at 96 h, there was a significant increase of IL-4 concentration in the SME treated with 50% L-PRG supernatant in comparison with the culture media from the same group at 48 h.

3.6. IL-1ra.

At 48 and 96 h, IL-1ra concentration was significantly ($P < 0.05_{[Tukey\ test]}$) higher in the SME group treated with 25% L-PRG supernatant in comparison to synovial fluid and the culture media from the SME control group and those groups treated with 50% L-PRG and 25% P-PRG supernatants (Figures 5(a) and 5(b)).

3.7. HA.

At 1 and 49 h, HA concentration was significantly ($P < 0.05_{[Tukey\ test]}$) lower in all culture media of the SME groups treated with PRG supernatants (Figure 6). At 48 and 96 h a significant ($P < 0.05_{[t\text{-paired test}]}$) increase in the concentration of this molecule was evident in all SME

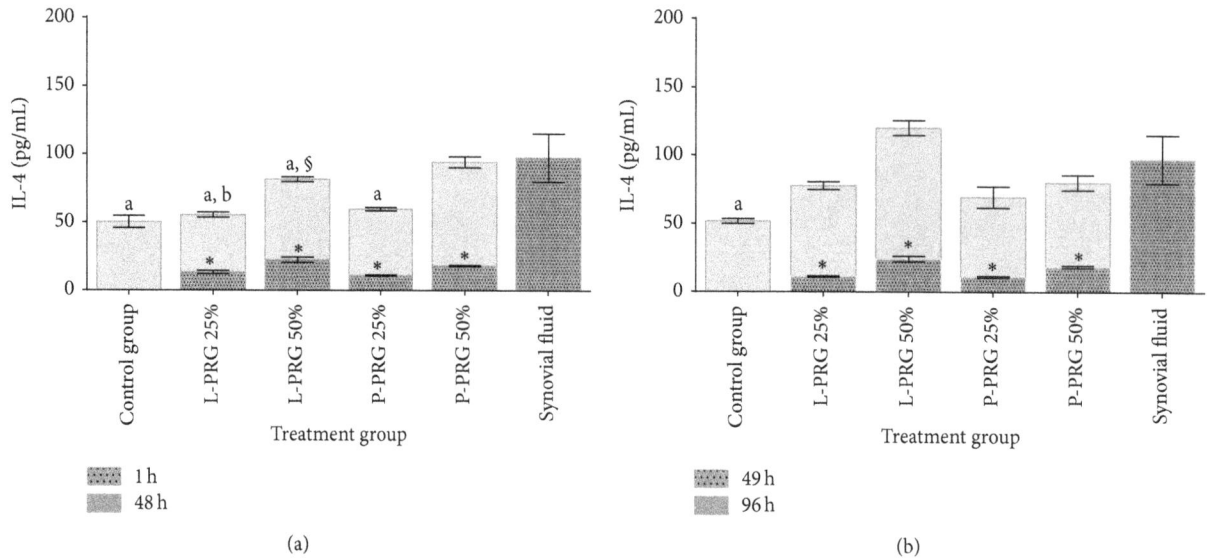

FIGURE 4: (a) [a-b]Lowercase letters denote significant ($P < 0.05$) differences between groups in the same column by Tukey test at 48 h. Significantly different with a: SF and b: P-PRG 50%. (b) [a]Lowercase letters denote significant ($P < 0.05$) differences between groups in the same column by Tukey test at 96 h. Significantly different with a: SF. *Significant differences ($P < 0.05$) between the same variable at 1 h and 48 h and at 49 h and 96 by t-paired test. [§]Significant differences ($P < 0.05$) between the same variable at 48 and 96 h by Tukey test.

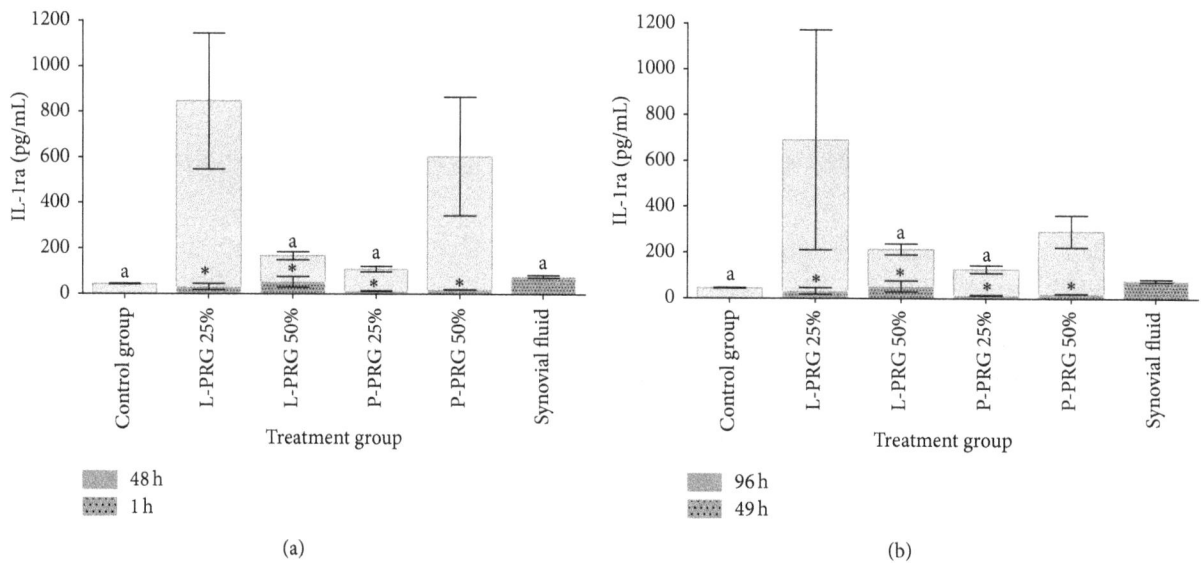

FIGURE 5: (a) [a-b]Lowercase letters denote significant ($P < 0.05$) differences between groups in the same column by Tukey test at 48 h. Significantly different with a: L-PRG 25%. (b) [a]Lowercase letters denote significant ($P < 0.05$) differences between groups in the same column by Tukey test at 96 h. Significantly different with a: L-PRP 25%. *Significant differences ($P < 0.05$) between the same variable at 1 h and 48 h and at 49 h and 96 by t-paired test.

groups evaluated respect to 1 and 46 h. However, HA synovial fluid concentration was significantly ($P < 0.05_{[Tukey\ test]}$) higher in comparison with the culture media from all SME evaluated groups (Figure 6). At 96 h, there was a significant increased HA concentration in culture medium from SME group treated with 50% L-PRG supernatant in comparison with the HA concentration of the same group at 48 h.

Notably, 50% L-PRG supernatant stimulated (although not significantly) the highest HA release to the culture media of the SME treated in comparison with the rest of the SME evaluated (Figure 6).

3.8. Correlations. No significant correlations were found between the variables studied.

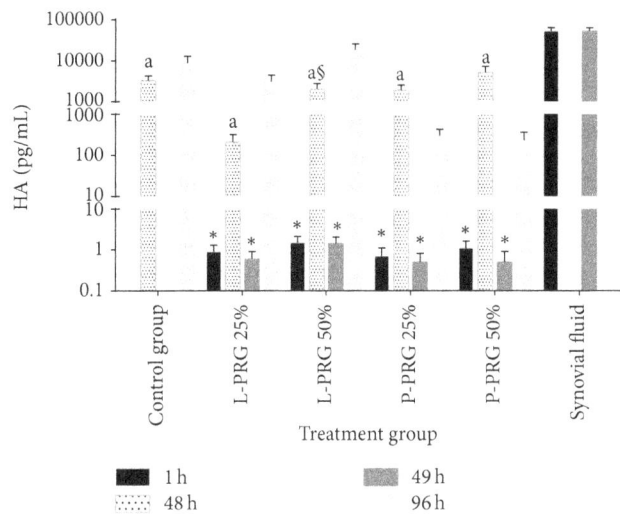

FIGURE 6: [a]Lowercase letters denote significant ($P < 0.05$) differences between groups in the same column by Tukey test at 48 h. Significantly different with a: SF. [*]Significant differences ($P < 0.05$) between the same variable at 1 h and 48 h and at 49 h and 96 by t-paired test. [§]Significant differences ($P < 0.05$) between the same variable at 48 and 96 h by Tukey test.

4. Discussion

The present study was aimed at knowing the *in vitro* effect of two PRG supernatants at 25 and 50% concentrations on both production and loss (degradation) in SME of some key molecules closely associated with the pathophysiology of OA [3]. TGF-β_1 and PDGF-BB were evaluated in this research, because they have been demonstrated for their important anabolic effects on joint tissues. In general, both proteins increase ECM cartilage synthesis, diminish both joint pain and inflammation, and promote the differentiation of synovial membrane cells in chondrocytes [23]. Both GF are mainly stored in platelet alpha granules, the reason why many of the therapeutic effects of PRP have been attributed to these proteins [19]. TNF-α was selected as a proinflammatory cytokine, because this protein and IL-1 represent the cornerstone proteins associated with the typical catabolic unbalance from OA [24]. This protein is also important in synovial inflammation and its upregulation in synovial tissue is associated with a more aggressive clinical picture of erosive arthritis [25]. In addition, recently a clinical study revealed that TNF-α is a useful biomarker for discriminating OA severity in horses in comparison to IL-1 [26].

IL-4 and IL-1ra were chosen because there are important anti-inflammatory cytokines related directly with OA pathophysiology [3]. IL-4 is associated with chondroprotection because it increases the synthesis of ECM cartilage [27]. However, the role for this cytokine in arthritis is more anti-inflammatory than anabolic because it increases the synthesis of IL-1ra and downregulates TNF-α [28–30]. On the other hand, IL-1ra is a natural antagonist of IL-1 effects, because it blocks the cellular receptors necessary for inducing joint inflammation and cartilage catabolism mediated by this last cytokine [31].

One of the most important aspects of the present study was that all the molecules evaluated were measured in PRG supernatants, culture media (at different time points), and synovial fluid. This methodological approach allowed establishing that SME groups attempted to reach in their culture media molecular environment to be similar to those observed in synovial fluid samples. However, in general, the SME groups treated with PRG supernatants showed a more robust physiological response related with a higher release to the culture media of all molecules evaluated in comparison with SME control group.

TGF-β_1 and PDGF-BB reached culture media concentrations at 48 and 96 h in a similar pattern to those observed after PRP joint injection in horses at different time points [17]. This could indicate that the synovial membrane cells equilibrate the concentration of TGF-β_1 and PDGF-BB, either by protein production or degradation, in order to reach a natural proportion of these proteins in synovial fluid.

The results from this study allow identifying that both L-PRG supernatants presented better anti-inflammatory and anabolic effects than both P-PRG supernatants. 25% L-PRG supernatant produced a robust and sustained release over time of IL-1ra and a gradual increased release of HA, whereas 50% L-PRG supernatant produced a sustained increase over time in the production of IL-4 and HA. In contrast, 50% P-PRG supernatant produced an anti-inflammatory effect manifested by an increased and sustained production of IL-1ra and IL-4. However, although not significant, the HA concentration tended to diminish over time. Moreover, a 25% P-PRG supernatant could be considered the treatment with the worst results, because it produced the lowest release of anti-inflammatory cytokines and progressive diminution (but not significant) in HA concentration in the time.

The results from this study are contradictory to previous *in vitro* studies evaluating the effect of several PRP preparations on equine cartilage and meniscus explants [15] and equine tendon explants [32, 33]. In general, these studies demonstrated that leukoreduced PRP (P-PRP) preparations produced an anabolic state in these tissues in comparison to L-PRP preparations, which induced upregulation of catabolic molecules, such as matrix metalloproteinases and proinflammatory cytokines [15, 32, 33]. Our findings are not also in agreement with *in vitro* studies that evaluated the effect of PRP preparations on human cartilage explants and synoviocytes in coculture [16] and synoviocytes alone [30].

Some explanations could be proposed to explain the discrepancies in the results from our research and the findings of the aforementioned studies [15, 16, 30, 32, 33]. We believe that different technical and methodological conditions of every study in particular could affect the final results and compromise a direct comparison between all studies. In our study, two concentrations of L-PRG and P-PRG supernatants were evaluated; however, this particular situation was not performed in the mentioned studies [15, 16, 30, 32, 33]. In addition, two culture media changes every 48 h were performed in the present research; in contrast, no culture media changes were performed in these studies [15, 16, 30, 32, 33]. Moreover, we used PRG supernatants for the experiments, whereas PRP preparations were employed in these studies [15, 16, 30, 32, 33].

The results from the present study could indicate that not only the cellular concentration (particularly leukocytes) in PRP but also its concentration on culture media could affect the molecular profile of the tissues treated with this substance. Our findings could also indicate the necessity to establish an adequate volume of PRP or PRG supernatant for the treatment of every specific joint affected by OA or traumatic arthritis. Moreover, these results open the question about which substance, either PRP or PRG supernatant, could be more indicated for OA or traumatic arthritis treatment.

The present study had several limitations. First of all, this was an *in vitro* study, which means that it is only useful for proposing and not for extrapolating the basic mechanisms underlying the PRP based treatment of OA [10–13]. Studies using *in vitro* systems of joint components, like this one, fail to demonstrate the tremendous role of the immunology system and their regulatory action in joint disease [34]. On the other hand, many molecules directly implicated in the OA pathophysiology, such as IL-1, IL-6, and matrix metalloproteinases, amongst others, were not included in this study by budget limitations; this situation logically limits the capacity for understanding the effect of the PRG supernatants evaluated in this study. Finally, further, *in vitro* studies are necessary in order to determine whether the synovial membrane response to PRG supernatants could be affected by inflammation induced by lipopolysaccharide or catabolic cytokines or whether the use of either PRP or PRG supernatant could induce different synovial membrane responses.

5. Conclusions

L-PRG and P-PRG supernatants at 25 and 50% concentrations influenced the molecular anti-inflammatory and anabolic profile of SME groups cultured with these substances. Twenty-five % and 50% L-PRG supernatants and 50% P-PRG supernatant produced the best anti-inflammatory and anabolic effects when compared to the SME control group and the SME group treated with 25% P-PRG supernatant. Additional *in vitro* research is necessary to determine if the synovial membrane response to PRG supernatants could be affected by an induced inflammatory state.

Conflict of Interests

The authors declare no competing interests related to this paper.

Authors' Contribution

This paper represents a part of a Ph.D. thesis submitted by Diana L. Ríos to the Biomedical Sciences Doctoral Program of the Universidad de Caldas, Manizales, Colombia. Jorge U. Carmona conceived the study, participated in its design, and coordination and revised the paper. Diana L. Ríos and Catalina López acquired data, participated in their analysis and interpretation, and drafted the paper. All authors read and approved the final paper.

Acknowledgments

Diana L. Ríos thanks COLCIENCIAS by her Ph.D. scholarship. The authors thank Wilson Gómez and Fabio Robayo for their assistance. This project was supported by Grant no. 397-2011 of the National Program of Biotechnology from COLCIENCIAS, Bogotá D.C., and by Grant no. 0250911 of the Vicerrectoría de Investigaciones y Postgrados of the Universidad de Caldas, Manizales, Colombia.

References

[1] P. D. Rossdale, R. Hopes, N. J. Digby, and K. offord, "Epidemiological study of wastage among racehorses 1982 and 1983," *Veterinary Record*, vol. 116, no. 3, pp. 66–69, 1985.

[2] S. Björnsdóttir, T. Árnason, and P. Lord, "Culling rate of icelandic horses due to bone spavin," *Acta Veterinaria Scandinavica*, vol. 44, no. 3-4, pp. 161–169, 2003.

[3] J. U. Carmona and M. Prades, "Pathophisiology of osteoarthritis," *Compendium Equine*, vol. 4, pp. 28–40, 2009.

[4] C. W. McIlwraith, "General pathobiology of the joint and response to injury," in *Joint Disease in the Horse*, C. W. McIlwraith and G. W. Trotter, Eds., pp. 40–70, Saunders, Philadelphia, Pa, USA, 1996.

[5] L. R. Goodrich and A. J. Nixon, "Medical treatment of osteoarthritis in the horse—a review," *Veterinary Journal*, vol. 171, no. 1, pp. 51–69, 2006.

[6] T. H. Hraha, K. M. Doremus, C. W. Mcilwraith, and D. D. Frisbie, "Autologous conditioned serum: the comparative cytokine profiles of two commercial methods (IRAP and IRAP II) using equine blood," *Equine Veterinary Journal*, vol. 43, no. 5, pp. 516–521, 2011.

[7] A. L. Bertone, A. Ishihara, L. J. Zekas et al., "Evaluation of a single intra-articular injection of autologous protein solution for treatment of osteoarthritis in horses," *American Journal of Veterinary Research*, vol. 75, no. 2, pp. 141–151, 2014.

[8] D. D. Frisbie and M. C. Stewart, "Cell-based therapies for equine joint disease," *Veterinary Clinics of North America—Equine Practice*, vol. 27, no. 2, pp. 335–349, 2011.

[9] J. A. Sandoval, C. López, and J. U. Carmona, "Therapies intended for joint regeneration in the horse," *Archivos de Medicina Veterinaria*, vol. 45, no. 3, pp. 229–236, 2013.

[10] J. U. Carmona, D. Argüelles, F. Climent, and M. Prades, "Autologous platele t concentrates as a treatment of horses with osteoarthritis: a preliminary pilot clinical study," *Journal of Equine Veterinary Science*, vol. 27, no. 4, pp. 167–170, 2007.

[11] F. Pichereau, M. Décory, and G. C. Ramos, "Autologous platelet concentrate as a treatment for horses with refractory fetlock osteoarthritis," *Journal of Equine Veterinary Science*, vol. 34, no. 4, pp. 489–493, 2014.

[12] A. Khoshbin, T. Leroux, D. Wasserstein et al., "The efficacy of platelet-rich plasma in the treatment of symptomatic knee osteoarthritis: a systematic review with quantitative synthesis," *Arthroscopy*, vol. 29, no. 12, pp. 2037–2048, 2013.

[13] R. F. Silva, J. U. Carmona, and C. M. F. Rezende, "Intra-articular injections of autologous platelet concentrates in dogs with surgical reparation of cranial cruciate ligament rupture,"

Veterinary and Comparative Orthopaedics and Traumatology, vol. 26, no. 4, pp. 285–290, 2013.

[14] B. Cuervo, M. Rubio, J. Sopena et al., "Hip osteoarthritis in dogs: a randomized study using mesenchymal stem cells from adipose tissue and plasma rich in growth factors," *International Journal of Molecular Sciences*, vol. 15, no. 8, pp. 13437–13460, 2014.

[15] J. D. Kisiday, C. W. McIlwraith, W. G. Rodkey, D. D. Frisbie, and J. R. Steadman, "Effects of platelet-rich plasma composition on anabolic and catabolic activities in equine cartilage and meniscal explants," *Cartilage*, vol. 3, no. 3, pp. 245–254, 2012.

[16] E. A. Sundman, B. J. Cole, V. Karas et al., "The anti-inflammatory and matrix restorative mechanisms of platelet-rich plasma in osteoarthritis," *The American Journal of Sports Medicine*, vol. 42, no. 1, pp. 35–41, 2014.

[17] J. A. Textor, N. H. Willits, and F. Tablin, "Synovial fluid growth factor and cytokine concentrations after intra-articular injection of a platelet-rich product in horses," *Veterinary Journal*, vol. 198, no. 1, pp. 217–223, 2013.

[18] D. M. D. Ehrenfest, T. Bielecki, A. Mishra et al., "In search of a consensus terminology in the field of platelet concentrates for surgical use: Platelet-Rich Plasma (PRP), Platelet-Rich Fibrin (PRF), fibrin gel polymerization and leukocytes," *Current Pharmaceutical Biotechnology*, vol. 13, no. 7, pp. 1131–1137, 2012.

[19] J. U. Carmona, C. López, and J. A. Sandoval, "Review of the currently available systems to obtain platelet related products to treat equine musculoskeletal injuries," *Recent Patents on Regenerative Medicine*, vol. 3, no. 2, pp. 148–159, 2013.

[20] C. E. Giraldo, C. López, M. E. Álvarez, I. J. Samudio, M. Prades, and J. U. Carmona, "Effects of the breed, sex and age on cellular content and growth factor release from equine pure-platelet rich plasma and pure-platelet rich gel," *BMC Veterinary Research*, vol. 9, article 29, 2013.

[21] B. P. Donnelly, A. J. Nixon, J. L. Haupt, and L. A. Dahlgren, "Nucleotide structure of equine platelet-derived growth factor-A and -B and expression in horses with induced acute tendinitis," *American Journal of Veterinary Research*, vol. 67, no. 7, pp. 1218–1225, 2006.

[22] M. N. Penha-Goncalves, D. E. Onions, and L. Nicolson, "Cloning and sequencing of equine transforming growth factor-beta 1 (TGFβ-1) cDNA," *Mitochondrial DNA*, vol. 7, no. 6, pp. 375–378, 1997.

[23] L. A. Fortier, J. U. Barker, E. J. Strauss, T. M. McCarrel, and B. J. Cole, "The role of growth factors in cartilage repair," *Clinical Orthopaedics and Related Research*, vol. 469, no. 10, pp. 2706–2715, 2011.

[24] F. David, J. Farley, H. Huang, J.-P. Lavoie, and S. Laverty, "Cytokine and chemokine gene expression of IL-1β stimulated equine articular chondrocytes," *Veterinary Surgery*, vol. 36, no. 3, pp. 221–227, 2007.

[25] L. Eder, A. Thavaneswaran, V. Chandran, and D. D. Gladman, "Tumour necrosis factor α blockers are more effective than methotrexate in the inhibition of radiographic joint damage progression among patients with psoriatic arthritis," *Annals of the Rheumatic Diseases*, vol. 73, no. 6, pp. 1007–1011, 2014.

[26] J. L. Kamm, A. J. Nixon, and T. H. Witte, "Cytokine and catabolic enzyme expression in synovium, synovial fluid and articular cartilage of naturally osteoarthritic equine carpi," *Equine Veterinary Journal*, vol. 42, no. 8, pp. 693–699, 2010.

[27] S. J. Millward-Sadler, M. O. Wright, L. W. Davies, G. Nuki, and D. M. Salter, "Mechanotransduction via integrins and interleukin-4 results in altered aggrecan and matrix metalloproteinase 3 gene expression in normal, but not osteoarthritic,

human articular chondrocytes," *Arthritis & Rheumatism*, vol. 43, no. 9, pp. 2091–2099, 2000.

[28] C. I. Westacott, J. T. Whicher, I. C. Barnes, D. Thompson, A. J. Swan, and P. A. Dieppe, "Synovial fluid concentration of five different cytokines in rheumatic diseases," *Annals of the Rheumatic Diseases*, vol. 49, no. 9, pp. 676–681, 1990.

[29] S.-G. Lee, E.-J. Lee, W.-D. Park, J.-B. Kim, E.-O. Kim, and S.-W. Choi, "Anti-inflammatory and anti-osteoarthritis effects of fermented Achyranthes japonica Nakai," *Journal of Ethnopharmacology*, vol. 142, no. 3, pp. 634–641, 2012.

[30] H. J. Braun, H. J. Kim, C. R. Chu, and J. L. Dragoo, "The effect of platelet-rich plasma formulations and blood products on human synoviocytes: implications for intra-articular injury and therapy," *The American Journal of Sports Medicine*, vol. 42, no. 5, pp. 1204–1210, 2014.

[31] M. Rutgers, D. B. F. Saris, W. J. A. Dhert, and L. B. Creemers, "Cytokine profile of autologous conditioned serum for treatment of osteoarthritis, in vitro effects on cartilage metabolism and intra-articular levels after injection," *Arthritis Research & Therapy*, vol. 12, no. 3, article R114, 2010.

[32] S. G. Boswell, L. V. Schnabel, H. O. Mohammed, E. A. Sundman, T. Minas, and L. A. Fortier, "Increasing platelet concentrations in leukocyte-reduced platelet-rich plasma decrease collagen gene synthesis in tendons," *American Journal of Sports Medicine*, vol. 42, no. 1, pp. 42–49, 2014.

[33] T. M. McCarrel, T. Minas, and L. A. Fortier, "Optimization of leukocyte concentration in platelet-rich plasma for the treatment of tendinopathy," *The Journal of Bone & Joint Surgery—American Volume*, vol. 94, no. 19, pp. e143.141–e143.148, 2012.

[34] I. Andia and N. Maffulli, "Anti-inflammatory and matrix restorative mechanisms of platelet-rich plasma in osteoarthritis: letter to the editor," *The American Journal of Sports Medicine*, vol. 42, no. 6, p. NP32, 2014.

4

Histomorphometric Evaluation of Superovulation Effect on Follicular Development after Autologous Ovarian Transplantation in Mice

Amin Tamadon,[1] Alireza Raayat Jahromi,[2] Farhad Rahmanifar,[3] Mohammad Ayaseh,[2] Omid Koohi-Hosseinabadi,[4] and Reza Moghiminasr[5]

[1]Transgenic Technology Research Center, Shiraz University of Medical Sciences, Shiraz, Iran
[2]Department of Clinical Sciences, School of Veterinary Medicine, Shiraz University, P.O. Box 1731-71345, Shiraz, Iran
[3]Department of Basic Sciences, School of Veterinary Medicine, Shiraz University, P.O. Box 1731-71345, Shiraz, Iran
[4]Laboratory Animal Center, Shiraz University of Medical Sciences, Shiraz, Iran
[5]Department of Stem Cells and Developmental Biology, Cell Science Research Center,
 Royan Institute for Stem Cell Biology and Technology, ACECR, Tehran, Iran

Correspondence should be addressed to Alireza Raayat Jahromi; raayat@shirazu.ac.ir
and Farhad Rahmanifar; rahmanifar@shirazu.ac.ir

Academic Editor: Sumanta Nandi

The effect of superovulation by pregnant mare serum gonadotropin (PMSG) on autologous transplanted ovaries in the lumbar muscles of mice was histomorphometrically evaluated using the indices of number and volume of different kind of follicles and volume of corpora lutea, ovary, and stroma. Angiogenesis was observed after mouse ovarian transplantation on days 14 and 21 after ovarian grafting. After transplantation, the total number and volume of primary and secondary follicles reduced, while PMSG superovulation increased the total number and total volume of tertiary follicles and also the ovarian volume after transplantation. Transplantation increased the average size of primary, secondary, and tertiary follicles. Therefore, primary and secondary follicles can survive after autologous transplantation but their reservations diminished by increasing the time of transplantation. However, number of tertiary follicles and their response to superovulation increased over time after transplantation.

1. Introduction

Ovary transplantation is a method for preservation of endangered and valuable species [1]. On the other hand, ovarian transplantation has the potential application for maintaining the fertility after chemotherapy and radiotherapy in women [2]. As a result of the ovarian transplantation, the possible depletion of follicle reserve and limitation of fertility restoration exist [3]. The major concern in grafting is that the graft survival is completely dependent on the establishment of neovascularization [4]. A number of follicles may be lost because of hypoxia and ischemia. For evaluation of the effect of ischemia after ovarian transplantation, whole or piece of small ovaries of laboratory rodents can be used [5]. To prevent ischemia and increase the rate of angiogenesis, surgery must

be rapid and the ovarian tissue should be placed in a highly vascular tissue [6]. It is shown that ischemia may cause disappearance of 50% or even greater percentage of primary follicles and almost all of the growing follicles 3 to 7 days after transplantation and before development of angiogenesis [7].

Steroidogenesis, proliferation, and differentiation of follicular granulosa cells of growing preovulatory stages of ovarian follicles are induced by follicle-stimulating hormone (FSH). However, primordial follicles' initial development is FSH independent [8], but FSH acts as survival factor in serum-free ovarian cortical tissue culture and during primordial follicular transition to primary and secondary follicles [9]. In addition, coordination of germ line and somatic compartments of follicle development in mouse is done by FSH [10]. FSH action in adult mouse can be induced using

TABLE 1: Groups and procedures for evaluation of superovulation effect on follicular development after autologous ovarian transplantation in mice.

Groups	Transplantation	PMSG injection and time	Day of sampling
Negative control	−	−	In the estrus phase
PMSG	−	+ (In the diestrus phase)	2 d after injection
Graft (14 d)	+	−	14 d after transplantation
Graft (21 d)	+	−	21 d after transplantation
Graft + PMSG (14 d)	+	+ (12 d after transplantation)	14 d after transplantation
Graft + PMSG (21 d)	+	+ (19 d after transplantation)	21 d after transplantation

pregnant mare serum gonadotropin (PMSG), a chorionic gonadotropin hormone of pregnant mare. PMSG superovulation can serve as a good model to understand the probable mechanism of FSH action in follicular development [11].

With that in mind that harvesting of mature oocytes for in vitro fertilization process increases the chances of reproductive success, PMSG is currently used for production of mature superovulated oocytes for in vitro fertilization of valuable species including endangered ones. In addition, it is not known if the transplanted preserved ovaries can respond to the superovulation to achieve this goal of harvesting higher number of matured oocytes. The aim of the present study was to (1) assess superovulation with PMSG on transplanted ovary as an indicator of posttransplantation normal activity of antral follicles, (2) evaluate histomorphometrically the effect of posttransplantation ischemia on different follicular stages, and (3) evaluate the effect of recovery time on follicular growth after autologous transplantation of murine ovaries by the induction of superovulation using PMSG.

2. Materials and Methods

2.1. Animals. The experimental study was approved by Ethics Committee of School of Veterinary Medicine, Shiraz University. Thirty-six female adult Balb/c mice weighing approximately 25–30 g were provided from Laboratory Animal Center, Shiraz University of Medical Sciences. The animals were kept at $23 \pm 1°C$ and $55 \pm 5\%$ relative humidity with 12 h light/dark cycle. They were given standard pellet and water *ad libitum* during experimental period.

The mice were randomly divided into 6 equal groups ($n = 6$), four transplantation groups and two control groups (Table 1). The transplantation groups included two transplantation (14 and 21 d) groups and two PMSG/transplantation (14 and 21 d) groups. The control groups were subdivided to a positive control PMSG group and a negative control group. The mice were entered into study on day of diestrus using vaginal smears. In PMSG positive control group, the mice received single intraperitoneal injection of PMSG (5 IU, Pregnecol, Bioniche Animal Health (A/Asia) Pty Ltd., Armidale, NSW, Australia) and 48 h later the animals were euthanized with ether and cervical dislocation. In the transplantation groups (14 and 21 d), the ovarian autotransplantation was done on both sides of spinal cord during the diestrus phase. After 14 d and 21 d, the mice of transplantation groups were sacrificed. In the PMSG/transplantation groups (14 and 21 d),

the same autotransplantation procedure was performed and after 12 d in the first group and 19 d in the second one PMSG (5 IU) was intraperitoneally injected and 48 h later the mice were euthanized. In the negative control group, surgery was not performed and the mice were sacrificed in the estrus phase. Stages of estrus cycle were determined based on vaginal smear method [12].

2.2. Ovarian Autotransplantation Surgical Method. Surgical procedures were performed under sterile conditions and in a $24°C$ temperature operating room. The diestrus mice were weighed and anesthetized with an IP injection of ketamine (100 mg/kg, Alfasan, Woerden, Netherland) and xylazine (10 mg/kg, Alfasan, Woerden, Netherland). Surgical area of abdomen and lateral lumbar region of the mice were surgically prepared. Both ovaries of the mice were removed from a midline abdominal incision and transferred to a sterile dish filled with prewarmed ($39°C$) sterile saline. Adipose and connective tissues were carefully removed from ovary using a stereomicroscope (SZM, Optika, Italy). The abdominal muscles and skin were sutured with a standard two-layer closure using a simple continuous suture pattern. Then, paralumbar incisions were made on both sides, parallel to the lumbar spinal cord. The ovaries were then grafted into the dorsal lumbar muscles and skin was routinely closed. Oxytetracycline spray was applied on the incision site. Animals were placed in individual controlled $25°C$ temperature recovery cages.

2.3. Histological Evaluation of Ovaries. On the day of sampling, animals were euthanized with ether and ovaries of control and PMSG groups and the transplanted ovarian tissues with their surrounding muscles of transplanting groups were removed. The tissues were fixed in fresh 10% buffered formalin solution in room temperature. After that they were implanted in paraffin. Ethanol and xylene were used for dehydration step. Samples were embedded in paraffin wax and serial sections at thicknesses of 20 μm were performed. During the block sectioning, serial sections were checked until the ovarian tissues appeared in the paraffin section. That was selected as the first section of ovary and the 10th section of every 10 consecutive slices were selected until the observation of the last section with ovarian tissue in the paraffin block. Selected sections were deparaffinized at $60°C$ and dehydrated in graded concentrations of xylene and ethanol rehydrated in room temperature and stained with hematoxylin and eosin stain.

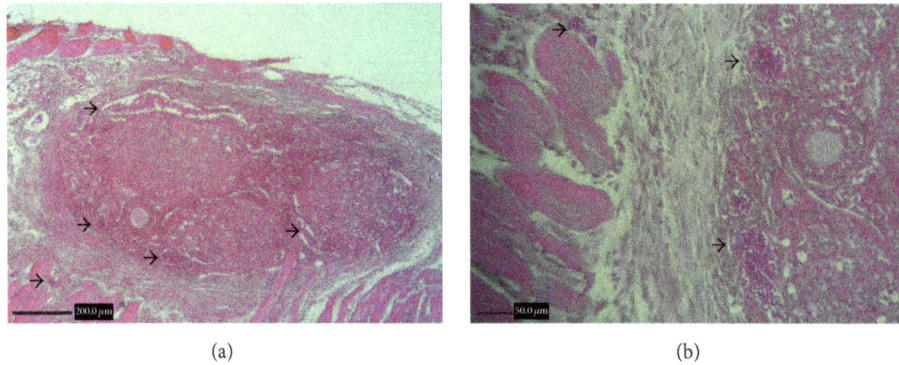

(a)   (b)

FIGURE 1: (a) Corpora lutea and secondary follicle in the section confirm ovarian function and folliculogenesis after 21 days' autologous ovarian transplantation in lateral lumbar muscles of mice without superovulation. (b) Angiogenesis, arrows show presence of blood cells in vessels of transplanted ovary and surrounding skeletal muscles. H&E staining.

2.4. Histomorphometric Analysis. Follicle types in ovarian sections were defined as previously explained [13] and the numbers of primary, secondary, and tertiary follicles were counted on light microscope (CX21, Olympus, Japan). Sections were also microscopically photographed with an adjusted digital camera (AM423U Eyepiece Camera, Dino-Eye, Taiwan) and Dino Capture 2.0 software (AnMo Electronics Corporation, New Taipei City, Taiwan). The area of total ovary, corpora lutea, and total follicles of each section were measured by drawing their scope using Digimizer software (MedCalc Software bvba; Mariakerke, Belgium).

Moreover, the volume of the ovary, developing follicles of all stages, and corpora lutea of all groups (V) were calculated according to the elliptical cone volume formula: $V = \pi D^2 h/6$, where π is equivalent to 3.14, D indicates the larger diameter, and h indicates the smaller diameter of the ovary, follicles, and corpora lutea. The mean follicle volume (v) was measured by taking the average of volume of ovarian tertiary follicles of all stages, according to the following formula: $v = V/N$, where N indicates the numbers of ovarian developing follicles of all stages. Furthermore, stromal volume (V_S) was calculated according to the following formula: $V_S = V_O - V_F$, where V_O is the volume of the ovary and V_F is the volume of the follicles.

2.5. Statistical Analysis. The data of histological indices of ovary were subjected to Kolmogorov-Smirnov test of normality and analyzed by one-way ANOVA and LSD post hoc test (SPSS for Windows, version 22, SPSS Inc., Chicago, Illinois). The P value of less than 0.05 was considered to be statistically significant. Group means and their standard error were reported in the text and graphs (GraphPad Prism version 5.01 for Windows, GraphPad software Inc., San Diego, CA, USA).

3. Results

Histological evaluation showed angiogenesis and folliculogenesis after grafting in ovaries in the transplantation and PMSG/transplantation groups (Figure 1). Moreover, in microscopic evaluation of ovaries in the PMSG group and the PMSG/transplantation (14 and 21 d) groups numerous large tertiary follicles were observed, but in the transplantation (14 and 21 d) groups and the control group the number and the size of tertiary follicles were smaller (Figure 2).

Histomorphometric analysis showed that there was a significant reduction in the number and total volume of primary follicles in the transplantation (14 and 21 d) and PMSG/transplantation (14 and 21 d) groups compared with the control and PMSG groups ($P < 0.05$, Figures 3(a) and 3(b)). The mean primary follicle volume in the transplantation (14 d) group was more than that in the other groups except for the PMSG/transplantation (14 d) group ($P < 0.05$, Figure 3(c)). Also there was a significant decrease in the mean primary follicle volume in the PMSG group in comparison with the other groups ($P < 0.05$).

Same as primary follicles, there was a significant reduction in the number of secondary follicles in the transplantation (14 and 21 d) and PMSG/transplantation (14 and 21 d) groups compared with the control and PMSG groups ($P < 0.05$, Figure 4(a)). Moreover, the total volume of secondary follicles in the PMSG group was more than the PMSG/transplantation (21 d) group ($P < 0.05$, Figure 4(b)). The mean secondary follicle volume in the transplantation (14 d) group was significantly more than the control, PMSG, and PMSG/transplantation (21 d) groups ($P < 0.05$, Figure 4(c)).

The number of tertiary follicles in the transplantation (21 d) and PMSG/transplantation (21 d) groups was significantly more than the control group ($P < 0.05$, Figure 5(a)). The total volume of tertiary follicles in the PMSG/transplantation (21 d) group was significantly greater than the control, PMSG, and transplantation (14 d) groups ($P < 0.05$, Figure 5(b)). The mean tertiary follicle volume in the PMSG/transplantation (14 and 21 d) group was more than the control and PMSG groups ($P < 0.05$, Figure 5(c)).

Ovary volume in the PMSG/transplantation (21 d) group was more than the control and transplantation (14 d) groups ($P < 0.05$, Figure 6(a)). Ovarian stromal volume in the PMSG group was more than the transplantation (14 and 21 d) groups ($P < 0.05$, Figure 6(b)).

Histomorphometric Evaluation of Superovulation Effect on Follicular Development after Autologous Ovarian...

27

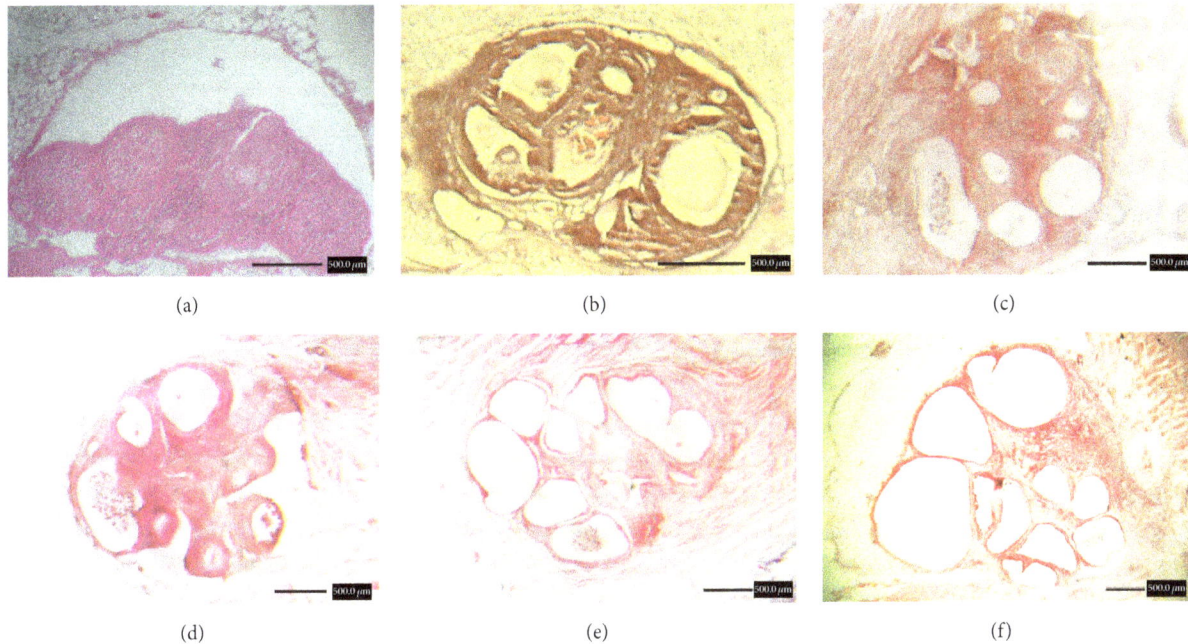

FIGURE 2: Comparison of the superovulatory effect of pregnant mare serum gonadotropin (PMSG) after autologous ovarian transplantation in mice. Ovaries of groups of (a) control, (b) PMSG, (c) transplantation (14 d), (d) transplantation (21 d), (e) PMSG/transplantation (14 d), and (f) PMSG/transplantation (21 d). H&E staining.

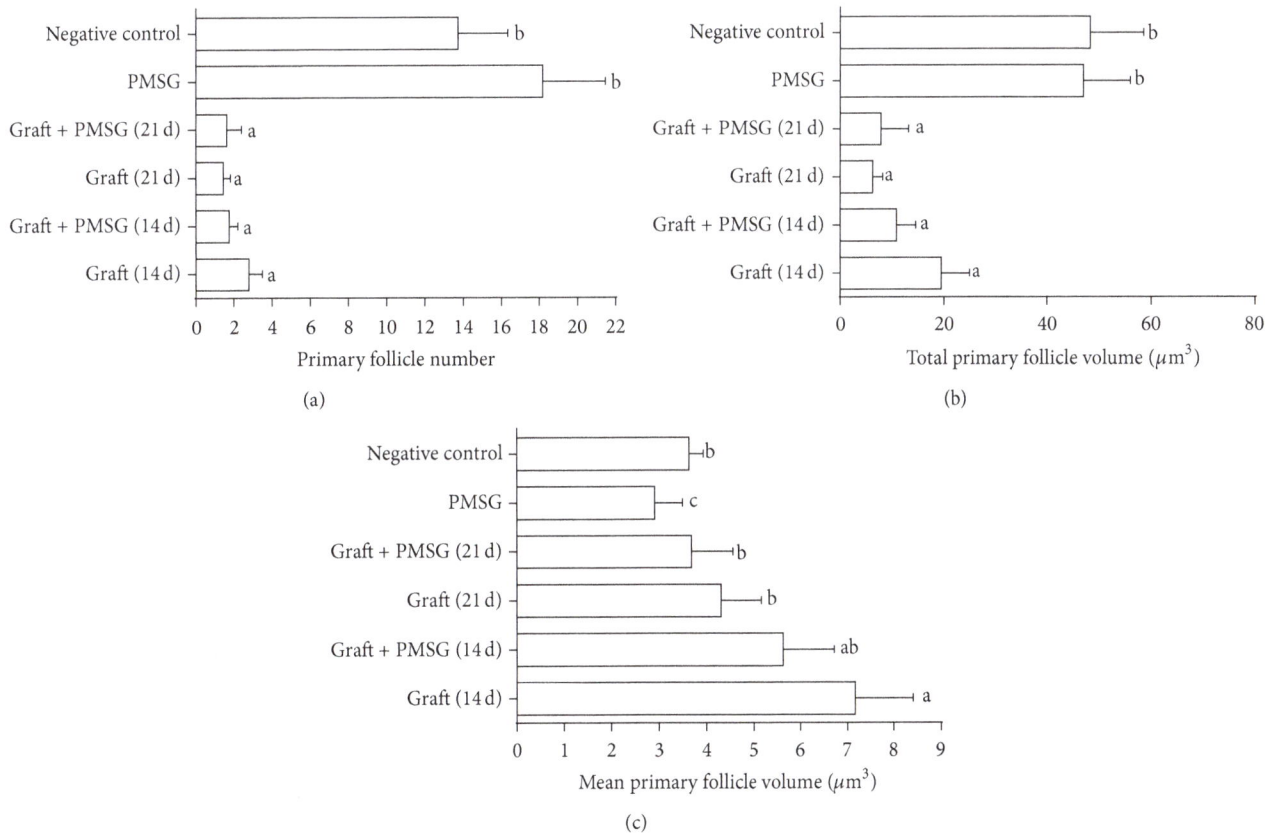

FIGURE 3: Mean and standard error of histomorphometric analysis of primary follicles (a) total number, (b) total volume, and (c) mean follicle volume in control group, pregnant mare serum gonadotropin (PMSG) group, transplantation (14 and 21 d), and PMSG/transplantation (14 and 21 d) groups after autologous ovarian transplantation and superovulatory effect of PMSG. [a, b, c] Different superscript letters show significant difference between different groups ($P < 0.05$).

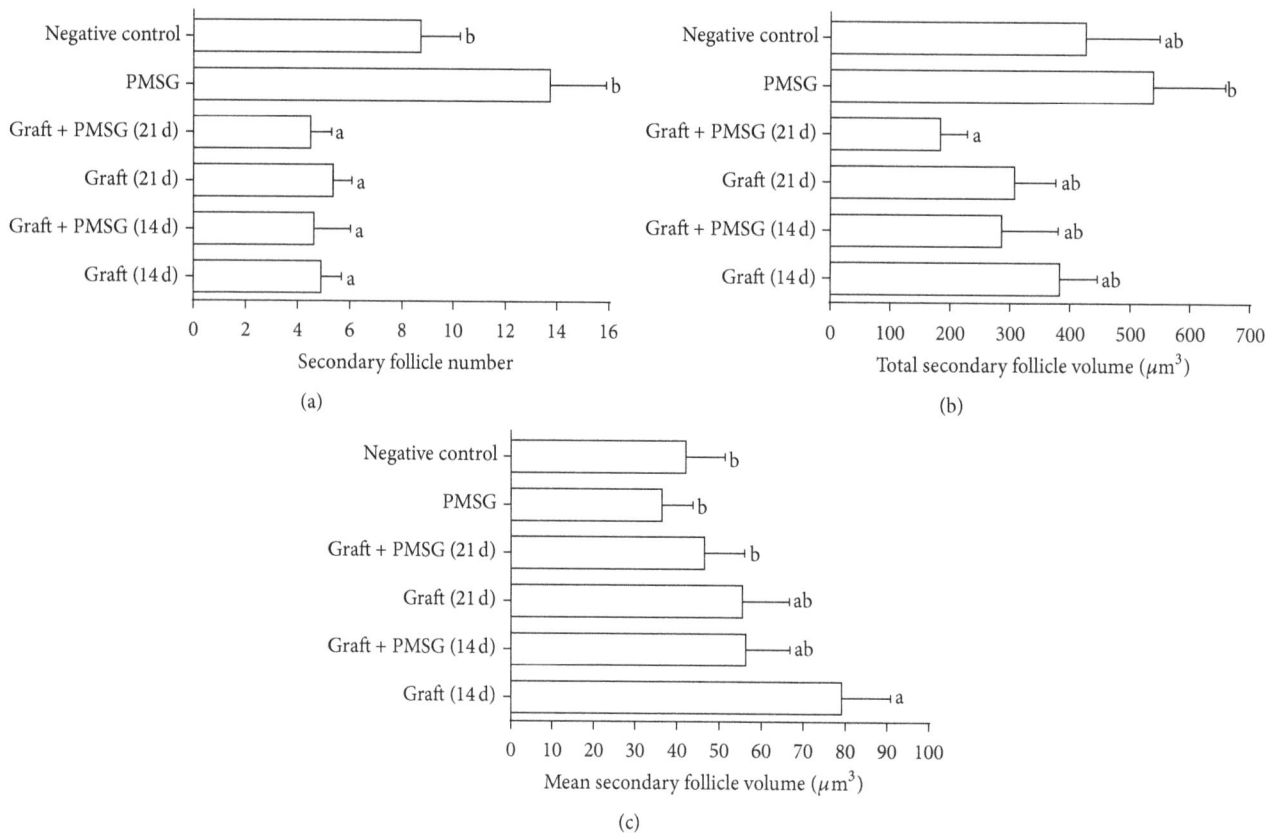

FIGURE 4: Mean and standard error of histomorphometric analysis of secondary follicles (a) total number, (b) total volume, and (c) mean follicle volume in control group, pregnant mare serum gonadotropin (PMSG) group, transplantation (14 and 21 d), and PMSG/transplantation (14 and 21 d) groups after autologous ovarian transplantation and superovulatory effect of PMSG. [a,b] Different superscript letters show significant difference between different groups ($P < 0.05$).

4. Discussion

In the present study, the impact of transplantation ischemia on survival and development of different follicular stages following whole ovary heterotopic autotransplantation were histomorphometrically evaluated after 14 and 21 d. The results indicated that survival and development of different follicular types were influenced by ischemia. Reduction in the number of primary and secondary follicles in the transplantation and PMSG/transplantation groups after 14 and 21 d showed the effect of ischemia on these follicular stages. However, the number and volume of these follicles decreased after grafting but estimated individual size of both types was increased after 14 days and again was decreased on day 21. Simultaneously, during the same period, increase of the number and volume of tertiary follicles showed follicular growth continued and was enhanced after heterotopic transplantation. Consistent with our findings, Xie et al. [3] recently showed that healthy rate of follicles and the number of follicles with positive proliferating cell nuclear antigen in primary follicles decreased 1 month after orthotopic autografting of the rabbit ovaries. Early follicular development is regulated by ovarian autocrine/paracrine regulators and interactions between oocyte-granulosa cells, ovarian stromal cells, and theca cells affect this process [14]. Grafting could induce deactivation of primordial follicles [15]. Therefore, decrease in number of primary follicles can be affected by cessation of primordial follicle growth. Our findings indirectly and directly may indicate that follicular growth and development in early stage (primordial and primary follicles) were more influenced by ischemia in comparison with late stages (secondary and tertiary follicles), and follicle reservoirs in primordial and primary stages cannot be well replaced after transplantation ischemia.

In this study, we observed that ovarian tissue survived and follicles grew in muscular spaces of back muscle. A rapid blood supply can prevent loss of follicular pool and cessation of folliculogenesis after ovarian transplantation may reduce the follicular quality and response to hormonal alterations. Therefore, in this study the effect of intraperitoneal injection of PMSG on follicular growth after ovarian transplantation was evaluated as an index of presence of ovarian blood supply, angiogenesis, and folliculogenesis especially after primordial follicular stage. Significant differences in the primary, secondary, and tertiary follicle number and volume after transplantation and superovulation, which indicated the time despite the positive role in follicular survival and better angiogenesis, have a significant impact on follicular growth and maturation in response to superovulation. Anatomically, primary follicles in rodents are small and located very close

(a)

(b)

(c)

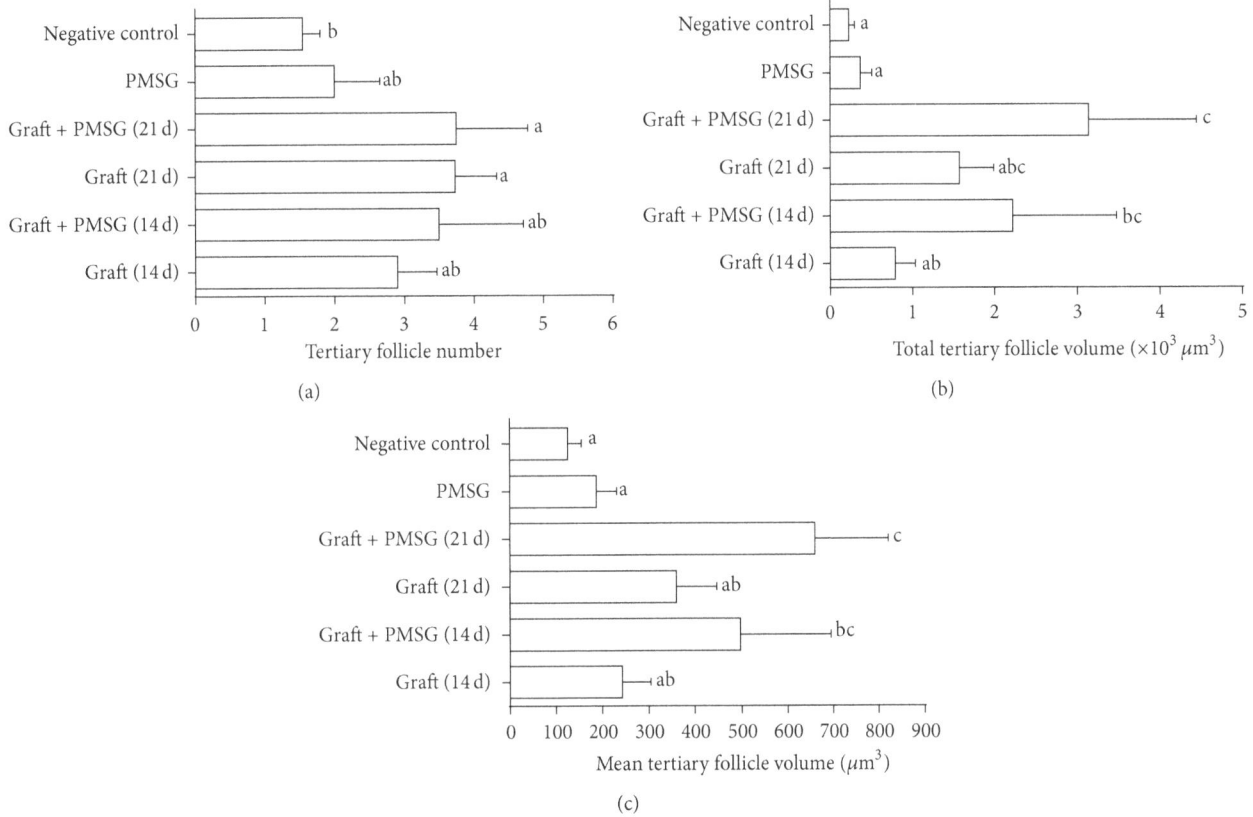

FIGURE 5: Mean and standard error of histomorphometric analysis of tertiary follicles (a) total number, (b) total volume, and (c) mean follicle volume in control group, pregnant mare serum gonadotropin (PMSG) group, transplantation (14 and 21 d), and PMSG/transplantation (14 and 21 d) groups after autologous ovarian transplantation and superovulatory effect of PMSG. [a,b,c]Different superscript letters show significant difference between different groups ($P < 0.05$).

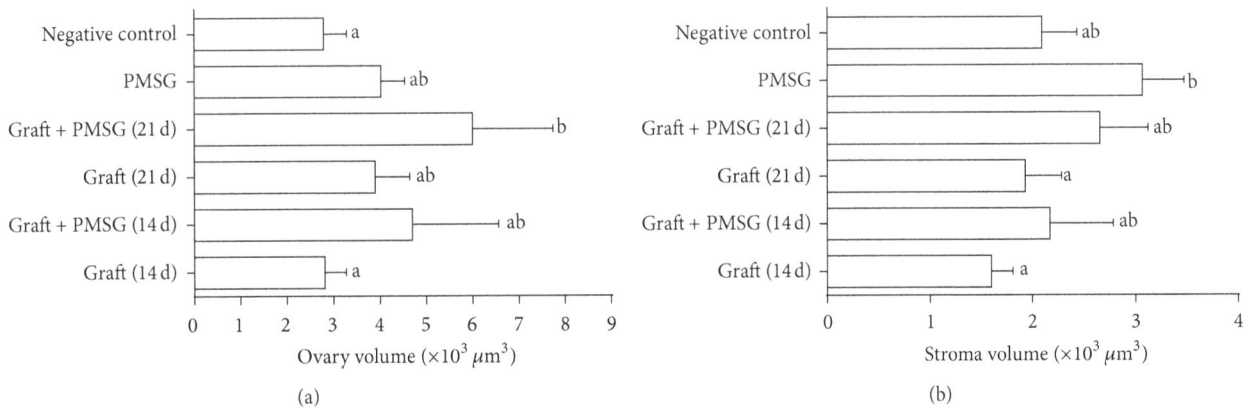

(a)

(b)

FIGURE 6: Mean and standard error of histomorphometric analysis of (a) ovarian volume and (b) stroma volume in control group, pregnant mare serum gonadotropin (PMSG) group, transplantation (14 and 21 d), and PMSG/transplantation (14 and 21 d) groups after autologous ovarian transplantation and superovulatory effect of PMSG. [a,b]Different superscript letters show significant difference between different groups ($P < 0.05$).

to the surface of ovary [16]. On the other hand, oocyte metabolism was higher in primary follicles than at any subsequent stage [17]. Therefore, more reduction of primary follicles than secondary ones after one week (time between two samplings) may be the result of the effect of posttransplantation ischemia on reduction of early stages of follicles.

Complete removal of ovarian fat tissue before transplantation enhanced revascularization via facilitation of cell infiltration from the high blood supply muscular tissue. Formation of new blood vessels was initiated by elongation, sprouting, intussusception, or the incorporation of circulating endothelial cells of preexisting vasculature [18]. Most of these processes can be involved in angiogenesis of ovary [19]. Ischemic damage of ovarian tissue is unavoidable during postgrafting period and its effect is reduced after neo- and revascularization. Vascular connections between the murine ovary and transplanted site were observed 5 days after transplantation [20].

A cohort of primordial follicles within 10 to 12 d reaches the secondary follicle stage and by 6 to 12 d develop to the large antral stage in mice [21]. Considering the 5 d of posttransplantation angiogenesis, in the first sampling of 14 d, the evaluated tertiary follicles were the developed follicles from the primary and secondary follicles which suffered from posttransplantation ischemia, while in the second sampling of 21 d the sectioned tertiary follicles were related to the developed follicles from the primary and secondary follicles after angiogenesis. Therefore, the increase in mean of number or volume of tertiary follicles after 21 d in comparison with 14 d sampling in transplantation groups can be explained.

5. Conclusions

Primary and secondary follicles can survive after autologous transplantation but their reservoirs gradually get diminished by increasing the time of transplantation. However, number of tertiary follicles and their response to superovulation increased over time after transplantation. Therefore, it seems that early collection or superovulation of transplanted ovaries may result in more tertiary follicles.

Conflict of Interests

The authors declare that there is no conflict of interests regarding the publication of this paper.

References

[1] R. R. Santos, C. Amorim, S. Cecconi et al., "Cryopreservation of ovarian tissue: an emerging technology for female germline preservation of endangered species and breeds," *Animal Reproduction Science*, vol. 122, no. 3-4, pp. 151–163, 2010.

[2] P. Ghadjar, V. Budach, C. Köhler, A. Jantke, and S. Marnitz, "Modern radiation therapy and potential fertility preservation strategies in patients with cervical cancer undergoing chemoradiation," *Radiation Oncology*, vol. 10, no. 1, p. 50, 2015.

[3] S. Xie, X. Zhang, W. Chen et al., "Developmental status: impact of short-term ischemia on follicular survival of whole ovarian transplantation in a rabbit model," *PLoS ONE*, vol. 10, no. 8, Article ID e0135049, 2015.

[4] A. R. Rajabzadeh, H. Eimani, H. Mohseni Koochesfahani, A.-H. Shahvardi, and R. Fathi, "Morphological study of isolated ovarian preantral follicles using fibrin gel plus platelet lysate after subcutaneous transplantation," *Cell Journal*, vol. 17, no. 1, pp. 145–152, 2015.

[5] E. Torrents, I. Boiso, P. N. Barri, and A. Veiga, "Applications of ovarian tissue transplantation in experimental biology and medicine," *Human Reproduction Update*, vol. 9, no. 5, pp. 471–481, 2003.

[6] I. Demeestere, P. Simon, S. Emiliani, A. Delbaere, and Y. Englert, "Orthotopic and heterotopic ovarian tissue transplantation," *Human Reproduction Update*, vol. 15, no. 6, pp. 649–665, 2009.

[7] R. G. Gosden, "Ovary and uterus transplantation," *Reproduction*, vol. 136, no. 6, pp. 671–680, 2008.

[8] R. Garor, R. Abir, A. Erman, C. Felz, S. Nitke, and B. Fisch, "Effects of basic fibroblast growth factor on in vitro development of human ovarian primordial follicles," *Fertility and Sterility*, vol. 91, no. 5, pp. 1967–1975, 2009.

[9] C. S. Wright, O. Hovatta, R. Margara et al., "Effects of follicle-stimulating hormone and serum substitution on the in-vitro growth of human ovarian follicles," *Human Reproduction*, vol. 14, no. 6, pp. 1555–1562, 1999.

[10] I. Demeestere, A. K. Streiff, J. Suzuki et al., "Follicle-stimulating hormone accelerates mouse oocyte development in vivo," *Biology of Reproduction*, vol. 87, no. 1, p. 3, 2012.

[11] D. Bhartiya, K. Sriraman, P. Gunjal, and H. Modak, "Gonadotropin treatment augments postnatal oogenesis and primordial follicle assembly in adult mouse ovaries?" *Journal of Ovarian Research*, vol. 5, no. 1, article 32, 2012.

[12] M. S. Salehi, M. R. J. Shirazi, M. J. Zamiri et al., "Hypothalamic expression of KiSS1 and RFamide-related peptide-3 mRNAs during the estrous cycle of rats," *International Journal of Fertility and Sterility*, vol. 6, no. 4, pp. 304–309, 2013.

[13] M. Azarnia, H. Koochesfahani, M. Rajabi, Y. Tahamtani, and A. Tamadon, "Histological examination of endosulfan effects on follicular development of BALB/C mice," *Bulgarian Journal of Veterinary Medicine*, vol. 12, no. 1, pp. 33–41, 2008.

[14] M. Qiu, F. Quan, C. Han et al., "Effects of granulosa cells on steroidogenesis, proliferation and apoptosis of stromal cells and theca cells derived from the goat ovary," *The Journal of Steroid Biochemistry and Molecular Biology*, vol. 138, pp. 325–333, 2013.

[15] A. David, A. Van Langendonckt, S. Gilliaux, M.-M. Dolmans, J. Donnez, and C. A. Amorim, "Effect of cryopreservation and transplantation on the expression of kit ligand and anti-Müllerian hormone in human ovarian tissue," *Human Reproduction*, vol. 27, no. 4, pp. 1088–1095, 2012.

[16] J. B. Kerr, R. Duckett, M. Myers, K. L. Britt, T. Mladenovska, and J. K. Findlay, "Quantification of healthy follicles in the neonatal and adult mouse ovary: evidence for maintenance of primordial follicle supply," *Reproduction*, vol. 132, no. 1, pp. 95–109, 2006.

[17] S. E. Harris, H. J. Leese, R. G. Gosden, and H. M. Picton, "Pyruvate and oxygen consumption throughout the growth and development of murine oocytes," *Molecular Reproduction and Development*, vol. 76, no. 3, pp. 231–238, 2009.

[18] G. D. Yancopoulos, S. Davis, N. W. Gale, J. S. Rudge, S. J. Wiegand, and J. Holash, "Vascular-specific growth factors and blood vessel formation," *Nature*, vol. 407, no. 6801, pp. 242–248, 2000.

[19] G. Macchiarelli, J.-Y. Jiang, S. A. Nottola, and E. Sato, "Morphological patterns of angiogenesis in ovarian follicle capillary networks. A scanning electron microscopy study of corrosion cast," *Microscopy Research and Technique*, vol. 69, no. 6, pp. 459–468, 2006.

[20] A.-S. Van Eyck, B. F. Jordan, B. Gallez, J.-F. Heilier, A. Van Langendonckt, and J. Donnez, "Electron paramagnetic resonance as a tool to evaluate human ovarian tissue reoxygenation after xenografting," *Fertility and Sterility*, vol. 92, no. 1, pp. 374–381, 2009.

[21] J. J. Eppig, K. Wigglesworth, and F. L. Pendola, "The mammalian oocyte orchestrates the rate of ovarian follicular development," *Proceedings of the National Academy of Sciences of the United States of America*, vol. 99, no. 5, pp. 2890–2894, 2002.

5

Studies on Antimicrobial and Immunomodulatory Effects of Hot Aqueous Extract of *Acacia nilotica* L. Leaves against Common Veterinary Pathogens

Arvind Kumar Sharma,[1] Amit Kumar,[1] Sharad Kumar Yadav,[1] and Anu Rahal[2]

[1] *Department of Veterinary Microbiology, College of Veterinary Sciences and Animal Husbandry, Uttar Pradesh Pandit Deen Dayal Upadhyaya Pashu Chikitsa Vigyan Vishwavidyalaya Evam Go Anusandhan Sansthan (DUVASU), Mathura 281001, India*

[2] *Department of Veterinary Pharmacology and Toxicology, College of Veterinary Sciences and Animal Husbandry, Uttar Pradesh Pandit Deen Dayal Upadhyaya Pashu Chikitsa Vigyan Vishwavidyalaya Evam Go Anusandhan Sansthan (DUVASU), Mathura 281001, India*

Correspondence should be addressed to Amit Kumar; balyan74@gmail.com

Academic Editor: Suresh Tikoo

Acacia nilotica is a plant species that is almost ubiquitously found in different parts of the world. Various preparations of it have been advocated in folk medicine for the treatment of tuberculosis, leprosy, smallpox, dysentery, cough, ophthalmia, toothache, skin cancer as astringent, antispasmodic, and aphrodisiac since immemorial times. The present study investigates the antibacterial, antifungal, antiviral, and immunomodulatory potential of hot aqueous extract (HAE) of *Acacia nilotica* leaves. On dry matter basis, the filtered HAE had a good extraction ratio (33.46%) and was found to have carbohydrates, glycosides, phytosterols, phenolic compounds, saponins, and flavonoids as major constituents. HAE produced dose dependent zone of inhibition against *Klebsiella pneumoniae, Pseudomonas aeruginosa, E. coli, Bacillus cereus, Staphylococcus aureus,* and *Streptococcus uberis* and fungal pathogens *Aspergillus niger* and *Aspergillus fumigates*; however, no antiviral activity was recorded against IBR virus. HAE of *A. nilotica* revealed both proliferative and inhibitory effects on the rat splenocytes and IL-10 release depending on the dose. Detailed studies involving wide spectrum of bacterial, fungal, and viral species are required to prove or know the exact status of each constituents of the plant extract.

1. Introduction

The genus *Acacia* is the second largest in the family Leguminosae, with about 1350 species. It is distributed throughout tropical and warm temperate areas of the world, with the largest concentration of species in Australia (957 species), The Americas (185 species), Africa (144 species), and Asia (89 species) [1]. Out of these, *Acacia nilotica* is one of the species that has been effectively utilized in folk medicine for the treatment of tuberculosis, leprosy, smallpox, dysentery, cough, ophthalmia, toothache, skin cancer as astringent, antispasmodic, and aphrodisiac by rural population [2, 3]. *Acacia nilotica* leaves are protein rich and highly digestible. Leaves of Acacia plants, in general, possess a significant level of antibacterial activity against a wide range of bacterial pathogens, although the extent of antibacterial activity varies depending upon the type of extract [4–8]. Various extracts in water, methanol, ethanol, n-hexane, Chloroform, and petroleum ether are reported with variable antibacterial activity against Gram-positive and Gram-negative bacteria [7–12], common fungal pathogens [13–17], and viruses [18–21]. Different preparations of *A. nilotica* leave have been reported with different phytoconstituents [7, 22, 23]. These constituents of extracts also revealed variable potential for blood cells proliferation [24] and immunomodulation [25–27]. However, a complete composite study on all the potential activities of aqueous extract of *A. nilotica*, the most commonly used extract in households, is lacking against common yet potential veterinary pathogens. Thus, the present study was planned to evaluate common phytochemical constituents of aqueous extract with antimicrobial activity against common pathogens of veterinary importance and its role in splenocyte stimulation to influence immune response and cytokine induction.

2. Materials and Methods

2.1. Collection and Processing of A. nilotica Leaves. The authenticated and verified plant leaves were included in the study. Procured leaves were washed with single glass distilled water and dried at 37°C in incubator. The dried plants samples were ground to prepare a coarse powder. The powdered samples were used for preparation of HAE using soxhlet apparatus [23].

2.1.1. Extracts Preparation. Triple glass distilled water was used as solvent for HAE preparation using Soxhlet apparatus as per previously described method [28].

2.1.2. Determination of Yields of Extract. The evaporated dried extracts (on dry weight basis) were calculated by the following equation [29]:

$$\text{Yield}\left(\frac{g}{100\,g \text{ of dry plant material}}\right) = \frac{(W_1 \times 100)}{W_2}, \quad (1)$$

where W_1 was the weight of the extract after the solvent evaporation and W_2 was the weight of the dry plant material loaded for extraction.

2.1.3. Phytochemical Studies. Qualitative phytochemical analysis of crude hot aqueous extract was carried out as per the standard methods [30, 31] to detect the presence or absence of different phytochemical constituents, namely, alkaloids, glycosides, flavonoids, resins, tannins, saponins, fixed oils, reducing sugars, proteins, and amino acids.

2.1.4. Disc Preparation. Blank sterile discs (Himedia, Mumbai, India) of 6 mm diameter were loaded with HAE of different concentrations (1000 mg/mL, 500 mg/mL and 250 mg/mL) to prepare discs containing 20 mg, 10 mg, 5 mg, 2.5 mg, and 1.25 mg extracts. Discs impregnated with sterilized triple distilled water were taken as negative control. Discs were allowed to dry at 40°C for 30 minutes [23]. Dried discs were tested for their sterility on nutrient and Sabouraud Dextrose agar (SDA).

2.2. Antimicrobial Activities

2.2.1. Bacterial, Fungal, and Virus Isolates. Bacterial cultures of *Staphylococcus aureus, Bacillus cereus, Streptococcus uberis, Escherichia coli, Pseudomonas aeruginosa,* and *Klebsiella pneumonia* and fungal cultures of *Candida albicans, Aspergillus niger,* and *Aspergillus fumigatus* were obtained from the Department of Microbiology and Immunology, UP Pt. Deen Dayal Upadhyaya Pashu Chikitsa Vigyan Vishwavidyalaya Evam Go Anusandhan Sansthan (DUVASU), Mathura, to determine *in vitro* antibacterial and antifungal

activity of HAE. Prior to use, the bacterial and fungal isolates were recharacterized on the basis of morphological, cultural, and biochemical characteristics as per standard methods [32]. For antiviral activity, Infectious Bovine Rhinotracheitis (IBR) virus was obtained from the Department of Epidemiology, UP Pt. Deen Dayal Upadhyaya Pashu Chikitsa Vigyan Vishwavidyalaya Evam Go Anusandhan Sansthan, (DUVASU), Mathura. Before its use, IBR virus was subcultured and characterized by cytopathic effect in Madin-Darby Bovine Kidney (MDBK) cell line.

2.2.2. In Vitro Study of Antibacterial Susceptibility. Bacterial cell concentration of the bacterial cultures was determined on Muller Hinton Agar [HiMedia, Mumbai] by Spread Plate Method and colony forming unit per mL (CFU/mL) were calculated by multiplying the number of colonies counted with respective dilution factor [33]. Antibacterial activity was carried out by disc diffusion method as per standard procedure [34]. Standard discs of antibiotic Tetracycline (30 µg) and Amikacin (30 µg) [Hi Media, Mumbai] were used as positive control for Gram-positive and Gram-negative bacteria, respectively.

2.2.3. In Vitro Antifungal Effect. The concentration of CFU of fungus was determined as per the method used for bacterial count except for the use of Sabouraud's Dextrose Agar (SDA) [HiMedia, Mumbai] in place of Muller Hinton Agar. *In vitro* study of antifungal susceptibility of plant extract was performed by standard disc diffusion method [34]. Standard antimycotic discs of Fluconazole (10 µg) [Hi Media, Mumbai] were used as positive control for fungal agents.

2.2.4. In Vitro Antiviral Effect against IBR Virus. MDBK cell lines were obtained from the Department of Epidemiology, UP Pt. Deen Dayal Upadhyaya Pashu Chikitsa Vigyan Vishwavidyalaya Evam Go Anusandhan Sansthan, (DUVASU) Mathura. These were maintained at 37°C, 5% CO_2, and 80% relative humidity using Dulbecco's Modified Eagle's Medium (DMEM) growth medium supplemented with 10% inactivated fetal calf serum, antibiotic antimycotic solution, sodium pyruvate, and sodium bicarbonate [35] to study the antiviral effect of HAE. To assess the antiviral effect the cellular toxicity of plant extract on MDBK cell line was carried by MTT {3-(4,5-Dimethylthiazolyl)-2,5-diphenyl tetrazolium bromide} dye method [36] in 96-well cell culture plates. The concentration at which there was no reduction of viable cells was considered as maximum nontoxic dose (MNTD) of the extract [37]. The concentrations of aqueous extract lower than MNTD were screened for antiviral property against $TCID_{50}$ virus challenge dose of IBR virus in MDBK cell lines. The antiviral effect was determined by cytopathic inhibition effect in MDBK cell lines and reduction in virus induced cytotoxicity was measured by using MTT dye uptake method [36] in the form of optical densities (O.D) [37]. The virus suspension and dilution medium without plant extract were also used as the virus control and cell control, respectively. Cell viability was evaluated by adding 10 µL MTT dye (5 mg/mL) and then extracting the dye with

TABLE 1: *In vitro* antibacterial effects.

S. no.	Name of bacteria	Quantity of extract (mg/disc)	Zone of inhibition (mm) after		
			24 hrs	36 hrs	48 hrs
1	*Staphylococcus aureus*	1.25	9	8	8
		2.5	10	9	9
		5	17	15	15
		10	20	19	19
		20	20	20	20
	Positive control	Tetracycline (30 μg)	30	30	30
2	*Bacillus cereus*	1.25	8	8	7
		2.5	12	10	9
		5	15	15	14
		10	18	17	17
		20	19	19	18
	Positive control	Tetracycline (30 μg)	23	23	23
3	*Streptococcus uberis*	1.25	9	9	9
		2.5	12	12	12
		5	16	16	16
		10	19	19	18
		20	22	22	22
	Positive control	Tetracycline (30 μg)	27	27	27
4	*Escherichia coli*	1.25	0	0	0
		2.5	8	8	7
		5	9	8	8
		10	11	10	10
		20	15	14	14
	Positive control	Amikacin (30 μg)	24	24	24
5	*Pseudomonas aeruginosa*	1.25	8	8	7
		2.5	10	9	8
		5	13	12	12
		10	15	13	13
		20	15	13	12
	Positive control	Amikacin (30 μg)	18	18	18
6	*Klebsiella pneumoniae*	1.25	9	9	8
		2.5	10	9	8
		5	13	12	12
		10	13	13	13
		20	13	13	13
	Positive control	Amikacin (30 μg)	25	25	25
7	Negative control	0	—	—	—

DMSO and measuring optical density (O.D.) at 560 nm–670 nm as described previously. The percentage protection was calculated by the following formula:

$$\frac{(ODt)\,v - (ODc)\,v}{(ODc)\,m - (ODc)\,v} \times 100, \qquad (2)$$

where $(ODt)v$, $(ODc)v$, and $(ODc)m$ correspond to absorbance in virus infected cells with plant extracts, virus infected cells without plant extracts, and cells without virus and plant extract, respectively [35, 37].

2.3. Immunomodulatory Activities

2.3.1. Experimental Animals. Wistar Albino Rats (Av wt-120 gm) were procured from the Department of Lab Animal Resource (LAR) of IVRI, Izatnagar, UP. The spleen cells were collected aseptically from the rats and used for spleenocyte proliferation and cytokine IL-10 analysis [35].

2.3.2. In Vitro Effect on Splenocytes Proliferation/Inhibition. The effect of HAE on splenocyte proliferation was evaluated

TABLE 2: *In vitro* antifungal effects.

S. no.	Name of fungus	Quantity of extract (mg/disc)	Zone of inhibition (mm) after		
			24 hrs	36 hrs	48 hrs
1	*Candida albicans*	2.5	—	—	—
		5	—	—	—
		10	10	—	—
		20	11	—	—
		Fluconazole (10 μg)	28	28	28
2	*Aspergillus niger*	2.5	—	—	—
		5	8	—	—
		10	8	8	7
		20	12	11	11
		Fluconazole (10 μg)	21	21	21
3	*Aspergillus fumigatus*	2.5	—	—	—
		5	8	—	—
		10	9	8	8
		20	13	13	12
		Fluconazole (10 μg)	23	23	23
4	Negative control	0	—	—	—

with wells containing only spleen cells as negative control and wells containing spleen cells with Con-A as positive control [35]. After incubation, 20 μL of MTT solution (5 mg/mL) was added in each well for formazione crystal formation. The plate was reincubated at 37°C for 4 hrs in CO_2 incubator containing 5% CO_2 and 80% relative humidity. After incubation, supernatant was removed. The plate was air dried and 100 μL of DMSO was added to dissolve the formazione crystals. O.D was taken at dual wavelength 560–670 nm by ELISA reader [35]. Mean values were calculated in comparison to control and taken positive if ratio was of significant difference [38].

3. *In Vitro* Effect on IL-10 Cytokine Induction

Splenocytes were prepared as prescribed for splenocyte proliferation assay and cultured in absence and presence of Con-A (5 mg/mL) along with 0.45 μm membrane filtered HAE of plants (31.25, 62.5, 125, 250, and 500 μg/mL, extract) in the cell culture plate [39]. Procedure followed for IL-10 assay was similar to that for splenocytes proliferation assay. However, the spleen cells were incubated for 48 hrs and then supernatant was collected for the detection of IL-10 cytokine. The quantitation of IL-10 cytokine in spleen culture supernatant was done according to the protocol supplied in the kit by BIOSOURCE (USA).

4. Results

4.1. Percentage Yield. On dry matter basis, the filtered HAE of *Acacia nilotica* leaves was 33.46% of the total dry weight of the leaves.

4.2. Phytochemical Studies. Phytochemical studies of HAE revealed the presence of carbohydrates, glycosides,

phytosterols, phenolic compounds, saponins, and flavonoids as major constituents.

4.3. In Vitro Antibacterial Effects. All the bacterial pathogens revealed concentration dependent sensitivity against HAE. HAE was more effective against Gram-positive bacteria in comparison to Gram-negative bacteria (Table 1).

4.4. In Vitro Antifungal Effects. All the fungal pathogens revealed concentration dependant sensitivity against higher concentrations of HAE. The discs with 2.5 and 5 mg concentration of HAE revealed no inhibition or the inhibition of the growth for initial few hours (Table 2).

4.5. In Vitro Antiviral Activity against IBR Virus

4.5.1. MNTD Determination in MDBK Cell Line. On the basis of observation of cytotoxic effect (vacuole formation and detachment of cells) in MDBK cells and absorbance, 1.25 mg/mL conc. of aqueous extract was determined as nontoxic dose of HAE. For further investigation, 1.25, 0.625, and 0.3125 mg/mL were taken to study the antiviral activity of HAE of *A. nilotica* leaves against IBR virus (Figures 1 and 6).

4.5.2. $TCID_{50}$ for IBR Virus. The number of viable cells after virus challenge was assessed by using MTT dye uptake assay and the virus dilution required to cause 50% cell death was calculated from dose response curve and virus was expressed as $TCID_{50}$ (50% tissue culture infective dose). $TCID_{50}$ of IBR virus was determined at 10^{-1} virus dilution level (Figure 2).

4.5.3. Antiviral Effect against IBR Virus. HAE of *A. nilotica* leaves showed no antiviral property against IBR, showing no protection to the cell line against the virus (Figure 3).

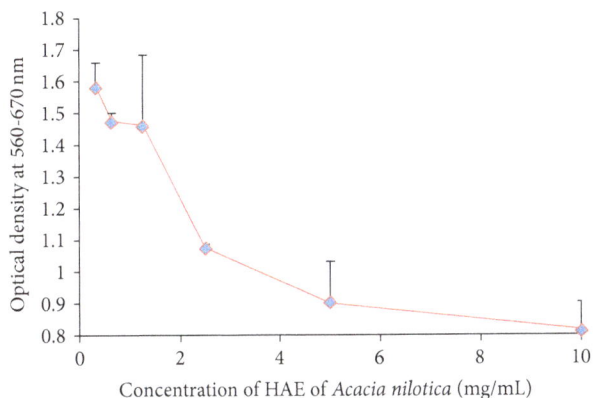

FIGURE 1: MNTD of HAE of *Acacia nilotica leaves* in MDBK cell line.

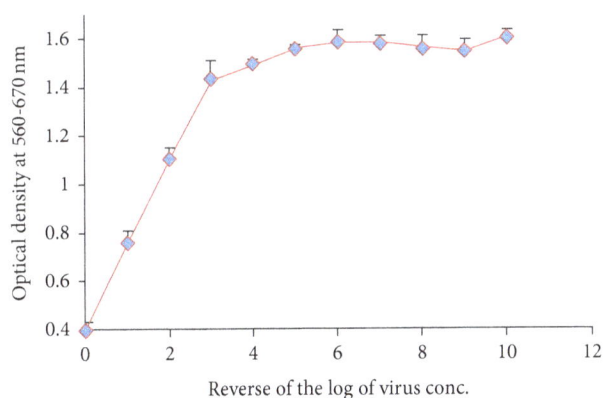

FIGURE 2: $TCID_{50}$ for Infectious Bovine Rhinotracheitis (IBR) virus.

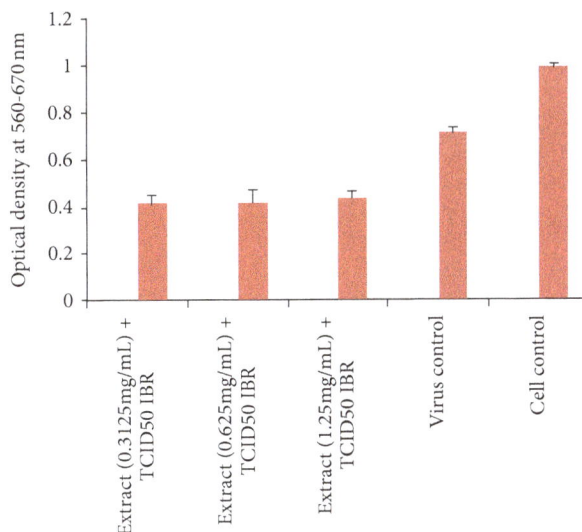

FIGURE 3: Antiviral effect of HAE of *Acacia nilotica* leaves against IBR virus.

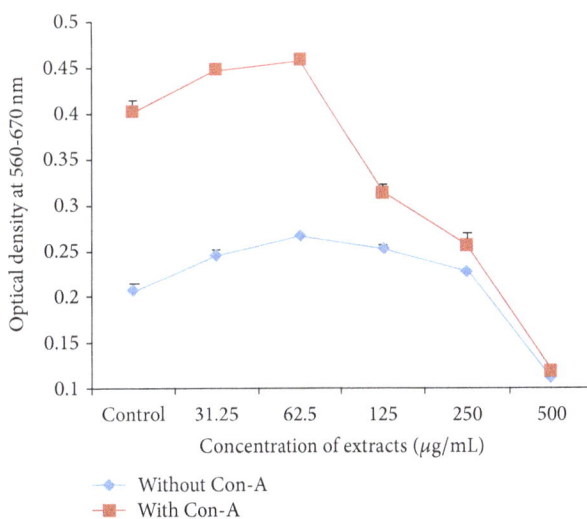

FIGURE 4: *In vitro* effect of HAE of *Acacia nilotica* leaves on Splenocyte proliferation in Wistar albino rats.

4.6. In Vitro Effect on Splenocytes Proliferation/Inhibition. HAE of *A. nilotica* leaves had a proliferative as well as inhibitory effect on splenocytes. In comparison to negative control, 18.27, 28.36, 21.63, and 9.61% increase in the proliferation of spleen cells were reported at the dose rate of 31.25, 62.5, 125, and 250 μg/mL of HAE, respectively, whereas 45.67% inhibition was reported at dose rate of 500 μg/mL HAE of *A. nilotica*. In comparison to positive control, spleen cells with HAE of *Acacia nilotica* leaves in presence of Con-A exhibited 11.17% and 13.18% increase in proliferation when splenocyte culture was treated with 31.25 and 62.5 μg/mL of HAE of *A. nilotica*, respectively. However, 22.33, 36.72, and 70.22% inhibition were observed when splenocyte culture treated with 125, 250, and 500 μg/mL HAE of *A. nilotica* with Con-A, respectively (Figures 4 and 7).

4.7. In Vitro Effect on Induction of IL-10 Cytokine. Splenocytes treated with HAE *in vitro* revealed 24.78, 6.21, 6.69, 8.15, and 11.86% reduction in the IL-10 secretion at dose rate of 31.25, 62.5, 125, and 500 μg/mL HAE of *A. nilotica* leaves, respectively, compared with negative control (only spleen cells). The minimum inhibition of cytokine secretion (6.21%) was observed with 62.5 μg/mL HAE in absence of Con-A (Figure 5).

Splenocytes treated with HAE and Con-A was compared with positive control (spleen cells + Con-A) and it was found that IL-10 secretion was reduced by 13.85, 2.42, 6.59, 10.78, and 21.09% when treated with 31.25, 62.5, 125, 250, and 500 μg/mL HAE, respectively. The minimum reduction 2.42% was observed with 62.5 μg/mL of HAE in presence of Con-A (Figure 5).

5. Discussion

A. nilotica is commonly located in Indian subcontinent [1] and is commonly used in folk medicine [40]. In traditional medicine, its role is well established [41]. However, in the era of increasing drug resistance to modern medicine in bacterial pathogens [42–44], it is to be validated scientifically.

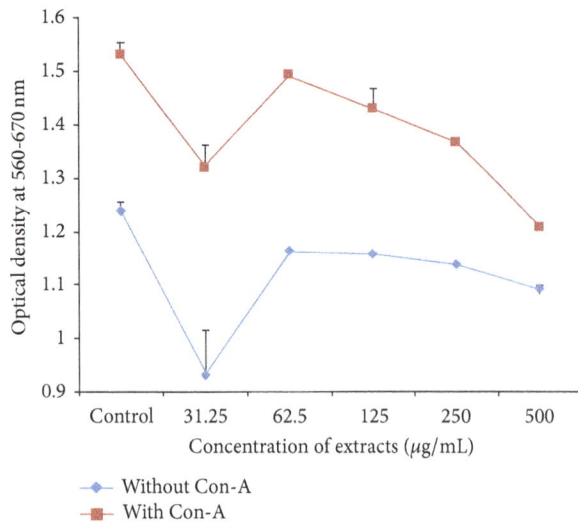

FIGURE 5: *In vitro* effect of HAE of *Acacia nilotica* leaves on Cytokine IL-10 induction.

Out of the numerous traditional therapeutic practices, the preparation of hot aqueous extract is the most common household means of herbal administration [33, 40]. Therefore, the antimicrobial potential along with immunomodulatory effects of hot aqueous extract of *A. nilotica* leaves was investigated in the present study.

The high yield of the plant leaves extract (33.46%) also supports its use and availability in folk medicine. The phytochemicals like tannins, flavonoids, phenols, and alkaloids are an important reflection of the pharmacological activities of a plant. The phytochemistry of the extract revealed the presence of carbohydrates, glycosides, phytosterols, phenolic compounds, saponins, and flavonoids as major constituents; the efficacy of these compounds is already well established for antimicrobial activities [8]. These findings are in agreement with earlier findings of phytoconstituents of different extracts of *Acacia nilotica*, namely, aqueous extract [22], methanolic, and ethanolic extracts [7, 23].

The HAE produced dose dependent zone of inhibition of variable size even after the incubation of 48 hours against both Gram-positive and Gram-negative bacteria (Table 1). These findings are in the concurrence with the earlier findings that reported better efficacy of *Acacia nilotica* extracts against Gram-positive cocci than Gram-negative bacilli [8]. The superior inhibition of bacterial growth against Gram-positive bacteria in comparison to Gram-negative bacteria might be because of the difference in cell wall composition of the bacteria [42]. Among Gram-negative bacteria, *Klebsiella pneumoniae* showed a little resistance to inhibition, perhaps due to the presence of a capsule [22]. The sensitivity of Gram-positive bacteria was in support to the use of HAE extracts in skin ailments and conditions like mastitis [45]. Similar to our findings, *E. coli* has been earlier found sensitive to hot aqueous, ethanolic, and methanolic extracts of *Acacia nilotica* [8, 9, 12, 14]. However, the alcoholic extracts are reported to have a better antibacterial activity against different bacterial

pathogens with significant inhibition of growth as compared to the aqueous extracts [10, 15].

Other than the bacterial pathogens, mycotic pathogens are always a clinical challenge to veterinarian and are very difficult to control [46]. The fungal manifestations are generally chronic in nature. Although an exhaustive range of antifungal drugs are available, the treatment becomes uneconomical particularly in the large animals due to large dose size. Therefore, to find out a suitable plant extract with antifungal activity was one of the key aims of the study. In this regard, HAE of *Acacia nilotica* plant leaves was tested against most common veterinary fungal pathogens, namely, *Candida albicans*, *Aspergillus fumigatus*, and *Aspergillus niger* (Table 2). The HAE showed good antifungal activity against all the fungal pathogens at higher concentration (Table 2). The inhibition was better against *Aspergillus fumigatus* and *Aspergillus niger* and was comparable to fluconazole, the reference antifungal drug. Our findings are also in agreement to the earlier findings against eight species of Aspergillus and other fungal pathogens [15–17, 47]. In contrast to our findings, some earlier reports have claimed absence of antifungal activity in HAE and other extracts of these plant parts [13, 14, 48]. This dissimilarity might be due to the difference in the collection season of plant material, extraction procedures, or geographical variations. The activity of HAE of *A. nilotica* leaves against *C. albicans* was only with higher concentration and only for 24 hours, while ethanolic extract of *A. nilotica* leaves were reported to be very effective [11]. This variation is commonly observed with the change of type of extract as phytoconstituents and their concentrations may vary significantly [8].

The severity of viral diseases and ability of virus to survive intracellularly pose a great challenge that is further aggravated by the nonavailability of specific antiviral chemical agents against veterinary pathogens [37]. Thus, the evaluation of antiviral effect of HAE of *A. nilotica* leaves was also attempted. The findings of the present study revealed no antiviral effect of HAE against IBR virus (Figure 3). There are no reports available on the antiviral activity of HAE of *A. nilotica* against IBR virus in the literature. However, variable antiviral activity of different extracts of different species of plant acacia have been reported, namely, *Acacia nilotica* (bark and pods) inhibitory effects against HIV-1 PR. [18]; *Acacia gummifera* inhibiting Sindbis virus [19]; *Acacia arabica*. var. *indica* against peste des petits ruminants virus (PPRV) [49]; *Acacia arabica* (babul) against Goat pox virus (GTPV) replication [21]; and *Acacia nilotica* (fruits) with mild virucidal to high activity against replication of Newcastle Disease virus and Fowl pox viruses [19, 21].

HAE of plant leaves revealed both proliferative and inhibitory effects on the splenocytes to be depending on the concentration of the extract (Figures 4 and 7). The proliferation of splenocyte occurred in dose dependent manner in the range of 9.61% to the 28.36%. These observations are in agreement with the *in vitro* findings of stimulation of rat pleural polymorphonuclear leukocytes (PMNs) [24] and proliferation of splenocyte [26]. Thus, the lower concentrations of the HAE of plants could be used to improve immune response or to combat the microorganisms causing immune-suppression

FIGURE 6: MNTD assessment with different concentrations of HAE of *A. nilotica* leaves in MDBK cell line, 10X.

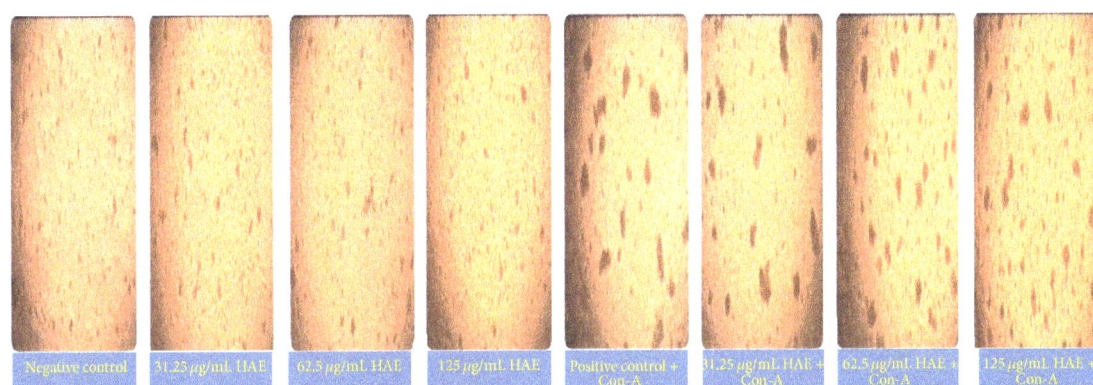

FIGURE 7: *In vitro* assessment of splenocyte proliferation with different concentrations of HAE of *A. nilotica* leaves on Wistar albino rat spleen cells, 10x.

as increase in the proliferation of splenocyte appeared to be an indicative of cellular immune response [50]. Moreover, oral feeding of *Acacia catechu* extract in mice produced a significant increase in the serum immunoglobulin levels, increase in the haemagglutination titre values, and decreased the mortality ratio in mice, suggesting its effect on the humoral arm of the immune system [27]. The inhibition of splenocytes proliferation observed at higher concentration of HAE (Figures 4 and 7) might be due to the accumulation of toxic constituents of plant extract which might be causing cytotoxic effects and ultimately inhibiting the cell proliferation [26]. The supernatants of splenocytes exposed to different concentrations of extract were assessed for the concentration of IL-10, an anti-inflammatory interleukin that plays important role in control of inflammatory process [40, 51]. The HAE of *Acacia nilotica* downregulated the IL-10 release from spleen cells in lower doses and maximum inhibition was 24.78%. Then inhibition was reduced with increase in HAE concentration, however further higher doses downregulated IL-10 release. Hence, dose dependent upregulation is observed in certain concentration which is again downregulated with increase in extract concentration (Figure 5). Thus, proliferation of splenocytes and upregulation of IL-10 can be observed for an optimum concentration of extract. No literature is available on IL-10 regulation

regarding this plant. Further, there are scanty reports available on the use of medicinal plants or the extracts of plant parts on the regulation of IL-10 as Fu-ling Chinese herb produced upregulation of IL-10 in murine spleen cell [52] and *Phyllanthus amarus* inhibited induction of interleukin (IL)-1β, IL-10, and interferon-γ in human whole blood [53]. Since cytokines regulate certain important biological functions such as cell growth, cell activation, immunity, inflammation, tissue repair, fibrosis, morphogenesis, and chemotaxis, thus the up- or downregulation of cytokines directly affect the body defense mechanism.

6. Conclusions

The study had tried to cover almost all the aspects of microbial pathogenesis and revealed that HAE of *Acacia nilotica* leaves had different effects upon bacteria, virus, and fungi with dose dependent variation in immunomodulatory and anti-inflammatory activities. HAE of *Acacia nilotica* leaves showed excellent antibacterial and antifungal activities with comparatively lesser antiviral and immunomodulatory activities. HAE of *Acacia nilotica* leaves had various active components that might have a role in variation in overall activities; therefore, further detailed studies involving wide spectrum of bacterial, fungal, and viral species are required to prove the exact statics of each constituent of the plant extract. However, study had shown an important level of the valuable effects of *Acacia nilotica* leaves.

Conflict of Interests

The authors of this paper do not have a direct financial relation that might lead to a conflict of interests for any of them.

Acknowledgments

The authors are thankful to the Dean of College of Veterinary Sciences and Vice Chancellor of UP Pt. Deen Dayal Upadhyaya Veterinary University & Gau Anusandhan Sansthan (DUVASU), Mathura, for providing the requisite facilities and support to carry out this investigation.

References

[1] B. R. Maslin, J. T. Miller, and D. S. Seigler, "Overview of the generic status of *Acacia* (Leguminosae: Mimosoideae)," *Australian Systematic Botany*, vol. 16, no. 1, pp. 1–18, 2003.

[2] J. A. Duke, *Medicinal Plants of the Bible*, Trado-Medic Book, Owerri, NY, USA, 1983.

[3] B. P. van Wky and B. E. van Wky, *PhoTographic Guide to Trees of Southern Africa*, Briza Publications, Pretoria, South Africa, 2000.

[4] T. R. New, *A Biology of Acacias*, Oxford University Press, New York, NY, USA, 1984.

[5] A. Kumar, A. Rahal, and A. K. Verma, "In vitro antibacterial activity of hot aqueous extract (HAE) of *Ocimum sanctum* (Tulsi) leaves," *Indian Journal of Veterinary Medicine*, vol. 31, no. 2, pp. 96–97, 2011.

[6] H. Upadhyay, A. Kumar, M. K. Gupta, A. Sharma, and A. Rahal, "Validation of medicinal values of traditionally used *Sonchus asper* (Prickly Sow Thistle) Leaves for the treatment of skin ailments," *Advancement in Medicinal Plant Research*, vol. 1, no. 3, pp. 29–35, 2013.

[7] G. O. Solomon-Wisdom and G. A. Shittu, "In vitro antimicrobial and phytochemical activities of *Acacia nilotica* leaf extract," *Journal of Medicinal Plant Research*, vol. 4, no. 12, pp. 1232–1234, 2010.

[8] N. K. Mustafa, M. O. M. Tanira, F. K. Dar, and H. Nsanze, "Antimicrobial activity of *Acacia nilotica subspp. nilotica* fruit extracts," *Pharmacy and Pharmacology Communications*, vol. 5, no. 9, pp. 583–586, 1999.

[9] M. E. Arias, J. D. Gomez, N. M. Cudmani, M. A. Vattuone, and M. I. Isla, "Antibacterial activity of ethanolic and aqueous extracts of *Acacia aroma* Gill. ex Hook et Arn," *Life Sciences*, vol. 75, no. 2, pp. 191–202, 2004.

[10] A. M. H. Ali and S. O. Yagoub, "Antimicrobial activity of *Acacia nilotica* extracts against some bacteria isolated from clinical specimen," *Research Journal of Medicinal Plants*, vol. 1, no. 1, pp. 25–28, 2007.

[11] R. Khan, B. Islam, M. Akram et al., "Antimicrobial activity of five herbal extracts against Multi Drug Resistant (MDR) strains of bacteria and fungus of clinical origin," *Molecules*, vol. 14, no. 2, pp. 586–597, 2009.

[12] J. D. Patel, D. K. Patel, A. K. Shrivastava, and V. Kumar, "Evaluation of some medicinal plants used in traditional wound healing preparations for antibacterial property against some pathogenic bacteria," *Journal of Clinical Immunology and Immunopathology Research*, vol. 1, no. 1, pp. 7–12, 2009.

[13] O. J. M. Hamza, C. J. P. van den Bout-van den Beukel, M. I. N. Matee et al., "Antifungal activity of some Tanzanian plants used traditionally for the treatment of fungal infections," *Journal of Ethnopharmacology*, vol. 108, no. 1, pp. 124–132, 2006.

[14] R. Dabur, A. Gupta, T. K. Mandal et al., "Antimicrobial activity of some medicinal plants," *African Journal of Traditional, Complementary and Alternative Medicines*, vol. 4, no. 3, pp. 313–318, 2007.

[15] B. Mahesh and S. Satish, "Antimicrobial activity of some important medicinal plant against plant and human pathogens," *World Journal of Agricultural Sciences*, vol. 4, pp. 839–843, 2008.

[16] R. K. Sahani and A. R. Saxena, "Fungitoxic properties of medicinal and aromatic plants against *Fusarium oxysporum* f.sp. *pisi*," *Annales of Plant Protection Sciences*, vol. 17, no. 1, pp. 146–148, 2009.

[17] R. M. Mariita, C. K. P. O. Ogol, N. O. Oguge, and P. O. Okemo, "Methanol extract of three medicinal plants from samburu in northern kenya show significant antimycobacterial, antibacterial and antifungal properties," *Research Journal of Medicinal Plant*, vol. 5, no. 1, pp. 54–64, 2011.

[18] G. Hussein, H. Miyashiro, N. Nakamura et al., "Inhibitory effects of Sudanese plant extracts on HIV-1 replication and HIV-1 protease," *Phytotherapy Research*, vol. 13, pp. 31–36, 1999.

[19] F. Mouhajir, J. B. Hudson, M. Rejdali, and G. H. N. Towers, "Multiple antiviral activities of endemic medicinal plants used by Berber peoples of Morocco," *Pharmaceutical Biology*, vol. 39, no. 5, pp. 364–374, 2001.

[20] V. Bhanuprakash, M. Hosamani, V. Balamurugan, R. K. Singh, and D. Swarup, "In vitro antiviral activity of *Eugenia jambolana* plant extract on Buffalopox virus: conventional and qPCR methods," *International Journal of Tropical Medicine*, vol. 2, no. 1, pp. 3–9, 2007.

[21] V. Bhanuprakash, M. Hosamani, V. Balamurugan et al., "In vitro antiviral activity of plant extracts on goatpox virus replication," *Indian Journal of Experimental Biology*, vol. 46, no. 2, pp. 120–127, 2008.

[22] T. Kalaivani, C. Rajasekaran, K. Suthindhiran, and L. Mathew, "Free radical scavenging, cytotoxic and hemolytic activities from leaves of *Acacia nilotica* (L.) Wild. ex. Delile subsp. *indica* (Benth.) Brenan," *Evidence-based Complementary and Alternative Medicine*, vol. 2011, Article ID 274741, 8 pages, 2011.

[23] M. P. Raghavendra, S. Satish, and K. A. Raveesha, "In vitro evaluation of anti-bacterial spectrum and phytochemical analysis of *Acacia nilotica*," *Journal of Agricultural Technology*, vol. 2, no. 1, pp. 77–88, 2006.

[24] A. El Abbouyi, M. Toumi, Y. El Hachimi, and A. Jossang, "In vitro effects of aqueous seeds extract of *Acacia cyanophylla* on the opsonized zymosan-induced superoxide anions production by rat polymorphonuclear leukocytes," *Journal of Ethnopharmacology*, vol. 91, no. 1, pp. 159–165, 2004.

[25] R. Kukhetpitakwong, C. Hahnvajanawong, P. Homchampa, V. Leelavatcharamas, J. Satra, and W. Khunkitti, "Immunological adjuvant activities of saponin extracts from the pods of *Acacia concinna*," *International Immunopharmacology*, vol. 6, no. 11, pp. 1729–1735, 2006.

[26] W. S. Koko, M. A. Mesaik, S. Yousaf, M. Galal, and M. I. Choudhary, "In vitro immunomodulating properties of selected

Sudanese medicinal plants," *Journal of Ethnopharmacology*, vol. 118, no. 1, pp. 26–34, 2008.

[27] S. Ismail and M. Asad, "Immunomodulatory activity of *Acacia catechu*," *Indian Journal of Physiology and Pharmacology*, vol. 53, no. 1, pp. 25–33, 2009.

[28] A. Goel, D. Kumar, and A. K. Bhatia, "Modulation of immune responses by aqueous extract of *Argemone maxicana* leaves," *Journal of Immunology and Immunopathology*, vol. 10, pp. 65–69, 2008.

[29] L. Stanojević, M. Stanković, V. Nikolić et al., "Antioxidant activity and total phenolic and flavonoid contents of *Hieracium pilosella* L. extracts," *Sensors*, vol. 9, no. 7, pp. 5702–5714, 2009.

[30] K. R. Brain and T. D. Turner, *The Practical Evaluation of Phytopharmaceuticals*, Wright Sciencetechnica, Bristol, UK, 2nd edition, 1975.

[31] W. C. Evans, *Trease and Evans Pharmacognosy*, WB Sauders, London, UK, 14th edition, 1996.

[32] R. Cruicshank, *Medical Microbiology*, Churchil Living stone, Edinburgh, UK, 11th edition, 1997.

[33] A. Kumar, A. K. Verma, A. K. Sharma, and A. Rahal, "Presence of extended spectrum β- lactamases producing α- haemolytic *E. coli* in Yellow-watteled lapwing (*Vanellus malabaricus*)," *Asian Journal of Animal Sciences*, vol. 7, no. 2, pp. 64–69, 2013.

[34] A. W. Bauer, W. M. Kirby, J. C. Sherris, and M. Turck, "Antibiotic susceptibility testing by a standardized single disk method," *The American Journal of Clinical Pathology*, vol. 45, no. 4, pp. 493–496, 1966.

[35] A. Goel, *Immumological studies on fileriaris* [Ph.D. thesis], Central Drug Research Institute (CDRI), Lucknow, Uttar Pradesh, India, 1991.

[36] F. Denizot and R. Lang, "Rapid colorimetric assay for cell growth and survival—modifications to the tetrazolium dye procedure giving improved sensitivity and reliability," *Journal of Immunological Methods*, vol. 89, no. 2, pp. 271–277, 1986.

[37] Jayati, A. K. Bhatia, A. Kumar, A. Goel, S. Gupta, and A. Rahal, "In vitro antiviral potential of *Ocimum sanctum* leaves extract against New Castle Disease Virus of poultry," *International Journal of Microbiology and Immunology Research*, vol. 2, no. 7, pp. 51–55, 2013.

[38] G. W. Snedecor and W. G. Cochran, *Statistical Methods*, The Iowa State University, Ames, Iowa, USA, 7th edition, 1981.

[39] A. Goel, D. K. Singh, S. Kumar, and A. K. Bhatia, "Immunomodulating property of *Ocimum sanctum* by regulating the IL-2 production and its mRNA expression using rat's splenocytes," *Asian Pacific Journal of Tropical Medicine*, vol. 3, no. 1, pp. 8–12, 2010.

[40] Mahima, A. Rahal, R. Deb et al., "Immunomodulatory and therapeutic potentials of herbal, traditional/indeginous and ethnoveterinary medicines," *Pakistan Journal of Biological Sciences*, vol. 15, no. 16, pp. 754–774, 2012.

[41] K. Dhama, S. Mani, S. Chakraborty et al., "Herbal remedies to combat cancers in humans and animals—a review," *International Journal of Current Research*, vol. 5, no. 7, pp. 1908–1919, 2013.

[42] A. Kumar, A. Rahal, S. K. Dwivedi, and M. K. Gupta, "Prevalence and antibiotic profile of bacterial isolates from bovine mastitis in Mathura," *Egyptian Journal of Dairy Sciences*, vol. 38, no. 1, pp. 31–34, 2010.

[43] K. Dhama, R. Tiwari, S. Chakraborty et al., "Global warming and emerging infectious diseases of animals and humans:current scenario, challenges, solutions and future

perspectives—a review," *International Journal of Current Research*, vol. 5, no. 7, pp. 1942–1958, 2013.

[44] S. Malik, A. Kumar, A. K. Verma et al., "Incidence and drug resistance pattern of collibacillosis in cattle and buffalo calves in Northwest part of Utter Pradesh in India," *Journal of Animal Health and Production*, vol. 1, no. 2, pp. 15–19, 2013.

[45] S. Vashney, P. Vashney, S. K. Dash et al., "Antibacterial activity of fruits of *Terminelia chebula* and *Terminalia belerica* against mastitis field isolates," *Medicinal Plants*, vol. 4, no. 3, pp. 167–169, 2012.

[46] K. Dhama, S. Chakraborty, A. K. Verma et al., "Fungal/Mycotic diseases of Poultry-diagnosis, treatment and control: a review," *Pakistan Journal of Biological Sciences*, vol. 16, no. 23, pp. 1626–1640, 2013.

[47] S. Satish, D. C. Mohana, M. P. Raghavendra, and K. A. Raveesha, "Antifungal activity of some plant extracts against important seed borne pathogens of *Aspergillus sp.*," *Journal of Agricultural Technology*, vol. 3, no. 1, pp. 109–119, 2007.

[48] A. Banso, "Phytochemical and antibacterial investigation of bark extracts of *Acacia nilotica*," *Journal of Medicinal Plant Research*, vol. 3, no. 2, pp. 82–85, 2009.

[49] V. Balamurugan, A. Sen, P. Saravanan et al., "Potential effect of *Acacia arabica* on peste des petits ruminants virus replication," *Pharmaceutical Biology*, vol. 46, no. 3, pp. 171–179, 2008.

[50] S. Singh, M. Taneja, and D. K. Majumdar, "Biological activities of *Ocimum sanctum* L. fixed oil—an overview," *Indian Journal of Experimental Biology*, vol. 45, no. 5, pp. 403–412, 2007.

[51] J. Kuby, *Book of Immunology*, W. H. Freeman and Company, New York, NY, USA, 5th edition, 2003.

[52] C. J. Liou and J. Tseng, "A Chinese herbal medicine, Fu-Ling, regulates interleukin-10 production by murine spleen cells," *The American Journal of Chinese Medicine*, vol. 30, no. 4, pp. 551–560, 2002.

[53] A. K. Kiemer, T. Hartung, C. Huber, and A. M. Vollmar, "*Phyllanthus amarus* has anti-inflammatory potential by inhibition of iNOS, COX-2, and cytokines via the NF-κB pathway," *Journal of Hepatology*, vol. 38, no. 3, pp. 289–297, 2003.

6

Effect of Propolis on Experimental Cutaneous Wound Healing in Dogs

Ashraf M. Abu-Seida

Department of Surgery, Anesthesiology & Radiology, Faculty of Veterinary Medicine, Cairo University, Giza 12211, Egypt

Correspondence should be addressed to Ashraf M. Abu-Seida; ashrafseida@cu.edu.eg

Academic Editor: Remo Lobetti

This study evaluates clinically the effect of propolis paste on healing of cutaneous wound in dogs. Under general anesthesia and complete aseptic conditions, two full thickness skin wounds (3 cm diameter) were created in each side of the chest in five dogs, one dorsal and one ventral, with 10 cm between them. These wounds were randomly allocated into two groups, control group (10 wounds) and propolis group (10 wounds). Both groups were represented in each dog. The wounds were cleaned with normal saline solution and dressed with macrogol ointment in control group and propolis paste in propolis group, twice daily till complete wound healing. Measurement of the wound area (cm^2) was monitored planimetrically at 0, 7, 14, 21, 28, and 35 days after injury. The data were analyzed statistically. The results revealed a significant reduction in the wound surface area in the propolis group after 14 and 21 days compared to control group. The wound reepithelization, contraction, and total wound healing were faster in propolis group than in control group during five weeks of study. In conclusion, propolis paste has a positive impact on cutaneous wound healing and it may be suggested for treating various types of wounds in animals.

1. Introduction

Wound healing results from a complex tissue repairing process to replace devitalized and missing cellular structures and tissue layers. This process is divided into four precisely and highly programmed phases including blood clotting, inflammation, the growth of new tissue (proliferation), and the remodeling of tissue (maturation). Several factors such as age, sex, nutrition, stress, infection, and medication can interfere with one or more phases of this process, thus causing improper or impaired wound healing. Although several wound healing agents are used in veterinary practice, new agents are usually discovered [1].

Propolis is a resinous material collected by bees from plants exudates and buds and mixed with wax and bee enzymes. It consisted of 30% beeswax, 50% resins and vegetable balsams, 10% essential oils, 5% pollen, and 5% other substances. Its color varies from green and red to dark brown. Propolis has a characteristic smell and shows adhesive properties because it strongly interacts with oils and proteins of the skin [2]. In contrast, geopropolis is produced by indigenous stingless bees and it is composed of resinous material of plants and soil or clay [3].

Etymologically, the Greek word propolis means *pro*, for or in defense, and *polis*, the city, that is, "defense of the hive." Propolis is a multifunctional material used by bees in the construction and maintenance of their hives. Bees use it to seal holes in their honeycombs, smooth out internal walls, and cover carcasses of intruders who died inside the hive in order to avoid their decomposition. Propolis also protects the colony from diseases because of its antiseptic efficacy and antimicrobial properties [4].

The use of propolis goes back to ancient times, at least to 300 BC, and it has been used as a medicine for internal and external uses in many parts of the world. Egyptians, Greeks, and Romans reported the use of propolis for its general healing qualities. Ancient Egyptians used it to embalm their dead, and more recently it was used during the Boer War for healing [5].

Propolis has been used empirically for centuries and it has several biological applications including acceleration of regenerating processes in the damaged cartilages and bones [6, 7], immunomodulatory [8], antimicrobial [9], antioxidant [10], analgesic, and anti-inflammatory agent [11], and antitumoral property [12]. Since propolis possesses these several biological properties, this study aims to evaluate clinically the potential therapeutic effects of propolis on cutaneous wound healing in dogs.

2. Materials and Methods

2.1. Animals. This study was approved by the Animal Use and Care Committee at Faculty of Veterinary Medicine, Cairo University, Egypt. All surgeries were performed under general anesthesia, and all efforts were made to minimize animal suffering and to reduce the number of animals used.

A total of five adult mongrel dogs (3 males and 2 females) aged approximately 1-2 years and weighing 20–25 kg were selected for this study. The animals were housed under standard environmental conditions ($23 \pm 1°C$, with $55 \pm 5\%$ humidity and a 12 h light/dark cycle) and maintained with free access to water and three meals per day, including dry food (Sportmix-Adult, USA) and milk.

2.2. Preparation of MP (Carrier). To prepare 100 g of Macrogol ointment, 40 g of polyethylene glycol 3350 (Ineos Manufacturing, Deutschland GmbH, Germany) was mixed with 60 g of polyethylene glycol 400 (DOW Chemical Company, USA). The two ingredients were heated in water bath at 65°C until complete melting and then allowed to cool down to room temperature while stirring until the mixture was congealed.

2.3. Formation of the Propolis Paste. To prepare 50 g of propolis paste, 15 g of propolis (Bee Propolis, Holistic Herbal Solutions, LLC, USA) was mixed well with 35 g of MP in a sterile mortar to obtain a creamy paste.

2.4. Creation of Skin Wounds. All dogs were premedicated with subcutaneous injection of atropine sulphate (Atropine, ADWIA, Egypt) at a dose of 0.05 mg/kg body weight and intravenous injection of xylazine HCl (Xylazine 2%, Alfasan, Belgium) 1 mg/kg body weight as a premedication. The dogs were generally anesthetized by using ketamine HCl (Ketamine 5%, TRITTAU, Germany) 5 mg/kg body weight given I.V. via a 20-gauge cannula. Then the general anesthesia was maintained by 25 mg/kg incremental doses of 2.5% solution of thiopental sodium (Thiopental Sodium, EPICO, Egypt).

Under complete aseptic conditions, four circular full thickness skin wounds (3 cm diameter) were created at both sides of the chest in each dog (2 wounds in each side, one dorsal and one ventral, with 10 cm between them). These wounds were left open to heal by the secondary intention. All dogs were given intramuscular cefotaxime sodium at a dose of 10 mg kg and diclofenac sodium at a dose of 1.1 mg kg once/day for 5 days after surgery for pain and infection control [13]. These wounds were divided randomly into two equal groups ($n = 10$) including group I (control group) and group II (treated group). In control group, the wounds

TABLE 1: Mean $\pm$ SD of wound surface area (cm^2) in both groups on different days after injury.

Days	Control group	Propolis group
7	5.54 ± 0.27	4.9 ± 0.36
14	3.38 ± 0.41^a	2.1 ± 0.27^b
21	1.1 ± 0.2^a	0.36 ± 0.1^b
28	0.28 ± 11	0.0 ± 0.0
35	0.0 ± 0.0	0.0 ± 0.0

Different letters in the same row are statistically significantly different at $P \leq 0.05$.

were cleaned with normal saline solution and dressed with macrogol ointment twice daily until complete wound healing. In treated group, the wounds were cleaned with normal saline solution and then dressed with 1 mL propolis paste twice daily. Measurement of the wound area (cm^2) was monitored planimetrically at 0, 7, 14, 21, 28, and 35 days after injury (DAI) according to the method described by Oryan et al. [14]. The measurement was carried out by another veterinarian who was blinded to the experimental design and group allocation.

2.5. Statistical Analysis. The data were expressed as mean and standard deviation. The one-way ANOVA followed by Turkey post hoc test were used for comparison of different parameters. The data were analyzed by SPSS software, version 16.0 (SPSS Inc., Chicago, IL, USA), and $P \leq 0.05$ was accepted as statistically significant.

3. Results

The surface area of all wounds was calculated and expressed in cm^2 as shown in Table 1.

The follow-up of wounds treated with propolis paste showed wound healing started at day three after injury and evident healing after seven days with significant difference compared to untreated wounds until the end of the study. The centre of the treated wounds became a scar and the total wound size appeared lesser than those of control group along the duration of the study. There was a significant reduction in the wound surface area in the propolis group on days 14 and 21 compared to those in the control group (Figure 1).

The wound reepithelization, contraction, and total wound healing were faster in propolis treated group than in control group during five weeks of study. In addition, no side effects were recorded after application of propolis paste during this study.

4. Discussion

Nonhealing wounds and wounds with secondary infection by multidrug resistant bacteria are a common challenge in veterinary practice. Therefore, several recent studies have been conducted to investigate various synthetic and biomaterials for enhancing wound healing in both humans and animals. These agents included glycerol, tripeptide copper complex (TCC) hydrogel, platelet rich plasma (PRP), zinc compounds,

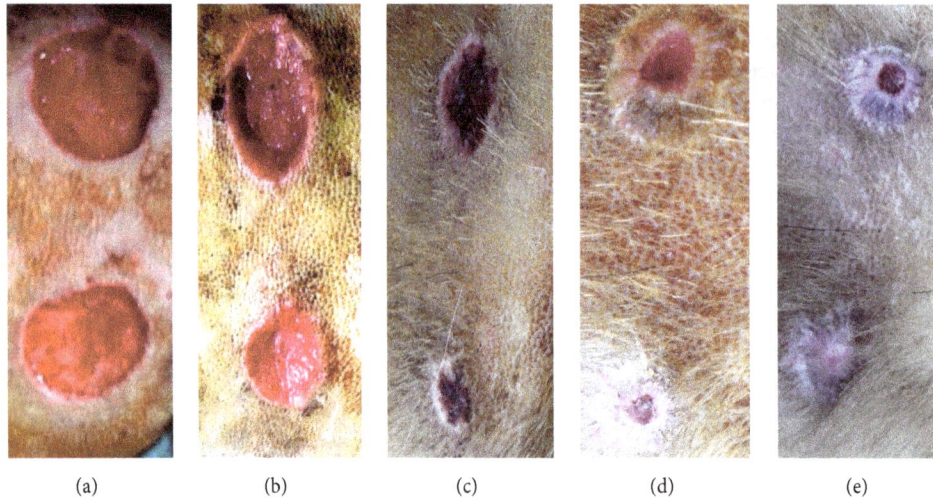

FIGURE 1: Representative skin wounds of the control group (upper wounds) and propolis group (lower wounds) at 0 (a), 7 (b), 14 (c), 21 (d), and 28 (e) days after surgery.

Aloe vera, sildenafil, tocopherol, pomegranate (*Punica granatum*), *Lantana* (*Lantana camara*), chitosan, stem cell therapy, honey, and hydroethanolic extract of ribwort plantain leaves [15, 16].

Cutaneous wound healing is a complex process involving the interplay of various cell types in the injured tissue, including inflammatory cells, keratinocytes, fibroblasts, and endothelial cells [17]. Wound healing is a natural body reaction initiated immediately after injury and occurs in four stages including coagulation, inflammation, reepithelization, and remodeling [18].

The skin is usually subjected to many injuries including chronic unhealed wounds, burns, and ulcers which do not heal at all or do so very slowly [19]. Moreover, acceleration of the healing of acute wounds is also required. The non-healing wounds are a large and growing problem, so several treatments were applied to enhance the wound healing, but wounds do not respond well to many of them. Therefore, there is a continuous need to develop agents that accelerate the healing of acute and chronic wounds and ulcers and regenerate of damaged tissue in burns.

The ideal topical wound treatment product must be biocompatible, nontoxic, and able to enhance the healing without adverse effects on the progress of the natural wound healing process [20]. To date, there is no single optimal treatment that enhances the resolution of problem wounds [21].

In the last decades, propolis has attracted researchers' interest because of several biological and pharmacological properties [22]. Therefore, propolis, as a natural product with useful biological properties and no recorded side effects, was selected in the present study to evaluate clinically its effect on healing of full thickness skin wound.

As regards the chemical composition of the used propolis in this study, the major constituents of propolis were flavonoids which contribute greatly to the pharmacological activities of propolis. Flavonoids have a broad spectrum of biological activities, such as anti-inflammatory, antibacterial, and antiviral effects. Moreover, the used propolis had phenylpropanoids, terpenoids, stilbenes, lignans, coumarins, and their prenylated derivatives. Terpenoids represented 10% of the propolis constituents and they exhibit antioxidant and antimicrobial effects. In addition, the used propolis had large amounts of caffeic acid phenethyl ester (CAPE), 3-methylbut-2-enyl caffeate, isopentyl ferulate, and moronic acid. The broad spectrum of biological properties of propolis is attributed to the variety of these major chemical constituents.

The present data showed that propolis helps the wound healing in a time-dependent manner. This could be attributed to immunomodulatory [8], antimicrobial [9], antioxidant [10], analgesic, and anti-inflammatory [11] effects of the propolis. These biological effects are essential for acceleration of the wound healing process. Caffeic acid phenethyl ester (CAPE) derived from the propolis has immunosuppressive activity in T-cells which play a key role in the onset of several inflammatory diseases. Moreover, CAPE specifically inhibited both interleukin- (IL-) 2 gene transcription and IL-2 synthesis in stimulated T-cells [23]. Data suggest an increase in the fungicidal activity of macrophages by propolis. In addition, propolis inhibits bacterial growth by preventing cell division, disorganizing the cytoplasm, the cytoplasmic membrane, and the cell wall, causing a partial bacteriolysis and inhibition of protein synthesis. Moreover, propolis contains 3-methyl-but-2-enyl caffeate, isopentyl ferulate, and moronic acid which have a significant antiviral activity [23].

In the present study, propolis paste was applied twice daily because it strongly interacts with oils and proteins of the skin resulting in good adhesion and prolonged action. Similarly, Burdock [2] mentioned that the use of products containing propolis has resulted in extensive dermal contact.

The results of this study demonstrated that topical application of propolis paste 30% enhanced wound contraction and reduced the healing time. In addition to its safety and effectiveness, propolis is an inexpensive topical wound treatment natural product. Therefore, propolis could be considered as a good alternative to several synthetic topical wound treatment products.

5. Conclusion

In conclusion, propolis paste 30% has a positive impact on cutaneous wound healing and it may be suggested for treating various types of wounds in animals.

Conflict of Interests

The author declares that there is no conflict of interests regarding the publication of this paper.

Acknowledgment

The author would like to acknowledge Dr. Oday S. Al-Abbadi for his assistance in the wounds measurement.

References

[1] D. Stavrou, "Neovascularisation in wound healing," *Journal of wound care*, vol. 17, no. 7, pp. 298–300, 2008.

[2] G. A. Burdock, "Review of the biological properties and toxicity of bee propolis (propolis)," *Food and Chemical Toxicology*, vol. 36, no. 4, pp. 347–363, 1998.

[3] N. C. Cinegaglia, P. R. O. Bersano, M. C. Búfalo, and J. M. Sforcin, "Cytotoxic action of Brazilian propolis in vitro on canine osteosarcoma cells," *Phytotherapy Research*, vol. 27, no. 9, pp. 1277–1281, 2013.

[4] A. Salatino, É. W. Teixeira, G. Negri, and D. Message, "Origin and chemical variation of Brazilian propolis," *Evidence-Based Complementary and Alternative Medicine*, vol. 2, no. 1, pp. 33–38, 2005.

[5] E. L. Ghisalberti, "Propolis: a review," *Bee World*, vol. 60, no. 2, pp. 59–84, 1979.

[6] S. Scheller, A. Stojko, I. Szwarnowiecka, J. Tustanowski, and Z. Obuszko, "Biological properties and clinical application of propolis. VI. Investigation of the influence of ethanol extracts of propolis (EEP) on cartilaginous tissue regeneration," *Arzneimittel-Forschung*, vol. 27, no. 11, pp. 2138–2140, 1977.

[7] A. Stojko, S. Scheller, I. Szwarnowiecka, J. Tustanowski, H. Ostach, and Z. Obuszko, "Biological properties and clinical application of propolis. VIII. Experimental observation on the influence of ethanol extract of propolis (EEP) on the regeneration of bone tissue," *Arzneimittel-Forschung*, vol. 28, no. 1, pp. 35–37, 1978.

[8] J. M. Sforcin, "Propolis and the immune system: a review," *Journal of Ethnopharmacology*, vol. 113, no. 1, pp. 1–14, 2007.

[9] R. L. Cardoso, F. Maboni, G. Machado, S. H. Alves, and A. C. de Vargas, "Antimicrobial activity of propolis extract against Staphylococcus coagulase positive and Malassezia pachydermatis of canine otitis," *Veterinary Microbiology*, vol. 142, no. 3-4, pp. 432–434, 2010.

[10] A. Ramadan, G. Soliman, S. S. Mahmoud, S. M. Nofal, and R. F. Abdel-Rahman, "Evaluation of the safety and antioxidant activities of *Crocus sativus* and *Propolis* ethanolic extracts," *Journal of Saudi Chemical Society*, vol. 16, no. 1, pp. 13–21, 2012.

[11] I. F. de Almeida Santo Ramos, M. T. Biz, N. Paulino et al., "Histopathological analysis of corticosteroid-antibiotic preparation and propolis paste formulation as intracanal medication after pulpectomy: an in vivo study," *Journal of Applied Oral Science*, vol. 20, no. 1, pp. 50–56, 2012.

[12] N. C. Cinegaglia, P. R. O. Bersano, M. J. A. M. Araújo, M. C. Búfalo, and J. M. Sforcin, "Anticancer effects of geopropolis produced by stingless bees on canine osteosarcoma cells *in vitro*," *Evidence-Based Complementary and Alternative Medicine*, vol. 2013, Article ID 737386, 6 pages, 2013.

[13] A. M. A. Abu-Seida, "Efficacy of diclofenac sodium, either alone or together with cefotaxime sodium, for control of postoperative pain, in dogs undergoing ovariohysterectomy," *Asian Journal of Animal and Veterinary Advances*, vol. 7, no. 2, pp. 180–186, 2012.

[14] A. Oryan, A. T. Naeini, B. Nikahval, and E. Gorjlan, "Effect of aqueous extract of *Aloe vera* on experimental cutaneous wound healing in rat," *Veterinarski Arhiv*, vol. 80, no. 4, pp. 509–522, 2008.

[15] Z. B. Ismail, M. A. Alshehabat, W. Hananeh, M. Daradka, J. H. Ali, and E. K. El-Najjar, "Recent advances in topical wound healing products with special reference to honey: a review," *Research Opinion in Animals and Veterinary Sciences*, vol. 5, pp. 76–83, 2015.

[16] M. R. Farahpour and A. Heydari, "Wound healing effect of hydroethanolic extract of *Ribwort plantain* leaves in rabbits," *Research Opinions in Animal and Veterinary Sciences*, vol. 5, no. 3, pp. 143–147, 2015.

[17] M. W. Bohling, R. A. Henderson, S. F. Swaim, S. A. Kincaid, and J. C. Wright, "Cutaneous wound healing in the cat: a macroscopic description and comparison with cutaneous wound healing in the dog," *Veterinary Surgery*, vol. 33, no. 6, pp. 579–587, 2004.

[18] G. D. Phillips, R. A. Whitehead, and D. R. Knighton, "Initiation and pattern of angiogenesis in wound healing in the rat," *American Journal of Anatomy*, vol. 192, no. 3, pp. 257–262, 1991.

[19] A. M. Abu-Seida and M. M. Saleh, "A gigantic cutaneous fibroadenoma in a dog," *Asian Journal of Animal Sciences*, vol. 10, no. 1, pp. 113–119, 2016.

[20] B. S. Atiyeh, S. A. Dibo, and S. N. Hayek, "Wound cleansing, topical antiseptics and wound healing," *International Wound Journal*, vol. 6, no. 6, pp. 420–430, 2009.

[21] S. A. Sell, P. S. Wolfe, A. J. Spence et al., "A preliminary study on the potential of manuka honey and platelet-rich plasma in wound healing," *International Journal of Biomaterials*, vol. 2012, Article ID 313781, 14 pages, 2012.

[22] V. S. Bankova, S. L. de Castro, and M. C. Marcucci, "Propolis: recent advances in chemistry and plant origin," *Apidologie*, vol. 31, no. 1, pp. 3–15, 2000.

[23] M. Lotfy, "Biological activity of bee propolis in health and disease," *Asian Pacific Journal of Cancer Prevention*, vol. 7, no. 1, pp. 22–31, 2006.

7

Social Network Analysis of Cattle Movement in Sukhothai Province, Thailand: A Study to Improve Control Measurements

Supot Noopataya,[1,2] **Sukanya Thongratsakul,**[1] **and Chaithep Poolkhet**[1]

[1]*Department of Veterinary Public Health, Faculty of Veterinary Medicine, Kasetsart University, Kamphaeng Saen Campus, Nakhon Pathom 73140, Thailand*
[2]*Department of Livestock Development, Ministry of Agriculture and Cooperatives, Bangkok 10400, Thailand*

Correspondence should be addressed to Chaithep Poolkhet; fvetctp@ku.ac.th

Academic Editor: Shane R. Raidal

The aim of this study is to analyse the pattern of cattle movement in Sukhothai province, Thailand. A validated questionnaire was applied to 308 respondents related to cattle farming using one-step snowball sampling. The results showed that most of the nodes are farmers who move their animals in the province. The average normalized degree centrality and normalized closeness centrality were low (<0.01 and 0.04, resp.). We found that traders are the nodes with a high value of centrality. This corresponds with the cutpoint analysis results that traders are outstanding. In conclusion, the relevant authorities should focus on the nodes such as traders for controlling disease. However, a measure to detect disease in the early stages needs to be implemented.

1. Introduction

One of the most important steps for cattle farming is the transport of cattle from place to place. These movements provide possible modes of transmitting infectious disease. For this reason, many countries have taken measures to control disease, such as restricting animal movement in the controlled areas during occurrence of disease [1]. However, these measures may not be taken in controlling the epidemic because of lack of real understanding about the movement patterns of animals [2–4]. Therefore, it would be valuable to understand the movement patterns of cattle in a developing country such as Thailand. The main point is to know the origin and destination of animal movement. This information can help the relevant authorities to improve disease control measures based on the analysis of scientific data. One of the best tools is the responses from Social Network Analysis (SNA).

SNA is a tool which defines the relationship between units of interest. A unit of interest might be an animal, human, or object, either individually or in a group. In terms of SNA, we usually call the unit of interest a "node." The "tie" is the term used to explain the relationship between one node and another. In this way, SNA uses the adjacency matrix and graph theory for the method of calculation [5]. Many researchers used the SNA to describe the pattern of diseases widely spreading in human and veterinary medicine [6–9]. Interesting work describes the network of cattle movement in Argentina, which relates to disease spreading. This study indicates that the relevant authorities should focus on the cattle moving out from the highlands to other areas [10]. A study in Great Britain found that the auction market plays an important role in Foot-and-Mouth Disease (FMD) outbreaks [11]. Moreover, Natale et al. showed that the live cattle market is the hub for disease spreading in Italy [12]. This result is similar to that found in a study in Denmark [13].

The aim of this study is to analyse the pattern of cattle movement in Thailand. We selected an area of Sukhothai province because this province is one of the places for cattle husbandry displayed at the live cattle market. Cattle husbandry activity in this area could provide answers about how disease is possibly spread. Additionally, Sukhothai is a perfect place for the study of cattle movement because there are slaughterhouses, backyard cattle farms, and commercial cattle farms in the province. The output from this study can be used to improve or design the control measures. In addition, knowledge of this study might be useful for the authorities in developing countries that have a similar pattern of cattle movement, such as countries in the Mekong subregion of Southeast Asia.

2. Materials and Methods

2.1. Study Framework and Data Collection. A retrospective and longitudinal study was performed using a validated questionnaire. The questionnaire was presented to respondents involved in the cattle movement network of Sukhothai province, Thailand. In this study, we have focused on beef and dairy movements. All questions of this study focused on cattle movements from January 2011 to December 2011. In this study, we define the node as the farmer, trader, collector, the owner of a slaughterhouse (or slaughterman), and the owner or worker of a live cattle market. For the cattle farms and slaughterhouses, we applied the questionnaire to one person from each location. For the remaining locations, we applied the questionnaires to as many people as we could during the date of data collection (more than 30% of the workers in each location). The tie in this study is the cattle movement among the pair of nodes. It is possible that this movement may or may not pass through the live cattle market. Our calculations did not account for cattle that were sent to a new location but did not arrive and were returned to the old location.

We applied the partial network method with one-step snowball sampling [5]. Data collection activities were started at the live cattle market on June 2012. Then, the information from our respondents about the places they got or bought the animal from (origin) and the places they sold the animal to (destination) pointed to the next locations for data collection. In cases where the original places or destination places were located out of the border of Sukhothai province, we did not follow the link for data collection. Two months later, we collected data at the initial place again. The process of data collection was repeated. At this point, the same respondents from the first data collection were excluded from the analysis. We finished our work on March 2013. A sample size was estimated by Yamane's methods [14]. Based on the suggestion of local authorities, we assumed there are 1,000 stakeholders in this network. We set the alpha error and precision at 5%. As a calculation, we needed the responses of more than 286 people in our study, and we successfully collected 308 responses to our work.

2.2. Questionnaire Design. The questionnaire used in the study was clarified by epidemiology experts and tested by asking farmers in the study area for any corrections or modifications. The approved questionnaire was discussed with our teams to clarify the questions before starting the data collection. The questionnaire contained both open and closed questions asked to the respondents in face-to-face interviews. The questions aimed to ask the respondents about general information, their role in cattle farming, trade activities, and movement patterns of the animals. The direction of the cattle movement (where the animal moves from and where the animal moves to) and number of animals moved each time were asked in the questionnaire but were excluded from our analysis to avoid analytical bias from respondents.

2.3. Data Analysis. A descriptive statistical analysis was used to explain the basic information of respondents related to their cattle activities. Network analysis was calculated based on the undirected binary network using Ucinet6 (Analytical Technologies, USA) as follows [5, 15].

Degree Centrality. It is the normalized value accounted for by analysing the number of ties in each node. The node with the high value of these reflects the high number of ties or the channel of node connection.

Betweenness Centrality. It is the Freeman normalized value which is considered the shortest path between two nodes. The node with a high value of these indicated a high frequency of animal movement through the node.

Closeness Centrality. It is the normalized value which is considered the geodesic distance from one node to all remaining nodes. A node with a high value indicated that it was easy to move animals to the linking node.

Component. It is considered a group of nodes connected to one another by at least one tie.

Cutpoint. It is a node whose removal causes the disconnected graph (i.e., creating two or more components).

Clustering Coefficient. It is calculated from three connected nodes. This results in a group of nodes forming a triangle shape (transitivity) in the network. The network with the highest probability number of clustering coefficient means that many node triangles are present.

Density. It reflects the actual ties that are present in the network compared to possible ties, and calculating density gives us the results of the probability number.

An Exponential Random Graph Model (ERGM) was calculated by using StOCNET [16]. These methods examined the network for possible alternative network based on observed uncertainty data. The features, such as transitive triplets (the amount of transitivity) and dyad (the number of pairwise relations between nodes) count, were examined with the 10,000 iterations of the Monte Carlo Simulation.

Mapping display of all nodes in these networks with ties was performed by using ArcGIS 10.2.1 (ESRI, USA). The respondents' nodes were recorded using their geographical coordinates from handheld GPS devices (Garmin, USA). For nodes unable to have their geographical coordinates located, their position was estimated based on the centroid from the border of subdistricts of Thailand's map using ArcGIS.

3. Results

3.1. General Information. According to our interviews with 308 respondents, 224 of them were animal owners, 82 were

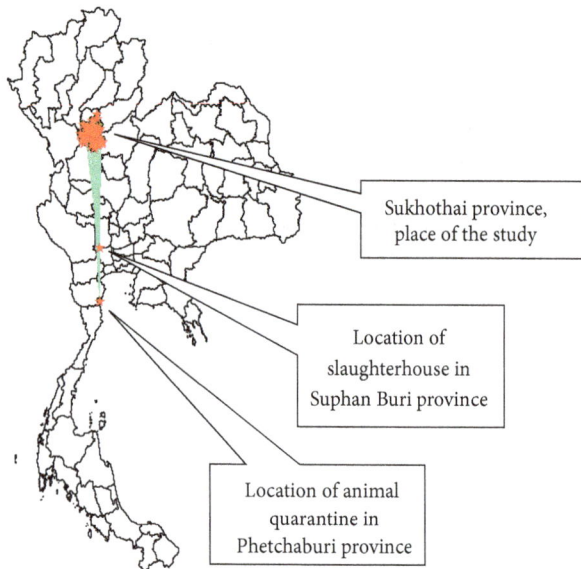

FIGURE 1: A map of Sukhothai's cattle movement in the year 2012.

slaughterhouse staff, 1 was an owner of a private animal quarantine station, and 1 was the owner of a live cattle market. We found that the respondents' average age was 52.72 years (SD = 8.32). Most of them (99.67%) graduated with compulsory education from elementary school, and some respondents held higher academic certificates. Most respondents (93.18%) were living in Sukhothai province. Only 6.82% were traders living in other provinces. For movement distances, the median of these activities was 39.60 kilometres (range = 0–550 kilometres). They usually moved their cattle to farms, slaughterhouses, or live cattle markets. For respondents, like the traders, who moved their animals farther distances, the cattle were moved and quarantined at the government quarantine station in Phetchaburi province. Some of the respondents who moved their cattle to a slaughterhouse were located in Suphan Buri province (Figure 1).

The results show that the animals mostly move within the province, and the number of animals moving is within the range of 1–5 heads. In cases of respondents who move their animals longer distances, they might be capable of increasing the number of cattle up to 30, depending on how many cattle they bought.

3.2. Network Analysis. The results show that this network has 2,367 nodes with 3,150 ties. We found that most of the nodes have connections with the others through a few links. The nodes were mostly connected to each other by dyad. The mean (and standard deviation) of normalized degree centrality was less than 0.01 (SD = 0.05), and the highest value and the lowest value of these parameters were 0.13 and 0, respectively. The nodes with the highest normalized degree centrality were a farmer and a trader in Sukhothai province. The node with the lowest normalized degree centrality was a farmer in this area in the cattle market who did not have any transactions during the study and moved the cattle back to the original location. In addition, we found that some farmers

raised their animals beside the market for transaction activities to occur in the next week. This meant they lived near the market and took care of their animals until the market opened the following week. The analysis of normalized closeness centrality in this network showed that the average was 0.04 (SD < 0.01). The maximum and minimum values were 0.04, and all were from farmers. Moreover, all nodes represented the null value of normalized betweenness centrality.

The analysis of the network component found that this network has seven components (Figure 2(a)). A main component contained most of the nodes and was located as a core network when multidimensional scaling was used for analysing network representation. This means that most of the nodes were similar. The five remaining components were small and disconnected from each other. We found that one node was identified as an isolator (separate node). The analysis found that the nodes in this network were the cutpoints at 1,565 (66.18%) and there were massive links between cutpoints (Figures 2(b) and 2(c)).

The average network density was 0.003 (SD = 0.109), which reflects the notion that the real movement activities in this network were only 0.3 per cent comparing to all possible movements in the theorem. This correlated with the result of centrality in this network, which had a low value. The clustering coefficient of this network was 0.009. The network density and clustering coefficient were low. This showed that this network had a random pattern. A calculation using ERGMs with Monte Carlo Simulation confirms that all possible dyads in this network should be 2,800,564 nodes or significantly represent 99.93% of the maximum value of dyads ($p < 0.01$). This reflects the notion that this network represents a dense social relationship structure like a dyad. It also proves that this network represents a significant triangle relationship (15; $p < 0.01$).

4. Discussion

Based on the respondents' answers and our observation, some participants do not pay much attention to farm biosecurity. The relevant authorities should regularly educate the stakeholders about risk factors, measures of biosecurity, measures for disease monitoring or surveillance, and measures for disease control. This is one way to successfully control and prevent disease in developing countries. Therefore, the relevant authorities must be educating them with easy-to-understand media, such as broadcast media.

We found that the farmers mostly move their cattle within the province and take less than 40 km to transport them each time; however, when cattle are moved to another province, the distances reached would be 550 kilometres. This study shows that the respondents do not move their animals to the neighboring province of Sukhothai, because the movement of animals across the border of province must be allowed by the authorities. They may feel not free to obtain approval documents from the authorities. The control measure of restricting animal movement between the provinces is a tool to help the authorities control the occurrence and spread of disease. If diseases such as FMD occur and spread through cattle movement, it would seem that there are dominant

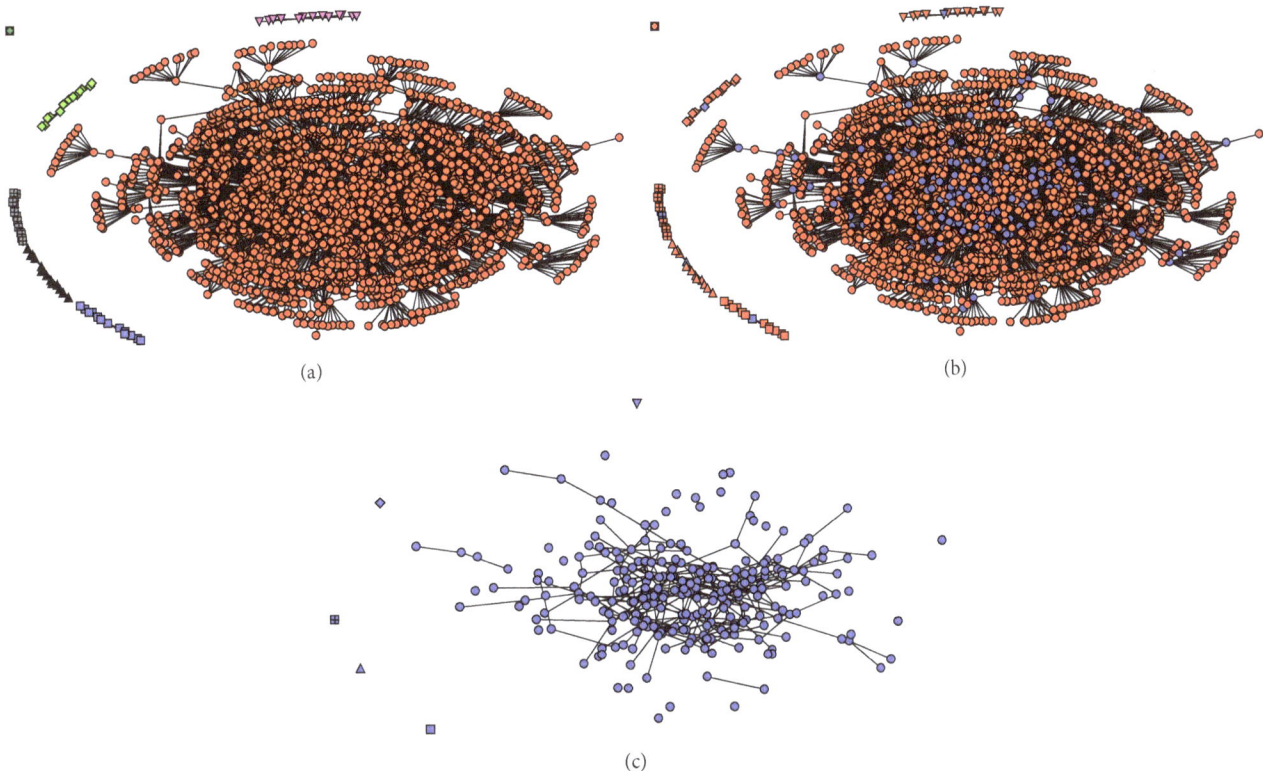

FIGURE 2: A sociogram of cattle movement in Sukhothai province during 2011. (a) represents the components separated by colour and shape. (b) represents all nodes in the network which were ordinary nodes (red) and cutpoint (blue). (c) only presents cutpoints showing their connections.

local occurrences within the province because of shorter movement distances. This coincides with the previous studies [17], which look at backyard farmer's behaviour. Another work found that most livestock premises in Peru are infected by the local spread of FMD [18].

Likewise, the disease can spread over long distances, and the pattern of disease distribution possibly jumps to provinces which are disconnected from Sukhothai province. From Figure 1, the disease possibly moved to the upper zone of the southern part of Thailand. From this analysis, we show that if the disease is present in countries with disconnecting geographic patterns of the infected areas, then the vehicle or carrier must be considered. To address these problems, the Department of Livestock Development of Thailand imposed the disease control measures to prevent and control animal diseases such as FMD. They have a system named "e-Movement, an electronic documentation for livestock movement approvals" for animal movement recording, which was designed for recording when the stakeholders move their animals between the provinces. The stakeholders must ask the authorities for permission by documentation and then the authorities will electronically record the data. However, they lack a routine analysis of this data, so we suggested that the analysis of network data is necessary. Moreover, the "e-Movement" does not cover the movement within the province and the Thai authorities need to consider that for effective analysis. For example, if the disease occurs in the area, the farmers or traders are free to move infected animals

to other areas within the province. We suggested that a system be designed to fulfil these gaps by extending the documentation for animal movement within the province. Thus, in Thailand, restricting animal movement is a key measurement for disease control during the outbreak situation. It is an administrative measurement at the provincial level only. We recommended that the authorities should improve the system by making it available at the district level.

We found that the majority of activities occurred at the farm, because Sukhothai has only one cattle market open once a week and this might not be enough for slaughtering. Therefore, the traders or other relevant players in the cattle market are looking for more animals. Thai authorities should think about this information for disease prevention and control.

In this study, we used the one-step snowball approach for sampling, which reflects the behaviour of the network as well, and we found that there were problems with complete node identification. In other words, some respondents could not remember exactly the name of the person who sold or bought their animal. This affects the identification of connecting nodes for data collection. We corrected these problems by using the demographic data (we collected the data from nodes who live in the same village) instead of name identification. Then, the nodes that the respondents refer to are possibly different from the data collected nodes. This explains why we found many components in this network. However, this sampling problem was less than 10% of the total data.

From our experience, we believe that the results might not be any different between a one-step and a more-than-one-step snowball approach, because most stakeholders have a few links of pair's connections. On the other hand, if we carry out a two-step approach, there will be more recall bias or lying.

For centrality value of network analysis, normalized degree centrality is low, which means the node has moved cattle through a few connections. This is consistent for most respondents, who are small stakeholders or backyard farmers who always sell or buy the animals with familiar people. In the network with high degree centrality, it is hard to control the disease spread compared to the network with low degree centrality [5]. In the network with low connection, the probability of detection will be low because not a lot of nodes will be infected. For this reason, active surveillance or education of farmers on the signs of FMD should be done. On the other hand, the standard deviation of degree centrality is low. This indicates that almost all the nodes in this network are homogeneous, and the multidimensional scaling confirmed this. Thus, there is no hub in this network [12]. The normalized closeness centrality in this network is low. This feature reflects the speed of the message flow [15]. Thus, if the disease occurs in the network, the speed of infection does not move rapidly. This is good for authorities to control the disease. The normalized Freeman betweenness centrality in this network is null, which consequently affects a high number of dyad node relationships. Thus, these statistics might not fit for this kind of network. We suggested that the centrality measures in a network representing a few steps, the degree centrality and closeness centrality, might be useful for centrality measurements. Moreover, the nodes as traders have the highest degree of centrality and they play an important role in spreading disease. The relevant authorities should focus on these nodes to control disease in cattle farming and should implement the active surveillance system on them. In this way, the authorities should request that they notify them of any diseases identified in the early stages to prevent further spreading. However, previous studies show different results in Denmark and Great Britain [11, 13]. They found that the animal market plays a key role in the continued spread of infectious disease. However, this depends on the nature of each country. We had expected that the other developing countries would present network's behaviour similar to Thailand.

As a cutpoint analysis, traders were densely connected together. If the disease spreads in the area, it is possible that traders influence the increase of infectious nodes. It seems appropriate that these nodes need to be under surveillance and control; however, these people are always a hidden population and the authorities need to handle them gently. The researchers were determined that an efficient surveillance system needs good cooperation between the local veterinarian and the relevant people such as farmers [19]. In this study, some farmers also played the role of traders. The trader is a key person for disease control. In addition, the result of cutpoint analysis showed that all traders are the cutpoint nodes which indicate that we can break the infectious network by controlling them. With good control of these nodes, the magnitude of disease during an outbreak can be minimized. It is similar to our previous study in Laos and Cambodia

[Authors; in preparation for publishing]. The results of clustering coefficient and density are low. We consider this network to be close to a random network, meaning that a node is connected to the others without a regular pattern. This corresponds with the standard deviation of degree centrality in which the hub is not present. Therefore, a connection from node to node could not predict a certain path [11].

Moreover, the ERGMs showed that the relationship in this network is significantly dominated by a dyad. In terms of infectious control, the dyad relationship is easier to control compared to others [5]. In this network, the triangle relationship is significantly present. In fact, triangle relationship is typically more stable than a dyad [15]. As we described above, Thai authorities need to develop an active surveillance system to detect the early stages of infectious disease with restrictions on current control measurements. This will help the authorities improve effective control measurements. The other developing countries can use this knowledge to develop their control measurements effectively. For further investigation, the influence of risky premises, such as shared grazing areas or other locations, needs to be studied.

5. Conclusion

The study of cattle movement using the SNA in Sukhothai province found that traders were the key players in this network. We found that the patterns of spreading diseases, such as FMD, are more locally spread than faraway spread. In this study, the results suggested a need to improve control measurements based on these nodes. We recommended that the following control measurements be developed: a database for animal movement within the provinces; an improvement in the quarantine station for lengthy movements; zoning regulations for cattle farming; control of trader activities; and the development of a highly sensitive disease detection system in the early stages. All of our suggestions are based on the results of descriptive statistics, our experiences, and SNA. These will help us to understand the possible patterns of disease spreading and to improve the control measurements for better control in Thailand and other developing countries which have the same cattle farming behaviours. An analysis of the network with a mathematic model such as SIR model needs to be conducted in further studies.

Conflict of Interests

The authors have declared no conflict of interests.

Acknowledgments

The authors would like to thank the officers of Sukhothai's Provincial Livestock Veterinary Office for their involvement and support. This study was granted by the Graduate Study Research scholarship for International Publication of the Graduate School, Kasetsart University, Thailand.

References

[1] World Health Organisation for Animal Health, *Foot and Mouth Disease Portal*, World Health Organisation for Animal Health,

2015, http://www.oie.int/animal-health-in-the-world/fmd-portal/prevention-and-control/.

[2] M. D. F. Shirley and S. P. Rushton, "Where diseases and networks collide: lessons to be learnt from a study of the 2001 foot-and-mouth disease epidemic," *Epidemiology and Infection*, vol. 133, no. 6, pp. 1023–1032, 2005.

[3] C. Dubé, C. Ribble, D. Kelton, and B. McNab, "A review of network analysis terminology and its application to foot-and-mouth disease modelling and policy development," *Transboundary and Emerging Diseases*, vol. 56, no. 3, pp. 73–85, 2009.

[4] A. L. Rivas, F. O. Fasina, J. M. Hammond et al., "Epidemic protection zones: centred on cases or based on connectivity?" *Transboundary and Emerging Diseases*, vol. 59, no. 5, pp. 464–469, 2012.

[5] S. Borgatti, G. Everett, and C. Johnson, *Analyzing Social Networks*, SAGE Publications, 2013.

[6] R. Curtis, S. R. Friedman, A. Neaigus, B. Jose, M. Goldstein, and G. Ildefonso, "Street-level drug markets: network structure and HIV risk," *Social Networks*, vol. 17, no. 3-4, pp. 229–249, 1995.

[7] D. C. Bell, J. S. Atkinson, and J. W. Carlson, "Centrality measures for disease transmission networks," *Social Networks*, vol. 21, no. 1, pp. 1–21, 1999.

[8] M. Bigras-Poulin, R. A. Thompson, M. Chriél, S. Mortensen, and M. Greiner, "Network analysis of Danish cattle industry trade patterns as an evaluation of risk potential for disease spread," *Preventive Veterinary Medicine*, vol. 76, no. 1-2, pp. 11–39, 2006.

[9] A. Ortiz-Pelaez, D. U. Pfeiffer, R. J. Soares-Magalhães, and F. J. Guitian, "Use of social network analysis to characterize the pattern of animal movements in the initial phases of the 2001 foot and mouth disease (FMD) epidemic in the UK," *Preventive Veterinary Medicine*, vol. 76, no. 1-2, pp. 40–55, 2006.

[10] M. N. Aznar, M. A. Stevenson, L. Zarich, and E. A. León, "Analysis of cattle movements in Argentina, 2005," *Preventive Veterinary Medicine*, vol. 98, no. 2-3, pp. 119–127, 2011.

[11] S. E. Robinson and R. M. Christley, "Exploring the role of auction markets in cattle movements within Great Britain," *Preventive Veterinary Medicine*, vol. 81, no. 1-3, pp. 21–37, 2007.

[12] F. Natale, A. Giovannini, L. Savini et al., "Network analysis of Italian cattle trade patterns and evaluation of risks for potential disease spread," *Preventive Veterinary Medicine*, vol. 92, no. 4, pp. 341–350, 2009.

[13] M. M. Mweu, G. Fournié, T. Halasa, N. Toft, and S. S. Nielsen, "Temporal characterisation of the network of Danish cattle movements and its implication for disease control: 2000–2009," *Preventive Veterinary Medicine*, vol. 110, no. 3-4, pp. 379–387, 2013.

[14] T. Yamane, *Elementary Sampling Theory*, Prentice-Hall, Englewood Cliffs, NJ, USA, 1967.

[15] C. Prell, *Social Network Analysis: History, Theory and Methodology*, SAGE Publications, 2011.

[16] P. Boer, M. Huisman, B. Snijders, C. Steglich, Y. Wichers, and H. Zeggelink, *StOCNET: An Open Software System for the Advanced Statistical Analysis of Social Networks. Version 1.7*, ICS/SciencePlus, Groningen, The Netherlands, 2006.

[17] C. Poolkhet, P. Chairatanayuth, S. Thongratsakul et al., "Social network analysis for assessment of Avian influenza spread and trading patterns of backyard chickens in Nakhon Pathom, Suphan Buri and Ratchaburi, Thailand," *Zoonoses and Public Health*, vol. 60, no. 6, pp. 448–455, 2013.

[18] B. Martínez-López, B. Ivorra, E. Fernández-Carrión et al., "A multi-analysis approach for space-time and economic evaluation of risks related with livestock diseases: the example of FMD in Peru," *Preventive Veterinary Medicine*, vol. 114, no. 1, pp. 47–63, 2014.

[19] S. Rautureau, B. Dufour, and B. Durand, "Vulnerability of animal trade networks to the spread of infectious diseases: a methodological approach applied to evaluation and emergency control strategies in Cattle, France, 2005," *Transboundary and Emerging Diseases*, vol. 58, no. 2, pp. 110–120, 2011.

8

Evaluation of Analgesic Effect of Caudal Epidural Tramadol, Tramadol-Lidocaine, and Lidocaine in Water Buffalo Calves (*Bubalus bubalis*)

Ayman Atiba,[1] **Alaa Ghazy,**[1] **Naglaa Gomaa,**[2] **Tarek Kamal,**[3] **and Mustafa Shukry**[4]

[1]*Department of Surgery, Anesthesiology and Radiology, Faculty of Veterinary Medicine, Kafrelsheikh University, Kafrelsheikh 33516, Egypt*
[2]*Department of Animal Medicine, Faculty of Veterinary Medicine, Kafrelsheikh University, Kafrelsheikh 33516, Egypt*
[3]*Department of Biochemistry, Faculty of Veterinary Medicine, Kafrelsheikh University, Kafrelsheikh 33516, Egypt*
[4]*Department of Physiology, Faculty of Veterinary Medicine, Kafrelsheikh University, Kafrelsheikh 33516, Egypt*

Correspondence should be addressed to Ayman Atiba; atiba_2003@yahoo.co.uk

Academic Editor: William Ravis

Aim of this study was to compare the analgesic effect of tramadol and a combination of tramadol-lidocaine with that produced by lidocaine administration in the epidural space in buffalo calves. In a prospective randomized crossover study, ten male buffalo calves were used to compare the epidural analgesic effect of tramadol (1 mg/kg) and tramadol-lidocaine combination (0.5 mg/kg and 0.11 mg/kg, resp.) with that produced by 2% lidocaine (0.22 mg/kg). Loss of sensation was examined by pin-prick test. Onset time, duration, and degree of analgesia and ataxia were recorded after each treatment. Heart rate (HR), respiratory rate (RR), rectal temperature, and haematobiochemical parameters were recorded after all treatments. Time to onset and duration of analgesia, respectively, were as follows: tramadol 11 ± 2 min and 208 ± 15 min; tramadol-lidocaine 6 ± 2 min and 168 ± 9 min; lidocaine 4 ± 1 min and 67 ± 13 min. Onset time and duration were significantly longer with tramadol than the other treatments. Duration was significantly longer with tramadol-lidocaine than lidocaine. Ataxia was mildly observed in tramadol-lidocaine and was moderate in lidocaine. HR, RR, and rectal temperature did not differ significantly from baseline after any treatment. Haematobiochemical parameters returned to basal levels by 24 h after all treatments. This combination might be clinically useful to provide analgesia in buffalo for long-duration surgical procedures.

1. Introduction

Caudal epidural analgesia is frequently used in large animals for surgical procedures in the perineal region [1]. Lidocaine is the most commonly used local anesthetic drug in epidural analgesia but has a relatively short duration of action and may require readministration of the drug to allow completion of the procedure [2]. Epidural administration of a drug or a combination results in a much longer duration of action which will be more appropriate for procedures requiring long-duration analgesia [3].

Recently, tramadol as an adjuvant to local anesthetics has been found to improve the quality and extend the duration of analgesia in humans [4, 5]. Tramadol is a synthetic analogue of codeine that has been demonstrated to provide prolonged epidural analgesia in human [6]. Moreover, epidural tramadol has been used alone or in combination with lidocaine to produce longer analgesia in many animal species, including horses, cattle, goats, and donkeys [7–10]. To date, epidural injection of tramadol has not yet been reported in buffalo. Therefore, the purpose of this study was to determine and compare the time of onset and the duration of analgesia produced by tramadol and tramadol-lidocaine combination with that produced by lidocaine administration in the epidural space of buffalo calves.

2. Materials and Methods

In this study, the experimental protocol was approved by the Animal Care Committee of Kafrelsheikh University.

2.1. Animals. Ten male water buffalo calves (*Bubalus bubalis*) aged 7–10 months, weight 78–112 kg, were selected. All calves were deemed healthy by physical examination. The animals were fasted for 24 hours, and water was withheld for 6 hours prior to the start of the experiment.

The animals were restrained in standing position in the stanchion. The sacrococcygeal (S5-Co1) area of each calf was shaved and prepared aseptically. Epidural injection was made using a 20-gauge, 4-cm long hypodermic needle. Confirmation of proper epidural injection was based on the standard technique of loss of resistance to injection of 2 mL of air and the hanging drop technique. In crossover study, calves were randomly assigned to receive each of the three treatment protocols, with a period of at least 10-day interval between them in a Latin square design. Treatment 1 was tramadol (1 mg/kg) (Amadol, 100 mg/1 mL, injectable sterilized solution; Adwia Co., 10th of Ramadan City, Egypt). Treatment 2 was a combination of tramadol (0.5 mg/kg) and 2% lidocaine hydrochloride without epinephrine (0.11 mg/kg) (Debocaine 2% Al-Debeiky Pharmaceutical Industries Co., Egypt). Treatment 3 was 2% lidocaine (0.22 mg/kg). The volume of the drug was expanded to 4.0 mL by adding 0.9% normal saline solution. All drugs were injected slowly over a period of approximately 40 seconds.

Time to the onset, duration, anatomical distribution, and degree of the analgesia were recorded. Analgesia was assessed by a pin-prick test (using a 21-gauge needle inserted through the skin into the underlying tissues) applied at the perineal region, tail base, and upper hind limb area (Figure 1). Time to the onset of analgesia was defined as a time interval (in minute) from the epidural injection of the drug to loss of response to pin-prick in the perineal region. The duration time of analgesia was defined as a time interval (in minute) from loss and reappearance of pain response to pin-prick in the perineal region. In the stanchions, the response was measured each minute until no reaction occurred, and then at 10-minute intervals until a response was observed. The degree of analgesia was graded subjectively by observing the response of the animal to the pin-prick test on a scale from 0 to 3 according to the following scoring system: 0 = no analgesia (strong avoidance response to pin-prick); 1 = mild analgesia (weak avoidance response to pin-prick); 2 = moderate analgesia (occasional mild avoidance response to pin-prick); 3 = complete analgesia (no avoidance response to pin-prick). To avoid any bias or potential manipulation of data, the same investigator assessed the analgesia in all calves and was blind to the treatment given.

The presence of ataxia was examined by walking animals out of the stanchions at 10-minute intervals until the end of the study. The ataxia was graded on a 0 to 3 scale according to Grubb et al. 2002 [11], using the following scoring system: 0 = normal (walking without staggering); 1 = mild (slight stumbling, easily able to continue walking); 2 = moderate (marked stumbling, walking but very ataxic); 3 = severe

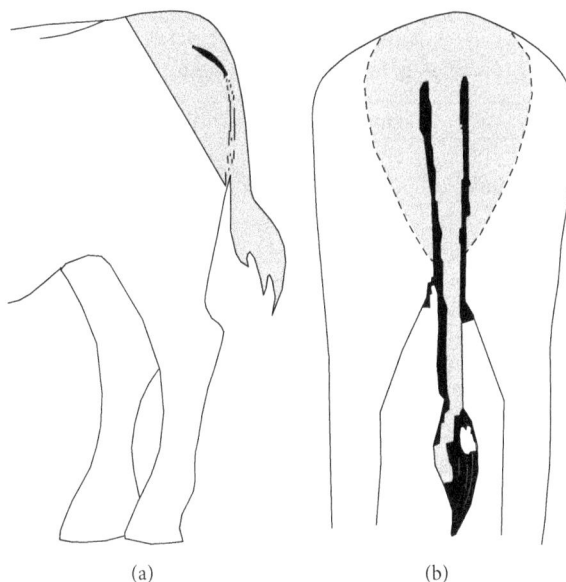

FIGURE 1: Schematic diagram from the left lateral view (a) and caudal view (b) of a buffalo calf showing the area was tested by a pin-prick test (applied at the perineal region, tail base, and upper hind limb area).

(animal unable to stand and falling). Person, unaware of the drugs used, made the observations.

Heart rate (HR) was measured by counting the heart beats over the cardiac area using a stethoscope. Respiratory rate (RR) was measured by counting chest movements per minute and rectal temperature (°C) was measured with a digital thermometer. HR, RR, and rectal temperature were recorded before (baseline, 0) and at 10-minute intervals for 2 hours after the administration of each treatment protocol. Blood samples were collected from the jugular vein for haematobiochemical parameters before (0 minute), at 30, 60, 90, 120, minutes, and 24-hour intervals after administration of drugs. For haematology, 3 mL venous blood was collected in test tubes containing EDTA. Hematological parameters including haemoglobin (Hb), packed cell volume (PCV%), total erythrocytes count (RBCs), and total leukocyte count (TLC) were examined. For biochemical parameters, 7 mL venous blood was collected in test tubes and serum was separated. Biochemical parameters including blood glucose, blood urea nitrogen (BUN) alanine aminotransferase (ALT), and alkaline phosphatase (ALP) were examined.

2.2. Statistical Analyses. All data were presented as mean ± SD. The data for time of onset and duration of analgesia, HR, RR, rectal temperature, and haematobiochemical parameters were analyzed by ANOVA (analysis of variance) and Duncan's test as a post hoc. Statistical analysis was undertaken using Graphpad Prism version 5 software program. A value of $p < 0.05$ was considered significant.

3. Results

Onset time of analgesia was significantly ($p < 0.05$) longer after tramadol than after the tramadol-lidocaine combination

TABLE 1: Anesthetic indices of epidurally administered tramadol (1.0 mg/kg), tramadol-lidocaine (0.5 and 0.11 mg/kg, resp.), and lidocaine (0.22 mg/kg) in buffalo calves (mean ± SD; $n = 10$).

Indices	Tramadol	Tramadol-lidocaine	Lidocaine
Onset of analgesia (min)	11 ± 2^a	6 ± 2	4 ± 1
Duration of analgesia (min)	208 ± 15	168 ± 9^c	67 ± 13^b

[a]Significant differences between onset of tramadol alone with lidocaine and tramadol-lidocaine combination. [b]Significant differences between duration of lidocaine alone with tramadol-lidocaine combination and tramadol alone. [c]Significant differences between duration of tramadol-lidocaine combination and lidocaine alone.

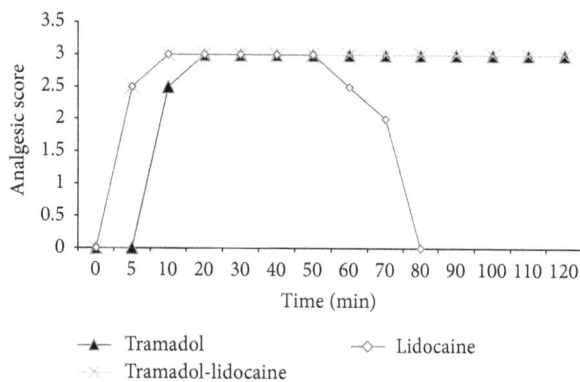

FIGURE 2: Degree of analgesia at the perineal region and tail base after epidural analgesia of tramadol, tramadol-lidocaine combination, and lidocaine in buffalo calves.

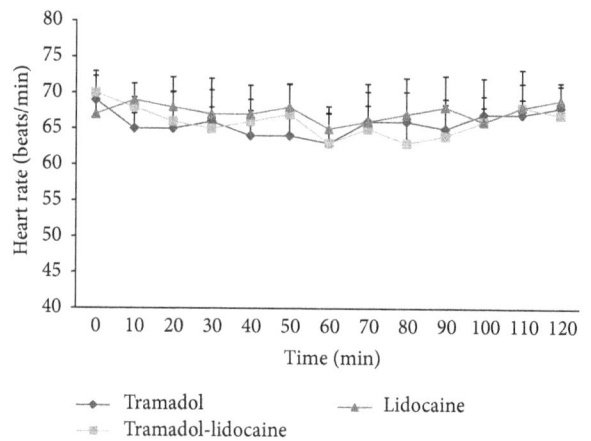

FIGURE 3: Mean heart rate (beats/minute) after epidural analgesia of tramadol, tramadol-lidocaine combination, and lidocaine in buffalo calves (mean ± SD in 10 calves). Error bars indicate the standard deviation of the mean.

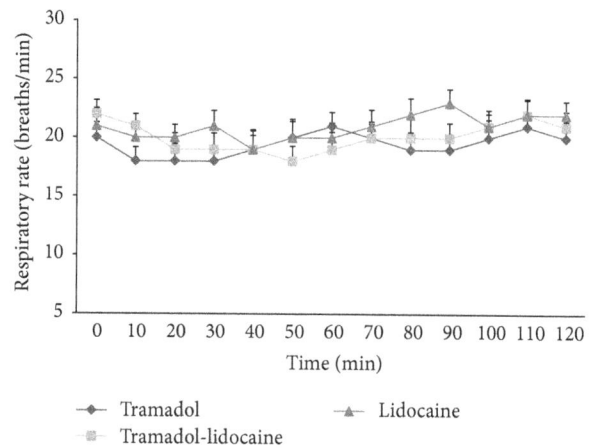

FIGURE 4: Mean respiratory rate (breaths/minute) after epidural analgesia of tramadol, tramadol-lidocaine combination, and lidocaine in buffalo calves (mean ± SD in 10 calves). Error bars indicate the standard deviation of the mean.

or lidocaine alone (Table 1). The duration of analgesia was significantly longer in animals that received tramadol ($p = 0.038$) or the combination of tramadol-lidocaine ($p = 0.043$) as compared with animals that received lidocaine alone and the duration of action of the tramadol was significantly greater than for tramadol-lidocaine combination ($p = 0.044$) (Table 1).

The results of this study demonstrated that all of the three treatments were effective in producing analgesia in the perineal region, tail base, and upper hind limb regions in all experimental animals but at different times. Analgesia at the perineal region and tail base (Figure 2) increased gradually and complete analgesia (score 3) was recorded from 10 minutes in lidocaine and tramadol-lidocaine groups while recorded from 20 minutes onwards in tramadol group. Analgesia started to wean off gradually and was lost by 80 minutes in lidocaine group. Analgesia of tramadol and tramadol-lidocaine groups showed complete analgesia until the end of the observation time. Analgesia at upper hind limb region was ranged from mild to moderate (score 1 to 2) and was observed from 10 to 60 minutes in lidocaine group. In animal of tramadol-lidocaine and tramadol groups moderated analgesia (score 2) was observed 20 and 30 minutes onwards, respectively, until the end of the observation time.

Ataxia was observed in all calves following epidural administration of lidocaine and a tramadol-lidocaine combination. All animals in the lidocaine group showed moderate ataxia (score 2) which started after 15 minutes and lasted for 35 minutes, while animals in tramadol-lidocaine combination group showed mild ataxia (score 1) which started after 20 minutes and lasted for 60 minutes from the time of injection. Animals of the tramadol group showed no signs of ataxia and animals of all groups remained in standing position all over the time of observation.

The HR (Figure 3), RR (Figure 4), and rectal temperatures did not differ significantly ($p > 0.05$) from baseline values following any treatment. Hematological parameters: a significant decrease in Hb, PCV%, RBCs, and TLC was recorded after 30 minutes, which persisted up to 120-minute intervals as compared to base value in all groups. However, values returned to basal level by 24 hours (Table 2). Biochemical parameters: a significant ($p < 0.01$) increase in glucose concentration from 30- to 120-minute intervals was recorded. A significant increase in BUN levels was observed in all animals after different treatments. ALP level concentration showed

TABLE 2: Hematobiochemical parameters after caudal epidural administration of tramadol alone (T), tramadol-lidocaine combination (TL), and lidocaine alone (L) in buffalo calves (mean ± SD, $n = 10$).

Parameter	Group	Time interval					
		0 min	30 min	60 min	90 min	120 min	24 h
Hb (gm/dL)	T	10.25 ± 1.3[a]	8.4 ± 1.2[b]	7.2 ± 1.3[c]	6.1 ± 0.3[cd]	6.2 ± 1.0[cd]	10.4 ± 0.3[a]
	TL	10.1 ± 1.8[a]	8.0 ± 0.7[b]	7.15 ± 1.2[c]	6.75 ± 1.0[c]	6.81 ± 0.7[c]	10.5 ± 0.3[a]
	L	9.7 ± 1.4[a]	7.24 ± 1.2[c]	7.20 ± 1.1[c]	6.82 ± 0.8[c]	6.05 ± 1.2[cd]	9.9 ± 0.5[a]
PCV%	T	26.8 ± 1.3[ab]	23.7 ± 2.1[c]	22.1 ± 1.3[c]	20.9 ± 0.3[d]	20.2 ± 1.1[d]	26.9 ± 1.2[ab]
	TL	28.2 ± 1.2[a]	24.0 ± 1.4[c]	22.02 ± 0.8[c]	20.4 ± 0.2[d]	20.0 ± 1.5[d]	28. 2 ± 0.2[a]
	L	28.8 ± 0.7[a]	23.24 ± 0.4[c]	21.9 ± 0.2[cd]	21.20 ± 0.8[d]	22.03 ± 0.6[c]	28.01 ± 1.0[a]
RBCs (10^6/mm^3)	T	6.4 ± 0.5[a]	5.5 ± 0.1[ab]	5.0 ± 0.3[b]	4.7 ± 0.1[b]	4.3 ± 0.1[b]	6.6 ± 0.2[a]
	TL	5.7 ± 0.3[ab]	4.9 ± 0.3[b]	4.4 ± 0.5[b]	4.1 ± 0.2[b]	3.75 ± 0.4[bc]	5.6 ± 0.5[ab]
	L	6.4 ± 0.3[a]	4.9 ± 0.5[b]	4.5 ± 0.2[b]	4.01 ± 0.2[b]	4.04 ± 0.5[b]	6.2 ± 0.2[a]
TLC (10^3/mm)	T	8.79 ± 0.52[ab]	7.7 ± 0.02[b]	7.91 ± 0.23[b]	7.0 ± 0.3[bc]	6.9 ± 0.02[bc]	9.25 ± 0.52[a]
	TL	9.22 ± 0.31[a]	8.5 ± 0.2[b]	7.5 ± 0.6[bc]	6.2 ± 1.1[c]	6.0 ± 0.2[c]	9.5 ± 0.2[a]
	L	9.5 ± 0.6[a]	8.1 ± 0.4[b]	7.3 ± 0.3[bc]	6.1 ± 0.2[c]	6.0 ± 0.5[c]	9.3 ± 0.7[a]
Blood glucose (mg/dL)	T	70.2 ± 1.5[d]	75.1 ± 0.2[b]	76.2 ± 0.6[ab]	76.5 ± 0.3[ab]	79.1 ± 0.1[a]	69.6 ± 1.0[d]
	TL	69.5 ± 1.5[d]	73.1 ± 2.3[c]	78.2 ± 1.1[a]	79.2 ± 0.4[a]	79.5 ± 1.5[a]	69.7 ± 0.8[d]
	L	70.5 ± 2.0[d]	75.2 ± 2.5[b]	75.4 ± 2.1[b]	77.3 ± 0.2[ab]	78.7 ± 2.5[a]	69.7 ± 2.0[d]
BUN (mg/dL)	T	29.2 ± 2.2[a]	29.7 ± 1.2[a]	29.9 ± 0.3[a]	29.9 ± 0.2[a]	30.4 ± 1.0[a]	28.3 ± 2.5[a]
	TL	24.2 ± 2.3[c]	25.1 ± 2.1[c]	27.2 ± 0.1[ab]	29.3 ± 0.4[a]	29.5 ± 0.9[a]	23.5 ± 2.2[c]
	L	25.4 ± 1.2[c]	26.2 ± 1.2[b]	27.5 ± 1.2[ab]	29.3 ± 1.1[a]	29.5 ± 1.3[a]	25.4 ± 1.4[c]
ALP (Unit/mL)	T	84.2 ± 2.2[a]	84.1 ± 1.2[a]	85.1 ± 2.2[a]	85.0 ± 0.2[a]	85.3 ± 1.2[a]	84.1 ± 2.0[a]
	TL	83.3 ± 1.2[ab]	84.1 ± 2.3[a]	85.0 ± 2.1[a]	85.5 ± 1.2[a]	85.5 ± 2.2[a]	83.4 ± 2.0[ab]
	L	83.2 ± 1.4[ab]	84.5 ± 2.2[a]	85.4 ± 2.0[a]	85.3 ± 0.6[a]	85.1 ± 2.5[a]	82.2 ± 1.0[ab]
ALT (Unit/mL)	T	27.2 ± 0.2[bc]	28.9 ± 0.2[a]	28.91 ± 0.3[a]	28.95 ± 0.3[a]	29.01 ± 0.2[a]	26.2 ± 0.1[a]
	TL	24.3 ± 0.3[c]	27.5 ± 1.0[bc]	28.9 ± 0.5[a]	29.01 ± 0.2[a]	29.2 ± 0.5[a]	23.9 ± 0.4[c]
	L	25.4 ± 0.7[c]	26.5 ± 1.6[c]	28.1 ± 0.4[ab]	28.5 ± 0.3[a]	28.9 ± 0.3[a]	25.2 ± 0.5[c]

Values with different letters differ significantly ($p < 0.05$) among groups.

no significant difference among different groups, while ALT level concentration showed a significant increase at different time points of treatment. However, biochemical parameters returned to basal levels after 24 hours of treatments (Table 2).

4. Discussion

There are currently only few published studies about epidural analgesia in buffalo [12–15]. Epidural use of tramadol has been reported in human and different animal species to provide prolonged duration of analgesia without serious side effects [4, 7, 16]. The present study is the first to investigate the analgesic effect of tramadol and tramadol-lidocaine combination given by an epidural injection to buffalo calves. The dose of tramadol chosen was based on the previous studies, where tramadol was used epidurally in horses, cattle, goats, and donkeys at doses of 1 mg/kg [7–10].

In the current study, the onset time of analgesia was prolonged with tramadol alone, compared with tramadol-lidocaine combination and lidocaine alone. Similar findings have been reported previously in horses, cattle, goats, and donkeys [7–10]. Moreover, epidural tramadol alone or tramadol-lidocaine combination produced significantly longer duration of analgesia in buffalo calves compared with lidocaine alone. These results are in agreement with the

previous reports that assessed the use of tramadol with the local anesthetic agents. They concluded that the duration of analgesia was significantly extended following the administration of epidural tramadol without any side effects [7–10].

Vasoconstrictors (mainly epinephrine) were used to increase the depth or duration of local anesthetics for epidural block [17]. However, all the previous studies compared the analgesic effect of epidural tramadol with plain lidocaine without epinephrine [8–10]. Similarly, the current study compared tramadol with plain lidocaine. Further studies are required to compare epidural tramadol with lidocaine-epinephrine.

Tramadol is an opioid analgesic with central effects like codeine and morphine [6]. Mechanism of action by which tramadol induced analgesia could be its action on opioid receptors and through inhibition of the reuptake of norepinephrine and serotonin [6, 16]. Tramadol alone produced longer duration of analgesia than tramadol-lidocaine combination. The vasodilatation due to sympathetic nerve block produced by epidurally injected lidocaine decreased the duration of analgesia [18]. In the present study, also shortened duration of analgesia in the tramadol-lidocaine combination compared with tramadol alone may be related to the possibility of vasodilation due to presence of lidocaine and/or the half dose of tramadol used in this combination

[8, 10]. Further research is necessary to determine the effect of various doses of tramadol in epidural administration in buffalo calves.

Complete analgesia at the perineal region and tail base was recorded after all treatments plausibly due to higher concentrations of the drugs in the sacrococcygeal space (site of epidural injection of drugs). Mild to moderate degree of analgesia at upper hind limb was probably attributed to the decreased concentration of the drugs anteriorly. In this study, mild to moderate ataxia was observed in buffalo following epidural administration of lidocaine and tramadol-lidocaine combination, which is as expected due to the blocking effect of lidocaine on both the sensory and motor nerves [2], while no ataxia was observed after epidural tramadol administration. These results are similar to those previously reported in cattle and other species [7–9].

The HR, RR, and rectal temperature were not significantly different in comparison with baseline values throughout the study in all treatments. This is in agreement with previous results reported following extradural tramadol in combination with lidocaine in cattle [8].

The measurement of haematobiochemical parameters following epidural tramadol has not yet been estimated in the previous animal studies. In the present study, the decrease in hematological parameters including Hb, PCV%, RBCs, and TLC after epidural analgesia might be due to shifting of fluids from extravascular compartment to intravascular compartment to compensate normal cardiac output [19] and might be due to pooling of blood cells in the reservoir organs like spleen, secondary to decrease sympathetic activity [12]. The present finding is similar to previous findings after epidural xylazine combined with lignocaine in cow calves [20] and with our previous study after epidural lidocaine-neostigmine combination in buffalo calves [13]. A significant increase in glucose levels was observed from 30- to 120-minute time points after all treatments. But, at 24 hours, glucose levels returned to basal levels. The exact mechanism of hyperglycaemia induced after epidural tramadol, tramadol-lidocaine combination, and lidocaine was not investigated in the current study. Mirakhur et al. 1984 [14] suggested that hyperglycaemia may be due to a rise in adrenocortical hormones during stress. The increase in BUN levels in all animals after all treatments may be as a result of increased hepatic urea production from amino acid degradation as reported earlier [15]. Similar changes in BUN levels have also been reported after epidural lidocaine-neostigmine in buffalo calves [13]. A significant increase in ALP and ALT levels after all treatments might be related to some alterations in cell membrane permeability, which may permit these enzymes to leak from the cells with intact membranes [21]. As the values returned to baseline levels at 24 hours of observation, the possibility of pathological changes in the liver could therefore be ruled out. Similar findings were reported after xylazine, lignocaine, and their combination for lumbar epidural analgesia in water buffalo calves [15].

In conclusion, the results of this study suggested that the combination of tramadol-lidocaine produced good analgesia with relatively rapid onset compared with tramadol alone and a longer duration compared with lidocaine alone in the perineal area. This combination may be useful in clinical practice for longer duration of surgical and obstetrical procedures. However, further studies are required to determine the utility of this combination for surgical procedures before final recommendations can be made.

Conflict of Interests

The authors declare that there is no conflict of interests regarding the publication of this paper.

Acknowledgment

The authors are grateful to Professor Samy Darwish, the manager of Mahalet-Mosa Farm for Buffalo Production, for the donation of animals used in this study.

References

[1] R. G. Elmore, "Food animal regional anesthesia. Bovine blocks: epidural," *Veterinary Medicine, Small Animal Clinician*, vol. 75, pp. 1017–1029, 1980.

[2] T. K. Day and R. T. Skarda, "The pharmacology of local anesthetics," *The Veterinary Clinics of North America: Equine practice*, vol. 7, no. 3, pp. 489–500, 1991.

[3] R. T. Skarda and W. J. Tranquil, "Local and regional anesthetic and analgesic techniques: ruminants and swine," in *Lumb and Jones' Veterinary Anesthesia and Analgesia*, W. J. Tranquilli, J. C. Thurmon, and K. A. Grimm, Eds., pp. 643–675, Blackwell Publishing, Ames, Iowa, USA, 4th edition, 2007.

[4] M. Gunduz, M. Ozalevli, H. Ozbek, and D. Ozcengiz, "Comparison of caudal ketamine with lidocaine or tramadol administration for postoperative analgesia of hypospadias surgery in children," *Paediatric Anaesthesia*, vol. 16, no. 2, pp. 158–163, 2006.

[5] A. C. Senel, O. Ukinc, and A. Timurkaynak, "Does the addition of tramadol and ketamine to ropivacaine prolong the axillary brachial plexus block?" *BioMed Research International*, vol. 2014, Article ID 686287, 5 pages, 2014.

[6] R. B. Raffa, E. Friderichs, W. Reimann, R. P. Shank, E. E. Codd, and J. L. Vaught, "Opioid and nonopioid components independently contribute to the mechanism of action of tramadol, an 'atypical' opioid analgesic," *Journal of Pharmacology and Experimental Therapeutics*, vol. 260, no. 1, pp. 275–285, 1992.

[7] C. C. Natalini and E. P. Robinson, "Evaluation of the analgesic effects of epidurally administered morphine, alfentanil, butorphanol, tramadol, and U50488H in horses," *American Journal of Veterinary Research*, vol. 61, no. 12, pp. 1579–1586, 2000.

[8] A. S. Bigham, S. Habibian, F. Ghasemian, and S. Layeghi, "Caudal epidural injection of lidocaine, tramadol, and lidocaine-tramadol for epidural anesthesia in cattle," *Journal of Veterinary Pharmacology and Therapeutics*, vol. 33, no. 5, pp. 439–443, 2010.

[9] S. H. Dehkordi, A. Bigham-Sadegh, and R. Gerami, "Evaluation of anti-nociceptive effect of epidural tramadol, tramadol-lidocaine and lidocaine in goats," *Veterinary Anaesthesia and Analgesia*, vol. 39, no. 1, pp. 106–110, 2012.

[10] M. A. Marzok and S. A. El-Khodery, "Comparative analgesic and sedative effects of tramadol, tramadol-lidocaine and lidocaine for caudal epidural analgesia in donkeys (*Equus asinus*),"

Veterinary Anaesthesia and Analgesia, vol. 42, no. 2, pp. 215–219, 2015.

[11] T. L. Grubb, T. W. Riebold, R. O. Crisman, and L. D. Lamb, "Comparison of lidocaine, xylazine, and lidocaine-xylazine for caudal epidural analgesia in cattle," *Veterinary Anaesthesia and Analgesia*, vol. 29, no. 2, pp. 64–68, 2002.

[12] R. Sharda, G. K. Dutta, S. K. Tiwari, and N. Sharda, "Effect of xylazine, ketamine and their combination as epidural anaesthesia in buffalo calves," *Indian Veterinary Journal*, vol. 85, no. 6, pp. 608–610, 2008.

[13] A. Ghazy, A. Atiba, M. Shukry, and T. Kamal, "Comparison of Lidocaine and Lidocaine-Neostigmine for epidural analgesia in water buffalo calves (Bubalus Bubalis)," *Alexandria Journal of Veterinary Sciences*, vol. 46, no. 1, pp. 177–181, 2015.

[14] K. K. Mirakhur, V. K. Sobti, and J. M. Nigam, "Effect of thiopentone anaesthesia on plasma catecholamine and cortisol in buffalo calves (Bubalus bubalis)," *Indian Journal of Veterinary Surgery*, vol. 3, no. 2, pp. 86–88, 1984.

[15] P. Singh, K. Pratap, Amarpal, P. Kinjavdekar, H. P. Aithal, and G. R. Singh, "Effects of xylazine, lignocaine and their combination for lumber epidural analgesia in water buffalo calves (*Bubalus bubalis*)," *Journal of the South African Veterinary Association*, vol. 76, no. 3, pp. 151–158, 2005.

[16] Y. Majid and K. Mohammad, "A comparison of caudally administered single dose bupivacaine and bupivacaine-tramadol combination for postoperative analgesia in children," *JK Science*, vol. 6, no. 1, pp. 19–22, 2004.

[17] S. Ghadirian and N. Vesal, "Brachial plexus block using lidocaine/epinephrine or lidocaine/xylazine in fat-tailed sheep," *Veterinary Research Forum*, vol. 4, no. 3, pp. 161–167, 2013.

[18] I. A. Gómez de Segura, I. Vazquez, and E. De Miguel, "Antinociceptive and motor-blocking action of epidurally administered IQB-9302 and bupivacaine in the dog," *Regional Anesthesia and Pain Medicine*, vol. 25, no. 5, pp. 522–528, 2000.

[19] A. E. Wagner, W. W. Muir III, and K. W. Hinchcliff, "Cardiovascular effects of xylazine and detomidine in horses," *American Journal of Veterinary Research*, vol. 52, no. 5, pp. 651–659, 1991.

[20] B. A. Moulvi, J. D. Parrah, M. O. Kalim, H. Athar, and F. H. Dedmari, "Haemato-biochemical response to lignocaine alone or in combination with xylazine for epidural analgesia in cow calves," *Journal of Advanced Veterinary Research*, vol. 1, pp. 17–20, 2011.

[21] K. Koichev, D. Golemanov, H. Houbenov, and B. Aminkov, "Experimental study on the effect of "Domosedan" in sheep and cattle," *Veterinary Anaesthesia and Analgesia*, vol. 15, no. 1, pp. 114–126, 1988.

9

Molecular Detection, Phylogenetic Analysis, and Identification of Transcription Motifs in Feline Leukemia Virus from Naturally Infected Cats in Malaysia

Faruku Bande,[1,2] Siti Suri Arshad,[1] Latiffah Hassan,[3] and Zunita Zakaria[1]

[1] *Department of Veterinary Pathology and Microbiology, Faculty of Veterinary Medicine, Universiti Putra Malaysia, 43400 UPM Serdang, Selangor, Malaysia*

[2] *Department of Veterinary Services, Ministry of Animal Health and Fisheries Development, PMB 2109, Usman Faruk Secretariat, 840221 Sokoto, Sokoto State, Nigeria*

[3] *Department of Veterinary Laboratory Diagnostics, Faculty of Veterinary Medicine, Universiti Putra Malaysia, 43400 UPM Serdang, Selangor, Malaysia*

Correspondence should be addressed to Siti Suri Arshad; suri@upm.edu.my

Academic Editor: Philip H. Kass

A nested PCR assay was used to determine the viral RNA and proviral DNA status of naturally infected cats. Selected samples that were FeLV-positive by PCR were subjected to sequencing, phylogenetic analysis, and motifs search. Of the 39 samples that were positive for FeLV p27 antigen, 87.2% (34/39) were confirmed positive with nested PCR. FeLV proviral DNA was detected in 38 (97.3%) of p27-antigen negative samples. Malaysian FeLV isolates are found to be highly similar with a homology of 91% to 100%. Phylogenetic analysis revealed that Malaysian FeLV isolates divided into two clusters, with a majority (86.2%) sharing similarity with FeLV-K01803 and fewer isolates (13.8%) with FeLV-GM1 strain. Different enhancer motifs including NF-GMa, Krox-20/WT1I-del2, BAF1, AP-2, TBP, TFIIF-beta, TRF, and TFIID are found to occur either in single, duplicate, triplicate, or sets of 5 in different positions within the U3-LTR-gag region. The present result confirms the occurrence of FeLV viral RNA and provirus DNA in naturally infected cats. Malaysian FeLV isolates are highly similar, and a majority of them are closely related to a UK isolate. This study provides the first molecular based information on FeLV in Malaysia. Additionally, different enhancer motifs likely associated with FeLV related pathogenesis have been identified.

1. Introduction

Feline leukaemia virus (FeLV) is a gammaretrovirus associated with anaemia, immunodeficiency, leukaemia, and lymphoma in cats [1]. FeLV has been studied extensively as a model for human immunodeficiency virus (HIV) and human T-cell lymphoma virus (HTLV) infections [2]. FeLV is distributed worldwide; however, prevalence varies greatly with geography and with risk factors that include age, health status, and population density [3, 4]. A recent study reported FeLV seroprevalence of 5.1% and 18.9% in healthy and sick Malaysian cats, respectively [4]. On the other hand, studies carried out in other Asian regions reported 0% FeLV prevalence in Vietnam [5]; 14.7% among cats in Singapore [6]; 2.9%

in Japan [7]; and 6% each from Taiwan and Thailand [8, 9]. In non-Asian countries, FeLV prevalence has been reported to be 4.8% on Prince Edward Island, Canada [10]; 5.3% and 3.7% in Raleigh and Gainesville, USA, respectively [11]; 3.4% in all Canada [12]; and 4.6% in Egypt [13]. These discrepancies in prevalence of FeLV may arise due to differences in cat's lifestyle and FeLV vaccination practices in different countries [4].

Diagnosis of FeLV is usually performed by detection of p27 antigen [14]. However, demonstrating p27 antigen is difficult during early viraemia and with latent infections. Studies have shown that FeLV viral RNA and provirus DNA are better predictors of progressive and latent infections, respectively [15, 16].

Apart from the envelope gene of FeLV, the long terminal repeats (LTRs) play important role in determining disease outcome and in differentiating exogenous from endogenous FeLV [15, 17]. Vaccination against FeLV is not carried out in Malaysia and, to date, FeLV clinical status of Malaysian cats has not been investigated using molecular assays. Additionally, unlike the ubiquitous feline infectious peritonitis (FIP) [18] sequence and phylogenetic characteristics of the Malaysian FeLV isolates have not been elucidated. The objectives of this study are to evaluate the presence of FeLV viral RNA and provirus DNA in selected antigenaemic and nonantigenaemic cats, respectively. Sequence characteristics, enhancer motifs as well as phylogenetic relationships of the Malaysian FeLV also were determined.

2. Materials and Methods

2.1. Animals and Sampling. Heparinized blood samples were collected from cats presented at University Veterinary Teaching Hospital, Universiti Putra Malaysia (UVH-UPM). The samples were tested for the presence of FeLV p27 viral antigen using a commercially available test kit [4]. These cats were divided into p27 antigen positive and p27 antigen-negative groups. From each group, 39 cats were selected by convenience sampling method and the samples were subjected to PCR analysis. All cats had no history of vaccination against FeLV as vaccination against FeLV is not practiced in Malaysia. All samples were collected by the attending veterinary clinicians, as part of routine practices. In addition, consent for evaluation was obtained from the cat owners, prior to sampling.

2.2. Nucleic Acid and PCR Amplification. Viral RNA was extracted from the plasma of p27-positive cats, using high pure viral RNA purification kit (Roche, Germany). On the other hand, genomic DNA was isolated from whole blood of p27-negative cats, using QIAGEN DNA extraction kits (QIAGEN, Germany). All nucleic acid extraction procedures were carried out according to manufacturers' instructions. RNA was reverse transcribed and subjected to nested PCR, using a one-step access RT PCR (Promega, USA). Genomic DNA was amplified by nested PCR assay.

Two sets of primers (outer and inner primers) were synthesised (1st BASE, Malaysia) and used to amplify a 601 bp segment of FeLV-U3LTR and partial *gag* regions. This segment recognises exogenous but not endogenous FeLV segments presence in cat genome; thus the primers used in this study are specific for exogenous FeLV detection. Outer PCR reaction was carried out using U3-F(1) ($5'$-ACA GCA GAA GTT TCA AGG CC -$3'$) and G-R(1) ($5'$-GAC CAG TGA TCA AGG GTG AG-$3'$) primers. The inner PCR reaction was carried out with U3-F(2) ($5'$-GCT CCC CAG TTG ACC AGA GT-$3'$) and G-R(2) ($5'$-GCT TCG GTA CCA AAC CGA AA-$3'$) primers [15].

The PCR mixture was prepared in 25 μL reaction volume containing 10 mM each of dNTPs mix, 0.2 mM *Tfl* DNA polymerase (5 U/μL), 0.1 U AMV (5 U/μL), 0.1 U recombinant RNasin ribonuclease inhibitor (400 U/μL), 0.8 U MgSO$_4$

(25 mM), 20 pmol of each of the forward and reverse primer, 5.0 μL of 1 times buffer, and 1 μL RNA or DNA template. Nuclease-free water was used to bring the mixture to its final volume of 25 μL. AMV reverse transcriptase enzymes and RNasin ribonuclease inhibitor were included only when RNA was a starting template for the PCR assay. In the nested PCR step, 1 μL of outer PCR product was used as template.

In both inner and outer PCR steps, the target gene regions were amplified using the following conditions: reverse transcription: 45°C (45 min) (only in the case of RNA), initial denaturation: 94°C (2 min), denaturation: 94°C (45 sec), annealing: 58°C (30 sec), extension: 72°C (1 min), 35 cycles of repeats, and final extension: 72°C (7 min). PCR product was electrophoresed using 1.5% agarose (SeaKem LE USA), stained with 0.5 μg/mL ethidium bromide (Bio-Rad USA), and visualised under UV light (Geldoc system, Bio-Rad, USA). Extraction and amplification procedures were carried out in separate hood to reduce chances of contamination.

2.3. Sequence and Phylogenetic Analyses. In order to gain insight on the characteristics of Malaysian FeLV sequences, 29 nested PCR-positive samples (RNA *n* = 14; DNA provirus *n* = 15) were selected and purified using an Accuprep purification kit (Bioneer, Daejeon, Korea). Sequencing was carried out based on the amplified U3LTR-gag segment using a standard ABI Big Dye terminator version 3.1 sequence kit (Applied Biosystem). The obtained sequences were analysed for homology using the NCBI Basic Local Alignment Search Tool (BLAST: http://www.ncbi.nlm.nih.gov). In addition, multiple sequence alignment was carried out using ClustalW and the percentage nucleotide identity was determined using DNA identity matrix [19, 20]. On the other hand, single nucleotide polymorphism (SNP), DNA distance matrix, and transcription binding proteins prediction analyses were carried out using geneious software version R7 [20]. A neighbour-joining (NJ) phylogenetic tree was constructed based on the U3LTR-gag sequences using MEGA5 software. The tree reliability was assessed using 100 bootstrap replicates [21]. All nucleotide sequences were deposited with the NCBI GenBank (Table 1).

3. Results and Discussion

FeLV infection is of concern to cat owners due to its ability to induce tumours and immunodeficiency, thus predisposing cats to other secondary diseases. In this study, a U3-LTR and gag regions of exogenous without endogenous FeLV sequences were amplified by nested PCR methods. Post-PCR analysis using electrophoresis revealed an expected amplicon size of 770 bp in the outer PCR and 601 bp in the nested inner PCR assay (Figure 1). Overall, it was found that 97.4% (38/39) of p27 antigen-negative cats were positive for FeLV provirus DNA suggesting that this category of cats likely goes undetected when only p27 detection is used to judge their FeLV clinical status. Similar studies reported high prevalence of FeLV provirus DNA in Brazilian cats [22]. However, Hofmann-Lehmann et al. [23] reported a lower provirus DNA rate in cats in Switzerland. The observed differences

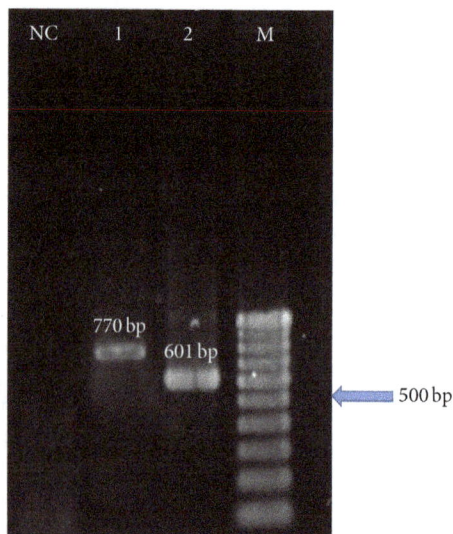

FIGURE 1: Nested RT-PCR assay used to detect FeLV U3LTR-gag sequence from naturally infected cats in Malaysia. The outer PCR reaction was performed using primer pair U3-F(1) and G-R(1) and amplified 770 bp (lane 1) whilst inner PCR reaction was performed using primer pair U3-F(2) and G-R(2) and amplified 601 bp (lane 2). Lane NC: negative control, lane M: 100 bp DNA marker (iDNA, Malaysia).

TABLE 1: List of local and reference sequences used in phylogenetic analysis of Malaysian FeLV isolates.

Isolate	Accession number	Country	Source
FeLV-UPM01	HQ197367	Malaysia	This study
FeLV-UPM02	HQ197368	Malaysia	This study
FeLV-UPM03	HQ197369	Malaysia	This study
FeLV-UPM04	HQ197370	Malaysia	This study
FeLV-UPM05	HQ197371	Malaysia	This study
FeLV-UPM06	HQ197372	Malaysia	This study
FeLV-UPM07	HQ197373	Malaysia	This study
FeLV-UPM08	HQ197374	Malaysia	This study
FeLV-UPM09	HQ197375	Malaysia	This study
FeLV-UPM10	HQ197376	Malaysia	This study
FeLV-UPM11	HQ197377	Malaysia	This study
FeLV-UPM12	HQ727890	Malaysia	This study
FeLV-UPM13	HQ727891	Malaysia	This study
FeLV-UPM14	HQ727892	Malaysia	This study
FeLV-UPM15	JF815538	Malaysia	This study
FeLV-UPM16	JF815539	Malaysia	This study
FeLV-UPM17	JF815540	Malaysia	This study
FeLV-UPM18	JF815541	Malaysia	This study
FeLV-UPM19	JF815542	Malaysia	This study
FeLV-UPM20	JF815543	Malaysia	This study
FeLV-UPM21	JF815544	Malaysia	This study
FeLV-UPM22	JF815545	Malaysia	This study
FeLV-UPM23	JF815546	Malaysia	This study
FeLV-UPM24	JF815547	Malaysia	This study
FeLV-UPM25	JF815548	Malaysia	This study
FeLV-UPM26	JF815549	Malaysia	This study
FeLV-UPM27	JF815550	Malaysia	This study
FeLV-UPM28	JF815551	Malaysia	This study
FeLV-UPM29	JF815552	Malaysia	This study
FeLV-914MG	EU048352	Brazil	GenBank
FeLV-1235MG	EU43664	Brazil	GenBank
FeLV-843MG	DQ821500	Brazil	GenBank
FeLV-887MG	DQ821501	Brazil	GenBank
FeLV-922MG	EU48356	Brazil	GenBank
FeLV-1286MG	EU090948	Brazil	GenBank
FeLV-328MG	AY745878	Brazil	GenBank
FeLV-Rickard	AF052723	USA	GenBank
FeLV-FAIDS	M18247	USA	GenBank
FeLV-GM1	D13922	UK	GenBank
FeLV-K01803	K01803	UK	GenBank
FeLV-TWK25	GQ465833	Taiwan	GenBank
FeLV-TW-K30	GQ327961	Taiwan	GenBank

Note: FeLV01–FeLV14 sequences were amplified from plasma viral RNA while the remaining local sequence (FeLVUPM13–FeLVUPM29) were amplified from proviral DNA.

in prevalence among different countries could be associated with cat lifestyle, as well as variations in factors known to favour FeLV transmission [3, 4]. Provirus DNA detection rate observed in this study could be associated with regressive or latent FeLV infection, which is characterized by integration of DNA provirus into the host cell genome and absence of viral antigen in circulation [1, 15].

The consequence of latent FeLV infection is that provirus DNA could reactivate to an infectious state, especially following stress and/or immunosuppression. Thus, cats that are p27 antigen-negative, but provirus DNA positive, could serve as sources of infection of FeLV-naïve cats [24]. A previous study has established an association between feline lymphoma and provirus DNA positivity in p27 antigen-negative cats, though this has not been evaluated in the present study [25]. Moreover, transmission of FeLV has been shown to occur in cats following blood transfusion from cats with provirus DNA, thus highlighting the importance of screening blood donor cats for provirus DNA [26].

Viral RNA was detected in 87.2% (34/39) of p27 antigen-positive cats whereas 13% (5/39) tested negative using RT-PCR assay. Since plasma viral RNA is an indicator of FeLV viraemia, cats that are positive for FeLV p27 antigen and viral RNA are likely to harbour replicating virus [27]. Cats in this category may progress to a persistent viraemic stage, succumbing to FeLV-associated illness [28].

Failure to detect FeLV viral RNA in about 13% p27 antigen-positive cats (p27-positive/viral RNA-negative) could result from atypical infection, wherein the virus is sequestered and replicates locally in tissues such as salivary gland, mammary gland, and urinary epithelium, causing intermittent or low-grade antigenaemia, although there is no detectable viraemia [28, 29]. Our findings are consistent with the results of an earlier study that failed to isolate FeLV from about 10% of p27 antigen-positive cats, irrespective of the antigen detection methods used. Such cats were considered as

TABLE 2: Predicted transcription binding motifs found within the LTR-gag sequence of Malaysian FeLV isolates.

Motifs	Sequence	Seq length	Coverage	Occurrence in local sequence	Occurrence in reference FeLV
NF-GMa	GAGGTTTCAT	10	523–532	All local seq except UPM08	FeLV-Rickard; FeLV-FAIDs
E1A-F	CGGATGT	7	521–527	UPM08	NA
E1A-F	CGGATGT	7	70–76	UPM18	NA
ELP	CAAGGTC	7	523–527	UPM03, 14, 18, 20	NA
Sp1	GGGGCTAGG	7	521–527	UPM03, 18, 20	NA
C\EBPbeta	CTGGAAA	7	387–393	UPM18, 20	NA
Krox-20/WT1I-del2	CGCCCCCGC	9	374–382	All local seq	FeLV-Rickard; FeLV-FAIDs
E2F	TTTTGGCGG	9	334–342	UPM03, 14, 18, 20	FeLV-Rickard; FeLV-FAIDs
BAF1	TCCTTGTATACG	12	301–312	All except UPM03, 14, 18, 20	NA
BAF1	TCCTTGTATACG	12	158–169	All local seq	NA
AP-2	CCCAACCG	8	243–250	All local seq	FeLV-Rickard; FeLV-FAIDs
AP-2	CCCAACCG	8	59–66	All local seq except UPM17	FeLV-Rickard; FeLV-FAIDs
AP-2	CCCAACCG	8	58–65	UPM03, 14, 18, 20, 25	NA
AP-2	CCCAACCG	8	4 to 11	All except UPM03, 14	NA
AP-2	CCCAACCG	8	3 to11	All local seq	FeLV-Rickard
GCF	CCGCCCC	7	93–99	All local seq	FeLV-Rickard, FeLV-FAIDs
GCF	CCGGCGC	7	64–70	All local seq except UPM03, UPM 14	NA
GCF	GCGCGCC	7	26–32	UPM27	NA
HNF-3	TGTTTGC	7	129–135	All local seq except UPM06	NA
PEA3	GCGGAAGT	8	69–76	UPM18	NA
TBP	TATAAAA	7	39–45	All local seq	FeLV-Rickard, FeLV-FAIDs
TFIIF-beta	TATAAAA	7	39–45	All local seq	FeLV-Rickard, FeLV-FAIDs
TRF	TATAAAA	7	39–45	All local seq	FeLV-Rickard, FeLV-FAIDs
TFIID	TATAAAA	7	39–45	All local seq	FeLV-Rickard, FeLV-FAIDs
TFIID	CTTCTCGC	8	10 to 17	UPM03, 14, 20	NA
MEP-1	TATAAAA	7	23–29	All local seq except UPM03, 14, 18, 20	FeLV-Rickard
MBF-I	TATAAAA	7	23–29	All local seq except UPM03, 14, 18, 21	FeLV-Rickard
MTF-1	TATAAAA	7	23–29	All except UPM03, 14, 18, 22	FeLV-Rickard

NA: not applicable or not present; seq: sequences.

"discordant," suggesting that p27 antigen-positive status may not always correlate with viraemia [30]. Another potential explanation for p27-positive-RNA-negative status might be false positive antigen or false negative RNA tests that arise occasionally because of low positive predictive value of p27 antigen tests in regions with low FeLV prevalence [31]. Clinical relevance of atypical FeLV infection is not well-understood, and it has been recommended to monitor the status of discordant cats over time [27, 28]. No additional follow-up was carried out in the present study, because most owners were not willing to subject cats to repeated venepunctures [4].

Based on the U3LTR and partial *gag* regions, nucleotide sequence analyses revealed homology of 91–100% among Malaysian FeLV isolates. However, homology decreased to 84.6% when local isolates were compared with reference isolates. Previous studies reported strong sequence conservation (>97%) among FeLV isolates of different geographic and temporal clusters [32, 33]. In agreement with Jackson et al. [17], we do observe point mutations and nucleotide deletion in Malaysian FeLV isolates (see Supplementary Material available online at http://dx.doi.org/10.1155/2014/760961).While U3LTR is conserved in FeLV, field isolates have been reported to exhibit sequence variation within the terminally repeated LTRs regions [17, 33]. Mutational changes in the LTR regions have been implicated with enhanced transcriptional and/or insertion activities of FeLV, thus supporting T-cell lymphomagenesis [34, 35].

In this study, several transcription binding motifs were predicted within the amplified U3LTR-gag region (Table 2). Of these, NF-GMa, Krox-20/WT1I-del2, BAF1, AP-2, TBP, TFIIF-beta, TRF, and TFIID motifs were found to be conserved between local FeLV isolates and the two characterized FeLV-Rickard subgroup A and FeLV-FAIDS reference

TABLE 3: Distance matrix showing sequence relationship among local FeLV isolates.

(a)

	FeLV-Rickard [AF052723]	FeLV-FAIDS [MI8247]	FeLV-UPM03 [HQ197369]	FeLV-UPM18 [JF815541]	FeLV-UPM20 [JF815543]	FeLV-UPM29 [JF815552]	FeLV-UPM28 [JF815551]	FeLV-UPM12 [HQ727890]	FeLV-UPM06 [HQ197372]
FeLV-Rickard [AF052723]		98.12	94.925	93.609	93.797	96.805	96.805	96.992	96.617
FeLV-FAIDS [MI8247]	98.12		95.301	93.985	94.173	96.429	96.429	96.617	96.617
FeLV-UPM03 [HQ197369]	94.925	95.301		96.429	98.496	94.737	94.737	94.925	94.549
FeLV-UPM18 [JF815541]	93.609	93.985	96.429		96.053	93.797	93.797	93.985	93.609
FeLV-UPM20 [JF815543]	93.797	94.173	98.496	96.053		93.609	93.609	93.797	93.421
FeLV-UPM29 [JF815552]	96.805	96.429	94.737	93.797	93.609		100	99.812	99.436
FeLV-UPM28 [JF815551]	96.805	96.429	94.737	93.797	93.609	100		99.812	99.436
FeLV-UPM12 [HQ727890]	96.992	96.617	94.925	93.985	93.797	99.812	99.812		99.624
FeLV-UPM06 [HQ197372]	96.617	96.617	94.549	93.609	93.421	99.436	99.436	99.624	
FeLV-UPM23 [JF815546]	96.805	96.429	94.737	93.797	93.609	99.248	99.248	99.436	99.06
FeLV-UPM21 [JF815544]	96.805	96.429	94.737	93.797	93.609	99.248	99.248	99.436	99.06
FeLV-UPM24 [JF815547]	96.805	96.429	94.737	93.797	93.609	99.248	99.248	99.436	99.06
FeLV-UPM26 [JF815549]	96.805	96.429	94.737	93.797	93.609	99.248	99.248	99.436	99.06
FeLV-UPM09 [HQ197375]	96.805	96.429	94.737	93.797	93.609	99.248	99.248	99.436	99.06
FeLV-UPM17 [JF815540]	96.617	96.241	94.549	93.609	93.421	99.06	99.06	99.248	98.872
FeLV-UPM16 [JF815539]	96.617	96.241	94.549	93.609	93.421	99.06	99.06	99.248	98.872
FeLV-UPM25 [JF815548]	96.429	96.053	94.549	93.797	93.421	98.872	98.872	99.06	98.684
FeLV-UPM19 [JF815542]	95.865	95.489	93.797	92.857	92.669	98.308	98.308	98.496	98.12
FeLV-UPM27 [JF815550]	96.617	95.865	94.173	93.233	93.045	98.684	98.684	98.872	98.496
FeLV-UPM22 [JF815545]	96.617	96.053	94.361	93.421	93.233	98.872	98.872	99.06	98.684
FeLV-UPM10 [HQ197376]	96.429	96.053	94.361	93.421	93.233	99.248	99.248	99.436	99.06
FeLV-UPM15 [JF815538]	96.992	96.617	94.925	93.985	93.797	99.436	99.436	99.624	99.248
FeLV-UPM11 [HQ197377]	96.992	96.617	94.925	93.985	93.797	99.436	99.436	99.624	99.248
FeLV-UPM13 [HQ727891]	96.805	96.429	94.737	93.797	93.609	99.624	99.624	99.812	99.436
FeLV-UPM05 [HQ197371]	96.429	96.053	94.361	93.421	93.233	99.248	99.248	99.436	99.06
FeLV-UPM07 [HQ197373]	96.805	96.429	94.737	93.797	93.609	99.624	99.624	99.812	99.436
FeLV-UPM02 [HQ197368]	96.805	96.429	94.737	93.797	93.609	99.624	99.624	99.812	99.436
FeLV-UPM01 [HQ197367]	96.805	96.429	94.737	93.797	93.609	99.624	99.624	99.812	99.436
FeLV-UPM04 [HQ197370]	96.617	96.241	94.549	93.609	93.421	99.06	99.06	99.248	98.872
FeLV-UPM08 [HQ197374]	94.737	93.985	92.669	91.729	91.541	97.18	97.18	97.368	96.992
FeLV-UPM14 [HQ727892]	95.865	96.241	99.06	96.992	97.932	95.677	95.677	95.865	95.489

(b)

	FeLV-UPM23 [JF815546]	FeLV-UPM21 [JF815544]	FeLV-UPM24 [JF815547]	FeLV-UPM26 [JF815549]	FeLV-UPM09 [HQ197375]	FeLV-UPM17 [JF815540]	FeLV-UPM16 [JF815539]	FeLV-UPM25 [JF815548]	FeLV-UPM19 [JF815542]	FeLV-UPM27 [JF815550]
FeLV-Rickard [AF052723]	96.805	96.805	96.805	96.805	96.805	96.617	96.617	96.429	95.865	96.617
FeLV-FAIDS [M18247]	96.429	96.429	96.429	96.429	96.429	96.241	96.241	96.053	95.489	95.865
FeLV-UPM03 [HQ197369]	94.737	94.737	94.737	94.737	94.737	94.549	94.549	94.549	93.797	94.173
FeLV-UPM18 [JF815541]	93.797	93.797	93.797	93.797	93.797	93.609	93.609	93.797	92.857	93.233
FeLV-UPM20 [JF815543]	93.609	93.609	93.609	93.609	93.609	93.421	93.421	93.421	92.669	93.045
FeLV-UPM29 [JF815552]	99.248	99.248	99.248	99.248	99.248	99.06	99.06	98.872	98.308	98.684
FeLV-UPM28 [JF815551]	99.248	99.248	99.248	99.248	99.248	99.06	99.06	98.872	98.308	98.684
FeLV-UPM12 [HQ727890]	99.436	99.436	99.436	99.436	99.436	99.248	99.248	99.06	98.496	98.872
FeLV-UPM06 [HQ197372]	99.06	99.06	99.06	99.06	99.06	98.872	98.872	98.684	98.12	98.496
FeLV-UPM23 [JF815546]		100	100	100	100	99.812	99.812	99.624	99.06	99.436
FeLV-UPM21 [JF815544]	100		100	100	100	99.812	99.812	99.624	99.06	99.436
FeLV-UPM24 [JF815547]	100	100		100	100	99.812	99.812	99.624	99.06	99.436
FeLV-UPM26 [JF815549]	100	100	100		100	99.812	99.812	99.624	99.06	99.436
FeLV-UPM09 [HQ197375]	100	100	100	100		99.812	99.812	99.624	99.06	99.436
FeLV-UPM17 [JF815540]	99.812	99.812	99.812	99.812	99.812		99.624	99.436	98.872	99.248
FeLV-UPM16 [JF815539]	99.812	99.812	99.812	99.812	99.812	99.624		99.436	98.872	99.248
FeLV-UPM25 [JF815548]	99.624	99.624	99.624	99.624	99.624	99.436	99.436		98.684	99.06
FeLV-UPM19 [JF815542]	99.06	99.06	99.06	99.06	99.06	98.872	98.872	98.684		98.496
FeLV-UPM27 [JF815550]	99.436	99.436	99.436	99.436	99.436	99.248	99.248	99.06	98.496	
FeLV-UPM22 [JF815545]	99.624	99.624	99.624	99.624	99.624	99.436	99.436	99.248	98.684	99.248
FeLV-UPM10 [HQ197376]	99.624	99.624	99.624	99.624	99.624	99.436	99.436	99.248	98.684	99.06
FeLV-UPM15 [JF815538]	99.812	99.812	99.812	99.812	99.812	99.624	99.624	99.436	98.872	99.248
FeLV-UPM11 [HQ197377]	99.812	99.812	99.812	99.812	99.812	99.624	99.624	99.436	98.872	99.248
FeLV-UPM13 [HQ727891]	99.624	99.624	99.624	99.624	99.624	99.436	99.436	99.248	98.684	99.06
FeLV-UPM05 [HQ197371]	99.248	99.248	99.248	99.248	99.248	99.06	99.06	98.872	98.308	98.684
FeLV-UPM07 [HQ197373]	99.624	99.624	99.624	99.624	99.624	99.436	99.436	99.248	98.684	99.06
FeLV-UPM02 [HQ197368]	99.624	99.624	99.624	99.624	99.624	99.436	99.436	99.248	98.684	99.06
FeLV-UPM01 [HQ197367]	99.624	99.624	99.624	99.624	99.624	99.436	99.436	99.248	98.684	99.06
FeLV-UPM04 [HQ197370]	99.06	99.06	99.06	99.06	99.06	98.872	98.872	98.684	98.12	98.496
FeLV-UPM08 [HQ197374]	96.805	96.805	96.805	96.805	96.805	96.617	96.617	96.429	96.053	96.617
FeLV-UPM14 [HQ727892]	95.677	95.677	95.677	95.677	95.677	95.489	95.489	95.489	94.737	95.113

(c)

	FeLV-UPM22 [JF815545]	FeLV-UPM10 [HQ197376]	FeLV-UPM15 [JF815538]	FeLV-UPM11 [HQ197377]	FeLV-UPM13 [HQ727891]	FeLV-UPM05 [HQ197371]	FeLV-UPM07 [HQ197373]	FeLV-UPM02 [HQ197368]	FeLV-UPM01 [HQ197367]	FeLV-UPM04 [HQ197370]	FeLV-UPM08 [HQ197374]	FeLV-UPM14 [HQ727892]
FeLV-Rickard [AF052723]	96.617	96.429	96.992	96.992	96.805	96.429	96.805	96.805	96.805	96.617	94.737	95.865
FeLV-FAIDS [M18247]	96.053	96.053	96.617	96.617	96.429	96.053	96.429	96.429	96.429	96.241	93.985	96.241
FeLV-UPM03 [HQ197369]	94.361	94.361	94.925	94.925	94.737	94.361	94.737	94.737	94.737	94.549	92.669	99.06
FeLV-UPM18 [JF815541]	93.421	93.421	93.985	93.985	93.797	93.421	93.797	93.797	93.797	93.609	91.729	96.992
FeLV-UPM20 [JF815543]	93.233	93.233	93.797	93.797	93.609	93.233	93.609	93.609	93.609	93.421	91.541	97.932
FeLV-UPM29 [JF815552]	98.872	99.248	99.436	99.436	99.624	99.248	99.624	99.624	99.624	99.06	97.18	95.677
FeLV-UPM28 [JF815551]	98.872	99.248	99.436	99.436	99.624	99.248	99.624	99.624	99.624	99.06	97.18	95.677
FeLV-UPM12 [HQ727890]	99.06	99.436	99.624	99.624	99.812	99.436	99.812	99.812	99.812	99.248	97.368	95.865
FeLV-UPM06 [HQ197372]	98.684	99.06	99.248	99.248	99.436	99.06	99.436	99.436	99.436	98.872	96.992	95.489
FeLV-UPM23 [JF815546]	99.624	99.624	99.812	99.812	99.624	99.248	99.624	99.624	99.624	99.06	96.805	95.677
FeLV-UPM21 [JF815544]	99.624	99.624	99.812	99.812	99.624	99.248	99.624	99.624	99.624	99.06	96.805	95.677
FeLV-UPM24 [JF815547]	99.624	99.624	99.812	99.812	99.624	99.248	99.624	99.624	99.624	99.06	96.805	95.677
FeLV-UPM26 [JF815549]	99.624	99.624	99.812	99.812	99.624	99.248	99.624	99.624	99.624	99.06	96.805	95.677
FeLV-UPM09 [HQ197375]	99.624	99.624	99.812	99.812	99.624	99.248	99.624	99.624	99.624	99.06	96.805	95.677
FeLV-UPM17 [JF815540]	99.436	99.436	99.624	99.624	99.436	99.06	99.436	99.436	99.436	98.872	96.617	95.489
FeLV-UPM16 [JF815539]	99.436	99.436	99.624	99.624	99.436	99.06	99.436	99.436	99.436	98.872	96.617	95.489
FeLV-UPM25 [JF815548]	99.248	99.248	99.436	99.436	99.248	98.872	99.248	99.248	99.248	98.684	96.429	95.489
FeLV-UPM19 [JF815542]	98.684	98.684	98.872	98.872	98.684	98.308	98.684	98.684	98.684	98.12	96.053	94.737
FeLV-UPM27 [JF815550]	99.248	99.06	99.248	99.248	99.06	98.684	99.06	99.06	99.06	98.496	96.617	95.113
FeLV-UPM22 [JF815545]		99.248	99.436	99.436	99.248	98.872	99.248	99.248	99.248	98.684	96.617	95.301
FeLV-UPM10 [HQ197376]	99.248		99.436	99.436	99.436	99.248	99.624	99.624	99.624	99.06	97.18	95.301
FeLV-UPM15 [JF815538]	99.436	99.436		100	99.812	99.436	99.812	99.812	99.812	99.248	96.992	95.865
FeLV-UPM11 [HQ197377]	99.436	99.436	100		99.812	99.436	99.812	99.812	99.812	99.248	96.992	95.865
FeLV-UPM13 [HQ727891]	99.248	99.624	99.812	99.812		99.624	100	99.624	100	99.436	97.18	95.677
FeLV-UPM05 [HQ197371]	98.872	99.248	99.436	99.436	99.624		99.624	99.624	99.624	99.06	96.805	95.301
FeLV-UPM07 [HQ197373]	99.248	99.624	99.812	99.812	100	99.624		100	100	99.436	97.18	95.677
FeLV-UPM02 [HQ197368]	99.248	99.624	99.812	99.812	100	99.624	100		100	99.436	97.18	95.677
FeLV-UPM01 [HQ197367]	99.248	99.624	99.812	99.812	100	99.624	100	100		99.436	97.18	95.677
FeLV-UPM04 [HQ197370]	98.684	99.06	99.248	99.248	99.436	99.06	99.436	99.436	99.436		96.617	95.489
FeLV-UPM08 [HQ197374]	96.617	97.18	96.992	96.992	97.18	96.805	97.18	97.18	97.18	96.617		93.609
FeLV-UPM14 [HQ727892]	95.301	95.301	95.865	95.865	95.677	95.301	95.677	95.677	95.677	95.489	93.609	

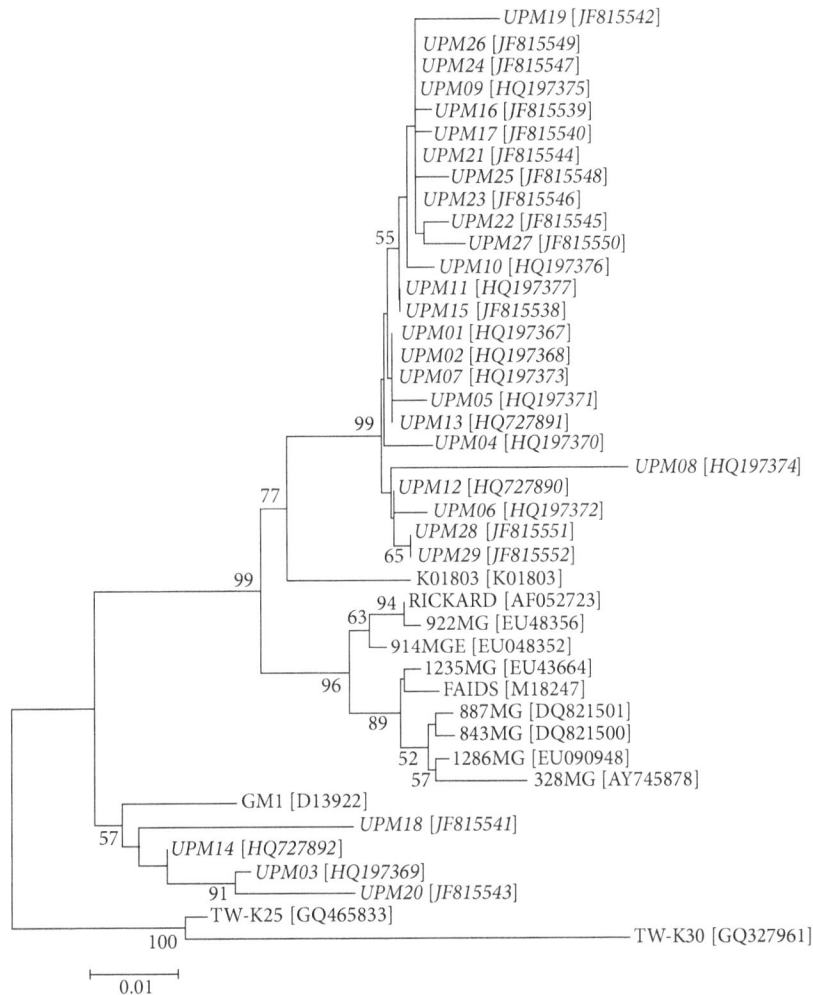

FIGURE 2: Neighbour-joining phylogenetic relationship of Malaysian FeLV isolates. The percentage of replicate trees in which the associated taxa clustered together in the bootstrap test (100 replicates) is shown next to the branches. Malaysian FeLV isolates are indicated in italic. Evolutionary analyses were conducted in MEGA5.

isolates. On the other hand, E1A-F, ELP, Sp1, C\EBPbeta, BAF1, GCF, HNF-3, and PEA3 motifs are found in some local isolates but were absent in reference sequences. These motifs may have implication for viral oncogenicity or probably favours viral replication. For example, an Sp1 enhancer, a member of Sp/Kruppel-like factor, was reported to activate gene transcription and contribute to abnormal metabolism of cancer cells [36, 37] whereas C\EBPbeta regulates the growth and differentiation of myeloid as well as lymphoid cells [38]. Studies have shown that, the U3-LTR sequence contains multiple transcription binding sites that aid viral replication and pathogenesis. Interactions of different transcription binding factors, via the U3-LTRs, may contribute to cellular gene transactivation and viral leukemogenesis [39, 40]. Enhancer motifs observed in this study appeared in multiple locations such as in the case of E1A-F, BAF1, and TFIID, each occurring in duplicate; GCF appeared in triplicate while AP-2 is repeated 5 times at different positions. An enhancer duplication and triplication has been reported in naturally occurring cases of FeLV-induced T-cell lymphomas

[41, 42]. The clinical relevance of multiple enhancers in cats used in the present study is not determined, although some FeLV positive cats had evidence of different tumour forms at post-mortem (result not shown). Previous studies reported that E1A-F, a member *ets*-oncogene family transcription factor, upregulates the multiple matrix metalloproteinase (MMP) genes thus contributing to the malignant phenotypic activity by increasing the invasion and metastatic activities of cancerous cells [43]. TFIID, a potential protooncogene with TATA-box protein and a TBP-associated factor also plays role in transcription initiation and genome expression [44]. On the other hand, AP2 and SP1 are known to activate epidermal growth factor receptor (EGFR) gene. In addition, overexpression of these gene has been reported to cause cellular transformation [45, 46]. Surprisingly we also identified a triplicate of GCF binding factor that has suppressor effect on EGR gene; these discrepancies, however, need further elucidation with quantitative real-time PCR [47].

Absence of length mutation (nucleotide position 473–481) in Malaysian FeLV isolates, as observed in FeLV isolates from Taiwan (FeLV-TW-25 and FeLV-TW-30) and a European isolate (FeLV-GM1), might suggest limited influence of geography in evolutionary patterns of FeLV, unlike its lentiviral counterpart, feline immunodeficiency virus [33, 48].

Phylogenetic analysis based on the U3LTR-gag sequence revealed that Malaysian FeLV isolates are closely related (Tables 3(a), 3(b), and 3(c)) but when compared with reference isolates, separated into two distinct clusters, with the majority (86.2%) being closely related to FeLV-K01803 isolate from UK. The remaining local FeLV isolates (13.8%) clustered with FeLV-GM1 (Figure 2). The reason for the observed similarity between local FeLV isolates and European isolates, but not with Taiwanese isolates, may suggest the lack of geographical influence, this should be explored further. It is possible also that FeLV might have been introduced into Malaysia as a result of translocation of domestic pets from Europe. Due to a somewhat conserved nature of the U3LTR region, conclusion about the FeLV subgroup requires further investigations of FeLV envelope protein gene.

4. Conclusion

This study revealed the occurrence of FeLV viral RNA and provirus DNA among naturally infected Malaysian cats. Based on the U3LTR-gag sequence, Malaysian FeLV isolates are highly conserved and more closely related to K01803 isolate from UK compared to Taiwanese and other reference isolates. Presence of multiple enhancers some of which have been linked with FeLV induced tumours may contribute to the development of poor prognostic outcome in naturally infected Malaysian cats although this needs further investigation. Overall, this is the first molecular study for evidence of FeLV in Malaysia. We also identified several motifs that have potential implications in FeLV-induced leukemogenesis. Future studies need to explore association between FeLV positive status and occurrence of feline tumour in Malaysian cats. The present findings is useful in designing molecular diagnostics for clinical applications and for improved understanding of FeLV infection outcome and epidemiology.

Conflict of Interests

The authors declare that there is no conflict of interests regarding the publication of this paper.

Acknowledgments

The authors thank cat owners and clinicians for their support, Dr. Dennis F. Lawler for proof reading the paper, and Saeid Kadkhodaei for assistance in sequence analysis. This project was funded by Science Fund, Ministry of Science and Technology and Innovation, Project no. 02-01-04-SF1070.

References

[1] J. L. Rojko, E. A. Hoover, L. E. Mathes, R. G. Olsen, and J. P. Schaller, "Pathogenesis of experimental feline leukemia virus infection," *Journal of the National Cancer Institute*, vol. 63, no. 3, pp. 759–768, 1979.

[2] O. Jarrett, "The relevance of feline retroviruses to the development of vaccines against HIV," *AIDS Research and Human Retroviruses*, vol. 12, no. 5, pp. 385–387, 1996.

[3] S. E. Gleich, S. Krieger, and K. Hartmann, "Prevalence of feline immunodeficiency virus and feline leukaemia virus among client-owned cats and risk factors for infection in Germany," *Journal of Feline Medicine and Surgery*, vol. 11, no. 12, pp. 985–992, 2009.

[4] F. Bande, S. S. Arshad, L. Hassan et al., "Prevalence and risk factors of feline leukaemia virus and feline immunodeficiency virus in peninsular Malaysia," *BMC Veterinary Research*, vol. 8, article 33, 2012.

[5] T. Miyazawa, Y. Ikeda, K. Maeda et al., "Seroepidemiological survey of feline retrovirus infections in domestic and leopard cats in Northern Vietnam in 1997," *Journal of Veterinary Medical Science*, vol. 60, no. 11, pp. 1273–1275, 1998.

[6] M. Chew-Lim, N. Fong, and S. Y. Chong, "A survey of the feline leukaemia virus in Singapore," *Annals of the Academy of Medicine Singapore*, vol. 18, no. 6, pp. 646–648, 1989.

[7] S. Maruyama, H. Kabeya, R. Nakao et al., "Seroprevalence of Bartonella henselae, toxoplasma gondii, FIV and FeLV infections in domestic cats in Japan," *Microbiology and Immunology*, vol. 47, no. 2, pp. 147–153, 2003.

[8] A. Litster and P. Nilkumhang, "Prevalence of feline leukaemia virus and feline immunodeficiency virus infection in Thailand," in *Proceedings of the 28th Congress of World Small Animal Association*, Bangkok, Thailand, 2003.

[9] J. A. Lin, M. C. Cheng, Y. Inoshima et al., "Seroepidemiological survey of feline retrovirus infections in cats in Taiwan in 1993 and 1994," *The Journal of Veterinary Medical Science*, vol. 57, no. 1, pp. 161–163, 1995.

[10] K. L. Gibson, K. Keizer, and C. Golding, "A trap, neuter, and release program for feral cats on Prince Edward Island," *Canadian Veterinary Journal*, vol. 43, no. 9, pp. 695–698, 2002.

[11] I. T. Lee, J. K. Levy, S. P. Gorman, P. C. Crawford, and M. R. Slater, "Prevalence of feline leukemia virus infection and serum antibodies against feline immunodeficiency virus in unowned free-roaming cats," *Journal of the American Veterinary Medical Association*, vol. 220, no. 5, pp. 620–622, 2002.

[12] S. Little, W. Sears, J. Lachtara, and D. Bienzle, "Seroprevalence of feline leukemia virus and feline immunodeficiency virus infection among cats in Canada," *Canadian Veterinary Journal*, vol. 50, no. 6, pp. 644–648, 2009.

[13] Y. M. Al-Kappany, M. R. Lappin, O. C. H. Kwok, S. A. Abu-Elwafa, M. Hilali, and J. P. Dubey, "Seroprevalence of *Toxoplasma gondii* and concurrent *Bartonella* spp., Feline immunodeficiency virus, feline leukemia virus, and *Dirofilaria immitis* infections in egyptian cats," *Journal of Parasitology*, vol. 97, no. 2, pp. 256–258, 2011.

[14] K. Hartmann, P. Griessmayr, B. Schulz et al., "Quality of different in-clinic test systems for feline immunodeficiency virus and feline leukaemia virus infection," *Journal of Feline Medicine and Surgery*, vol. 9, no. 6, pp. 439–445, 2007.

[15] T. Miyazawa and O. Jarrett, "Feline leukaemia virus proviral DNA detected by polymerase chain reaction in antigenaemic but non-viraemic ("discordant") cats," *Archives of Virology*, vol. 142, no. 2, pp. 323–332, 1997.

[16] V. Cattori and R. Hofmann-Lehmann, "Absolute quantitation of feline leukemia virus proviral DNA and viral RNA loads by

TaqMan real-time PCR and RT-PCR," in *Anonymous Molecular Beacons: Signalling Nucleic Acid Probes, Methods, and Protocols*, p. 73, 2008.

[17] M. L. Jackson, D. M. Haines, and V. Misra, "Sequence analysis of the putative viral enhancer in tissues from 33 cats with various feline leukemia virus-related diseases," *Veterinary Microbiology*, vol. 53, no. 3-4, pp. 213–225, 1996.

[18] A. Amer, A. Siti Suri, O. Abdul Rahman et al., "Isolation and molecular characterization of type I and type II feline coronavirus in Malaysia," *Virology Journal*, vol. 9, article 278, 2012.

[19] T. A. Hall, "BioEdit: a user-friendly biological sequence alignment editor and analysis program for windows 95/98/NT," *Nucleic Acids Symposium*, vol. 41, pp. 95–98, 1999.

[20] M. Kearse, R. Moir, A. Wilson et al., "Geneious Basic: an integrated and extendable desktop software platform for the organization and analysis of sequence data," *Bioinformatics*, vol. 28, no. 12, pp. 1647–1649, 2012.

[21] J. Felsenstein, "Confidence limits on phylogenies: an approach using the bootstrap," *Evolution*, vol. 39, no. 4, pp. 783–791, 1985.

[22] F. M. Coelho, M. R. Q. Bomfim, F. D. A. Caxito et al., "Naturally occurring feline leukemia virus subgroup A and B infections in urban domestic cats," *Journal of General Virology*, vol. 89, no. 11, pp. 2799–2805, 2008.

[23] R. Hofmann-Lehmann, J. B. Huder, F. Boretti, B. Sigrist, and H. Lutz, "Feline leukaemia provirus load during the course of experimental infection and in naturally infected cats," *Journal of General Virology*, vol. 82, no. 7, pp. 1589–1596, 2001.

[24] B. R. Madewell and O. Jarrett, "Recovery of feline leukaemia virus from non-viraemic cats," *Veterinary Record*, vol. 112, no. 15, pp. 339–342, 1983.

[25] L. J. Gabor, M. L. Jackson, B. Trask, R. Malik, and P. J. Canfield, "Feline leukaemia virus status of Australian cats with lymphosarcoma," *Australian Veterinary Journal*, vol. 79, no. 7, pp. 476–481, 2001.

[26] S. Nesina, A. K. Helfer-Hungerbuehler, F. Boretti et al., "Transmission of FeLV infection by provirus positive blood," in *Proceedings of the 11th International Feline Retrovirus Research Symposium Anonymous*, Leipzig, Germany, August 2012.

[27] H. Lutz, D. Addie, S. Belák et al., "Feline leukaemia ABCD guidelines on prevention and management," *Journal of Feline Medicine and Surgery*, vol. 11, no. 7, pp. 565–574, 2009.

[28] E. A. Hoover and J. I. Mullins, "Feline leukemia virus infection and diseases," *Journal of the American Veterinary Medical Association*, vol. 199, no. 10, pp. 1287–1297, 1991.

[29] K. A. Hayes, J. L. Rojko, and L. E. Mathes, "Incidence of localized feline leukemia virus infection in cats," *The American Journal of Veterinary Research*, vol. 53, no. 4, pp. 604–607, 1992.

[30] O. Jarrett, M. C. Golder, and K. Weijer, "A comparison of three methods of feline leukaemia virus diagnosis," *Veterinary Record*, vol. 110, no. 14, pp. 325–328, 1982.

[31] J. A. Beatty, S. Tasker, O. Jarrett et al., "Markers of feline leukaemia virus infection or exposure in cats from a region of low seroprevalence," *Journal of Feline Medicine and Surgery*, vol. 13, no. 12, pp. 927–933, 2011.

[32] P. R. Donahue, E. A. Hoover, G. A. Beltz et al., "Strong sequence conservation among horizontally transmissible, minimally pathogenic feline leukemia viruses," *Journal of Virology*, vol. 62, no. 3, pp. 722–731, 1988.

[33] C. Chandhasin, P. Lobelle-Rich, and L. S. Levy, "Feline leukaemia virus LTR variation and disease association in a geographical and temporal cluster," *Journal of General Virology*, vol. 85, no. 10, pp. 2937–2942, 2004.

[34] Y. Fujino, K. Ohno, and H. Tsujimoto, "Molecular pathogenesis of feline leukemia virus-induced malignancies: insertional mutagenesis," *Veterinary Immunology and Immunopathology*, vol. 123, no. 1-2, pp. 138–143, 2008.

[35] L. S. Levy, "Advances in understanding molecular determinants in FeLV pathology," *Veterinary Immunology and Immunopathology*, vol. 123, no. 1-2, pp. 14–22, 2008.

[36] M. C. Archer, "Role of sp transcription factors in the regulation of cancer cell metabolism," *Genes and Cancer*, vol. 2, no. 7, pp. 712–719, 2011.

[37] R. Pal, M. Janz, D. L. Galson et al., "C/EBPβ regulates transcription factors critical for proliferation and survival of multiple myeloma cells," *Blood*, vol. 114, no. 18, pp. 3890–3898, 2009.

[38] A. Amer, A. Siti Suri, O. Abdul Rahman et al., "Isolation and molecular characterization of type I and type II feline coronavirus in Malaysia," *Virology Journal*, vol. 9, article 278, 2012.

[39] S. K. Ghosh and D. V. Faller, "Feline leukemia virus long terminal repeat activates collagenase IV gene expression through AP-1," *Journal of Virology*, vol. 73, no. 6, pp. 4931–4940, 1999.

[40] A. L. Abujamra, D. V. Faller, and S. K. Ghosh, "Mutations that abrogate transactivational activity of the feline leukemia virus long terminal repeat do not affect virus replication," *Virology*, vol. 309, no. 2, pp. 294–305, 2003.

[41] Y. Matsumoto, Y. Momoi, T. Watari, R. Goitsuka, H. Tsuilmoto, and A. Hasegawa, "Detection of enhancer repeats in the long terminal repeats of feline leukemia viruses from cats with spontaneous neoplastic and nonneoplastic diseases," *Virology*, vol. 189, no. 2, pp. 745–749, 1992.

[42] G. B. Athas, P. Lobelle-Rich, and L. S. Levy, "Function of a unique sequence motif in the long terminal repeat of feline leukemia virus isolated from an unusual set of naturally occurring tumors," *Journal of Virology*, vol. 69, no. 6, pp. 3324–3332, 1995.

[43] M. Shindoh, F. Higashino, and T. Kohgo, "E1AF, an ets-oncogene family transcription factor," *Cancer Letters*, vol. 216, no. 1, pp. 1–8, 2004.

[44] M. Purrello, C. Di Pietro, A. Viola et al., "Genomics and transcription analysis of human TFIID," *Oncogene*, vol. 16, no. 12, pp. 1633–1638, 1998.

[45] R. Kageyama, G. T. Merlino, and I. Pastan, "Nuclear factor ETF specifically stimulates transcription from promoters without a TATA box," *Journal of Biological Chemistry*, vol. 264, no. 26, pp. 15508–15514, 1989.

[46] T. J. Velu, L. Beguinot, W. C. Vass et al., "Epidermal growth factor-dependent transformation by a human EGF receptor proto-oncogene," *Science*, vol. 238, no. 4832, pp. 1408–1410, 1987.

[47] Y. Kitadai, H. Yamazaki, W. Yasui et al., "GC factor represses transcription of several growth factor/receptor genes and causes growth inhibition of human gastric carcinoma cell lines," *Cell Growth & Differentiation*, vol. 4, no. 4, pp. 291–296, 1993.

[48] J. Pecon-Slattery, J. L. Troyer, W. E. Johnson, and S. J. O'Brien, "Evolution of feline immunodeficiency virus in Felidae: implications for human health and wildlife ecology," *Veterinary Immunology and Immunopathology*, vol. 123, no. 1-2, pp. 32–44, 2008.

10

Effect of Three Colostrum Diets on Passive Transfer of Immunity and Preweaning Health in Calves on a California Dairy following Colostrum Management Training

Deniece R. Williams,[1] Patrick Pithua,[2] Angel Garcia,[3] John Champagne,[1] Deborah M. Haines,[4,5] and Sharif S. Aly[1,6]

[1] Veterinary Medicine Teaching and Research Center, School of Veterinary Medicine, University of California, Davis, 18830 Road 112, Tulare, CA 93274, USA

[2] Department of Veterinary Medicine & Surgery, Veterinary Medicine Teaching Hospital, College of Veterinary Medicine, University of Missouri, 900 E. Campus Drive, Columbia, MO 65211, USA

[3] Departamento de Producción y Sanidad Animal, Facultad de Veterinaria, Universidad CEU Cardenal Herrera, Moncada, 46113 Valencia, Spain

[4] Department of Veterinary Microbiology, Western College of Veterinary Medicine, University of Saskatchewan, Saskatoon, SK, Canada S7N 5B4

[5] The Saskatoon Colostrum Co. Ltd., 30 Molaro Pl, Saskatoon, SK, Canada S7K 6A2

[6] Department of Population Health and Reproduction, School of Veterinary Medicine, University of California, One Shields Avenue, Davis, CA 95616, USA

Correspondence should be addressed to Sharif S. Aly; saly@ucdavis.edu

Academic Editor: Alexander Rodriguez-Palacios

Following colostrum management training, a randomized field trial was conducted on a California dairy to determine the effect of supplementing pooled colostrum with either colostrum-derived replacer (CDR) or second-milking colostrum (transition milk) on failure of passive transfer (FPT) and preweaning morbidity risks. A total of 166 calves were randomly assigned to 4L first-milking pooled colostrum (treatment 1), 2L first-milking pooled colostrum and 2L of CDR (treatment 2), or 2L first-milking pooled colostrum and 2L second-milking pooled colostrum (treatment 3). Mean 24-hour serum TP and IgG for treatments 2 (TP 5.2 g/dL, IgG 15.9 g/L) and 3 (TP 5.4 g/dL, IgG 18.3 g/L) did not statistically differ but were significantly lower than for treatment 1 (TP 5.9 g/dL, IgG 24.6 g/L). Risk of FPT did not differ for treatments 1, 2, and 3 (0.0%, 9.3%, and 1.9%, resp.). Similarly, the preweaning risk of diarrhea (81.0%, 92.5%, and 87.0%, resp.) or pneumonia (6.9%, 13.2%, and 18.5%, resp.) did not differ between treatments. Feeding 4L first-milking pooled colostrum resulted in adequate passive transfer. When first-milking pooled colostrum quantity is inadequate, CDR or second-milking pooled colostrum can be used to supplement the required colostrum volume and IgG mass without adversely affecting the risks of FPT or preweaning diarrhea and pneumonia.

1. Introduction

Timely ingestion of high quality colostrum is one of the most important factors affecting both short and long term calf performance. Calves that ingest >2 L of high quality colostrum or that have higher levels of serum IgG in the first week of life have lower morbidity and mortality than calves with lower serum IgG levels or that ingest insufficient quantities of high quality colostrum. Adequate passive transfer of immunity has been associated with lower preweaning veterinary costs, improved weight gain, and increased milk production and longevity in the milking herd [1–4]. Current recommendations to reduce the incidence of failure of passive transfer of immunity (FPT), defined as serum

IgG < 10 mg/mL in the first 1 to 7 days of life, include feeding 3 to 4 L of colostrum containing a minimum of 50 mg/mL IgG within the first 1 to 2 hours of birth [3, 5–8]. Additionally, studies have shown that colostrum with bacterial counts <100,000 cfu/mL has a superior apparent efficiency of absorption (AEA) of immunoglobulins than colostrum with higher bacterial counts, when fed to calves [5, 9]. Despite these recommendations, a recent survey of US dairies reported that, among those tested, 40.7% of dairies had at least one calf with FPT and that 19.2% of all calves fail to achieve adequate passive transfer of immunity, with calves in the Western USA experiencing a higher FPT rate than calves in the Eastern USA [10, 11]. Understanding the underlying factors contributing to FPT on dairies is essential to reduce the occurrence of this condition and to improve short term calf performance and long term dairy productivity.

A management practice contributing to FPT may be pooling colostrum. Based on a 2007 National Animal Health Monitoring survey of US dairy herds, Beam and others estimated that calves fed pooled colostrum were more than twice as likely to have FPT as calves fed colostrum from an individual cow [10, 11]. In addition, a recent study conducted on a California dairy showed that calves fed pooled colostrum with a low IgG concentration (21.1 g/L) had significantly lower 24-hour serum total protein and IgG concentrations and a significantly higher risk of FPT compared to calves fed colostrum-derived replacer (CDR) [12]. The California study also showed that both the colostrum IgG concentration and the IgG mass fed were significantly higher in the CDR compared to the pooled colostrum [12]. Pooling can maintain an adequate supply of colostrum but may result in lower quality due to dilution of IgG, as cows producing higher volumes often contribute colostrum with a lower concentration of immunoglobulins [3]. Immunoglobulins are present at high concentrations in colostrum, the initial secretion from the mammary gland following parturition. While the levels of immunoglobulins decrease rapidly with each milking, they remain at higher levels than found in milk for 5–7 days after calving, as the cow transitions to production of normal milk [13–18]. Intentional or accidental addition of colostrum from the second or later milkings (also known as transition milk), to the colostrum pool can, therefore, lead to dilution of the IgG concentration of the pooled colostrum. Furthermore, it is common practice on California dairies to house recently calved cows in the hospital pen. As such, sick cows, newly admitted into the hospital pen, may be misidentified in the parlor, allowing milk from nonfresh cows to be harvested into the colostrum supply, further contributing to dilution of the IgG in the colostrum pool. In a recent national study of colostrum quality in the USA, only 25.6% of pooled colostrum samples met industry standards for both IgG concentration and bacterial count compared with 41.2% of nonpooled samples [19]. Pooling colostrum also increases the risk of exposure to infectious disease organisms, such as *Mycobacterium avium* subsp. *paratuberculosis*, bovine leukosis virus, and bovine viral diarrhea virus [20]. Despite the recognized biosecurity risks and negative effect on passive transfer of immunity associated with feeding pooled colostrum, calves in 16% of US

herds with <100 cows and approximately 57% of herds with >500 cows continue to be fed pooled colostrum [11].

A second, related management factor contributing to FPT on dairies is a shortage in colostrum supply and, in response, commercial colostrum supplements and replacer products have been developed from bovine plasma, serum, or colostrum [20]. Results of studies evaluating the efficacy of these products on serum IgG concentrations, rates of FPT, and preweaning health outcomes in calves are mixed. Colostrum replacers and supplements derived from plasma or serum that provided higher doses of IgG (>170 g IgG) were shown to prevent FPT; however, those with lower IgG doses were not [21–26]. Similarly, colostrum-derived replacers with high doses of IgG (>170 g IgG) were shown to prevent FPT; however, some but not all colostrum-derived replacers and supplements with lower doses of IgG also prevented FPT [8, 12, 25, 27–31]. Studies of plasma-derived replacers have shown either no difference or an increased risk of health events in calves compared to colostrum, whereas studies of colostrum-derived replacers have shown both a decreased and increased risk of health events in calves compared to colostrum [23, 25, 26, 32]. Feeding pooled colostrum in conjunction with a CDR has not been evaluated and could be an effective approach to address colostrum shortages on dairies.

The first objective of this study was to evaluate the effect of implementing colostrum management training regarding the collection and pooling of colostrum on the IgG concentration in pooled colostrum, on a dairy previously shown to have low quality, pooled colostrum [12]. For the purposes of this study, colostrum is defined as the lacteal secretion produced for the first 5 days of lactation [13, 15–17]; however, only first- and second-milking colostrum pools were used based on the milking number from which they were obtained. The second objective was to conduct a randomized field trial to compare the effect of feeding first-milking pooled colostrum or first-milking pooled colostrum followed by either a reconstituted CDR or second-milking pooled colostrum on the risk of FPT, morbidity, and mortality in preweaning Jersey and Holstein calves. Results of this study will help veterinarians and dairy producers more effectively manage colostrum supply, ultimately improving calf performance on dairies.

2. Materials and Methods

2.1. Study Herd and Experimental Design. This study was approved by the University of California at Davis Institutional Animal Care and Use Committee (approval date 2/22/2012). The trial was conducted on a Central California Holstein and Jersey dairy in Tulare County which milked 3,600 cows and fed unpasteurized pooled colostrum to calves. The dairy was selected because of its large size, records availability through the California Dairy Herd Improvement Association's milk testing program, and the owner's interest and willingness to participate in the study.

In a previous study, pooled colostrum collected from the study herd had lower IgG concentrations (mean 21.1 g/L, SD 9.76) than the reported average for Southwestern US dairies

(64.3 g/L, SE = 2.9) which may explain the high proportion of FPT in the dairy's calves [12, 19]. Hence, the herd provided a unique opportunity for colostrum management training to improve the IgG concentration of pooled colostrum.

2.2. Pretrial Training Period

2.2.1. Colostrum Management Training.
Between November 2011 and January 2012, training was provided to the dairy staff by the study veterinarians to prevent misidentification of fresh and sick cows in the hospital pen and to eliminate mixing first- and second-milking colostrum within the same pool. All cows were milked twice a day and the dairy's protocols regarding timing of milking or parlor hygiene remained unaltered. After calving and prior to the first milking, maternity pen staff used a degradable color wax stick to mark each cow's hind limb with a line from above the hock to below the tarsal joint. Only cows with a line contributed to the first-milking pooled colostrum supply. After the first milking, a single cross hatch was placed over this line by the milking staff. Only cows with the single cross hatch supplied the second-milking colostrum. After the second milking, another cross hatch was placed to indicate that these cows were excluded from further colostrum collection. First- and second-milking pooled colostrum were collected into receiver containers that had been permanently marked with the labels "1" and "2", respectively.

2.2.2. Baseline Estimation of Herd-Level Colostrum IgG Concentration.
Prior to initiation of the current trial and while colostrum management training was ongoing, colostrum samples were collected between November 2011 and January 2012 to evaluate the effect of the colostrum management training on baseline IgG concentration of the colostrum. Herd personnel collected a colostrum sample (50 mL) from the first- and second-milking colostrum containers after each milking. These colostrum samples were frozen on the dairy at $-20°C$ and were transported on a weekly basis to the University of California at Davis, Veterinary Medicine Teaching and Research Center (VMTRC, Tulare, CA). The samples were stored at $-80°C$ until the end of the pretrial period, at which point all samples were sent to the testing laboratory (The Saskatoon Colostrum Co. Ltd., Saskatoon, Canada) for estimation of IgG (g/L) concentration using radial immunodiffusion.

2.3. Trial Period

2.3.1. Estimation of Sample Size.
Sample size for a significant difference in 24-hour serum IgG among the three groups of calves estimated for multiple comparisons using the Tukey-Kramer (Pairwise) method, at a power of 95%, an alpha of 0.05, a minimal detectable difference of 1 unit, and a SD = 2 resulted in a sample size of 50 calves per group. Adding an additional 20% to account for attrition, the total sample size of 60 calves per group was estimated.

2.3.2. Colostrum and Feeding Treatments.
Cows within the last 2 weeks of pregnancy were monitored by trained dairy staff and moved to a group maternity pen upon showing signs of impending parturition. Calves were separated from the dam as soon as possible after birth to prevent suckling and moved to a group pen where they were ear-tagged, had their navels dipped with 7% iodine tincture, and were fed colostrum. Jersey heifer calves, Holstein heifer calves, and Holstein bull calves were enrolled between February and March, 2012. Jersey bull calves, all cross-breeds, and calves born between 5 pm and 9 pm, Monday through Thursday, and between 5 pm Friday and 9 pm Sunday were excluded from enrollment into the study.

Calves were randomly assigned to one of three treatments using a list of random numbers pregenerated in Excel 2010 (Microsoft, Redmond, WA). The randomization list was sealed with opaque adhesive notes that were sequentially removed only at each calf's birth to reveal treatment assignment. In treatment 1, calves were fed 4 L of raw, first-milking pooled colostrum. In treatment 2, calves were fed 2 L of raw, first-milking pooled colostrum followed immediately by 2 L of CDR (Calf's Choice Total HiCal, Alta Genetics Inc.). In treatment 3, calves were fed 2 L of raw, first-milking pooled colostrum followed immediately by 2 L of raw, second-milking pooled colostrum.

Colostrum was harvested and stored as described for the pretrial period. First- and second-milking pooled colostrum were divided into individual plastic nipple bottles, stored at 4°C until feeding, and warmed prior to feeding. Calves were fed colostrum harvested on the day of their birth. The CDR powder was reconstituted according to the manufacturer's instruction by dissolving 700 g of the powder in 1.25 L of warm water (46–57°C), ensuring a solvent that provided 100 g of IgG per dose. Holstein calves that did not suckle after multiple attempts or failed to ingest the entire volume within 3 hours were fed the remaining volume via an esophageal tube feeder. Jersey heifer calves that did not voluntarily ingest 4 L of colostrum were instead tube-fed a volume of 3 L of their assigned colostrum treatment.

2.3.3. Preweaning Calf Management.
All study calves were housed in individual, elevated wooden hutches, and given free choice water and starter grain until weaning at approximately 60 to 75 days of age. Calves were fed 2 L of pasteurized waste milk supplemented with milk replacer containing 20% protein and 20% fat, twice a day. In April 2012, the dairy's management implemented changes to the calf feeding program. Changes affected the type and quantity of milk fed and the number of feedings per day. The youngest study calf affected by these changes was 20 days old.

2.4. Data Collection and Laboratory Analysis of Samples.
Information recorded for each calf included herd identification number, sex, breed, birthdate, dam identification, birth weight (kg), time to separation from dam (hrs), and time to colostrum feeding (hrs).

Immediately before and 24 hours after colostrum was fed, a blood sample (5 mL) from each calf was collected by jugular venipuncture, allowed to clot, and centrifuged (Model E8, LW Scientific, Lawrenceville, GA) at 3300 rpm within 30 minutes of collection. Serum samples were harvested, divided into two aliquots, and labeled with the calf ID and whether the sample was collected before or after feeding colostrum.

A sample of pooled colostrum (5 mL) fed to each calf was collected before feeding and labeled with calf ID and milking number. All samples were frozen at −20°C, transported on ice to the VMTRC, and stored at −80°C until shipment to the testing laboratory (The Saskatoon Colostrum Co. Ltd., Saskatoon, Canada) for further analyses. Serum samples were analyzed for total protein (g/dL) by digital refractometer. The IgG (g/L) of the colostrum and serum samples were analyzed using radial immunodiffusion [27]. All laboratory personnel were blinded to treatment.

2.4.1. Health Monitoring. Each calf was monitored twice daily by dairy staff and at least once daily by study personnel for signs of illness including lethargy, weakness, decreased appetite, dehydration, fever, abnormal fecal consistency, cough, increased respiratory rate, ocular or nasal discharge, drooping ears, and head tilt. All health events and medical treatments prescribed by the herd veterinarian were recorded on waterproof cards hanging on each calf hutch. Data on the health events and treatments for each calf was subsequently transferred daily to a standard database by study personnel until the end of follow-up for each calf at approximately 53 (±3) days of age. All personnel monitoring the calves were blinded to treatment.

The preweaning morbidity events of interest in this study were diarrhea and pneumonia. To ensure consistency, the Wisconsin Calf Health Scoring Chart was modified and used as a guide in the diagnosis of health events [33]. Diarrhea was defined as a calf passing abnormal, watery feces with a foul odor (score 2 or 3). Pneumonia was defined as a calf displaying signs of spontaneous cough and increased respiratory rate, with or without ocular and/or nasal discharge or otitis (score 2 or 3), except no attempt was made to induce a cough. A health event that occurred more than seven days following recovery from a previous health event was considered a new incident. Health events occurring within seven days of a previous health event with similar clinical signs were considered the same incident.

2.5. Statistical Analysis. All statistical analyses were performed using standard statistical software (IBM SPSS Statistics, version 22.0.0, Armonk, NY, IBM Corp.) and were considered significant if the P value was <0.05. Mean ± standard error of the mean (SE) pooled colostrum IgG concentrations for the study pretrial and trial periods were calculated and compared using a one-way ANOVA. For each treatment in the study, categorical baseline characteristics (sex, breed, time to separation from dam, and time to colostrum feeding) were compared using a Pearson chi-square test or Fischer's exact test. Continuous baseline characteristics (birth weight, precolostrum serum total protein, precolostrum serum IgG, first-milking colostrum IgG, and total IgG fed) were compared among treatments using one-way ANOVA. The AEA for each calf was calculated using the following formula:

$$\text{AEA} = \frac{\text{Serum IgG (g/L)} \times \text{Serum volume (L)}}{\text{IgG Intake (g)}} \quad (1)$$

with plasma volume estimated as 9.9% and 9.7% of birth weight for Holsteins and Jerseys, respectively [34]. Means of the AEA of IgG (%) for the treatments were compared using a one-way ANOVA. Proportions of calves with FPT (defined as 24-hour postfeeding serum IgG < 10 g/L), diarrhea, and pneumonia among the treatments were compared using a Z-test with the alpha level adjusted for multiple comparisons using the Bonferroni method.

Two separate Cox proportional hazard models were used to estimate and compare the preweaning hazards for both diarrhea and pneumonia among treatments. Follow-up time for all calves occurred from enrollment until just prior to weaning (53 ± 3 days of age). The proportional hazards assumption was evaluated graphically and using the Schoenfeld residuals. Violation in the proportional hazards assumption was addressed by estimating hazard ratios using an extended Cox model with time-dependent covariates. Variables considered in the models were treatment, sex, and breed. With the exception of treatment, which was forced into each model, all variables were entered into the Cox models using a backwards stepwise elimination procedure. Variables were selected for removal if the P value for the change in the log-likelihood ratio was greater than 0.10.

3. Results

3.1. Effect of Colostrum Management Training on Pooled Colostrum Quality. In the pretrial period, a total of 56 first-milking pooled colostrum and 66 second-milking pooled colostrum samples were analyzed. The mean (±SE) IgG concentrations in these samples were 56.3 g/L (±2.69) and 18.3 g/L (±1.72), respectively. In the trial, a total of 166 first-milking pooled colostrum and 53 second-milking pooled colostrum samples were tested. The mean (±SE) IgG concentrations in these samples were 65.1 g/L (±1.25) and 25.8 g/L (±1.81), respectively. The first-milking pooled colostrum from the trial period had a mean IgG concentration that was significantly higher than the first-milking pooled colostrum in the pretrial period ($P = 0.003$) and the second-milking pooled colostrum in both the pretrial and trial periods ($P < 0.001$). Similarly, the mean IgG concentration of the pretrial, first-milking pooled colostrum was significantly higher than the second-milking pooled colostrum from the pretrial and trial periods ($P = 0.003$). No statistical difference was noted between the mean IgG concentration of the second-milking pooled colostrum in the pretrial and trial periods ($P = 0.059$); however this comparison had low statistical power because of the small number of samples tested.

3.2. Effect of Colostrum Type on Passive Transfer of Immunity, Preweaning Health, and Survival. A total of 187 calves were enrolled in the study. Of these, 166 calves comprising 57 Holstein heifers, 85 Holstein bulls, and 24 Jersey heifers remained eligible for statistical analysis. Of those enrolled, 58, 54, and 54 calves were allocated to treatments 1, 2, and 3, respectively. Of the 21 calves excluded from the analysis, 16 had precolostrum serum IgG concentrations greater than 2.3 g/L (5, 7, and 4 calves from treatments 1, 2, and 3, resp.)

TABLE 1: Comparison of baseline characteristics among 3 treatments in a randomized field trial comparing the effects of feeding first-milking pooled colostrum alone or first-milking pooled colostrum followed by either a colostrum-derived replacer or second-milking pooled colostrum to newborn Holstein and Jersey calves.

Characteristic	Treatment 1[*] N = 58	Treatment 2[*] N = 54	Treatment 3[*] N = 54	P value
Sex: N (%)				0.167[†]
Female	23 (39.7)	27 (50.0)	31 (57.4)	
Male	35 (60.3)	27 (50.0)	23 (42.6)	
Breed: N (%)				0.544[†]
Holstein	52 (89.7)	45 (83.3)	45 (83.3)	
Jersey	6 (10.3)	9 (16.7)	9 (16.7)	
Time to separation from dam: N (%)				0.912[†]
<1 hour	41 (70.7)	42 (77.8)	39 (72.2)	
1–6 hours	15 (25.9)	11 (20.4)	14 (25.9)	
6–9 hours	2 (3.4)	1 (1.9)	1 (1.9)	
Time to colostrum feeding: N (%)				0.764[†]
<1 hour	4 (6.9)	3 (5.6)	4 (7.4)	
1–6 hours	44 (75.9)	37 (68.5)	41 (75.9)	
6–9 hours	10 (17.2)	14 (25.9)	9 (16.7)	
Birth weight (kg):				0.750[§]
mean (SE[‡])	39.02 (0.86)	38.68 (1.05)	37.99 (1.03)	
Precolostrum serum total protein (g/dL):				0.689[§]
mean (SE)	4.44 (0.04)	4.49 (0.04)	4.45 (0.06)	
Precolostrum serum IgG (g/L):				0.715[§]
mean (SE)	0.40 (0.05)	0.45 (0.06)	0.46 (0.06)	
First-milking colostrum IgG (g/L):				0.505[§]
mean (SE)	65.0 (2.16)	67.0 (2.01)	63.4 (2.35)	
Second-milking colostrum IgG (g/L):				—
mean (SE)	—	—	25.8 (1.81)	
Total IgG fed[‖] (g):				<0.001[§]
mean (SE)	255.9[a] (8.87)	222.1[b] (4.84)	172.2[c] (4.75)	

[*]Treatment 1: 4L 1st-milking pooled colostrum, treatment 2: 2L 1st-milking pooled colostrum followed by 2L colostrum-derived replacer, and treatment 3: 2L 1st-milking pooled colostrum followed by 2L 2nd-milking pooled colostrum.
[†]Pearson chi-square or Fischer's exact test with 5% level of significance.
[‡]SE: standard error.
[§]One-way ANOVA using the Tukey multiple comparison procedure with 5% level of significance. Means without a common superscript are significantly different.
[‖]Total IgG fed for treatment 2 estimated assuming 100 g IgG in colostrum-derived replacer.

due to possible colostrum ingestion prior to sampling [35]. The remaining 5 calves that were excluded consisted of four calves that died within 48 hours from atresia coli, which was not apparent at birth (treatment 2: one calf and treatment 3: three calves), and one calf (treatment 2) that had no 24-hour serum sample taken. An additional calf (treatment 2) was euthanized by the dairy at 9 days of age due to a leg injury and was excluded from analysis of health events. A second-milking colostrum sample for one calf was not collected; therefore, comparison of second-milking colostrum IgG concentration, total IgG fed, and AEA among treatments was based on 165 calves.

Of the baseline characteristics tested, only total IgG (g) fed was significantly different among treatments, with calves fed only first-milking pooled colostrum (treatment 1) having the highest and calves fed first- and second-milking pooled colostrum having the lowest (treatment 3) mean total IgG fed (Table 1). Calves that received only first-milking pooled colostrum had 24-hour serum TP and IgG that was significantly higher than calves in the other treatments ($P <$ 0.001); however, no difference was noted between the calves fed first-milking pooled colostrum followed by either CDR or second-milking pooled colostrum (Table 2). Calves that received first-milking pooled colostrum followed by CDR (treatment 2) had a significantly lower AEA than calves that received either first-milking pooled colostrum alone or a mixture of first- and second-milking pooled colostrum ($P <$ 0.001, Table 2). Although numerical differences existed, no statistical difference was noted in the risk of FPT as defined by serum IgG $<$ 10 g/L ($P \geq$ 0.05) among the treatments (Table 2). No statistical difference ($P \geq$ 0.05) was noted among treatments for the risk of preweaning diarrhea

TABLE 2: Effect of treatment on 24-hour serum total protein and IgG concentrations, apparent efficiency of IgG absorption, and passive transfer status of Holstein and Jersey calves in a randomized field trial comparing the effect of feeding either first-milking pooled colostrum alone or first-milking pooled colostrum followed by either a colostrum-derived replacer or second-milking pooled colostrum.

Item	Treatment 1[*] N = 58	Treatment 2[*] N = 54	Treatment 3[*] N = 54	P value
24-hour serum total protein (g/dL):				
mean (SE[†])	5.9[a] (0.08)	5.2[b] (0.07)	5.4[b] (0.06)	<0.001[‡]
24-hour serum IgG (g/L):				
mean (SE)	24.6[a] (1.06)	15.9[b] (0.78)	18.3[b] (0.66)	<0.001[‡]
Apparent efficiency of IgG absorption (%):				
mean (SE)	37.0[a] (1.14)	26.3[b] (1.01)	40.0[a] (1.29)	<0.001[‡]
Failure of passive transfer: % (95% CI)				
IgG (<10 g/L)	0.0[a] (—)	9.3[a] (1.53, 16.99)	1.9[a] (0, 5.45)	≥0.05[§]

[*]Treatment 1: 4L 1st-milking pooled colostrum, treatment 2: 2L 1st-milking pooled colostrum followed by 2L colostrum-derived replacer, and treatment 3: 2L 1st-milking pooled colostrum followed by 2L 2nd-milking pooled colostrum.
[†]SE: standard error.
[‡]One-way ANOVA using the Tukey multiple comparison procedure with 5% level of significance. Means without a common superscript are significantly different.
[§]Column proportions were compared using a z-test with the alpha adjusted for multiple comparisons using the Bonferroni method. Means without a common superscript are significantly different at the 5% level.

(treatment 1: 81.0%, $n = 58$, SE = 0.052, treatment 2: 92.5%, $n = 53$, SE = 0.037, and treatment 3: 87.0%, $n = 54$, SE = 0.046) or pneumonia (treatment 1: 6.9%, $n = 58$, SE = 0.034, treatment 2: 13.2%, $n = 53$, SE = 0.047, and treatment 3: 18.5%, $n = 54$, SE = 0.053). Two calves (treatment 2) died from diarrhea. No other deaths due to infectious disease occurred during the study period.

The final Cox model for diarrhea was adjusted for breed where Jersey calves' hazard rate ratio (HRR) for diarrhea was 2.13 times that of Holsteins (95% CI (1.35, 3.35), $P = 0.001$). In comparison, the best-fitting model for pneumonia was adjusted for gender; however, the hazard for bull compared to heifer calves was not significant (HRR = 0.39, 95% CI (0.151, 1.01), $P = 0.39$). In both models, the treatment variable violated the proportional hazard assumption and a treatment-time interaction term was forced into the model. The hazard for diarrhea was not significant for treatment 2 or 3 (HRR = 1.03, 95% CI (0.997, 1.07), $P = 0.074$; HRR = 1.02, 95% CI (0.98, 1.06), $P = 0.332$, resp.) compared to treatment 1. Similarly, the hazards for pneumonia for treatment 2 or 3 were not significant (HRR = 1.04, 95% CI (0.99, 1.09), $P = 0.100$; HRR = 1.04, 95% CI (0.99, 1.09), $P = 0.114$, resp.) compared to treatment 1.

4. Discussion

Feeding 4 L of first-milking pooled colostrum to calves ensured adequate passive transfer of immunity. However, dairies that properly manage the quality of pooled colostrum may, at times, experience a shortage of first-milking colostrum. The current study is the first to investigate the alternatives of feeding 2 L of first-milking pooled colostrum followed by either 2 L of CDR or 2 L of second-milking pooled colostrum. Although mean 24-hour serum

IgG levels were significantly lower in calves fed either alternative, mean IgG levels in all groups were excellent [36] and the risks of FPT and preweaning diarrhea or pneumonia were not significantly different from calves fed 4 L of first-milking pooled colostrum. The lack of significant differences in FPT or preweaning morbidity between treatments could have been due to a small sample size or the fact that all treatments delivered a mass of IgG that met or exceeded the current industry recommendation of feeding 150–200 g IgG in 3-4 L of colostrum [3, 5–8] and far exceeded the historical recommendation of 100 g IgG in 2 L of colostrum [37, 38].

In addition, feeding first-milking pooled colostrum followed by either CDR or second-milking pooled colostrum did not result in an increased hazard for either diarrhea or pneumonia compared to feeding first-milking pooled colostrum alone. However, these results should be interpreted with caution as it is possible that the diet changes implemented by the dairy management during the follow-up period affected the risk of diarrhea or pneumonia for the calves. Improved nutrient intake has been associated with improved immune function [39]. Therefore, the diet changes may have provided protection against diarrhea or pneumonia, biasing the results by decreasing disease incidence. However, at the onset of the diet changes, the youngest calf was 20 days of age, which is older than the mean age of onset reported for the major causes of preweaning calf diarrhea [40]. Therefore, it is possible that the calves had passed the period of highest risk for diarrhea prior to the onset of diet changes such that the hazard results for diarrhea were unaffected. Additionally, survival analysis for diarrhea in a subset of the data for calves from birth to 20 days of age showed a nonsignificant hazard for diarrhea (data not shown), which is in agreement with the results of the Cox extended model based on the entire follow-up period.

Feeding high quality colostrum is an important management tool for ensuring healthy and productive calves. Results from this study indicated that dairies with management practices similar to the study herd could significantly improve the IgG concentration of first-milking pooled colostrum by implementing colostrum management training to prevent misclassification of fresh cows. As with many large California dairies, the study dairy housed fresh and sick cows in the same pen. Before initiation of the colostrum management training in this herd, there was no formal method to distinguish the fresh cows in the milking parlor. Thus, colostrum from the third or later milkings and milk from nonfresh, sick cows may have been included in the colostrum supply prior to this study. Misclassification of cows was eliminated through the colostrum management training, which emphasized proper identification of cows at their first and second milking and likely contributed to the significant increase in the IgG concentration of the first-milking pooled colostrum between the pretrial and trial periods. However, the training of the dairy's staff was provided by veterinarians who were present on the dairy daily for the first 3 weeks of the pretrial period and for the duration of the trial period. The level of training and oversight is not likely to be repeated by veterinarians working with producers, which may limit the effectiveness of similar colostrum management training in a field setting. In addition, this study was conducted on a single dairy and, hence, may not be generalizable to other dairies.

The study herd offered a unique opportunity to contrast results of the current trial to results from a previous trial that compared the effect of CDR or undifferentiated pooled colostrum on FPT, morbidity, and mortality in preweaning calves [12, 32]. Calves fed first-milking pooled colostrum alone in the current study had higher 24-hour serum IgG concentrations than calves fed pooled colostrum in the previous study (24.6 g/L and 7.50 g/L, resp.), whereas calves fed first-milking pooled colostrum followed by CDR had similar 24-hour serum IgG concentrations to calves fed CDR in the previous study (15.9 g/L and 15.15 g/L, resp.) on this dairy [12]. In addition, the risk of FPT in calves fed first-milking pooled colostrum alone was lower in the current study (0.0%, n = 58) compared to in the earlier study (70%, n = 269) [12]. Differences in the 24-hour serum IgG concentrations and FPT between the two studies may have been due to the increased amount of IgG fed to the calves in the current study or to differences in apparent efficiency of IgG absorption between the studies. In the current study, the IgG concentration in the first-milking pooled colostrum after the colostrum management training was higher (65.1 g/L) than previous pooled colostrum IgG concentrations measured from the same dairy in the earlier study (21.1 g/L) [12] but similar to the average IgG concentration in pooled colostrum from dairies in the Southwest region of the USA (64.3 g/L) [19]. The increase in the IgG concentration of the pooled colostrum in the current study is likely due to the improved colostrum collection by the dairy personnel following the colostrum management training. However, colostrum samples were not obtained prior to the initiation of the colostrum management training making it impossible to assess the direct effect of training.

The results of this study indicated that feeding calves either first-milking pooled colostrum alone or first- and

second-milking pooled colostrum was associated with a significantly higher AEA than feeding calves first-milking pooled colostrum followed by CDR. These results are in contrast with the previous study conducted on this study dairy where the AEA of calves fed pooled colostrum (28.8%) was similar to the AEA of calves fed CDR (27.0%) [12]. However, the AEA of the calves fed first-milking pooled colostrum followed by CDR in the current study was similar to the AEA of calves fed CDR in the earlier study conducted on this dairy [12] but was lower than the AEA (35.5 to 38.8%) reported for calves fed CDR in other studies [8, 25]. Colostrum replacer products vary in the postcolostrum serum IgG concentrations which they can achieve in calves, despite providing similar amounts of IgG [20]. The use of different colostrum replacers among these studies may explain the variable AEA observed. Absorption of IgG across the intestinal epithelium is a saturable process [41, 42] and it is possible that other macromolecules present in the colostrum replacers may compete with the IgG absorption. Alternatively, differences in AEA observed among this and other studies may be due to differences in calf management practices among the studies, such as the amount of colostrum feedings provided, method of colostrum feeding, or time from birth to colostrum feeding that may have affected the calves' ability to absorb IgG from the colostrum [20, 43]. The results of this trial suggest that colostrum composition, in addition to volume and mass of IgG, is important in IgG absorption. Further research is needed to determine the effect of various macromolecules in colostrum and colostrum replacers on AEA and, in particular, the impact of supplementing maternal colostrum with colostrum replacers of varying composition.

Results of our study showed that dairies that feed high quality first-milking pooled colostrum can minimize or eliminate the risk of FPT in calves. Furthermore, during times of colostrum shortage, the colostrum supply can be extended by feeding 2 L of first-milking pooled colostrum combined with either 2 L of CDR or 2 L of second-milking pooled colostrum without significant differences in the risk of calves experiencing FPT and preweaning diarrhea or pneumonia.

Conflict of Interests

The Dairy Epidemiology Laboratory (Aly Lab) has previously received funding from The Saskatoon Colostrum Co. Ltd. for research on calf health and colostrum management. Dr. Haines is affiliated with The Saskatoon Colostrum Co. Ltd.; the manufacturer of the product kindly donated for the purpose of this study. Her participation did not influence or bias the performance or presentation of the research described in this paper in any way. No other authors are affiliated with or receive compensation or royalties from The Saskatoon Colostrum Co. Ltd.

Authors' Contribution

Sharif S. Aly, Patrick Pithua, and Deborah M. Haines designed the trial. Sharif S. Aly and JDC conducted the colostrum management training. Sharif S. Aly, Deniece R. Williams, and Angel Garcia conducted the study and contributed to data collection. Deniece R. Williams and Sharif S. Aly analyzed the data. Deniece R. Williams wrote the first paper draft. Sharif S. Aly and Patrick Pithua wrote the paper. All authors reviewed and provided comments on the paper. All authors approved the final version of the paper.

Acknowledgments

The authors acknowledge the in-kind donation of the colostrum product and testing of colostrum and serum samples by Saskatchewan colostrum Co. Ltd. The authors thank Drs. Jessica Davis and Mohamed Elramady for their technical assistance during the trial and the dairy management and staff for their cooperation. Funding was provided by Saskatoon Colostrum Co. Ltd. and the Dairy Epidemiology Laboratory (Aly Lab), Veterinary Medicine Teaching and Research Center, School of Veterinary Medicine, University of California, Davis. This paper represents the thesis submitted by Dr. Williams to the University of California at Davis, School of Veterinary Medicine, as partial fulfillment of the requirements for the Master of Preventive Veterinary Medicine Degree.

References

[1] S. K. DeNise, J. D. Robison, G. H. Stott, and D. V. Armstrong, "Effects of passive immunity on subsequent production in dairy heifers," *Journal of Dairy Science*, vol. 72, no. 2, pp. 552–554, 1989.

[2] S. Faber, N. Faber, T. McCauley et al., "Case study: effects of colostrum ingestion on lactational performance," *The Professional Animal Scientist*, vol. 21, no. 5, pp. 420–425, 2005.

[3] D. M. Weaver, J. W. Tyler, D. C. VanMetre, D. E. Hostetler, and G. M. Barrington, "Passive transfer of colostral immunoglobulins in calves," *Journal of Veterinary Internal Medicine*, vol. 14, no. 6, pp. 569–577, 2000.

[4] S. J. Wells, D. A. Dargatz, and S. L. Ott, "Factors associated with mortality to 21 days of life in dairy heifers in the United States," *Preventive Veterinary Medicine*, vol. 29, no. 1, pp. 9–19, 1996.

[5] S. M. McGuirk and M. Collins, "Managing the production, storage, and delivery of colostrum," *Veterinary Clinics of North America: Food Animal Practice*, vol. 20, no. 3, pp. 593–603, 2004.

[6] M. Chigerwe, J. W. Tyler, L. G. Schultz, J. R. Middleton, B. J. Steevens, and J. N. Spain, "Effect of colostrum administration by use of oroesophageal intubation on serum IgG concentrations in Holstein bull calves," *American Journal of Veterinary Research*, vol. 69, no. 9, pp. 1158–1163, 2008.

[7] S. M. Godden, D. M. Haines, K. Konkol, and J. Peterson, "Improving passive transfer of immunoglobulins in calves. II: interaction between feeding method and volume of colostrum fed," *Journal of Dairy Science*, vol. 92, no. 4, pp. 1758–1764, 2009.

[8] S. M. Godden, D. M. Haines, and D. Hagman, "Improving passive transfer of immunoglobulins in calves. I: dose effect of feeding a commercial colostrum replacer," *Journal of Dairy Science*, vol. 92, no. 4, pp. 1750–1757, 2009.

[9] J. L. Johnson, S. M. Godden, T. Molitor, T. Ames, and D. Hagman, "Effects of feeding heat-treated colostrum on passive transfer of immune and nutritional parameters in neonatal

dairy calves," *Journal of Dairy Science*, vol. 90, no. 11, pp. 5189–5198, 2007.

[10] A. L. Beam, J. E. Lombard, C. A. Kopral et al., "Prevalence of failure of passive transfer of immunity in newborn heifer calves and associated management practices on US dairy operations," *Journal of Dairy Science*, vol. 92, no. 8, pp. 3973–3980, 2009.

[11] NAHMS, *Heifer Calf Health and Management Practices on U.S. Dairy Operations, 2007*, USDA:APHIS:VS, 2010.

[12] P. Pithua, S. S. Aly, D. M. Haines et al., "Efficacy of feeding a lacteal-derived colostrum replacer or pooled maternal colostrum with a low IgG concentration for prevention of failure of passive transfer in dairy calves," *Journal of the American Veterinary Medical Association*, vol. 243, no. 2, pp. 277–282, 2013.

[13] P. Marnila and H. Korhonen, "Milk | Colostrum," in *Encyclopedia of Dairy Sciences*, J. W. Fuquay, Ed., pp. 591–597, Academic Press, 2nd edition, 2011.

[14] D. Levieux and A. Ollier, "Bovine immunoglobulin G, β-lactoglobulin, α-lactalbumin and serum albumin in colostrum and milk during the early post partum period," *Journal of Dairy Research*, vol. 66, no. 3, pp. 421–430, 1999.

[15] A. Tsioulpas, A. S. Grandison, and M. J. Lewis, "Changes in physical properties of bovine milk from the colostrum period to early lactation," *Journal of Dairy Science*, vol. 90, no. 11, pp. 5012–5017, 2007.

[16] G. H. Stott, W. A. Fleenor, and W. C. Kleese, "Colostral immunoglobulin concentration in two fractions of first milking postpartum and five additional milkings," *Journal of Dairy Science*, vol. 64, no. 3, pp. 459–465, 1981.

[17] O. O. Oyeniyi and A. G. Hunter, "Colostral constituents including immunoglobulins in the first three milkings postpartum," *Journal of Dairy Science*, vol. 61, no. 1, pp. 44–48, 1978.

[18] M. Chigerwe, M. E. Dawes, J. W. Tyler, J. R. Middleton, M. P. Moore, and D. M. Nagy, "Evaluation of a cow-side immunoassay kit for assessing IgG concentration in colostrum," *Journal of the American Veterinary Medical Association*, vol. 227, no. 1, pp. 129–131, 2005.

[19] K. M. Morrill, E. Conrad, A. Lago et al., "Nationwide evaluation of quality and composition of colostrum on dairy farms in the United States," *Journal of Dairy Science*, vol. 95, no. 7, pp. 3997–4005, 2012.

[20] S. Godden, "Colostrum management for dairy calves," *Veterinary Clinics of North America: Food Animal Practice*, vol. 24, no. 1, pp. 19–39, 2008.

[21] J. D. Arthington, M. B. Cattell, J. D. Quigley III, G. C. McCoy, and W. L. Hurley, "Passive immunoglobin transfer in newborn calves fed colostrum or spray-dried serum protein alone or as a supplement to colostrum of varying quality," *Journal of Dairy Science*, vol. 83, no. 12, pp. 2834–2838, 2000.

[22] A. P. Fidler, M. L. Alley, and G. W. Smith, "Short communication: serum immunoglobulin G and total protein concentrations in dairy calves fed a colostrum-replacement product," *Journal of Dairy Science*, vol. 94, no. 7, pp. 3609–3612, 2011.

[23] C. M. Jones, R. E. James, J. D. Quigley III, and M. L. McGilliard, "Influence of pooled colostrum or colostrum replacement on IgG and evaluation of animal plasma in milk replacer," *Journal of Dairy Science*, vol. 87, no. 6, pp. 1806–1814, 2004.

[24] K. P. Poulsen, A. L. Foley, M. T. Collins, and S. M. McGuirk, "Comparison of passive transfer of immunity in neonatal dairy calves fed colostrum or bovine serum-based colostrum replacement and colostrum supplement products," *Journal of

the American Veterinary Medical Association, vol. 237, no. 8, pp. 949–954, 2010.

[25] D. Priestley, J. H. Bittar, L. Ibarbia et al., "Effect of feeding maternal colostrum or plasma-derived or colostrum-derived colostrum replacer on passive transfer of immunity, health, and performance of preweaning heifer calves," *Journal of Dairy Science*, vol. 96, no. 5, pp. 3247–3256, 2013.

[26] H. Swan, S. Godden, R. Bey, S. Wells, J. Fetrow, and H. Chester-Jonest, "Passive transfer of immunoglobulin G and preweaning health in Holstein calves fed a commercial colostrum replacer," *Journal of Dairy Science*, vol. 90, no. 8, pp. 3857–3866, 2007.

[27] B. J. Chelack, P. S. Morley, and D. M. Haines, "Evaluation of methods for dehydration of bovine colostrum for total replacement of normal colostrum in calves," *The Canadian Veterinary Journal*, vol. 34, no. 7, pp. 407–412, 1993.

[28] J. D. Arthington, M. B. Cattell, and J. D. Quigley III, "Effect of dietary IgG source (colostrum, serum, or milk-derived supplement) on the efficiency of Ig absorption in newborn Holstein calves," *Journal of Dairy Science*, vol. 83, no. 7, pp. 1463–1467, 2000.

[29] D. M. Foster, G. W. Smith, T. R. Sanner, and G. V. Busso, "Serum IgG and total protein concentrations in dairy calves fed two colostrum replacement products," *Journal of the American Veterinary Medical Association*, vol. 229, no. 8, pp. 1282–1285, 2006.

[30] F. B. Garry, R. Adams, M. B. Cattell, and R. P. Dinsmore, "Comparison of passive immunoglobulin transfer to dairy calves fed colostrum or commercially available colostral-supplement products," *Journal of the American Veterinary Medical Association*, vol. 208, no. 1, pp. 107–110, 1996.

[31] G. W. Smith and D. M. Foster, "Short communication: absorption of protein and immunoglobulin G in calves fed a colostrum replacer," *Journal of Dairy Science*, vol. 90, no. 6, pp. 2905–2908, 2007.

[32] S. S. Aly, P. Pithua, J. D. Champagne et al., "A randomized controlled trial on preweaning morbidity, growth and mortality in Holstein heifers fed a lacteal-derived colostrum replacer or pooled maternal colostrum," *BMC Veterinary Research*, vol. 9, no. 1, article 168, 2013.

[33] School of Veterinary Medicine, University of Wisconsin and S. M. McGuirk, "Calf Health Scoring Chart," http://www.vetmed.wisc.edu/dms/fapm/fapmtools/8calf/calf_health_scoring_chart.pdf.

[34] J. D. Quigley III, J. J. Drewry, and K. R. Martin, "Estimation of plasma volume in Holstein and Jersey calves," *Journal of Dairy Science*, vol. 81, no. 5, pp. 1308–1312, 1998.

[35] M. Chigerwe, J. W. Tyler, D. W. Nagy, and J. R. Middleton, "Frequency of detectable serum IgG concentrations in precolostral calves," *American Journal of Veterinary Research*, vol. 69, no. 6, pp. 791–795, 2008.

[36] NAHMS, *Passive Transfer Status of Heifer Calves on U.S. Dairies, 1991-2007 Info Sheet*, USDA:APHIS:VS:CEAH:NAHMS, 2010.

[37] T. E. Besser, C. C. Gay, and L. Pritchett, "Comparison of three methods of feeding colostrum to dairy calves," *Journal of the American Veterinary Medical Association*, vol. 198, no. 3, pp. 419–422, 1991.

[38] G. H. Stott, D. B. Marx, B. E. Menefee, and G. T. Nightengale, "Colostral immunoglobulin transfer in calves II. The rate of absorption," *Journal of Dairy Science*, vol. 62, no. 11, pp. 1766–1773, 1979.

[39] M. A. Khan, D. M. Weary, and M. A. G. von Keyserlingk, "Invited review: effects of milk ration on solid feed intake, weaning, and performance in dairy heifers," *Journal of Dairy Science*, vol. 94, no. 3, pp. 1071–1081, 2011.

[40] P. C. Blanchard, "Diagnostics of dairy and beef cattle diarrhea," *Veterinary Clinics of North America: Food Animal Practice*, vol. 28, no. 3, pp. 443–464, 2012.

[41] T. E. Besser, A. E. Garmedia, T. C. McGuire, and C. C. Gay, "Effect of colostral immunoglobulin G1 and immunoglobulin M concentrations on immunoglobulin absorption in calves," *Journal of Dairy Science*, vol. 68, no. 8, pp. 2033–2037, 1985.

[42] G. H. Stott, D. B. Marx, B. E. Menefee, and G. T. Nightengale, "Colostral immunoglobulin transfer in calves. III. Amount of absorption," *Journal of Dairy Science*, vol. 62, no. 12, pp. 1902–1907, 1979.

[43] B. A. Hopkins and J. D. Quigley III, "Effects of method of colostrum feeding and colostrum supplementation on concentrations of immunoglobulin G in the serum of neonatal calves," *Journal of Dairy Science*, vol. 80, no. 5, pp. 979–983, 1997.

11

A Study on the Nature of Association between *Demodex* Mites and Bacteria Involved in Skin and Meibomian Gland Lesions of Demodectic Mange in Cattle

Mukhtar Taha Abu-Samra[1] and Yassir Adam Shuaib[2,3]

[1] *Department of Veterinary Medicine and Surgery, College of Veterinary Medicine (CVM), Sudan University of Science and Technology (SUST), P.O. Box 204, Hilat Kuku, Khartoum North, Sudan*
[2] *Department of Preventive Veterinary Medicine, College of Veterinary Medicine (CVM), Sudan University of Science and Technology (SUST), P.O. Box 204, Hilat Kuku, Khartoum North, Sudan*
[3] *Research Center Borstel, Parkallee 18, 23845 Borstel, Germany*

Correspondence should be addressed to Yassir Adam Shuaib; vet.aboamar@gmail.com

Academic Editor: Francesca Mancianti

The nature of association between *Demodex* mites and bacteria involved in bovine demodectic mange lesions and the normal flora inhabiting the skin of noninfected animals was investigated. *Demodex bovis* and *D. ghanensis* mites were isolated from the infected purulent material extracted from skin and meibomian gland lesions, respectively. The mites could not be demonstrated in skin brushings or impression smears from the eyes of noninfected cattle. Pathogenic bacteria (*Staphylococcus aureus* and *Streptococcus pyogenes* (Group A)) and opportunistic organisms (*Proteus vulgaris*, *Pseudomonas aeruginosa*, *Staphylococcus epidermidis*, and *Trueperella pyogenes*) were isolated from skin lesions of demodectic mange, and *Moraxella bovis* and *Staphylococcus aureus* were isolated from meibomian gland lesions. *Bacillus subtilis*, *Escherichia coli*, *Proteus vulgaris*, *Staphylococcus aureus*, *Staphylococcus epidermidis*, and *Streptococcus pyogenes* (Group A) were isolated from skin brushings from noninfected cattle. The nature of association between *Demodex* mites and bacteria in demodectic mange lesions is synergistic and of equal significance. Pathogenic and opportunistic bacteria facilitated the establishment of *Demodex* mites in the lesions produced and provided an excellent microclimate for the mites to propagate and reproduce, resulting in severe and progressive disease. The "high-turnover" granulomatous reaction which characterized the histopathological changes proved that *Demodex* mites and associated bacteria were persistent and immunogenic.

1. Introduction

Demodex belongs to a very specialized group of mites which live in the hair follicles and sebaceous glands of various mammals and man, causing demodectic or follicular mange [1–5]. Demodectic mange in cattle is caused by *Demodex bovis* (Stiles 1892) [1, 4]. Transmission usually occurs by direct contact from the dam to her offspring during nursing in the neonatal period and never between host animals of different species [6, 7].

The disease is characterized by the formation of papules, nodules, pustules, and cysts of varying sizes [3, 5, 8, 9].

The predilection sites of the lesions seemed to be the neck, withers, shoulders, and forequarters [3, 5, 9–11]. As the disease progressed, the lesions spread from their original sites to the rest of the body, and in severe infections, most of the skin became involved [7–9, 12]. Many cattle with demodectic mange might have no visible cutaneous lesions and the disease might pass unnoticed. In such cases, the lesions could only be detected by running the hand over the shoulders, axillae, brisket, and neck and by rolling the loose skin in the axillae and brisket between the thumb and other fingers [3, 5, 9, 13]. A satisfactory diagnosis of demodicosis could only be made by the demonstration of *Demodex* mites in the infected purulent material extracted from nodules and pustules [2, 5, 8, 9, 14].

Meibomian gland demodicosis was reported by a few workers [15–17]. Meibomian glands and eye infection with demodectic mange in cattle were associated with skin lesions of the disease and were never observed in cattle without skin lesions [16]. Some workers [15, 18–20] reported the occurrence of different species of *Demodex* mites in macerated or histological sections of the eyelids of clinically healthy cattle, while other workers [16, 17, 21] described a bilateral palpebral demodicosis with firm swellings in both eyelids. They added that the eyelids became thickened and resulted in blindness due to their physical closure.

The bacteria associated with the mites in demodectic mange lesions were regarded by some workers as secondary invaders [7, 9]. Some workers [22, 23] reported that the bacteria were introduced in the follicles by being carried on the exoskeleton or in the gut of the mite.

The invasion of a host by pathogenic bacteria may be aided by the production of bacterial extracellular substances (invasins) which act against the host by breaking down primary or secondary defenses of the body [24, 25]. Spreading factors are bacterial enzymes that affect the physical properties of tissue matrices and intercellular spaces, thereby promoting the spread of the pathogen [25].

Staphylococcus aureus and *Streptococcus pyogenes* were reported to produce a wide array of virulence factors in the form of exotoxins and enzymes that damaged host tissues; expressed many potential virulence factors such as surface proteins that promote colonization of host tissues; inhibit phagocytosis; provoke symptoms of disease; and possessed inherent and acquired resistance to antimicrobial agents [24–26].

Moraxella bovis caused infectious bovine keratoconjunctivitis, a devastating ocular disease of cattle which occurs worldwide [27]. The organism is an opportunistic pathogen whose virulence is influenced by both host and environmental factors. The virulence of *M. bovis* was attributed to fimbriae, which allowed adherence of the organisms to the cornea, and during replication, haemolysin and other lytic enzymes were produced playing a significant role in virulence [9, 24, 27–29].

Pseudomonas aeruginosa caused a wide range of opportunistic infections. Pathogenic strains of *P. aeruginosa* produced a variety of toxins and enzymes which promote tissue invasion and damage [24, 25]. Attachment to host cells is mediated by fimbriae. Colonization and replication are aided by antiphagocytic properties of exoenzyme S, extracellular slime, and outer membrane lipopolysaccharides. Resistance to complement-mediated damage and the ability to obtain iron from host tissues are additional virulence factors [24, 25].

Trueperella pyogenes (*Arcanobacterium pyogenes*) is one of the most common opportunistic pathogens of domestic ruminants, capable of producing suppurative lesions in any organ or tissue in animals. In farm animals, especially ruminants, it is the most common bacteria found in infected wounds and abscesses [30, 31]. *A. pyogenes* expressed several

known and putative virulence factors required for adherence, subsequent colonization, and host tissue damage [24, 31].

The pathology of the disease was described in different animals including man; in cattle [11, 32]; in the American bison [13]; in dogs [33, 34]; and in man [35, 36].

Previous workers have undermined the role played by bacteria in demodectic mange lesions by simply regarding them as secondary invaders. The current study is probably the first encounter on the nature of association of bacteria and *Demodex* mites in skin and meibomian gland lesions of demodectic mange. Studying the normal flora inhabiting the skin of normal noninfected cattle of the same herds is a crucial and prerequisite part of this investigation, as it represents an important integral part in the ecology of cattle skin. Moreover, the role played by bacteria in the severity and spread of the lesions of demodectic mange in relation to host parasite interactions is elucidated.

2. Materials and Methods

2.1. Animals. Three hundred cattle with skin and eye lesions suggestive of demodectic mange and 50 noninfected cattle belonging to the same herds were clinically examined and sampled to study the nature of association between *Demodex* mites and bacteria involved in the lesions of demodectic mange. Purulent infected material was extracted from skin and meibomian gland lesions using sterile techniques. Each specimen of infected material was divided into two parts. The first part of each specimen was kept in a sterile Bijou bottle and refrigerated for bacteriological investigations. The second part was kept in other Bijou bottles containing equal volumes of glycerol and ethanol for parasitological examination. Two sets of impression smears and swabs from the eyes of noninfected cattle were also collected and refrigerated. Bacteriological and parasitological investigations were also conducted on each of 200 specimens of skin brushings collected from noninfected cattle belonging to the same infected herds using a coarse brush. Skin biopsy specimens were collected from the infected and noninfected cattle following the technique described by Abu-Samra [37]. After being slaughtered, the upper and lower eyelids of the eyes from 25 cattle with eye infection and 10 noninfected ones were excised and removed. The biopsy and necropsy specimens were fixed in 10% formal saline.

2.2. Laboratory Investigations

2.2.1. Bacteriological Investigations. Two milliliters of sterile nutrient broth was added to the refrigerated infected material and skin brushings in each bottle, and two drops of sterile nutrient broth were placed on the swabs from the eyes of noninfected animals. The contents of the bottles were thoroughly mixed using a mechanical shaker. The procedures adopted for the preparation of culture media and media for biochemical tests were according to standard methods and techniques described by Barrow and Feltham [38]. Each of the specimens was cultured under aerobic, anaerobic, and increased carbon dioxide conditions at $37°C$ for 24–48 hours on the following media: nutrient agar [39], 5 percent sheep, bovine or horse blood enriched agar prepared from blood agar, McConkey's agar, and nutrient broth (Oxoid). Moreover, one set of the seeded blood enriched agar was incubated at $33°C$ in a humid chamber. Pure cultures were obtained through serial subcultures. The pure isolates were biochemically tested according to standard methods and techniques [38].

2.2.2. Parasitological Investigations. A small piece from each specimen of the infected purulent material was crushed between two microscope slides. Another piece from each specimen and a small amount of each specimen of skin brushings was placed in the middle of a microscope slide, a drop of 20 percent potassium hydroxide was added, and the preparations were gently heated and covered with coverslips. The two preparations were examined under the microscope. Individual mites were isolated and identified following the technique described by Abu-Samra et al. [40].

2.2.3. Histopathological Investigations. The biopsy and necropsy specimens were processed, embedded in paraffin wax, and sectioned at $5 \mu m$ prior to staining with Haematoxylin and Eosin stain and examined following standard methods and techniques described by Bancroft and Harry [41].

3. Results

3.1. Animals. Five forms of skin lesions were recognized. They were papules, nodules and papules, nodules and few pustules (Figure 1), pustules and few nodules or pustules, and crust-covered lesions (Figure 2). Table 1 summarizes the gross appearance of the five forms of skin lesions.

Themeibomian gland lesions were characterized by swelling of the eyelids, lacrimation, hyperaemia, and congestion of the mucous membranes, and in extreme cases by purulent exudation, swelling, and closure of the eyelids. Both eyelids showed 2–4 purulent nodules of 3-4 mm in diameter arranged in a linear fashion (Figure 3). Inspection of the eyes was much resented by the animals, and in the majority of animals, the lower eyelids were more affected and disfigured than the upper ones. Among the 300 cattle, 218 (72.7%) animals had simultaneous skin and meibomian gland lesions. The remaining 82 (27.3%) cattle had skin but no eye infection, and their eyes were free of any clinically detectable abnormality. None of the infected cattle had only meibomian gland lesions. All animals had severe pruritus and were persistently scratching, rubbing, licking or gnawing at the affected areas of the skin, and rubbing their eyes against their body.

Control noninfected cattle had no visible or palpable lesions after careful examination of the skin and eyes.

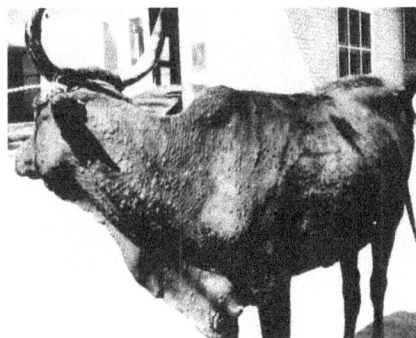

FIGURE 1: A cow infected with demodectic mange, showing pustules involving the neck, and nodules scattered over the whole body. Note folding of the skin at the base of the neck.

3.2. Laboratory Investigations

3.2.1. Bacteriological Findings

Skin Lesions. Culture of the 300 specimens of infected purulent material (Table 2) revealed growth of organisms from 252 specimens (84%) and no growth was obtained from the remaining 48 specimens (16%). Gram's stained smears from the cultures revealed the following: Gram-positive cocci in 136 cultures (54%), Gram-negative rods in 106 cultures (42%), and Gram-positive rods in the remaining 10 cultures (4%).

Meibomian Gland Lesions. Culture of 218 specimens of infected purulent material (Table 2) revealed growth of organisms from 128 specimens (58.7%) and no growth was obtained from the remaining 90 specimens (41.3%). Gram's stained smears from the cultures showed the following: Gram-negative diplobacilli occurring in pairs in 102 cultures (80%) and mixed Gram-negative diplobacilli and clusters of Gram-positive cocci in the remaining 26 cultures (20%).

Skin Brushings. Cultures of 200 skin brushings from noninfected cattle (Table 2) revealed growth of organisms from 156 specimens (78%) and no growth was obtained from cultures of the remaining 44 specimens (22%). Gram's stained smears from the cultures revealed Gram-positive cocci in 75 cultures (48%), Gram-positive rods in 57 cultures (36%), and Gram-negative rods in 24 cultures (16%).

Eye Impression Smears and Swabs. Gram's stained impression smears from the eyes of noninfected cattle showed insignificant numbers of microorganisms, and no growth was obtained from swab cultures.

Identification of the Isolates. The following bacteria were isolated and identified following the methods and techniques described by Barrow and Feltham [38]: *Bacillus subtilis, Escherichia coli, Moraxella bovis, Proteus vulgaris, Pseudomonas aeruginosa, Staphylococcus aureus, Staphylococcus epidermidis, Streptococcus pyogenes* (Group A), and *Trueperella (Arcanobacterium) pyogenes* (Table 2).

TABLE 1: Gross appearance of the five forms of skin lesions of demodectic mange in cattle.

Form of lesion	Gross appearance of lesions
Papules	Palpable papules, 1–3 mm in diameter, hard in consistency resembling sand grains, detected after running the hand over the shoulders, axillae, brisket, and neck and by rolling the loose skin in the axillae and brisket between the thumb and other fingers. When incised and squeezed, a small amount of white waxy material was expressed.
Nodules and papules	Visible nodules, 5–10 mm in diameter and 3-4 mm raised above the skin surface, and palpable papules. Nodules are in close association or scattered all over the body. Over some nodules small tufts of hair stood out from the general level of the hair coat. Nodules were firm in consistency and when squeezed a yellowish white material oozed in a single stream.
Nodules and few pustules	Visible nodules and few pustules. Pustules, 15–20 mm in diameter and 2-3 mm raised above the skin surface, majority devoid of hair, erythematous on unpigmented areas, less firm than nodules and when squeezed a yellowish white caseated or moist material tinged with blood oozed out in multiple streams.
Pustules and few nodules	Large indurated pustules and few nodules; pustules, 20–30 mm in diameter and 3-4 mm raised above the skin surface, devoid of hair, erythematous on unpigmented areas, fragile and when squeezed a yellowish white material tinged with blood oozed out in large amounts leaving tiny bleeding holes. The skin became thickened showing many wrinkles and folds.
Pustules and crust-covered lesions	Pustules, 20–40 mm in diameter and 2–4 mm raised above the skin surface, in close association, devoid of hair and covered with thin yellowish white crusts. Crust-covered lesions were typified by extensive patches covered with thin yellowish white or pale yellow crusts incorporated with tufts of matted hair. Crusts could easily be removed leaving tiny but visible holes in the skin. The skin became thickened showing many wrinkles and folds.

TABLE 2: Number of bacterial isolates from skin brushings from noninfected cattle and number of isolates from skin and meibomian gland lesions of demodectic mange.

Bacteria isolated	Noninfected cattle Skin brushings	Infected cattle Skin lesions	Meibomian gland lesions
Bacillus subtilis	57	—	—
Escherichia coli	9	—	—
Moraxella bovis	—	—	102
Proteus vulgaris	15	58	—
Pseudomonas aeruginosa	—	48	—
Staphylococcus aureus	33	80	26[*]
Staphylococcus epidermidis	16	34	—
Streptococcus pyogenes (Group A)	26	22	—
Trueperella pyogenes[**]	—	10	—
Total	156	252	128

[*] Mixed *Moraxella bovis* and *Staphylococcus aureus*.
[**] Formerly (*Arcanobacterium pyogenes*, *Actinomyces pyogenes*, and *Corynebacterium pyogenes*).

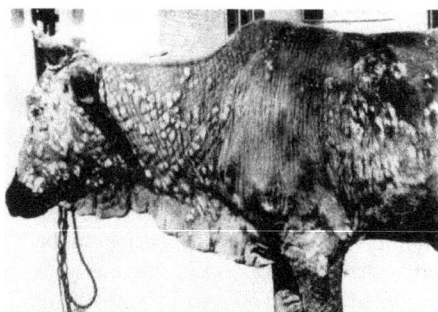

FIGURE 2: Pustules and crust-covered lesions of demodectic mange involving extensive areas of the body of a heifer. Note marked wrinkling and folding of the skin.

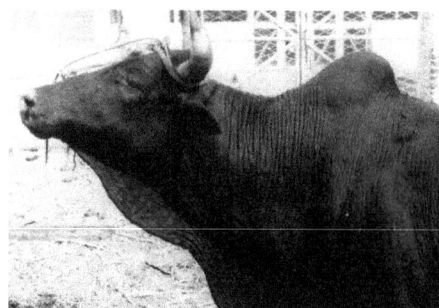

FIGURE 3: Simultaneous skin and meibomian gland demodicosis. Note swelling of the eyelids and nodules on the upper eyelid arranged in a linear fashion.

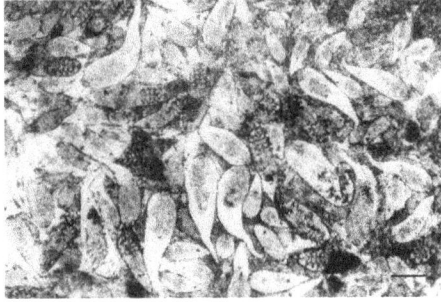

FIGURE 4: Numerous *Demodex bovis* mites and its different developmental stages, pus, and cell debris in a crushed specimen of infected purulent material extracted from skin lesions of demodectic mange. Scale bar: 70 μm.

3.2.2. Parasitological Findings

Skin Lesions. Examination of crushed infected material showed numerous different developmental stages of *Demodex* mites, pus, and cell debris (Figure 4). Eggs, larvae, nymphs, and adult mites were seen in 20 percent potassium hydroxide preparations. The mites were isolated and identified as *Demodex bovis*. They are elongated, gently tapered, and cigar-shaped.

Meibomian Gland Lesions. Findings similar to those recorded for skin lesions were observed. However, *Demodex* mites and their different developmental stages were much less than those observed in infected material from skin lesions. The mites were identified as *Demodex ghanensis* (Figure 5). They are long, slender, and gradually tapered to a sharp pointed terminus.

Skin Brushings. Examination of the 200 specimens of skin brushings from noninfected cattle, in 20 percent potassium hydroxide, was negative for *Demodex mites*.

Eye Impression Smears. Examination of the 50 eye impression smears from noninfected cattle in 20 percent potassium hydroxide was negative for *Demodex* mites.

3.2.3. Histopathological Findings.

Demodex bovis mites invaded the corium through the orifices of the hair follicles (Figure 6) and *D. ghanensis* invaded the meibomian glands through the orifices of the main collecting tubules (Figure 7). The mechanical movement of the mites through the hair follicles and meibomian glands caused severe irritation, the persistent cutting and feeding of the mite on the epithelium of hair follicles and main collecting tubules of the meibomian glands and their secretions, excretions, and somatic debris resulted in inflammation and dilatation of the orifices of the hair follicles and main collecting tubules of the meibomian glands. This paved the way for active or passive introduction of pathogenic bacteria in the hair follicles and meibomian glands (*Staphylococcus aureus*, *Moraxella bovis*, and *Streptococcus pyogenes* Group A). These pathogenic organisms produced an array of invasins (toxins and enzymes) that break down primary and secondary defenses and produced allergic reactions causing severe irritation and pruritus resulting in scratching, rubbing, licking, or gnawing at the affected areas of the skin and eyes. This produced more inflammation, wounds, and damage of the affected areas in the skin and meibomian glands. The reaction became more severe as the result of invasion of the devitalized structures in the skin and meibomian glands by commensal and opportunistic pathogens (*Proteus vulgaris*, *Pseudomonas aeruginosa*, and *Trueperella pyogenes*). These organisms also possessed an array of virulence factors, invaded damaged tissues, and produced a suppurative reaction. Thus, the bacteria had created a suitable microclimate for the establishment and rapid replication of *Demodex bovis* and *D. ghanensis* mites in the skin and meibomian gland lesions, respectively. Maximum distension of the hair follicles with mites, bacteria, pus, secretions, and excretions resulted in the transformation of the hair follicles to cylindrical or saccular bladder-like cysts (Figure 8) and dilatation of the main collecting tubules of the meibomian glands (Figure 7). This is exacerbated by the toxins and enzymes produced by the bacteria, and the continuous cutting and feeding of the epithelium of the distended hair follicles and main collecting tubules of the meibomian glands by the mites resulted in damage of these structures and liberation of the mites and primary pathogenic bacteria in the subepidermal and upper dermal layers of the skin and the glandular acini and surrounding connective tissue of the meibomian glands (Figure 9). This resulted in hemorrhage, infiltration by inflammatory cells, and evolved "high-turnover" granulomas with influx of macrophages and lymphocytes. Typical granulomas were seen in areas where mites, bacteria, and purulent exudate congregated (Figure 9). The damaged hair follicles and meibomian gland acini were surrounded by connective tissue, giant and epithelioid cells in the inner layers, and macrophages, lymphocytes, plasma cells, and few eosinophils in the outer layers. The degenerated mites and associated bacteria were engulfed and digested by the giant cells, resulting in regression and later healing of the lesions as judged by the progressive proliferation of connective tissue and degeneration of the granulomatous reaction in different areas of the same section or in different sections.

Sections from the skin and eyelids of noninfected cattle were normal and showed no histopathological changes.

4. Discussion

Demodex bovis and *D. ghanensis* mites had initiated infection by invading the skin through the orifices of the hair follicles and meibomian glands through the main collecting tubules of the meibomian glands, respectively. They caused inflammation that resulted in dilatation of the orifices of these structures and paved the way for active and/or passive introduction of primary pathogenic bacteria and opportunistic pathogens in the skin and meibomian glands, producing their deleterious damaging effects.

Bacillus subtilis and *Escherichia coli* were only isolated from skin brushings from noninfected cattle and seemed to

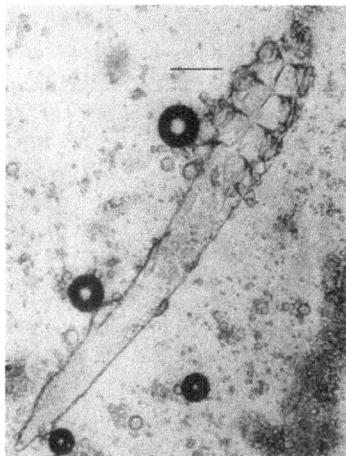

FIGURE 5: *Demodex ghanensis* mite in infected material extracted from meibomian gland lesions of demodectic mange in a cow. 20% potassium hydroxide solution. Scale bar: 50 μm.

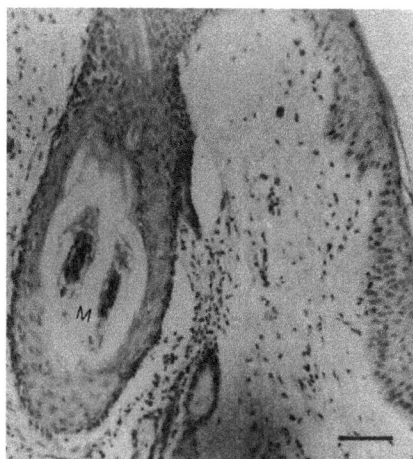

FIGURE 7: Sections from the eyelid of a cow, showing invasion of the meibomian gland with *Demodex ghanensis*. Note hemorrhage, exudation, and damage of the proximal part of the main collecting tubule (asterisks), marked infiltration with inflammatory cells, dilatation of the main collecting tubules, and *Demodex ghanensis* mite in the main collecting tubule (black arrow). Haematoxylin and Eosin. Scale bar: 120 μm.

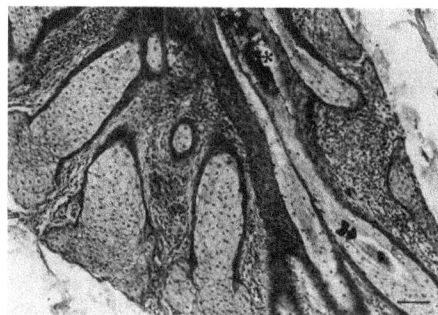

FIGURE 6: Section from the skin of a cow, showing invasion of a hair follicle with *Demodex bovis*. Note dilatation of the hair follicle bulb, mites (M), and slight infiltration by inflammatory cells in close proximity of the hair follicle. Haematoxylin and Eosin. Scale bar: 100 μm

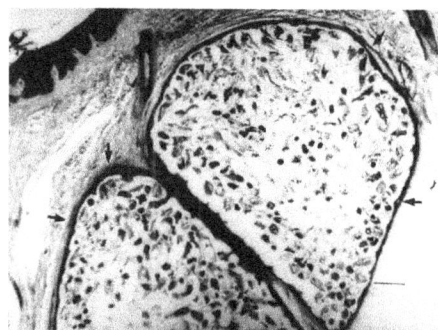

FIGURE 8: Saccular distension of adjacent hair follicles with *Demodex bovis* mites and associated bacteria, forming large colonies of demodectic mange (bladder-like cysts) in skin sections from an infected cow. Note extremely stretched and jagged epithelial lining (black arrows). Haematoxylin and Eosin. Scale bar: 200 μm.

have no role to play in demodectic mange lesions. The former organism is nonpathogenic and is naturally found in soil and vegetation, and the latter existed in the animals' surroundings as it is commonly found in the lower intestine of warm-blooded organisms [24, 25].

Proteus vulgaris, *Staphylococcus aureus*, *Staphylococcus epidermidis*, and *Streptococcus pyogenes* (Group A) were isolated from the infected purulent material extracted from skin lesions of infected cattle and from skin brushings from noninfected cattle. These bacteria had probably chosen the skin surface as a natural habitat, were intestinal flora existing in the animals' surroundings as reported by some workers [9, 24, 25], and/or originated from bladder cysts of demodectic mange which opened towards the exterior liberating their contents on the skin surface of infected animals and resulted

in spread of infection as well as contaminating the surroundings, as was reported by other workers [7, 9, 11, 42, 43]. After being actively or passively introduced in the inflamed and dilated hair follicles, pathogenic bacteria produced an array of invasins (toxins and enzymes) that broke down primary and secondary defenses of the body and produced allergic reactions causing severe irritation and pruritus resulting in scratching, rubbing, licking, or gnawing at the affected areas of the skin and evoked severe inflammation, wounds, and damage of the affected areas. These findings confirmed the reports of some workers [25, 26] who enumerated the toxins and enzymes (virulence factors) produced by these organisms which acted against the host by breaking down primary or secondary defenses of the body, aggravating the lesions, and caused marked deterioration of the skin.

Pseudomonas aeruginosa and *Trueperella* (*Arcanobacterium*) *pyogenes* were only isolated from skin lesions of demodectic mange and were not isolated from skin brushings of noninfected cattle. The former organism usually infected damaged tissues or tissues with reduced immunity, while the latter is one of the most common opportunistic pathogens of

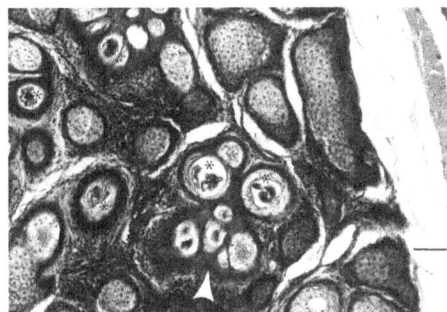

FIGURE 9: Section from an infected meibomian gland, showing *D. ghanensis* mites (asterisks) in the glandular acini, granulomatous reactions in the infected acini, and proliferation of connective tissue surrounding the granulomas (white arrow head). Haematoxylin and Eosin. Scale bar: 200 μm.

domestic ruminants capable of producing suppurative lesions in any organ or tissue in farm animals. Many workers [25, 30, 31] reported that these organisms produced a suppurative reaction and possessed multiple virulence factors that were instrumental in producing serious damage resulting in marked deterioration of tissues. These organisms caused more damage of the skin lesions and resulted in maximum distension and rupture of the hair follicles resulting in partial or complete liberation of their contents in the surrounding connective tissue resulting in severe pathological changes and evolved "high-turnover" granulomas with influx of macrophages and lymphocytes.

Moraxella bovis and *Staphylococcus aureus* were isolated from the infected material extracted from meibomian gland lesions. However, these organisms could not be demonstrated in impression smears or isolated in swab cultures from the eyes of noninfected cattle. This proved that the two organisms did not exist as natural inhabitants of the eyes of noninfected cattle. *Moraxella bovis* is an opportunistic pathogen whose virulence is influenced by both host and environmental factors. *Moraxella bovis* might have been acquired from the animals' surroundings being contaminated by ocular discharges from cattle infected with infectious keratoconjunctivitis, while *Staphylococcus aureus* might have been acquired from the skin when the animals scratched or rubbed their irritated eyes against their bodies. *Moraxella bovis* was reported to be of high morbidity (80%), reaching epizootic proportions when transmission agents (*Musca autumnalis* flies, dust and long grass contaminated by ocular discharges from infected cattle) became available [9]. The pathogenesis of this bacterium was described by many workers [27–29, 44] who reported that it adhered to the cells via its fimbriae and pili proteins, produced β-haemolysin toxins which lysed the corneal epithelial cells, and secreted cytotoxic toxin and pathogenic fibrinolysin, phosphatase, hyaluronidase, and aminopeptidases.

Failure to isolate bacteria from 48 specimens (16%) of purulent material extracted from skin lesions of demodectic mange and from 90 specimens (41.3%) of purulent material extracted from meibomian gland lesions was probably due to the destruction of the bacteria by the degenerative and

reparative reaction of the high turn-over granulomatous reaction (humoral and cellular responses). The isolation of the mites (*D. bovis* and *D. ghanensis*) from the same specimens was probably due to the chitinous exoskeleton of these mites making them resilient and resistant and would take a longer time to be destroyed, engulfed, and digested by the macrophages and giant cells.

Demodex bovis mites were demonstrated and isolated from all specimens of infected material extracted from skin lesions. However, the mite was not encountered in any of the skin brushings from noninfected animals. This finding proved that *Demodex bovis* mites did not exist as normal inhabitants of the skin of healthy normal cattle and was contrary to the findings of many workers [9, 13, 16, 22, 32, 33, 35, 45–47] who reported the existence of different species of *Demodex* mites in harmony with the host and/or commensals as part of the cutaneous flora on the skin of different species of animals and man. Similarly, *Demodex ghanensis* mites were isolated from all specimens of infected material extracted from meibomian gland lesions but could not be demonstrated in impression smears from the eyes or histological sections from the eyelids of noninfected cattle. This finding also proved that *D. ghanensis* mites did not exist as natural inhabitants of the eyes or eyelids of noninfected cattle and was also contrary to the findings of early investigators [15, 18–20, 48] who reported that the mites were demonstrated in macerated and histological sections of the eyelids of clinically healthy cattle.

The isolation of only *D. bovis* from skin lesions and only *D. ghanensis* from meibomian gland lesions of the same animal was of interest and was subject to speculation. The most probable explanation to this finding was that *Demodex* mites have remarkable adaptation to match their unique environment and that each species of mite possessed distinct anatomical structures that enabled them to pave their way through their habitat and become well established and reproduced. This finding disagreed with the findings of many workers [32, 48, 49] who isolated *D. ghanensis*, *D. bovis*, and a demodicid shorter than *D. bovis* from the meibomian glands of the same animal (cattle), thus establishing the phenomenon of synhospitality.

In both skin and meibomian gland lesions, the histopathological changes seen were compatible with cell-mediated immunity. This was in agreement with the report of a previous investigator [50] who reported that on the basis of histopathological investigations, an immunological response to the parasite seemed to be implied. In the current study the destruction caused by the mites and associated bacteria resulted in a typical granulomatous reaction. The central core of infection composed of mites, bacteria, and purulent exudate was infiltrated by neutrophils and a few eosinophils and surrounded by lymphocytes, macrophages, epithelioid, giant cells, and proliferation of connective tissue. The giant cells engulfed, destroyed, and digested the mites and bacteria, resulting in healing of the lesions as judged by the progressive proliferation of connective tissue and degeneration of the granulomatous reaction in different areas of the same sections or in different sections. This reaction proved that *Demodex* mites and associated bacteria were both persistent and immunogenic producing severe, progressive, and generalized disease as was observed in natural field cases. These findings were in agreement with other workers [51, 52] who reported that when the inflammatory agent was both persistent and antigenic a "high-turnover" granuloma evolved with influx of macrophages and lymphocytes.

5. Conclusion

It was concluded that the nature of association between *Demodex* mites and bacteria in demodectic mange lesions is synergistic and of equal significance. Most of the bacteria involved in the lesions possessed an array of virulence factors (toxins and enzymes) causing severe skin and meibomian gland deterioration and damage facilitating the establishment of *Demodex* mites in the lesions produced and provided an excellent microclimate for the mites to propagate and reproduce, resulting in a severe and progressive disease as observed in natural field cases. Furthermore, the "high-turnover" granulomatous reaction which characterized the histopathological changes proved that *Demodex* mites and associated primary pathogenic bacteria are both persistent and immunogenic.

Conflict of Interests

The authors declare that there is no conflict of interests regarding the publication of this paper.

Acknowledgments

The authors are indebted to the Agricultural Research Council, National Council for Research, Khartoum, Sudan, for the generous support of this work. Dr. W. N. Beesley, formerly Head of Department of Veterinary Parasitology, Liverpool School of Tropical Medicine, UK, is gratefully acknowledged for his interest in this work and for the confirmation of the identification of *Demodex bovis* mites. The confirmation of the identification of *D. bovis* and *D. ghanensis* mites by the late Professor W. B. Nutting, Department of Zoology, University of Massachusetts, USA, is highly appreciated and acknowledged with thanks.

References

[1] J. Kaufmann, *Parasitic Infections of Domestic Animals: A Diagnostic Manual*, Birkhäuser, Berlin, Germany, 1996.

[2] OIE, "Mange," Terrestrial Manual, Chapter 2. 9. 8., 2013.

[3] D. W. Scott, *Color Atlas of Farm Animal Dermatology*, Blackwell Australia Publishing, 1st edition, 2007.

[4] E. J. L. Soulsby, *Helminths, Arthropods and Protozoa of Domesicated Animals*, Bailliere Tindall, London, UK, 7th edition, 1982.

[5] G. M. Urquhart, J. Armour, J. L. Duncan, A. M. Dunn, and F. W. Jennings, *Veterinary Parasitology*, Blackwell, 2nd edition, 2010.

[6] W. F. Fisher, R. W. Miller, and A. L. Everett, "Natural transmission of Demodex bovis to dairy calves," *Veterinary Parasitology*, vol. 7, pp. 233–241, 1980.

[7] K. Y. Jubb, F. C. Kennedy, and C. Palmers, *Pathology of Domestic Animals*, vol. 1, Saunders Elsevier, 5th edition, 2007.

[8] M. T. Abu-Samra, A. K. Mahgoub, and W. N. Beesley, "Demodicosis in Sudanese cattle," *Transactions of the Royal Society of Tropical Medicine and Hygiene*, vol. 78, p. 271, 1984.

[9] O. M. Radostits, C. C. Gay, K. W. Hinchcliff, and P. D. Constable, *Veterinary Medicine: A Textbook of the Diseases of Cattle, Horses, Sheep, Pigs and Goats*, Elsevier Saunders, Edinburgh, Scotland, 10th edition, 2007.

[10] M. T. Abu-Samra, S. E. Imbabi, and E. S. Mahgoub, "Mange in domestic animals in the Sudan," *Annals of Tropical Medicine and Parasitology*, vol. 75, no. 6, pp. 627–637, 1981.

[11] H. F. Matthes, "Investigations of pathogenesis of cattle demodicosis: sites of predilection, habitat and dynamics of demodectic nodules," *Veterinary Parasitology*, vol. 53, no. 3-4, pp. 283–291, 1994.

[12] W. F. Fisher, "Natural transmission of Demodex bovis Stiles in cattle." *Journal of Parasitology*, vol. 59, no. 1, pp. 223–224, 1973.

[13] J. G. Vestweber, R. K. Ridley, J. C. Nietfeld, and M. J. Wilkerson, "Demodicosis in an American bison," *Canadian Veterinary Journal*, vol. 40, no. 6, pp. 417–418, 1999.

[14] A. Milnes, S. Mitchell, and S. Bell, "Emerging skin conditions in cattle," *In Practice*, vol. 34, no. 10, pp. 588–597, 2012.

[15] V. Bukva, "Demodex tauri sp.N. (Acari: Demodicidae), a new parasite of cattle," *Folia Parasitologica*, vol. 33, no. 4, pp. 363–369, 1986.

[16] T. Fantahun, T. Yigzaw, and M. Chanie, "Bovine demodecosis: treat to leather industry in Ethiopia," *Asian Journal of Agricultural Sciences*, vol. 4, pp. 314–318, 2012.

[17] M. S. Gearhart, J. W. Crissman, and M. E. Georgi, "Bilateral lower palpebral demodicosis in a dairy cow," *The Cornell Veterinarian*, vol. 71, no. 3, pp. 305–310, 1981.

[18] C. A. Himonas, J. T. Theodorides, and A. E. Alexakis, "Demodectic mites in eyelids of domestic animals in Greece," *Journal of Parasitology*, vol. 61, no. 4, p. 767, 1975.

[19] W. B. Nutting, P. R. Kettle, J. D. Tenquist, and L. K. Whitten, "Hair follicle mites (Demodex Spp.) in New Zealand," *New Zealand Journal of Zoology*, vol. 2, pp. 219–222, 1975.

[20] H. Rak and R. Rahgozar, "Demodectic mange in the eyelid of domestic ruminants in Iran," *Bulletin de la Societe de Pathologie Exotique et de ses Filiales*, vol. 68, no. 6, pp. 591–593, 1975.

[21] G. O. Esuruoso, "Bovine demodicosis in Southern Nigeria," *Bulletin of Animal Health and Production in Africa*, vol. 25, pp. 65–72, 1977.

[22] F. P. English, T. Iwamoto, R. W. Darrell, and A. G. DeVoe, "The vector potential of Demodex folliculorum," *Archives of Ophthalmology*, vol. 84, no. 1, pp. 83–85, 1970.

[23] W. B. Nutting, "Hair follicle mites (Demodex spp.) of medical and veterinary concern," *Cornell Veterinarian*, vol. 66, no. 2, pp. 214–231, 1976.

[24] P. J. Quinn, B. K. Markey, M. E. Carter, W. J. Donnelly, and F. C. Leonard, *Veterinary Microbiology and Microbial Disease*, Iowa State University Press, Ames, Iowa, USA, 1st edition, 2002.

[25] K. Todar, *Todar's Online Textbook of Bacteriology*, Wisconsin, Madison, Wis, USA, 2012.

[26] A. L. Bisno, M. O. Brito, and C. M. Collins, "Molecular basis of group A streptococcal virulence," *The Lancet Infectious Diseases*, vol. 3, no. 4, pp. 191–200, 2003.

[27] M. H. Brown, A. H. Brightman, B. W. Fenwick, and M. A. Rider, "Infectious bovine keratoconjunctivitis: a review," *Journal of Veterinary Internal Medicine*, vol. 12, no. 4, pp. 259–266, 1998.

[28] H. J. Davidson and G. L. Stokka, "A field trial of autogenous Moraxella bovis bacterin administered through either subcutaneous or subconjunctival injection on the development of keratoconjunctivitis in a beef herd," *Canadian Veterinary Journal*, vol. 44, no. 7, pp. 577–580, 2003.

[29] J. J. Webber and L. A. Selby, "Risk factors related to the prevalence of infectious bovine keratoconjunctivitis," *Journal of the American Veterinary Medical Association*, vol. 179, no. 8, pp. 823–826, 1981.

[30] M. D. Collins and C. S. Cummins, "Genus corynebacterium lehmann and neumann 1896, 350AL," in *Bergey's Manual of Systematic Bacteriology*, P. H. A. Sneath, N. S. Mair, M. E. Sharpe, and J. G. Holt, Eds., vol. 2, pp. 1266–1276, Williams & Wilkins, Baltimore, Md, USA, 1986.

[31] B. H. Jost and S. J. Billington, "*Arcanobacterium pyogenes*: molecular pathogenesis of an animal opportunist," *Antonie van Leeuwenhoeky*, vol. 88, no. 2, pp. 87–102, 2005.

[32] J. Slingenbergh, A. N. Mohammed, and S. A. Bida, "Studies on bovine demodecosis in Northern Nigeria," *The Veterinary Quarterly*, vol. 2, no. 2, pp. 90–94, 1980.

[33] R. S. Aujla, L. D. Singla, P. D. Juyal, and P. P. Gupta, "Prevalence and pathology of mange-mite infestations in dogs," *Journal of Veterinary Parasitology*, vol. 14, pp. 45–49, 2000.

[34] N. K. Sood, B. Mekkib, L. D. Singla, and K. Gupta, "Cytopathology of parasitic dermatitis in dogs," *Journal of Parasitic Diseases*, vol. 36, no. 1, pp. 73–77, 2012.

[35] B. Baima and M. Sticherling, "Demodicidosis revisited," *Acta Dermato-Venereologica*, vol. 82, no. 1, pp. 3–6, 2002.

[36] J. B. Bikowski and J. Q. Del Rosso, "Demodex dermatitis: a retrospective analysis of clinical diagnosis and successful treatment with topical crotamiton," *Journal of Clinical and Aesthetic Dermatology*, vol. 2, no. 1, pp. 20–25, 2009.

[37] M. T. Abu-Samra, "A new skin biopsy technique in domestic animals," *Zentralblatt für Veterinarmedizin A*, vol. 27, no. 7, pp. 614–617, 1980.

[38] G. I. Barrow and R. K. A. Feltham, *Cowan and Steel's Manual for the Identification of Medical Bacteria*, Cambridge University Press, 3rd edition, 1993.

[39] E. Y. Bridson, *Oxoid Manual Compiled*, Oxoid Ltd., 8th edition, 1998.

[40] M. Abu-Samra, M. A. R. Abdel Aziz, and A. K. M. M. Salih, "A new technique for the isolation of *Demodex bovis* from preserved infected material," *Annals of Tropical Medicine and Parasitology*, vol. 78, no. 3, pp. 319–321, 1984.

[41] J. D. Bancroft and C. C. Harry, *Manual of Histological Techniques and Their Diagnostic Application*, Longman, Singapore, 2nd edition, 1994.

[42] N. R. Krieg and L. G. Holt, "The Gram-negatives of general medical, or industrial importance," in *Bergyes Manual of Systematic Bacteriology*, vol. 1, Williams and Wilkins, Baltimore, Md, USA, 1984.

[43] P. H. A. Sneath, N. S. Mair, M. E. Sharpe, and J. G. Holt, "The Gram-positives other than Actinomyctes," in *Bergy's Manual of Systematic Bacteriology*, vol. 2, Williams and Wilkins, Baltimore, Md, USA, 1986.

[44] J. F. Hess and J. A. Angelos, "The *Moraxella bovis* RTX toxin locus mbx defines a pathogenicity island," *Journal of Medical Microbiology*, vol. 55, no. 4, pp. 443–449, 2006.

[45] M. J. Marples, *The Ecology of the Human Skin*, Charles C. Thomas, Springfield, Ill, USA, 1965.

[46] G. H. Muller and R. W. Kirk, *Small Animal Dermatology*, W.B. Saunders, Philadelphia, Pa, USA, 2nd edition, 1975.

[47] S. K. Singh, M. Kumar, R. K. Jadhav, and S. K. Saxenab, "An update on therapeutic management of canine demodicosis," *Veterinary World*, vol. 4, no. 1, pp. 41–44, 2011.

[48] K. P. Baker, "*Demodex* SPP. in the meibomian glands of Irish cattle," *Veterinary Record*, vol. 92, no. 26, pp. 699–700, 1973.

[49] E. N. W. Oppong, R. P. Lee, and S. A. Yasin, "*Demodex ghanensis Sp. Nov.* (Acari-Demodicidae) parasitic on West Africa cattle," *Ghana Journal of Science*, vol. 15, pp. 39–43, 1975.

[50] T. Rufli and Y. Mumcuoglu, "The hair follicle mites *Demodex folliculorum* and *Demodex* brevis: biology and medical importance. A review," *Dermatologica*, vol. 162, no. 1, pp. 1–11, 1981.

[51] H. M. Dick, P. Wilkinson, and S. Powis, "The normal immune system," in *Topley and Wilsons' Principles of Bacteriology, Virology and Immunity*, G. Wilson and H. M. Dick, Eds., vol. 1 of *General Micobiology and Immunity*, pp. 296–318, Edward Arnold, London, UK, 7th edition, 1983.

[52] R. G. Thomson, *General Veterinary Pathology*, W.B. Saunders, Philadelphia, Pa, USA, 1978.

12

A Retrospective Analysis of 5,195 Patient Treatment Sessions in an Integrative Veterinary Medicine Service: Patient Characteristics, Presenting Complaints, and Therapeutic Interventions

Justin Shmalberg[1] and Mushtaq A. Memon[2]

[1]Small Animal Clinical Sciences, College of Veterinary Medicine, University of Florida, Gainesville, FL 32608, USA
[2]Department of Veterinary Clinical Sciences, College of Veterinary Medicine, Washington State University, Pullman, WA 99164, USA

Correspondence should be addressed to Justin Shmalberg; shmalberg@ufl.edu

Academic Editor: Pedro J. Ginel

Integrative veterinary medicine, the combination of complementary and alternative therapies with conventional care, is increasingly prevalent in veterinary practice and a focus of clinical instruction in many academic teaching institutions. However, the presenting complaints, therapeutic modalities, and patient population in an integrative medicine service have not been described. A retrospective analysis of 5,195 integrative patient treatment sessions in a veterinary academic teaching hospital demonstrated that patients most commonly received a combination of therapeutic modalities (39% of all treatment sessions). The 274 patients receiving multiple modalities were most frequently treated for neurologic and orthopedic disease (50.7% versus 49.6% of all presenting complaints, resp.). Older neutered or spayed dogs (mean age = 9.0 years) and Dachshunds were treated more often than expected based on general population statistics. Acupuncture, laser therapy, electroacupuncture, and hydrotherapy were frequently administered (>50% patients). Neurologic patients were more likely to receive acupuncture, electroacupuncture, and therapeutic exercises but less likely than orthopedic patients to receive laser, hydrotherapy, or therapeutic ultrasound treatments ($P < 0.05$). The results suggest that the application of these specific modalities to orthopedic and neurologic diseases should be subjected to increased evidence-based investigations. A review of current knowledge in core areas is presented.

1. Introduction

Integrative medicine describes an increasingly popular form of medicine combining conventional medical practice with alternative or complementary therapies, which is based on the best available scientific evidence [1]. Alternative or complementary therapies are broadly defined in human medical practice but may include nutrition, acupuncture, laser therapy, hyperbaric oxygen, rehabilitation, and other interventions not typically considered mainstream medical practice. Integrative *veterinary* medicine is poorly described both in definition and in practice although the term occasionally appears in the scientific literature [2]. However, a similar definition as to that used in integrative human medical practice characterizes the concept in veterinary medicine. Alternate and historical terms used to describe unconventional therapies inadequately distort the purpose of such treatments. Alternative veterinary medicine suggests that certain therapies are a replacement or a mutually exclusive option to conventional care, which disregards the potential for synergistic effects. Complementary medicine implies that the therapies can and should only be used in tandem, when in some cases a modality may be the preferred or exclusive treatment available. Finally, holistic medicine suggests that conventional veterinary practice does not consider the impacts of treatment on the whole animal, an obviously flawed assumption.

The prevalence of integrative medical interventions in veterinary medicine has not been established. A survey of owners of veterinary oncology patients found a robust usage of therapies regarded as alternative or complementary [3]. A survey of one school's veterinary graduates identified that more than two-thirds of these veterinarians encountered clinical situations involving these therapies at least monthly and over 25% experienced them on a weekly or daily basis [4]. These findings served as a framework for that study's authors to suggest, with evidence from surveys of AVMA-accredited colleges of veterinary medicine, that a comprehensive curriculum should be available to veterinary students. The need for education and information in integrative medicine is highlighted by the fact that nearly one-third of the general population has used a complementary or alternative medical approach for their own health [5].

The purpose of this study was to retrospectively evaluate the caseload from within a busy academic integrative veterinary medicine service to determine the frequency with which specific modalities were used and the relationships of such modalities to presenting complaint, breed, age, and other factors. Study findings provide critical information to other integrative medicine services and for researchers investigating specific modalities within the scope of the service's practice. Future randomized controlled trials are needed to further evaluate a number of the modalities.

2. Material and Methods

The electronic medical records were collected from a mixed animal integrative medicine service at an academic teaching hospital over a 400-day period from July 2014 to August 2015. The total number of patient visits in each hospital service was tabulated. The presenting complaints for integrative medicine visits were recorded along with the species of patient, body condition score, outpatient or inpatient status, and the date of treatment.

The records of small animal patients receiving more than one therapeutic modality at a visit were further analyzed to determine whether each patient had seen another service in the 6 months before treatment and to calculate the number of integrative visits for each patient. If patients were seen more than once during the retrospective period, a visit was randomly selected to determine which therapeutic modalities the patient received.

The differences between groups were evaluated using one-way ANOVA and commercially available statistical software (Minitab 17.1). Results were considered statistically significant if the probability of error was less than 5% ($P <$ 0.05). Post hoc analysis was performed with Fisher's test for pairwise comparisons. Odds ratios were calculated, using commercial software (Microsoft Excel 2010), to assess if specific patient populations, grouped by condition or breed, had a different likelihood of receiving each modality or of presenting with a particular complaint. A result was considered statistically significant if the 95% confidence interval for the odds ratio excluded the value 1.0. The Pearson correlation coefficients (r) were calculated for the potential relationships between age, body weight, number of treatments, and the number of modalities used for each patient; results were considered significant if $P <$ 0.05.

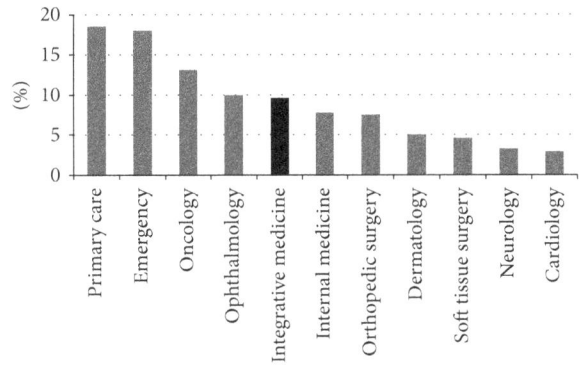

FIGURE 1: Comparative caseload of the study site's Academic Veterinary Hospital.

3. Results

The integrative medicine service attended to 5,195 patient treatment sessions during the study period. The distribution of species from greatest to least was as follows: dogs (95.6%), cats (3.0%), horses (0.8%), and exotic species or wildlife (0.6%). The majority of these cases were managed as outpatients (90.2%), with the remainder receiving inpatient treatment (9.8%) over an average inpatient rehabilitation period of 3.0 days. Recorded treatments included those performed during business hours (93.3%) and after hours (6.7%). The integrative medicine service received 9.6% of total hospital caseload (Figure 1).

A number of different therapies are included in the total treatment sessions. Outpatient integrative medicine sessions, which included multiple modalities, were the most prevalent (n = 2,042 or 39.3%), followed by rehabilitation-exclusive appointments (20.5%) and nutrition visits (11.1%). The complete distribution of service caseload is provided (Figure 2).

The patients who received multiple therapies were selected for additional analysis. The multiple modality treatment sessions were most commonly utilized for patients (n = 274) with neurological and orthopedic conditions (50.7% and 49.6%, resp.). 17.4% of patients presenting with primary neurologic disease had concurrent orthopedic abnormalities, and 15.6% of patients presenting with orthopedic disease had concurrent neurologic disorders. Patients also presented with issues related to internal medicine, oncology, soft tissue surgery, critical care, dermatology, and other conditions (Figure 3). Each patient receiving multiple modalities visited the service an average of 7.6 ± 10.5 times during the study period with a range of 1–106 visits. Orthopedic conditions were treated on average with more visits (10.1 ± 14.2) than were neurologic conditions (6.7 ± 8.9) (P = 0.007). The number of visits did not differ by breed (P = 0.128) or by age (P = 0.68).

The majority of small animal patients that presented for multiple modality visits were of ideal body condition (body condition score (BCS) = 4-5/9, 41.6%) but a significant number were classified as overweight (BCS = 6, 31.8%) or obese (BCS ≥ 7, 25%) (Figure 4). No statistical difference

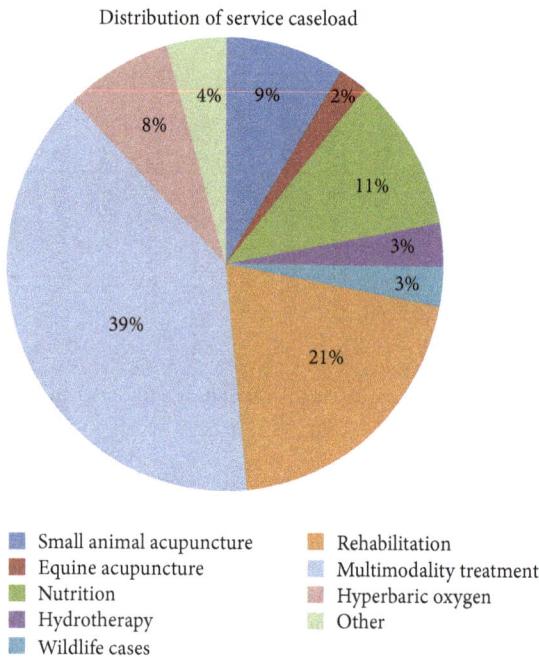

Distribution of service caseload

FIGURE 2: Distribution of integrative medicine patient visits of the study site's Academic Veterinary Hospital.

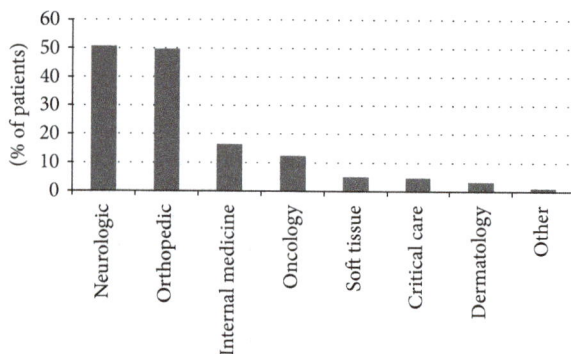

FIGURE 3: Presenting complaints of veterinary patients receiving multiple therapeutic modalities in the study site's integrative medicine service.

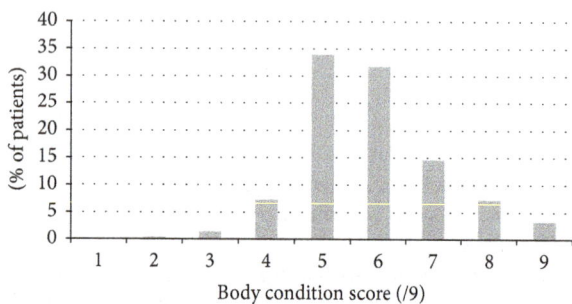

FIGURE 4: Body condition of veterinary patients receiving multiple integrative therapeutic modalities at the study site's Academic Veterinary Hospital.

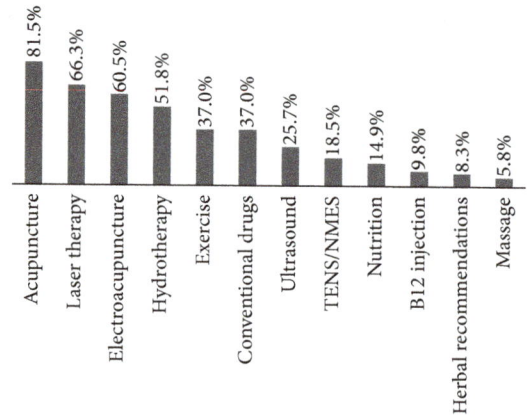

FIGURE 5: The percentage of patients receiving each integrative therapeutic modality at the study site's integrative medicine service.

was noted in the body condition scores of those patients presenting for neurologic, orthopedic, or other conditions ($P = 0.15$). A weak negative correlation was observed between the body condition score of the patient and the number of visits ($r = -0.12$, $P = 0.04$).

Patients receiving multiple modalities received 4.1 ± 1.6 different therapies at a visit, with a range of 1–11 modalities. No statistically significant differences were identified in the number of modalities used in patients with neurologic, orthopedic, or other conditions ($P = 0.19$). A weak positive correlation was identified between the number of modalities employed and the number of visits ($r = 0.21$, $P = 0.001$). No differences were detected in the number of modalities any breed category received ($P = 0.07$).

Four modalities were used in greater than half of the treatment sessions analyzed. These included acupuncture (81.5% of all treatment sessions), laser therapy (66.3%), electroacupuncture (60.5%), and hydrotherapy (51.8%). Eight other interventions were used for the mixed modality patients but less frequently (Figure 5).

Neurologic patients were significantly more likely to receive acupuncture, electroacupuncture, and rehabilitation exercises as compared to orthopedic patients ($P < 0.05$, Figure 6). These patients were less likely to receive laser therapy, hydrotherapy, and ultrasound. There was no difference in the odds of either group receiving transcutaneous electrical nerve stimulation (TENS) or neuromuscular electrical stimulation (NMES), nutritional or herbal recommendations, massage, conventional drugs, or cyanocobalamin injections.

Sixty-two breeds of dogs were treated. Mixed breed dogs were most commonly presented (27.0%). Both Dachshunds and Labrador retrievers were overrepresented in the patient population when compared to other breeds, amounting to 15.2% and 7.4% of the study population, respectively. German Shepherds comprised 3.3% of patients, and the remainder of breeds accounted for less than 2.2% of the dogs treated.

Analysis of the five major breed categories (Dachshunds, Labrador retrievers, mixed breeds, German Shepherds, and a group of all other breeds) did not show any statistically significant difference in age ($P = 0.12$). Labrador retrievers

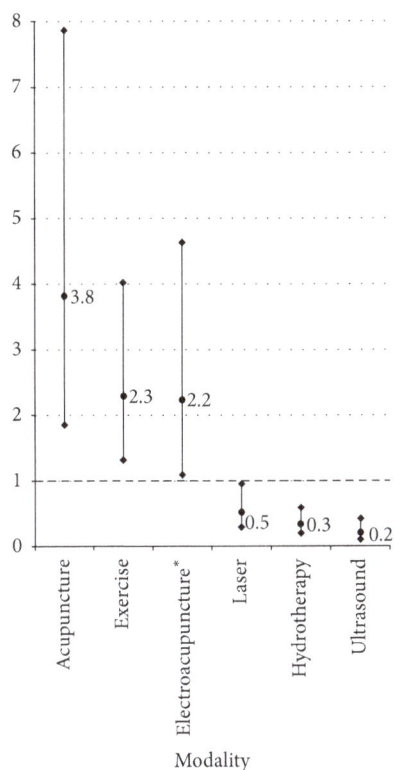

FIGURE 6: The odds of receiving six modalities were different in neurologic as compared to orthopedic patients (OR, 95% CI) of the veterinary patients at the study site's integrative medicine service. * The odds ratio was calculated by comparing the odds of neurologic patients with acupuncture receiving electroacupuncture as compared to orthopedic patients with acupuncture receiving electroacupuncture. Electroacupuncture was always performed with acupuncture, and therefore this comparison normalizes for the observed differences in the odds of receiving acupuncture alone.

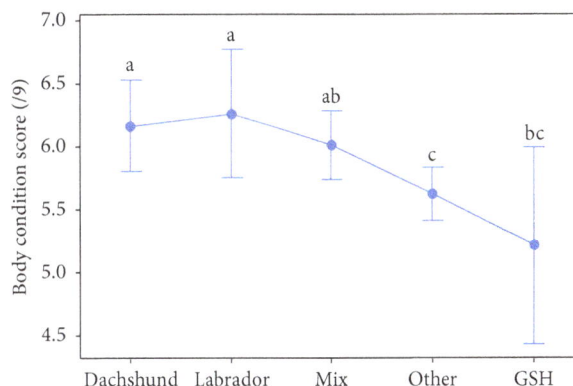

FIGURE 7: Breed differences in body condition score at the study site's integrative medicine service (breeds with different letters are statistically different).

and German Shepherds were heavier than mixed and other breeds in this study, and all four groups were more massive than Dachshunds. Statistically significant differences were noted between breeds and average body condition scores (P = 0.008, Figure 7).

Multiple modality treatments were employed primarily for dogs (n = 270) and also for cats (n = 4). The mean age of cats was 14.0 years (10–17) with a body weight of 4.6 kg (3.5–5.9). All cats were neutered males. The mean age for dogs (n = 270) was 9.0 ± 3.9 years (1–18) with a body weight of 19.2 kg ± 12.8 (1.2–63.2 kg). The genders of dogs were as follows: 23 intact males, 127 neutered males, 11 intact females, and 109 spayed females. The majority of the animals treated were seen either concurrently or within the previous six months by another service in the same academic teaching hospital (92.2%, n = 249).

Statistically significant differences were determined between dogs grouped by presenting condition. Dogs presenting for orthopedic conditions weighed less than those presenting for neurologic or for other conditions (14.9 ± 13.1 versus 23.3 ± 11.3 and 19.8 ± 12.5 kg, resp. P < 0.001). Dogs were younger if treated for orthopedic as opposed to other

conditions (8.3 ± 3.4 years versus 9.8 ± 3.6 years) (P = 0.048) but were not different in age from those treated for neurologic diseases. No difference was detected in the body condition scores of dogs when grouped by presenting complaint (P = 0.12). There was no difference in the number of modalities received for dogs presenting with orthopedic, neurologic, or other problems (P = 0.57).

Dachshunds were substantially more likely to present with a neurologic condition than with orthopedic or other conditions (OR 23.6; 7.47–74.5). Conversely, Labrador retrievers were more likely to be treated for a primary orthopedic complaint as opposed to a neurologic issue (OR 6.0; 1.46–24.7). Predictably, Dachshunds were more likely to present with neurologic conditions than were Labradors (OR 19.4; 4.96–76.1), mixed breed dogs (OR 14.8; 5.61–39.2), or other breeds (OR 7.48; 3.08–18.2). No Dachshunds presented with orthopedic complaints and they were therefore the least likely of the breeds to present with this condition.

The odds ratios for dogs receiving some modalities differed significantly among the breed categories (Dachshunds, Labradors, German Shepherds, mixed breed dogs, and the group of other dog breeds). Dachshunds were less likely to receive B12 injections than were German Shepherds (OR 0.10; 0.01–0.74) and were less likely to receive therapeutic ultrasound than mixed breed dogs (OR 0.21; 0.07–0.60). They were, however, more likely than other breeds to receive TENS/NMES (OR 2.51; 1.08–5.79) and also more likely than mixed breeds (OR 2.98; 1.33–6.68) and Labrador retrievers (OR 5.95; 1.51–23.5) to receive therapeutic exercises. Mixed breeds were more likely to receive therapeutic ultrasound than other breeds (OR 2.44; 1.30–4.60) and less likely to receive B12 injections than were German Shepherds (OR 0.15; 0.04–0.49). Other breeds were less likely than German Shepherds to receive conventional prescription drug recommendations (OR 0.21; 0.05–0.90).

4. Discussion

The integrative medicine service from which data was derived is unique in several respects. The academic mission of the veterinary college necessitates a model that incorporates student experiential learning, the training of house officers, and an emphasis on inter-specialty cooperation and on evidence-based medicine. The service was staffed during the study period by 1.25–2.25 full-time-equivalent faculty, 1-2 house officers, and two certified rehabilitation veterinary technicians. Four to five students were present in rotating two-week elective rotations for the entire year. The integrative nature of the service is supported by data in the present investigation; a large number of patients also presented to other hospital services (92%), and a recommendation of conventional therapies was made in 36.6% of multimodality treatment visits. Comparative data from integrative services at other institutions are unavailable, and no other service combines the same therapeutic options. Therefore, additional data and descriptions from other services are required before comparative conclusions can be made.

The service offers four of the five most commonly taught modalities in veterinary schools: nutrition, rehabilitation, acupuncture, and herbal therapy [4]. The notable exception is veterinary spinal manipulative therapy, also referred to as veterinary chiropractic. This practice, based on a principle that manually applied forces induce joint mobility and subsequent myofascial effects, has been objectively studied in horses but not in dogs [6]. Anecdotal concerns about mobilization and worsening of intervertebral discs exist, and practitioners of the modality do advise caution [7]. The absence of evidence-based testing and the lack of training by the service clinicians precluded the use of this technique. Other therapies discussed in the context of integrative medicine were also not a component of the service, including homeopathy, which is derived from foundational principles that "like treats like" and that serial dilutions of a compound increase the potency of a remedy. A recent meta-analysis of veterinary homeopathy found only scant data supporting its use in randomized controlled trials, and the two acceptable studies focused on bovine and porcine treatments [8]. Philosophical arguments surround the plausibility of the therapy, but nevertheless integration into a conventional veterinary hospital is both difficult and questionable given the competing tenets [9, 10].

The study data suggest that multimodality therapies were the most frequent treatment intervention elected by the attending clinicians. The patients receiving a multimodality therapy session were treated in the absence of the owners, from whom a brief history was obtained at the start of the visit and who were updated at the conclusion of the visit. The clients were charged a flat treatment fee irrespective of the number of modalities performed in order to eliminate the appearance of any financial incentive to expand a treatment protocol. Therefore, the patients in this study, which received a range of 1–11 modalities, were all charged equally, and patients on average received four of the available modalities based on clinician assessments. The students were permitted to assist with these patients, and the overall efficiency and case volume was managed by having the patients in the service for several hours.

4.1. Acupuncture, Electroacupuncture, and Vitamin B12 Injections.

Acupuncture and electroacupuncture were two of the four most frequently administered treatments. Acupuncture remains a source of significant controversy in veterinary medicine. Much of this controversy is derived from debates surrounding the antiquity of acupuncture, and available evidence suggests that modern veterinary acupuncture is a recent invention [11]. Veterinarians may place acupuncture needles based on traditional Chinese practices, on medical explanations and published studies of clinical effects or on a combination of the two approaches [12, 13]. A dated systematic review found there was insufficient evidence to recommend acupuncture in small animal patients like those of the study population [14]. Admittedly, two studies failed to document a significant benefit in dogs with both acute and chronic orthopedic injury [15, 16]. However, studies of varying methodological quality suggested an improvement in neurologic function of dogs affected by intervertebral disc disease when treated with electroacupuncture [17–19]. Interestingly, dogs treated in the retrospective period of this study were more likely to receive acupuncture and electroacupuncture when presenting with neurologic as opposed to orthopedic issues. Some studies of naturally occurring canine pain support an analgesic effect of acupuncture which could be beneficial for many conditions [20, 21]. A number of mechanisms have been postulated for the effects of acupuncture, including endogenous opioid release, substance P modulation, myofascial input, cannabinoid receptor modulation, and other cellular mediators. However, detailed evidence-based discussions should inform the location, effects, and utility of acupoints, several examples of which have been recently published [22, 23].

Cyanocobalamin injections (vitamin B12) were administered infrequently in patients (<10%). The technique has been recommended as an adjunctive method of acupoint stimulation [13], although it has not been scientifically validated. Cobalamin requires intrinsic factor, produced in the stomach and pancreas of dogs and in the pancreas of cats, for intestinal absorption and is a critical cofactor in enzymes for carbon rearrangement and methyl donation [24]. Cyanocobalamin injections have a wide margin of safety, and physiologic and cellular deficiencies have been reported in various conditions [24]. The finding that German Shepherds received B12 injections more commonly than some other breeds is likely unintentional. The fact that oncology patients accounted for the largest number of injections may suggest an intentional supplementation of this group due to perceived neoplasia-related true or relative deficiencies [25]. No animals were tested for their B12 status prior to supplementation so the effectiveness of such an approach remains unclear.

The application of electrical current to a patient's soft tissues is not unique to electroacupuncture. However, electroacupuncture has been shown in multiple species to augment therapeutic response by enhancing the release of endogenous opioids [26]. The best available data suggests that low frequency (2 Hz) acupuncture releases μ-acting opioids whereas high frequency stimulation (100 Hz) affects κ receptors. Veterinary studies frequently employ a mixed low and high frequency treatment of at least 20-minute duration [15,

17, 20]. Release of β-endorphins was documented three hours after treatment in dogs receiving an uncommon protocol of electroacupuncture (24 Hz and 43 Hz) [21]. Horses had a measurable rise of the same opioid in CSF for 2 hours following a 15–30 Hz treatment [27]. The most common protocol used in the present investigation was 2 Hz for 20 minutes in dogs, but additional studies are required to determine the optimal electroacupuncture frequency for the common neurologic and orthopedic conditions encountered during the study period.

4.2. TENS and NMES. Transcutaneous electrical nerve stimulation (TENS) utilizes conductive pads to activate sensory nerve fibers and to modulate pain. This therapy was employed in only about 18% of the study patients and was often used in Dachshunds. A recent meta-analysis of human patients found some favorable evidence for TENS treatment of the pain associated with knee osteoarthritis, but subsequent small studies were unable to confirm the effect [28]. TENS treatments set to a frequency of 70 Hz improved ground reaction forces in osteoarthritic dogs [29]. TENS was also employed in a canine physiotherapy program but at unknown settings [30]. TENS units frequently contain a different program for neuromuscular electrical stimulation, which is employed in the treatment of atrophy by recruiting motor fibers. Increased muscle mass was documented in dogs receiving this type of stimulation following surgical repair of a cranial cruciate ligament repair [31]. TENS or NMES could be theorized to be more beneficial for the treatment of large areas given the greater current dispersal area over the pads whereas electroacupuncture might more effectively treat deep tissues; neither suggestion has been scientifically evaluated. Whether the clinical patients in the present retrospective would have benefited more from one therapy as opposed to the other remains unknown.

4.3. Laser Therapy (Photobiomodulation). A therapeutic laser treatment was performed in a majority of the study population. The cellular effects of laser treatments, often referred to as photobiomodulation, are well established and include photonic changes to cytochrome c oxidase resulting in increased cellular energy (ATP) production, the release of nitric oxide, and the generation of free oxygen radicals which stimulates an endogenous antioxidant production [32]. The primary controversy of laser therapy is the dose needed to achieve such biologic effects given that water, melanin, and hemoglobin all absorb photons in a similar spectrum as the target cytochromes. Laser penetration has been poorly studied in dogs, although a study in horses showed consistent differences in penetration in shaved versus unshaved areas [33]. A single clinical trial of canine laser therapy found that dogs had a significantly reduced time to ambulation when treated with laser following a decompressive hemilaminectomy [34]. Therefore, the observation in this study that neurologic patients were less likely to receive laser therapy deserves attention because the strongest clinical evidence supports its use in these patients. Failure to provide this therapy may have been due to pragmatic considerations given

that a number of the postoperative patients treated by the service have an adhesive, absorbent, and poorly penetrable bandage over the surgical incision.

4.4. Hydrotherapy: Underwater Treadmill Walking and Swimming. Hydrotherapy was more commonly used for orthopedic than neurologic patients, which may be because the service treats a large number of paralyzed dogs with no motor function at the outset of treatment. Neurosurgical patients in the academic teaching hospital typically have intravenous catheters for approximately 48 hours after surgery, and urinary catheters are frequently placed for lower motor neuron bladder dysfunction. The presence of either catheter complicates hydrotherapy, but the degree to which this influenced the odds ratio of hydrotherapy in orthopedic as compared to neurologic patients could not be quantified from the retrospective data available. Additionally, the available evidence for hydrotherapy is presently limited to orthopedic pathology although some authors advocate introduction of the technique 3 to 5 days after surgery for intervertebral disc disease and other neurologic conditions [35]. Underwater treadmill therapy reduces concussive forces on joints and promotes increased joint flexion and full active extension [36]. It has been used for both weight loss protocols and for postoperative rehabilitation of dogs following a tibial plateau leveling osteotomy [37, 38]. Hydrotherapy was defined as either swimming or underwater treadmill therapy in this study, and the exact distribution of each was not collected. Swimming, however, can be used to maximize active range of motion; hip, stifle, and hock flexion were all increased in a pool as compared to a ground treadmill after cranial cruciate ligament repair and in healthy dogs [39]. Conversely, hip and stifle extension angles were reduced by about 13 and 19 degrees, respectively, in swimming dogs after cruciate repair as compared to healthy controls. This was not observed in the same dogs when walking at two speeds on a land (nonaquatic) treadmill [39]. Severely osteoarthritic dogs often exercised more comfortably in a pool because they are completely nonweight bearing. Additional data is required to better inform the optimal time for starting hydrotherapy and the clinical benefits, if any, in neurologic patients.

4.5. Therapeutic Exercise. Therapeutic exercises were performed less frequently than hydrotherapy, presumably because the service first exercises patients in water before advancing them to weight-bearing activities with the aid of ground treadmills or other interventions, such as cavaletti poles, weaves, balance ball, and related rehabilitation techniques. Several authors have advocated early limb use after injury in animals, and the kinematics of many techniques are described for dogs [40–43]. However, no study has yet independently associated any one particular exercise with any improvement in clinical outcome. Dachshunds and neurologic patients in the present study were interestingly more likely to receive therapeutic exercises than Labrador retrievers, mixed breeds, and those with orthopedic conditions. This may be due to the fact that many neurologic dogs were paretic and therefore more difficult for owners to exercise when compared to those with orthopedic pathology.

4.6. Therapeutic Ultrasound. Therapeutic ultrasound provides energy in the form of sound, which is absorbed by tissues of high protein content such as skeletal muscle, thereby providing deep heating to target tissues. Short-term (<10 minutes) heating of 1.6–4.6 degrees Celsius was reported in the caudal thigh muscles of dogs following ultrasound, with results dependent on the selected power (1–1.5 W/cm^2). Calcaneal tendon extensibility and tarsal flexion also increased for 5 minutes following a similar protocol in dogs [44]. The short-term effects of ultrasound are likely most beneficial when followed by range of motion exercises. Repeated and frequent administration may produce faster rates of healing in tendons and in other tissues, but this approach is often constrained by logistical and financial considerations in clinical practice [45]. The facilitation of tissue stretching and thermal heating was used more often in orthopedic as opposed to neurologic patients, likely due to the more severe range of motion restrictions noted in many orthopedic conditions, such as cranial cruciate ligament rupture [15].

4.7. Massage Therapy. Massage therapy may have similar effects as to the aforementioned modalities. The techniques and goals of such manipulations are similar to those described in humans, although there is minimal scientific literature regarding the efficacy of massage in dogs and cats [46]. The principles by which massage might benefit an integrative medicine patient, based on available human studies, include increased lymphatic flow, modulation of local pain mediators such as substance P and prostaglandins, positive cortical responses, increased local circulation, reductions in muscle spasms and pain, and reduction of tissue adhesions [46]. Massage was the least frequently applied therapeutic modality, which may be related to the time required for the treatment or to the perception that manual therapies are less effective than other interventions. The latter cannot be determined until further veterinary studies are performed.

4.8. Herbal Interventions. Herbal recommendations were made to a small number of clients for a number of different conditions. A discussion of the merits of herbal supplements is outside the scope of this investigation, but there are a number of herbs and herbal formulas suggested to impart a clinical effect in veterinary species [47, 48]. Unfortunately, herbal veterinary products have minimal regulatory oversight, as neither the Association of American Feed Control Officials (AAFCO) nor the United States Food and Drug Administration (FDA) controls these products. A previous study of Chinese herbal formulas identified variable amounts of minerals and potential contaminants, and some contain small amounts of potentially toxic compounds [49, 50]. The herbal recommendations in this study were made by the supervising clinician based on a review of the conventional therapies and with a risk-benefit discussion with the owner, recognizing that interactions with drugs or unpredictable reactions are of real concern [51].

4.9. Nutritional Recommendations and Obesity Prevalence. Nutritional recommendations were provided to the owners in approximately 15% of cases. This is in contrast to current recommendations that every patient receives a nutritional assessment and recommendation [52]. All audited patient records except for one contained a weight and body condition score, and the multiple modality visits were nearly all recheck examinations. Therefore, it is likely that the collected data underestimates the percentage of patients receiving nutritional recommendations in the service. The importance of communication is stressed in current consensus guidelines and as such a revision of the patient discharge form to reinforce nutritional plans and monitoring appears warranted.

More than half of the dogs treated were overweight or obese. This prevalence is consistent with a recent study in the United Kingdom but higher than a dated study performed in the United States [53, 54]. Nevertheless, the animals in this study do not appear to be more overweight than the general population. A limitation of the collected retrospective data is that the same clinician did not perform all body condition scoring, but a validated nine-point system was available to all service clinicians. Dachshunds and Labrador retrievers were both more likely to be overweight than were other breeds in this study. A previous study identified that both breeds had increased risk of being overweight (OR = 1.6) and that Dachshunds also displayed increased risk for obesity (OR = 1.7) [53]. An association between body condition score and the number of visits or the presenting complaint was not detected, suggesting either that body condition did not contribute to the observed pathologies or, more likely, that excess adiposity contributed equally to the patients' conditions.

4.10. Breed, Age, and Gender Distribution of the Study Population. The breed distributions observed in this study are remarkably similar to a previous survey of general breed prevalence [55]. Mixed breeds accounted for 27% of this patient population and the same amount was reported in a national survey. Labrador retrievers comprised 7.4% and German Shepherds 3.3% which is again similar to the 7.9% and 3%, respectively, reported in the previous population study. Therefore, only the Dachshund appears overrepresented when compared to available data; they were 15.2% of the treated dogs, which dramatically contrasts with published statistics that they are less than 1.5% of the general population.

The predisposition of Labradors to orthopedic disease in this study is consistent with previous reports [56, 57], as is the predisposition of Dachshunds to intervertebral disc disease [57, 58]. The Dachshund accounted for 31.8% of all cases with a primary neurologic complaint, and a previous report found that Dachshunds comprised 48.0% of all canine intervertebral disc disease cases [58]. In the present study, intervertebral disc disease was included in a broader category of all neurologic disease and therefore a definitive comparison between the reported prevalence data cannot be made. The average age of the treated Dachshunds (7.9 years) is older than the age of highest risk for IVDD in chondrodystrophic breeds of 4–6 years [58], which could represent an anomaly. The finding could also suggest that older Dachshunds are more likely to require rehabilitation or those owners are more likely to elect therapy for this population.

Treated dogs were older (median = 9) and more likely to be neutered when compared to general population statistics (median age = 4.8) [55]. Intact males comprised 8.5% of caseload, neutered males 47%, intact females 4%, and spayed females 40.5% as compared to 21.2%, 24.4%, 16.7%, and 37.1%, respectively. It is unclear if neutering is causally related to the orthopedic and neurologic diseases treated in this study although an association between early neutering and joint disorders has been suggested [59].

4.11. Treatment Differences between Orthopedic and Neurologic Patients. The present data demonstrates that more than 15% of patients presenting with orthopedic or neurologic disease will have concurrent pathology of the other type. Therefore, a thorough physical examination and inventory of all conditions should be performed in all integrative medicine patients. Given that neurologic and orthopedic patients received the same number of modalities, it is logical to suggest that the same amount of time can be dedicated to orthopedic and neurologic cases. However, orthopedic patients were treated with more sessions during the study period than were those with neurologic disease. It could be hypothesized that this is because some neurologic patients, particularly those with intervertebral disc disease, make a full and complete recovery whereas many orthopedic diseases are chronic. Identification of overweight and obese patients is equally important in both groups as neither was more predisposed to obesity than the other.

4.12. Study Limitations. The study is subject to several limitations. The medical record system did not allow for clear examination of efficacy across the range of conditions that were treated. Prospective studies of each modality are needed. As is true of most individualized patient rehabilitation protocols, the effectiveness of a combination protocol, as opposed to a single modality treatment, was not assessed. The combination of modalities selected by a clinician could act synergistically or could negate the benefits of other therapies. The reason for selection of modalities was not explored, and the bias of the different service clinicians may confound the presented results. Additionally, detailed data is not presented on other types of appointments although information on hyperbaric oxygen treatments performed by the service is available elsewhere [60].

The data are heavily skewed toward dogs, but this is not surprising given that more of the small animal publications in integrative medicine, especially rehabilitation, focus on dogs. Additional investigation is warranted in practices that support a higher feline caseload. Similarly, equine cases were insufficient to be compared to dogs and are likely different in the modalities elected and the patient demographics. A limitation of this study is that detailed data was only collected from one treatment sheet from each patient's record, and

therefore the audited data may not accurately reflect the characteristics of the patients despite randomization. However, the large volume of cases prohibited a more comprehensive analysis.

4.13. Controversies in Integrative Veterinary Medicine. General controversies regarding the efficacy and suitability of integrative medical practice exist, and this study may incite criticisms of the use of these modalities in integrative practice. The amount of evidence for each technique employed in this study is admittedly unknown. One prominent integrative medicine scholar in the human medical field has proposed that only 7.4% of complementary and alternative techniques have compelling evidence justifying their use [61]. No similar attempt has been made to characterize the evidence for integrative or conventional veterinary therapies. The veterinary profession has very few interventions which reach the highest evidence grade, and significant challenges of the application of evidence-based medicine to veterinary practice have been described [62]. These include the expense of randomized controlled trials, the reliance on retrospective studies, the smaller population of researchers and research funding, the inherent difficulties in searching available databases, and the veterinarian's reliance on clinical experience. Clearly, however, integrative veterinary medicine should adopt the recommendations of McKenzie that all interventions, whether integrative, complementary, alternative, or holistic, be subjected to the same investigative standards and that practitioners accept both the primacy of empirical evidence and willingness to modify their practice based on such evidence [63]. This conversely requires skeptics of integrative medicine to support evidence-based integrative medicine based on the available data and evidence rather than on a perceived scale of acceptability. The authors of this paper hope that the information contained herein can provide a starting point for continued research on the applicability of these and other modalities.

5. Conclusions

The collected data provide a foundation for future prospective evaluations of integrative veterinary medicine. The prevalence of acupuncture, laser, and hydrotherapy in this patient population suggests that these should be initial areas of research. Older dogs with neurologic or orthopedic diseases were the primary patient populations treated, and Dachshunds were overrepresented compared to national statistics. Therefore, these patients should likely serve as the target populations for additional study. The data further support that integrative medicine can be successfully incorporated into conventional multispecialty referral practices with a high degree of cooperation. Additional evidence-based outcome measures should be used to evaluate the efficacy of integrative therapies, and both veterinarians and veterinary students should be prepared to counsel owners in these areas.

Conflict of Interests

The authors declare that there is no conflict of interests regarding the publication of this paper.

Acknowledgments

The authors acknowledge participation of the University of Florida Integrative Medicine clinicians, interns, technicians, and veterinary students. The study was conducted during Dr. Memon's sabbatical leave from Washington State University to the University of Florida during July–December, 2015.

References

[1] B. Kligler, V. Maizes, S. Schachter et al., "Core competencies in integrative medicine for medical school curricula: a proposal," *Academic Medicine*, vol. 79, no. 6, pp. 521–531, 2004.

[2] D. M. Raditic and J. W. Bartges, "Evidence-based integrative medicine in clinical veterinary oncology," *Veterinary Clinics of North America: Small Animal Practice*, vol. 44, no. 5, pp. 831–853, 2014.

[3] S. E. Lana, L. R. Kogan, K. A. Crump, J. T. Graham, and N. G. Robinson, "The use of complementary and alternative therapies in dogs and cats with cancer," *Journal of the American Animal Hospital Association*, vol. 42, no. 5, pp. 361–365, 2006.

[4] M. A. Memon and L. K. Sprunger, "Survey of colleges and schools of veterinary medicine regarding education in complementary and alternative veterinary medicine," *Journal of the American Veterinary Medical Association*, vol. 239, no. 5, pp. 619–623, 2011.

[5] M. Frass, R. P. Strassl, H. Friehs, M. Müllner, M. Kundi, and A. D. Kaye, "Use and acceptance of complementary and alternative medicine among the general population and medical personnel: a systematic review," *The Ochsner Journal*, vol. 12, no. 1, pp. 45–56, 2012.

[6] K. K. Haussler, A. E. Hill, C. M. Puttlitz, and C. W. McIlwraith, "Effects of vertebral mobilization and manipulation on kinematics of the thoracolumbar region," *American Journal of Veterinary Research*, vol. 68, no. 5, pp. 508–516, 2007.

[7] L. L. Taylor and L. Romano, "Veterinary chiropractic," *The Canadian Veterinary Journal*, vol. 40, no. 10, pp. 732–735, 1999.

[8] R. T. Mathie and J. Clausen, "Veterinary homeopathy: meta-analysis of randomised placebo-controlled trials," *Homeopathy*, vol. 104, no. 1, pp. 3–8, 2015.

[9] D. Mastrangelo, "Hormesis, epitaxy, the structure of liquid water, and the science of homeopathy," *Medical Science Monitor*, vol. 13, no. 1, pp. SR1–SR8, 2007.

[10] C. Bayley, "Homeopathy," *Journal of Medicine and Philosophy*, vol. 18, no. 2, pp. 129–145, 1993.

[11] J. Shmalberg, *Acupuncture: History and Application*, Clinician's Brief, 2014.

[12] C. Chrisman and H. Xie, "Canine transpositional points," in *Xie's Veterinary Acupuncture*, V. Preast and H. Xie, Eds., pp. 129–216, Blackwell, Ames, Iowa, USA, 2007.

[13] S. L. Cantwell, "Traditional Chinese veterinary medicine: the mechanism and management of acupuncture for chronic pain," *Topics in Companion Animal Medicine*, vol. 25, no. 1, pp. 53–58, 2010.

[14] G. Habacher, M. H. Pittler, and E. Ernst, "Effectiveness of acupuncture in veterinary medicine: systematic review," *Journal of Veterinary Internal Medicine*, vol. 20, no. 3, pp. 480–488, 2006.

[15] J. Shmalberg and J. Burgess, "A randomized controlled blinded clinical trial of electro-acupuncture administered one month after cranial cruciate ligament repair in dogs," *American Journal of Traditional Chinese Veterinary Medicine*, vol. 9, no. 2, pp. 43–51, 2014.

[16] A. S. Kapatkin, M. Tomasic, J. Beech et al., "Effects of electrostimulated acupuncture on ground reaction forces and pain scores in dogs with chronic elbow joint arthritis," *Journal of the American Veterinary Medical Association*, vol. 228, no. 9, pp. 1350–1354, 2006.

[17] A. M. Hayashi, J. M. Matera, and A. C. B. de Campos Fonseca Pinto, "Evaluation of electroacupuncture treatment for thoracolumbar intervertebral disk disease in dogs," *Journal of the American Veterinary Medical Association*, vol. 231, no. 6, pp. 913–918, 2007.

[18] H.-J. Han, H.-Y. Yoon, J.-Y. Kim et al., "Clinical effect of additional electroacupuncture on thoracolumbar intervertebral disc herniation in 80 paraplegic dogs," *The American Journal of Chinese Medicine*, vol. 38, no. 6, pp. 1015–1025, 2010.

[19] J. G. F. Joaquim, S. P. L. Luna, J. T. Brondani, S. R. Torelli, S. C. Rahal, and F. P. De Freitas, "Comparison of decompressive surgery, electroacupuncture, and decompressive surgery followed by electroacupuncture for the treatment of dogs with intervertebral disk disease with long-standing severe neurologic deficits," *Journal of the American Veterinary Medical Association*, vol. 236, no. 11, pp. 1225–1229, 2010.

[20] A. Laim, A. Jaggy, F. Forterre, M. G. Doherr, G. Aeschbacher, and O. Glardon, "Effects of adjunct electroacupuncture on severity of postoperative pain in dogs undergoing hemilaminectomy because of acute thoracolumbar intervertebral disk disease," *Journal of the American Veterinary Medical Association*, vol. 234, no. 9, pp. 1141–1146, 2009.

[21] D. Groppetti, A. M. Pecile, P. Sacerdote, V. Bronzo, and G. Ravasio, "Effectiveness of electroacupuncture analgesia compared with opioid administration in a dog model: a pilot study," *British Journal of Anaesthesia*, vol. 107, no. 4, pp. 612–618, 2011.

[22] R. B. Koh, N. Isaza, H. Xie, K. Cooke, and S. A. Robertson, "Effects of maropitant, acepromazine, and electroacupuncture on vomiting associated with administration of morphine in dogs," *Journal of the American Veterinary Medical Association*, vol. 244, no. 7, pp. 820–829, 2014.

[23] N. Robinson, "The need for consistency and comparability of transitional acupuncture points across species," *American Journal of Traditional Chinese Veterinary Medicine*, vol. 1, no. 1, pp. 14–21, 2006.

[24] C. G. Ruaux, "Cobalamin in companion animals: diagnostic marker, deficiency states and therapeutic implications," *The Veterinary Journal*, vol. 196, no. 2, pp. 145–152, 2013.

[25] A. K. Cook, Z. M. Wright, J. S. Suchodolski, M. R. Brown, and J. M. Steiner, "Prevalence and prognostic impact of hypocobalaminemia in dogs with lymphoma," *Journal of the American Veterinary Medical Association*, vol. 235, no. 12, pp. 1437–1441, 2009.

[26] G. A. Ulett, S. Han, and J.-S. Han, "Electroacupuncture: mechanisms and clinical application," *Biological Psychiatry*, vol. 44, no. 2, pp. 129–138, 1998.

[27] R. T. Skarda, G. A. Tejwani, and W. W. Muir III, "Cutaneous analgesia, hemodynamic and respiratory effects, and β-endorphin concentration in spinal fluid and plasma of horses

after acupuncture and electroacupuncture," *American Journal of Veterinary Research*, vol. 63, no. 10, pp. 1435–1442, 2002.

[28] A. W. Rutjes, E. Nüesch, R. Sterchi et al., "Transcutaneous electrostimulation for osteoarthritis of the knee," *Cochrane Database of Systematic Reviews*, no. 4, Article ID CD002823, 2009.

[29] D. Levine, K. Johnson, M. Price et al., "The effect of TENS on osteoarthritic pain in the stifle of dogs," in *Proceedings of the 2nd International Symposium on Rehabilitation and Physical Therapy in Veterinary Medicine*, Knoxville, Tenn, USA, 2002.

[30] E. Mlacnik, B. A. Bockstahler, M. Müller, M. A. Tetrick, R. C. Nap, and J. Zentek, "Effects of caloric restriction and a moderate or intense physiotherapy program for treatment of lameness in overweight dogs with osteoarthritis," *Journal of the American Veterinary Medical Association*, vol. 229, no. 11, pp. 1756–1760, 2006.

[31] J. M. Johnson, A. L. Johnson, G. J. Pijanowski et al., "Rehabilitation of dogs with surgically treated cranial cruciate ligament-deficient stifles by use of electrical stimulation of muscles," *American Journal of Veterinary Research*, vol. 58, no. 12, pp. 1473–1478, 1997.

[32] H. Chung, T. Dai, S. K. Sharma, Y.-Y. Huang, J. D. Carroll, and M. R. Hamblin, "The nuts and bolts of low-level laser (Light) therapy," *Annals of Biomedical Engineering*, vol. 40, no. 2, pp. 516–533, 2012.

[33] T. Ryan and R. Smith, "An investigation into the depth of penetration of low level laser therapy through the equine tendon in vivo," *Irish Veterinary Journal*, vol. 60, no. 5, pp. 295–299, 2007.

[34] W. E. Draper, T. A. Schubert, R. M. Clemmons, and S. A. Miles, "Low-level laser therapy reduces time to ambulation in dogs after hemilaminectomy: a preliminary study," *Journal of Small Animal Practice*, vol. 53, no. 8, pp. 465–469, 2012.

[35] M. G. Drum, "Physical rehabilitation of the canine neurologic patient," *Veterinary Clinics of North America: Small Animal Practice*, vol. 40, no. 1, pp. 181–193, 2010.

[36] A. Jackson, D. Millis, M. Stevens et al., "Joint kinematics during underwater treadmill activity," in *Proceedings of the 2nd International Symposium on Rehabilitation and Physical Therapy in Veterinary Medicine*, Knoxville, Tenn, USA, 2002.

[37] M. L. Monk, C. A. Preston, and C. M. McGowan, "Effects of early intensive postoperative physiotherapy on limb function after tibial plateau leveling osteotomy in dogs with deficiency of the cranial cruciate ligament," *American Journal of Veterinary Research*, vol. 67, no. 3, pp. 529–536, 2006.

[38] A. Chauvet, J. Laclair, D. A. Elliott, and A. J. German, "Incorporation of exercise, using an underwater treadmill, and active client education into a weight management program for obese dogs," *Canadian Veterinary Journal*, vol. 52, no. 5, pp. 491–496, 2011.

[39] G. S. Marsolais, S. McLean, T. Derrick, and M. G. Conzemius, "Kinematic analysis of the hind limb during swimming and walking in healthy dogs and dogs with surgically corrected cranial cruciate ligament rupture," *Journal of the American Veterinary Medical Association*, vol. 222, no. 6, pp. 739–743, 2003.

[40] D. Millis and D. Levine, *Canine Rehabilitation and Physical Therapy*, Elsevier Health Sciences, 2013.

[41] R. P. Millard, J. F. Headrick, and D. L. Millis, "Kinematic analysis of the pelvic limbs of healthy dogs during stair and decline slope walking," *Journal of Small Animal Practice*, vol. 51, no. 8, pp. 419–422, 2010.

[42] M. G. Drum, D. J. Marcellin-Little, and M. S. Davis, "Principles and applications of therapeutic exercises for small animals," *Veterinary Clinics of North America: Small Animal Practice*, vol. 45, no. 1, pp. 73–90, 2015.

[43] P. J. Holler, V. Brazda, B. Dal-Bianco et al., "Kinematic motion analysis of the joints of the forelimbs and hind limbs of dogs during walking exercise regimens," *American Journal of Veterinary Research*, vol. 71, no. 7, pp. 734–740, 2010.

[44] J. Loonam, D. Millis, and M. Stevens, "The effect of therapeutic ultrasound on tendon heating and extensibility," in *Proceedings of the 30th Veterinary Orthopedic Society Conference*, Steamboat Springs, Colo, USA, February-March 2003.

[45] N. S. Saini, K. S. Roy, P. S. Bansal, B. Singh, and P. S. Simran, "A preliminary study on the effect of ultrasound therapy on the healing of surgically severed Achilles tendons in five dogs," *Journal of Veterinary Medicine Series A*, vol. 49, no. 6, pp. 321–328, 2002.

[46] A. Sutton and D. Whitlock, "Massage," in *Canine Rehabilitation and Physical Therapy*, D. Millis and D. Levine, Eds., pp. 464–483, Elsevier, Philadelphia, Pa, USA, 2014.

[47] D. C. Brown and J. Reetz, "Single agent polysaccharopeptide delays metastases and improves survival in naturally occurring hemangiosarcoma," *Evidence-Based Complementary and Alternative Medicine*, vol. 2012, Article ID 384301, 8 pages, 2012.

[48] K. A. Wirth, K. Kow, M. E. Salute, N. J. Bacon, and R. J. Milner, "In vitro effects of *Yunnan Baiyao* on canine hemangiosarcoma cell lines," *Veterinary and Comparative Oncology*, 2014.

[49] J. Shmalberg, R. C. Hill, and K. C. Scott, "Nutrient and metal analyses of Chinese herbal products marketed for veterinary use," *Journal of Animal Physiology and Animal Nutrition*, vol. 97, no. 2, pp. 305–314, 2013.

[50] J. Shmalberg, "Detection and quantification of neuroexcitatory alkaloids in modified Da Huo Luo Dan prescribed for paresis or paralysis in dogs," *American Journal of Traditional Chinese Veterinary Medicine*, vol. 10, no. 2, pp. 27–31, 2015.

[51] R. H. Poppenga, "Herbal medicine: potential for intoxication and interactions with conventional drugs," *Clinical Techniques in Small Animal Practice*, vol. 17, no. 1, pp. 6–18, 2002.

[52] K. Baldwin, J. Bartges, T. Buffington et al., "AAHA nutritional assessment guidelines for dogs and cats," *Journal of the American Animal Hospital Association*, vol. 46, no. 4, pp. 285–296, 2010.

[53] E. M. Lund, P. J. Armstrong, C. A. Kirk et al., "Prevalence and risk factors for obesity in adult dogs from private US veterinary practices," *International Journal of Applied Research in Veterinary Medicine*, vol. 4, no. 2, pp. 177–186, 2006.

[54] E. A. Courcier, R. M. Thomson, D. J. Mellor, and P. S. Yam, "An epidemiological study of environmental factors associated with canine obesity," *Journal of Small Animal Practice*, vol. 51, no. 7, pp. 362–367, 2010.

[55] E. M. Lund, P. J. Armstrong, C. A. Kirk, L. M. Kolar, and J. S. Klausner, "Health status and population characteristics of dogs and cats examined at private veterinary practices in the United States," *Journal of the American Veterinary Medical Association*, vol. 214, no. 9, pp. 1336–1341, 1999.

[56] J. M. Duval, S. C. Budsberg, G. L. Flo, and J. L. Sammarco, "Breed, sex, and body weight as risk factors for rupture of the cranial cruciate ligament in young dogs," *Journal of the American Veterinary Medical Association*, vol. 215, no. 6, pp. 811–814, 1999.

[57] E. LaFond, G. J. Breur, and C. C. Austin, "Breed susceptibility for developmental orthopedic diseases in dogs," *Journal of the*

American Animal Hospital Association, vol. 38, no. 5, pp. 467–477, 2002.

[58] W. A. Priester, "Canine intervertebral disc disease—occurrence by age, breed, and sex among 8,117 cases," *Theriogenology*, vol. 6, no. 2-3, pp. 293–303, 1976.

[59] B. L. Hart, L. A. Hart, A. P. Thigpen, and N. H. Willits, "Long-term health effects of neutering dogs: comparison of labrador retrievers with golden retrievers," *PLoS ONE*, vol. 9, no. 7, Article ID e102241, 2014.

[60] J. Shmalberg, W. Davies, S. Lopez, D. Shmalberg, and J. Zilberschtein, "Rectal temperature changes and oxygen toxicity in dogs treated in a monoplace chamber," *Undersea & Hyperbaric Medicine*, vol. 42, no. 1, pp. 95–102, 2015.

[61] E. Ernst, "How much of CAM is based on research evidence?" *Evidence-Based Complementary and Alternative Medicine*, vol. 2011, Article ID 676490, 3 pages, 2011.

[62] J.-M. Vandeweerd, N. Kirschvink, P. Clegg, S. Vandenput, P. Gustin, and C. Saegerman, "Is evidence-based medicine so evident in veterinary research and practice? History, obstacles and perspectives," *Veterinary Journal*, vol. 191, no. 1, pp. 28–34, 2012.

[63] B. A. McKenzie, "Is complementary and alternative medicine compatible with evidence-based medicine?" *Journal of the American Veterinary Medical Association*, vol. 241, no. 4, pp. 421–426, 2012.

13

Computed Tomographic Tenography of Normal Equine Digital Flexor Tendon Sheath: An Ex Vivo Study

Luca Lacitignola, Pasquale De Luca, Alessandro Guarracino, and Antonio Crovace

Sezione di Cliniche Veterinarie e P.A., Dipartimento delle Emergenze e Trapianti di Organo, Università degli Studi di Bari "Aldo Moro", s.p. per Casamassima km 3, Valenzano, 70010 Bari, Italy

Correspondence should be addressed to Luca Lacitignola; luca.lacitignola@veterinaria.uniba.it

Academic Editor: Nigel R. Perkins

Aim of this study was to document the normal computed tomographic tenography findings of digital flexor tendon sheath. Six ex vivo normal equine forelimbs were used. An axial approach was used to inject 185 mg/mL of iopamidol in a total volume of 60 mL into the digital flexor tendon sheaths. Single-slice helical scans, with 5 mm thickness, spaced every 3 mm, for a pitch of 0.6, and with bone algorithm reconstruction, were performed before and after injections of contrast medium. To obtain better image quality for multiplanar reconstruction and 3D reformatting, postprocessing retroreconstruction was performed to reduce the images to submillimetre thickness. Computed tomographic tenography of digital flexor tendon sheaths could visualize the following main tendon structures for every forelimb in contrast-enhanced images as low densities surrounded by high densities: superficial digital flexor tendon, deep digital flexor tendon, manica flexoria, mesotendons, and synovial recess. Results of this study suggest that computed tomographic tenography can be used with accuracy and sensitivity to evaluate the common disorders of the equine digital flexor tendon sheath and the intrathecal structures.

1. Introduction

Equine digital flexor tendon sheath (DFTS) lesions are usually investigated using radiography, ultrasonography, and tenoscopy; contrastography has also been successfully employed to detect pathologic conditions involving the DFTS of sport horses [1]. Normal radiographic anatomy of the DFTS using contrast tenography for the investigation of chronic tenosynovitis was described in 1986 [2, 3].

Deep digital flexor tendon (DDFT) or manica flexoria (MF) tears have been demonstrated to be the most frequently associated lesions of nonseptic tenosynovitis of digital tendon sheath in the horse [1, 3, 4].

Ultrasonography and contrast radiography of DFTS have been employed as principal diagnostic techniques, with different reported sensitivity [1, 3, 4]. The sensitivity of ultrasonography in diagnosing MF tears has been shown to be poor. In a retrospective analysis of 76 cases of nonseptic tenosynovitis of DFTS, the tears of the MF were predicted with a sensitivity of 38% compared with DDFT tears, which

were predicted with a sensitivity of 71% [4]. Contrast radiography was found to delineate the border of the MF accurately and, with a description of the normal orientation of the MF, evaluators were able to identify an abnormal appearance and therefore diagnose MF tears with a sensitivity which exceeds that of ultrasonography [1].

However, advances in ultrasound technology and operator experience led to a decline in the use of contrast radiography before these injuries were first recognised upon the advent of tenoscopy [1, 5].

Although computed tomography (CT) has been increasingly used in some veterinary institutions to evaluate the equine appendicular skeleton, including the stifle joint, carpus, hock, and fetlock [6–10], unfortunately, visualization of the soft tissues by CT is limited and commonly unrewarding without the use of intravascular or intrasynovial contrast.

Computed tomographic arthrography (CTR) was recently described as an imaging technique that uses intraarticular administration of contrast to improve visualization of the intrasynovial and perisynovial soft tissues [7, 9]. The contrast medium diffuses within the joint compartments, resulting in more conspicuous structures. The soft tissue structures appear as filling defects outlined by the contrast medium in the joint. CTR has been used to identify abnormalities of the articular surfaces, intrasynovial soft tissue structures, the synovial surface of joint capsules, and periarticular structures closely associated with the joint compartments.

At the time of writing, there were no published descriptions of DFTS tenography performed with the use of CT. The aim of this study was to determine the normal findings of DFTS using computed tomographic tenography on the ex vivo limbs of horses.

2. Material and Methods

2.1. Specimens. A cadaveric study was performed to evaluate a total of 6 equine distal forelimbs, collected at the slaughterhouse, from horses of unknown breed and age. The limbs were amputated at the level of the carpometacarpal joint and were examined to exclude limbs with any gross anatomical abnormalities or damage produced during the cutting process. The specimens were used fresh and the hair was clipped. The limbs were positioned with the palmar surface on the table, and one specimen was also scanned in lateral recumbency.

2.2. Contrast Medium (CM) Injection. Injection of DFTS was performed using the axial approach. With the metacarpophalangeal joint flexed to a 225° angle, the needle was inserted at the level of the midbody of the lateral proximal sesamoid bone, through the palmar annular ligament, and 3 mm axial to the palpable palmar or plantar border of the lateral proximal sesamoid bone, in the transverse plane, and directed 45° from the sagittal plane, angled toward the central intersesamoidean region, approximately 15 to 20 mm in depth [11]. The contrast medium iopamidol, 370 mg/mL (IOPAMIRO 370, Bracco; Rome, Italy), was diluted 1 : 1 with saline solution (0.9%) to a final concentration of 185 mg/mL, and a total of 60 mL was injected, except for 1 specimen that was injected with 30 mL to test the grade of synovial distension.

2.3. CT Scanning. A third generation single-slice CT scanner (GE Prospeed Power SX, GE Healthcare, Milwaukee, WI) was used for all procedures. The helical scan mode was used with the following parameters: 120 kVp, 130 mA, 1.0 sec scan time, 5 mm slice thickness, and 5 mm table advancement. The standard acquisition preset of a 25 cm field of view, matrix of 512 × 512 pixels, bone reconstruction algorithm, and WL of 300 and WW of 1000 was used. The raw dataset was retroreconstructed to a slice thickness of 0.3 mm. To obtain better reconstruction images, the overlapping technique, 5 mm slice thickness and 3 mm table advancement, pitch 0.6, (X-ray beam in overlapping) was also performed.

Images were visualized using PACS software (OsiriX DICOM Viewer, Pixmeo; Bernex, Switzerland), for transverse scanning, multiplanar reformatting (MPR), and 3D-rendering reconstruction.

CT images of each limb were analysed by 3 expert clinicians (L. L., A. G., and P. D. L.) and 2 students in veterinary medicine using the same software. An anatomical textbook [12] was used as reference for identifying normal anatomical structures in the CT tenography images. Each observer described the following normal structures for each specimen examined: in transverse scans, the proximal pouch of the DFTS synovial cavity, palmar aspect of the DFTS synovial cavity, synovial collateral recess, distal synovial fold, dorsal distal recess of the DFTS, superficial digital flexor tendon (SDFT), MF, DDFT, mesotendon, intersesamoidean ligament, straight sesamoidean ligament, and mesotendons; in MPR and 3D reformatted images, the dorsal proximal recess, palmar proximal recess, collateral recess, palmar distal recess, and dorsal distal recess. The observer assigned a score for each structure as follows: 0 if the structure was not identifiable, 1 if it is difficult to identify, and 2 if it is easy to identify; the total maximum score obtainable for a specimen was 34. The presence of artefacts (air bubbles, contrast medium leakage, reinforced beam, and inadequate distension) was also assigned a score as follows: 0 not appreciable, 1 slightly appreciable, and 2 highly appreciable.

2.4. Statistical Analysis. Data were analysed using Minitab 15.1 Statistical Software (Minitab, Inc.; State College, PA, USA). Data was analysed for normal distribution and analysis of variance (ANOVA) was performed to compare the scores assigned to the structures and artefacts by the expert versus the student observers and to compare the scores of the specimens. The significance level was set at $p < 0.05$.

3. Results

3.1. Transverse Scans. High-quality transverse scan images were obtained using either the contiguous or the overlapping scanning technique. The volume of CM used was adequate and provided intrathecal distension sufficient for separating anatomical structures and facilitating interpretation of the images. Intrathecal digital tendon structures were visualized at low density ranging from 150 to 240 Hounsfield Units (HU), and the synovial cavity was visualized with CM (>2000 HU). The MFs were also visible, especially if there was a high pressure of CM. Some artefacts were due to CM leakage that penetrated the subcutaneous tissue surrounding the point of injection and air bubbles that accumulated in the proximal DFTS pouch. In the specimen injected with 30 mL of CM solution, no leakage was verified, but less synovial distension was obtained, leading to difficulty in identifying the MF. Limb positioning (lateral or palmar recumbency) did not affect the distribution of CM in the synovial cavity; however, air bubbles were found in the uppermost regions of the cavity.

Figure 1 shows representative images obtained from the transverse scans. The intrathecal regions of the main tendon structures such as SDFT and DDFT were easy to identify, whereas the extrathecal regions were difficult to appreciate. High pressure of CM into the synovial cavity adequately separated the MF from the DDFT and synovial membrane,

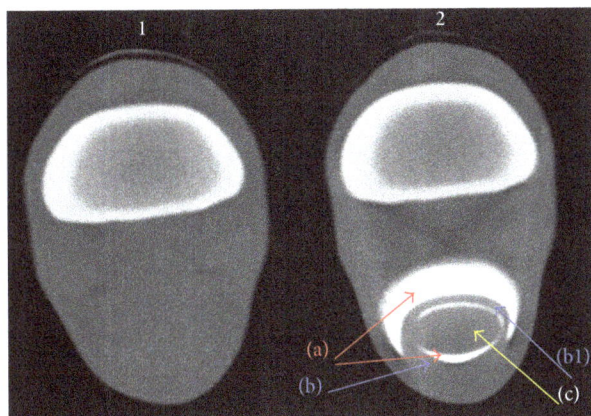

FIGURE 1: Normal representative images of transverse scans of direct CT (scan 1), and CT tenography (scan 2) of ex vivo forelimb of horses. (a) Proximal pouch of DFTS synovial cavity, (b) SDFT, (b1) manica flexoria, and (c) DDFT.

TABLE 1: Median of total scores assigned by observers for normal structures and artefacts for each specimen.

Specimen number	1	2	3	4	5	6
Median total score of structures	32	31	32	30	32	29
Median total score of artefacts	5	4	5	4	6	6

allowing accurate identification (Figures 2(a) and 2(b)). Transverse scans performed at the proximal sesamoid bones level showed a low volume of CM in the synovial cavity, whereas, in the pastern region, the distal DFTS pouch and synovial folds were clearly identified, because there was adequate distension by CM. The mesotendon was easily identified at this level in every specimen (Figure 2(b), scan 11, letter f).

3.2. MPR and 3D Reconstruction.

Figures 3 and 4 show representative images of MPR and 3D reconstructions of CT DFTS tenography. The image quality was considerably better using the overlapping scanning technique (pitch 0.6) with a retroreconstruction of a slice thickness < 1 mm.

3.3. Observer Scores of the Images.

Table 1 shows the median scores of all the observers' scores for each structure.

A comparison of the scores assigned to the structures and artefacts of each specimen showed that the MF and synovial collateral recess were more easily recognized ($p < 0.05$) by the expert observers (score median 2) than the students (score median 1.5). All the other structures were easily recognized by both the experts and students.

Comparison of the scores assigned to each specimen showed that observers had more difficulty ($p < 0.05$) identifying the SDFT, DDFT, and collateral recess of specimen 6 than for the other specimens.

Comparison of the artefact scores of each specimen showed that the expert observers assigned a significantly lower median score ($p < 0.05$) to the specimen that was insufficiently distended by CM than the students. Specimen

6 had a significantly higher score ($p < 0.05$) than the other specimens because of insufficient distension by CM.

4. Discussion

To the best of our knowledge, this is one of the first study reports to describe the normal CT tenographic anatomy of DFTS in the horse.

The results of this study indicate that the CT tenography of normal horse forelegs allowed easy identification of the entire DFTS and intrathecal digital tendons. In particular, the MF was identified in all the specimens that were investigated; the mesotendons and synovial recess were also identified.

CT tenographic images of the DFTS were acquired rapidly with high-quality images. Both images obtained with submillimetric thickness (obtained with retroreconstruction) and overlapping technique were very useful in reconstruction for MPR and 3D images, allowing improvement of quality, especially for images obtained in the sagittal and parasagittal planes, which were fundamental to visualizing normal tendon structures in this study. In fact, with the standard contiguous scanning technique (slice thickness = 3 mm), reconstruction of images in planes other than transverse image quality was very low. The use of novel 4- to 16-slice CT scanner will provide submillimetric thickness slice, resulting in improvement of the image quality, even in MPR and 3D, in order to diagnose very small defects, avoiding partial volume artefacts. Multislice CT scanners could improve also scanning time resulting in lower anaesthesia time. Anaesthesia is required to perform in vivo CT scanning of the horse; a shorter CT procedure could prevent intra- and postanaesthesia complications and reduce associated costs. Notwithstanding in this study we employed a single-slice CT scanner, the scanning procedure was performed in less than 10 min for each specimen.

The concentration of CM (185 mg/mL) was sufficient for visualizing intrathecal structures; the total volume should be larger than 30 mL but should not exceed 60 mL, in order to obtain adequate synovial distension while avoiding CM leakage from the puncture site. This artefact did not affect the anatomical assessments performed on transverse scans. Adequate synovial distension has been reported to improve the image quality of the equine stifle joint [9].

Analysis of score assignments showed that the main structures were easily identified by both expert and student observers, apart from the synovial collateral recess and MF. These two structures were recognized more easily by the experts, probably because they are normally thin and require a skilled observer for accurate identification.

Artefacts (air bubbles, CM leakage, and reinforced beam) were similarly recognised and scored by both observer categories, not influencing image interpretation. Inadequate distension was found to be the main factor that affected the interpretation of images. This was illustrated by the structure scores of specimen 6 compared with the other specimens. Injecting half volume (30 mL) of CM, SDFT, and DDFT at the intrathecal level and also collateral recess were distinguished more difficultly ($p < 0.05$) by observers. We therefore can speculate that a total CM volume of 60 mL was adequate for

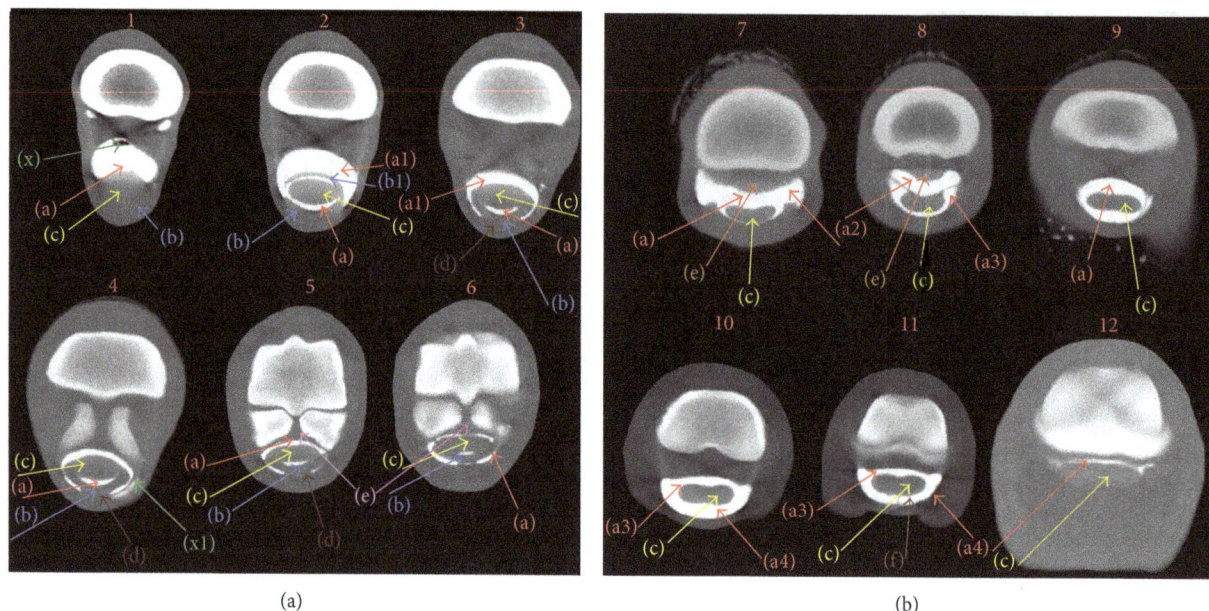

FIGURE 2: Computed tomographic tenography of ex vivo normal forelimbs of horses: representative images of transverse scans. Scans are shown proximally to distally: scans 1 to 6 of metacarpal region and 7 to 12 of pastern region. (a) Proximal pouch of digital flexor tendon sheath (DFTS) synovial cavity, (a1) palmar aspect of DFTS synovial cavity, (a2) synovial collateral recess, (a3) distal synovial fold, (a4) dorsal distal recess of DFTS, (b) superficial digital flexor tendon (SDFT), (b1) manica flexoria, (c) deep digital flexor tendon (DDFT), (d) mesotendon, (e) intersesamoidean ligament, (f) straight sesamoidean ligament, (g) mesotendon, (x) artefact and air bubbles, and (x1) subcutaneous contrast medium (CM) outflow after injection.

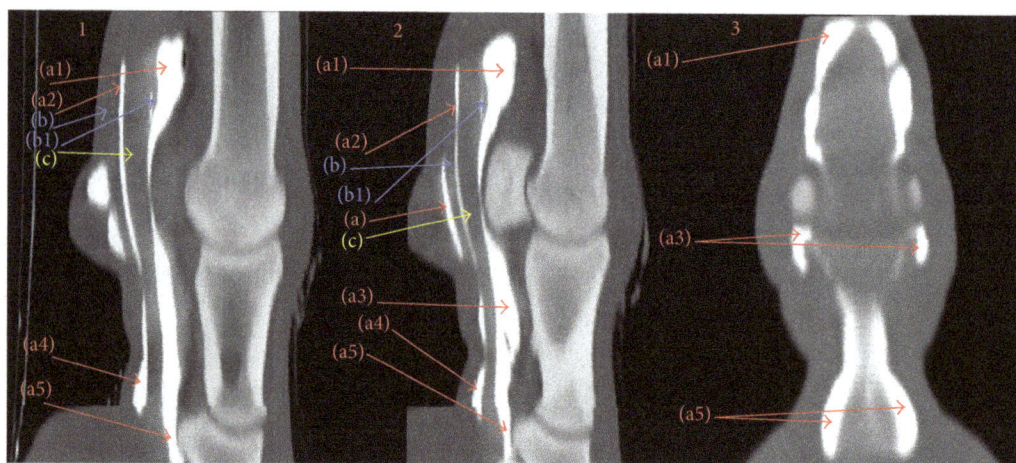

FIGURE 3: Multiplanar reconstruction (MPR). Computed tomographic tenography of ex vivo normal forelimbs of horses: representative images of sagittal (1), parasagittal (2), and dorsal (3) scans of DFTS. (a1) Dorsal proximal recess, (a2) palmar proximal recess, (a3) collateral recess, (a4) palmar distal recess, and (a5) dorsal distal recess. (b) SDFT and (b1) manica flexoria.

optimal filling of synovial cavity allowing proper separation of structures and distension of recess, helping in image interpretation.

In conclusion, CT tenography of equine DFTS has been evaluated as an alternative diagnostic technique to visualize intrathecal structures digital tendons in the horse. This imaging method could be employed with adequate technique and good knowledge of the normal tomographic anatomy to test specificity and accuracy in diagnosing specific conditions affecting the digital sheath, mesotendon, *manica flexoria* or SDFT, and DDFT.

Conflict of Interests

The authors declare that there is no conflict of interests regarding the publication of this paper.

Acknowledgments

This paper has been edited by native English-speaking experts of BioMed Proofreading. Students participating in the study are gratefully acknowledged.

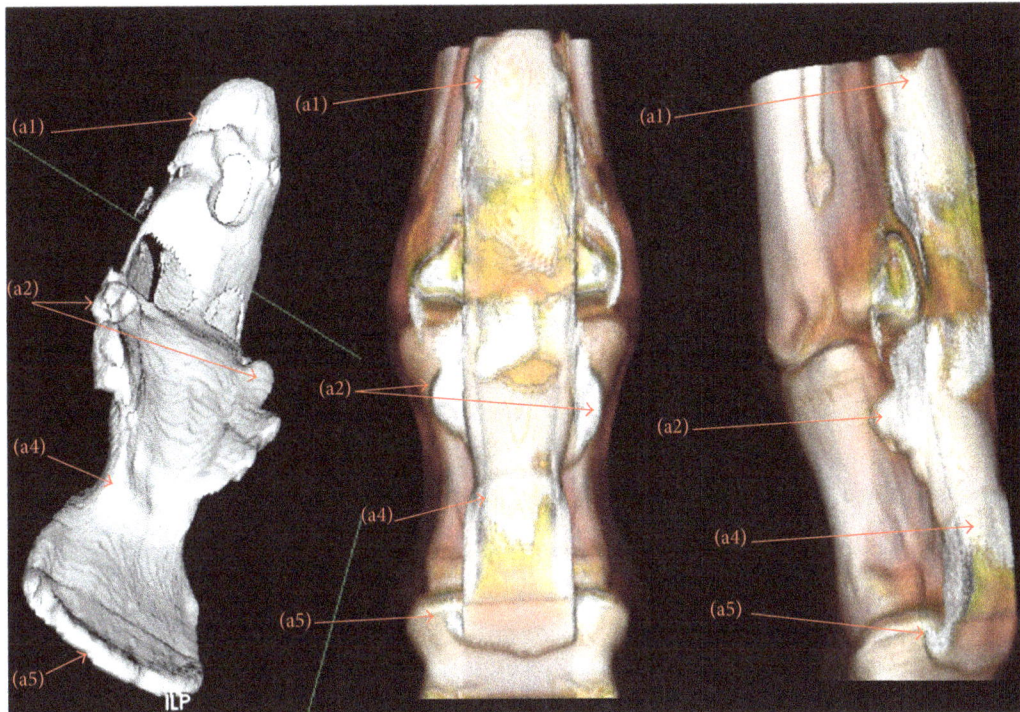

FIGURE 4: 3D reconstruction. (1) Surface rendering; (2) volume rendering. (a1) Dorsal proximal recess, (a2) palmar proximal recess, (a3) collateral recess, (a4) palmar distal recess, and (a5) dorsal distal recess.

References

[1] A. R. Fiske-Jackson, W. H. J. Barker, E. Eliashar, K. Foy, and R. K. W. Smith, "The use of intrathecal analgesia and contrast radiography as preoperative diagnostic methods for digital flexor tendon sheath pathology," *Equine Veterinary Journal*, vol. 45, no. 1, pp. 36–40, 2013.

[2] B. E. Hago and L. C. Vaughan, "Radiographic anatomy of tendon sheaths and bursae in the horse," *Equine Veterinary Journal*, vol. 18, no. 2, pp. 102–106, 1986.

[3] B. E. Hago and L. C. Vaughan, "Use of contrast radiography in the investigation of tenosynovitis and bursitis in horses," *Equine Veterinary Journal*, vol. 18, no. 5, pp. 375–382, 1986.

[4] M. R. Smith and I. M. Wright, "Noninfected tenosynovitis of the digital flexor tendon sheath: a retrospective analysis of 76 cases," *Equine Veterinary Journal*, vol. 38, no. 2, pp. 134–141, 2006.

[5] A. J. Nixon, "Endoscopy of the digital flexor tendon sheath in horses," *Veterinary Surgery*, vol. 19, no. 4, pp. 266–271, 1990.

[6] C. P. Crijns, I. M. V. L. Gielen, H. J. J. van Bree, and E. H. J. Bergman, "The use of CT and CT arthrography in diagnosing equine stifle injury in a Rheinlander gelding," *Equine Veterinary Journal*, vol. 42, no. 4, pp. 367–371, 2010.

[7] S. N. Gray, S. M. Puchalski, and L. D. Galuppo, "Computed tomographic arthrography of the intercarpal ligaments of the equine carpus," *Veterinary Radiology and Ultrasound*, vol. 54, no. 3, pp. 245–252, 2013.

[8] F. Hontoir, J.-F. Nisolle, H. Meurisse et al., "A comparison of 3-T magnetic resonance imaging and computed tomography arthrography to identify structural cartilage defects of the fetlock joint in the horse," *Veterinary Journal*, vol. 199, no. 1, pp. 115–122, 2014.

[9] A. Valdes-Martinez, "Computed tomographic arthrography of the equine stifle joint," *Veterinary Clinics of North America: Equine Practice*, vol. 28, no. 3, pp. 583–598, 2012.

[10] E. van der Vekens, E. H. J. Bergman, K. Vanderperren et al., "Computed tomographic anatomy of the equine stifle joint," *American Journal of Veterinary Research*, vol. 72, no. 4, pp. 512–521, 2011.

[11] M. Jordana, M. Oosterlinck, F. Pille, A. Valère, and A. Martens, "Comparison of four techniques for synoviocentesis of the equine digital flexor tendon sheath: a cadaveric study," *Veterinary and Comparative Orthopaedics and Traumatology*, vol. 25, no. 3, pp. 178–183, 2012.

[12] J. M. Denoix, *The Equine Distal Limb. An Atlas of Clinical Anatomy and Comparative Imaging*, Manson Publishing, London, UK, 2000.

14

The Effect of Different Types of Physical Exercise on the Behavioural and Physiological Parameters of Standardbred Horses Housed in Single Stalls

Barbara Padalino,[1] Paola Zaccagnino,[2] and Pietro Celi[3,4]

[1] Department of Veterinary Medicine, University of Bari, Str. prov. Per Casamassima, km 3, 70010 Valenzano (Bari), Italy
[2] Dipartimento di Scienze delle Produzioni Animali, Università degli Studi della Basilicata, Via dell'Ateneo Lucano 10, 85100 Potenza, Italy
[3] Faculty of Veterinary Science, University of Sydney, P.M.B. 4003, Narellan, NSW 2567, Australia
[4] Melbourne School of Land and Environment, The University of Melbourne, Parkville, VIC 3010, Australia

Correspondence should be addressed to Barbara Padalino; barbarapad@iol.it

Academic Editor: Pedro J. Ginel

The aim of this study was to investigate the impacts of three different physical exercises on the physiological and behavioural patterns of Standardbred trotters housed in single stalls. Twelve racing mares were observed twice during each different exercise: daily training (DT) consisted of forty minutes at slow trot (4-5 m/s) in a small track; maximal exercise (ME) consisted of 1600 m run at maximal velocity; race (R) was a real race of 1600 m. The mares were examined at rest in their stall (Time I), soon after the completion of the exercise (Time II), one hour (Time III), and two hours (Time IV) after the exercise. Their heart rate, respiratory rate, and rectal temperature were recorded and they were videotaped in order to complete a focal animal sampling ethogram. All physiological parameters increased after exercise, in accordance with its intensity. After R and ME horses spent more time drinking, eating, and standing. The incidence of abnormal behaviours was very low and it was not affected by the different types of exercise. Overall, the assessment of horse behaviour after physical exercise by means of a focal animal sampling ethogram represents a useful tool to monitor equine welfare.

1. Introduction

Although animal welfare has become more important in the equine industry, housing systems limiting natural behaviour patterns are still widespread [1]. Single stalls can confine social interaction and locomotion to a great extent, but, despite this, they are widely adopted in the equine industry, especially for Standardbred horses [2]. Housing horses in a single stall can influence equine welfare [3], with physical exercise being the only moment when horses can regularly move and express social behaviour. However, the possible consequences of prolonged confinement in stables on equine well-being have been studied [4] and group housing systems have been tested [5]. Animals can adapt to a new environment, but, when horses are kept alone on a flat, unstimulating square with nothing to do, some adaptative responses might include apathy and unresponsiveness, hyperresponsiveness, and stereotypic behaviour [6]. Apparently functionless, repetitive, stereotypic activities can be seen in stable horses [7–9] and equine stereotypies are primarily based on feeding and locomotory behaviours, due to management practices that limit foraging behaviour and social contact [10].

Although some researchers are investigating the relationships between exercise, housing and management, and the development of abnormal behaviour in horses [11], there is a lack of information about the effect of traditional training and racing on the Standardbred horse's behaviour. By understanding the behaviour modification that different kinds of exercise could induce, the management of racing horses could be improved especially in terms of their welfare status. Therefore, we sought to evaluate the effect of two different types of exercise, as well as racing, on some behavioural patterns of Standardbred horses kept in single boxes. Some physiological parameters, namely, heart rate (HR), respiratory rate (RR), and temperature (T), were also monitored.

2. Materials and Methods

2.1. Animals, Management, and Physical Exercises. Twelve Standardbred mares, homogeneous for live weight (450 ± 25 kg), body condition score (3 ± 0.25 arbitrary units; from 1 to 5 accordingly with Martin-Rosset [12]), and age (3.5 ± 0.5 years), were recruited in this study. All mares were in good health status and they all were qualified to race (mean record on 1600 m race track was $1'16'' ± 02''$). The research was carried out on a racetrack in Castelluccio dei Sauri, Foggia (Italy), during the summer months of June and July where the average maximum and minimum temperature and relative humidity were 31 ± 4°C, 16 ± 3°C, and 61 ± 5%, respectively. All mares were housed at the racetrack in a stable which contained 16 single stalls (3.00 m ∗ 3.50 m, 10.5 m^2) in two rows, with a central aisle (3 m wide). The front has sliding doors, divided in two parts with the bottom panel being always kept shut and the top one always open, when the mares were monitored for behavioural status.

The horses were fed with hay and concentrate three times a day: early in the morning (7 am), after the completion of the physical exercises (between 12 pm and 1 pm), and late in the afternoon (6 pm). The amount of feed, feed quality and type remained constant over the course of the experiment. Water was available in the stable at all times for each individual horse.

All mares were housed in the same horse stalls, trained and raced by the same trainer, and performed the following physical exercises at the same time of day during the whole study. (1) Daily training (DT): consisted of forty minutes at a slow trot (4-5 m/s) on the small track of the race track; mares would cover an average of 10,000 m. The mares were jugged to a heavy gig by Custom [13]. (2) Maximal exercise (ME): consisted of 1600 m at maximal velocity; the mares were jugged to a sulky and they were alone on the track. Before performing the ME, mares were warmed up with a 5,000 m trot at the speed of 6-7 m/s. (3) Race (R): consisted of a real race over a 1600 m distance. All races were in the morning from 11 am to 1 pm (matinee' race); DT and ME were also performed at a similar time of the day. The number of the horses in each race was about 14. Before the race, horses were warmed up with a 5000 m trot at the speed of 6-7 m/s. Immediately after each exercise the mares were showered, walked by an operator for 5 minutes, and then returned to their individual stalls. The weekly training regime consisted of three days of DT followed by one day of ME and then three days of DT again. Horses raced every fortnight and they rested the day after the race in paddocks. During DT and ME, horses performed the physical exercises in an empty racetrack, while during the race the racetrack had several spectators.

2.2. Behavioural and Physiological Parameters. The mares were examined at rest in their stalls (Time I) at 8 AM, within 10 ± 2 minutes after exercise, before washing and cooling down (Time II), one hour after exercise (Time III), and two hours after exercise (Time IV). Each examination included recording the heart rate (HR) by auscultation, respiratory rate (RR) through observation of chest-wall movement, and rectal temperature (RT) with an electronic thermometer in °C (Vedodigit II-PIC). All measures were taken by the same veterinarian. The mares were videotaped by a video camera (Sony) while they were in their stalls. Briefly, each observation cycle was 1 hour in duration for a total period of 4 hours, with one hour of observation before exercise and three hours observation after exercise: the first took place from 8 to 9 AM, before the training session (Time I), the second was when the horse came back to the stall after exercise (Time II), the third was one hour later (Time III), and the last one was two hours later (Time IV). Between the three observation periods after exercise there was a 5-minute break during which the physiological parameters described above were taken. One operator reviewed all the videos and compiled a "focal animal sampling ethogram" and the duration (sec) of the following behavioural states was calculated: lying, standing, drinking, hay and concentrate feeding, and walking, eliminative and explorative behaviours. Standing was defined as the time spent in station without doing other activities, such as feeding or drinking, while explorative behaviour was defined as the time that the mares spent sniffing each part of the box. Moreover, the duration of the following events was also calculated: urination, defecation, hay and concentrate feeding, and stereotypical and abnormal behaviour. Particular attention was placed on the possible identification of the following abnormal behaviours reported for Standardbreds: weaving, box-walking, crib-biting/wind sucking, and wood chewing [7]. All mares were observed twice for each exercise.

2.3. Ethical Guidelines. All the procedures were carried out in accordance with the Italian legislation on animal care (DL n. 116, 27/01/1992).

2.3.1. Statistical Analysis. All data were normally distributed and were analysed by using REML variance component analysis procedure for *GenStat version 14*, where the type of physical exercise (R, ME, and DT), the time of observation (Times I, II, III, and IV), and the interaction between physical exercise and time of observation were considered as fixed factors, while mares and replicate were considered as random factors. All data were expressed as mean ± SE. The effects were considered to be significant at $P < 0.05$; differences between means were tested using least significant difference.

3. Results

A significant effect of physical exercise ($P < 0.001$), time ($P < 0.001$), and their interaction ($P < 0.001$) was observed for both heart rate (HR) (Figure 1(a)) and respiratory rate (RR) (Figure 1(b)). Both HR and RR were similar before the commencement of physical exercise and as expected they increased significantly soon after the completion of physical exercise (Time II) and then returned to preexercise levels by the end of the observation period (Time IV). A significant effect of the interaction time of observation × physical exercise was noted on both HR and RR ($P < 0.001$), with horses that undertook the race (R) presenting higher HR and RR levels than the horse that performed the daily training (DT) or maximal velocity (ME) exercises at Time II. HR levels were still higher in horses that performed the R exercise compared to those that performed the DT and ME exercises at Time III; at Time IV, horses that performed the R exercise had higher HR values than horses that performed the DT exercise. Differences in RR values between the race and the other two exercises disappeared after 1 h (Time III) from the completion of physical exercise. A significant effect of physical exercise ($P < 0.001$), time ($P < 0.001$), and their interaction ($P < 0.05$) was observed for rectal temperature (RT) with its values increasing soon after completion of the three different physical exercises (Time II) (Figure 1(c)). This increase was more pronounced in horses that performed the race. RT levels returned to preexercise levels 1 h (Time III) from the completion of physical exercise.

A significant effect of physical exercise ($P < 0.05$) and physical exercise × time interaction ($P < 0.01$) was observed on standing activity (Figure 2(a)). Standing behaviour was significantly lower in horses that performed the R and ME exercises than in horses that performed the DT exercise on Times II and IV. A significant effect of time ($P < 0.01$) and physical exercise × time interaction ($P < 0.05$) was observed on resting behaviour (lying) (Figure 2(b)). Resting behaviour was significantly lower in horses that performed the R and ME exercises than in horses that performed the DT exercise on Times II and III.

A significant effect of time ($P < 0.001$) was observed for drinking activity with horses spending a higher amount of time drinking soon after the completion of physical exercise (Figure 3(a)). A significant effect of physical exercise ($P < 0.05$), time ($P < 0.001$), and their interaction ($P < 0.05$) was noted for eating activity (Figure 3(b)). One hour after the completion of physical exercises (Time II), horses that undertook the R and ME exercises spent more time eating than horses that performed the DT exercise. On Time III horses that undertook the R exercise spent more time eating than horses that performed the DT and ME exercises.

Eliminative behaviours (urinating and defecating) were significantly affected by time ($P < 0.01$ and $P < 0.05$, resp.) only. Defecating activity was significantly higher before the commencement of physical exercise (Time I; Figure 4(b)), while urinating activity was significantly higher during Time II compared to the other times of observation (Figure 4(a)).

Among the abnormal behaviours, crib-biting was the only one that was observed and only in two mares. No effect of physical exercise, time, and their interaction was observed for this stereotypic behaviour (Figure 5(a)) and explorative behaviours (Figure 5(b)).

4. Discussion

The good health of the horses recruited in this study was substantiated by the rapid return of the physiological parameters (HR, RR, and RT) measured to baseline levels after the completion of the different physical exercises. As expected the increase in HR induced by DT was lower than that induced by ME and R. In particular, the HR increase was higher in horses that participated in the race event than those that performed ME, even though the horses covered the same distance at a similar speed, as the race not only represents a maximal exercise, but it also produces a stronger emotional response and mental stress [14]. Moreover, during a race event the presence of the audience might also have resulted in increased stress levels [15] and thus this emotional influence might explain the higher increase in HR observed in horses after the race. As expected, changes in RR were proportional to the intensity of the physical exercises. Horses rely primarily on sweating for heat loss, but the respiratory tract contributes to heat loss especially during exercise [16, 17]. Similarly, Miraglia et al. [18] found a positive correlation between the increase of RT and exercise intensity. Since it is well known that thermoregulation is impaired in poorly trained horses [17], we can conclude that our horses were in good health as their RT returned to preexercise levels within one hour from completion of the physical activity.

The duration of drinking activity was higher in horses after the race event than after ME and DT exercises; this behaviour was particularly evident during the first hour of observation, in accordance with Carson and Wood-Gush [19], who also reported an increase in the drinking activities soon after an intense exercise. In our study urinations occurred predominantly during the second hour of observation after exercise; a likely consequence of the increase in drinking activity was observed during the first hour after exercise, which indicates that the horses in this study quickly achieved a good state of hydration. Eating behaviour was particularly frequent during the first observation period after the race event and ME. Our findings are in agreement with those of Caanitz et al. [20], who proposed that the observed increase in time spent eating might have been a physiological consequence of the high energy expenditure during intense exercise. Increase in eating behaviour and in appetite has also been reported in trotters after a three-hour journey to restore the energy lost during transport [21]. However, our observations might also have been influenced by that fact that in this study horses were fasted for two hours prior to the race and ME events; therefore, the motivation to eat after these exercises could have been stronger.

Resting behaviour, such as lying down or standing while resting was less frequent in horses after R and ME than after DT. Usually horses only lie down only in a quiet environment [19]; however, in this study, when horses performed a race or ME, there were people, trainers, and drivers in their stable and therefore the horses might have been more alert, particularly after the race when the race track was usually very noisy [22]. Alternately, the horses might have been more active in their stalls in response to catecholamines released during the strenuous exercise [23].

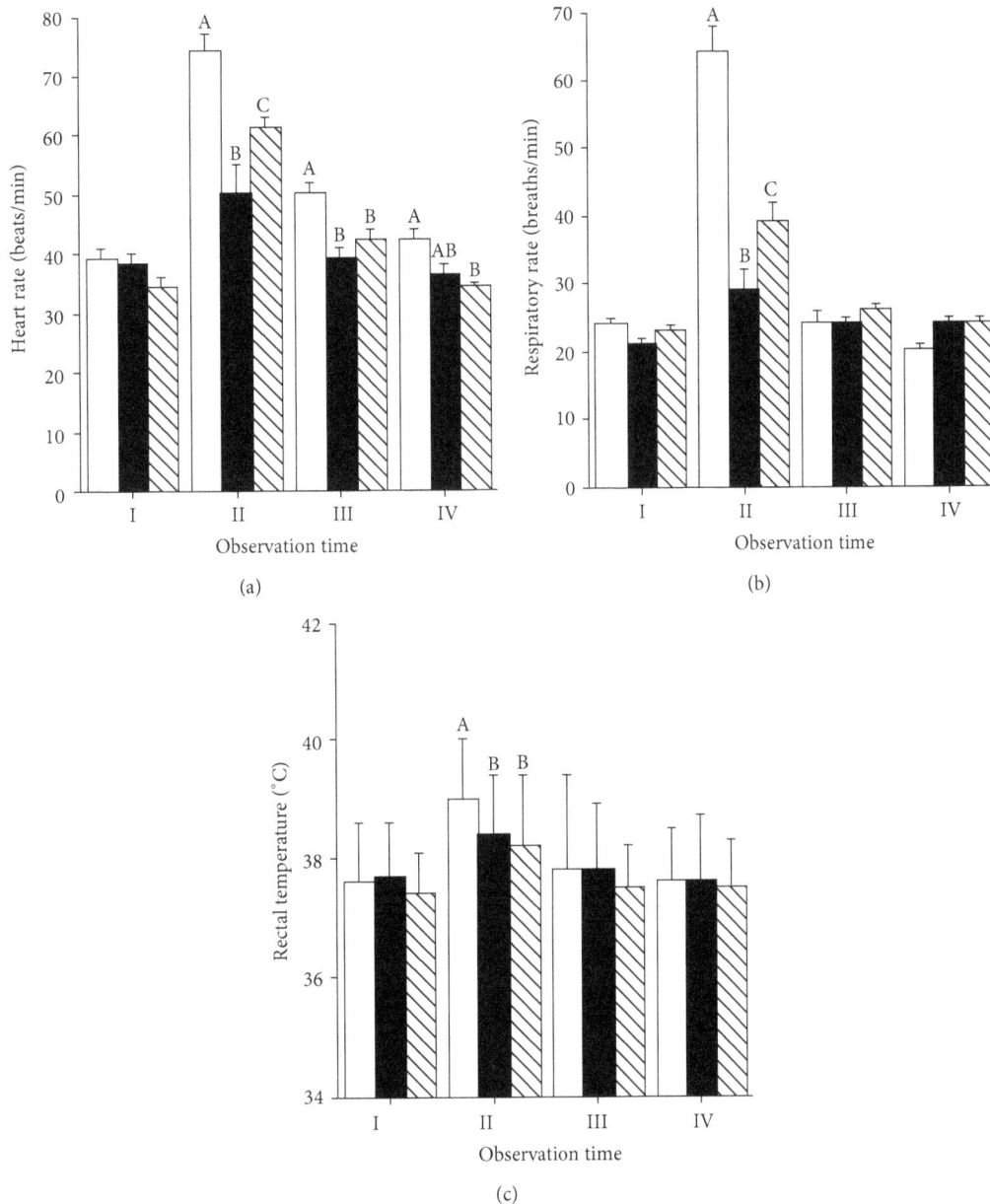

FIGURE 1: Effect of different types of physical exercise (race blank; maximal exercise shaded; daily exercise lined) on heart rate (a), respiratory rate (b), and rectal temperature (c) of Standardbred horses housed in single stalls. Mares were examined at rest in their stalls (Time I), immediately after exercise (Time II), one (Time III), and two hours (Time V) after the completion of exercise. Values are expressed as means ± SE. For parameters where a significant effect of type of exercise × time interaction was noted, means with different capital letters indicate significant difference ($P < 0.01$) between types of exercises.

There was no effect of type of exercise on explorative behaviour. Horses exhibit explorative behaviour to investigate new situations and environments [24], whereas horses well adapted to their environment and in good welfare present decreased explorative behaviour [25]; therefore, our findings suggest that in this study horses were well accustomed to their environment. It is important to note that explorative behaviour did not show any statistical difference between exercise types, but all horses showed explorative behaviours within the normal range and did not manifest any atypical posture. Therefore, in accordance with that reported by

Fureix et al. [26] we can infer that the mares enrolled in this study did not suffer from depression.

Furthermore, our findings indicate that the incidence of abnormal behaviours in the horses recruited in this study was extremely low and that it was not affected by the type of physical exercise. One explanation for this observation is that our horses were quite young and therefore less prone to show stereotypies in agreement with Bachmann et al. [27]. Another explication could be that the horses were well managed and accustomed to the training regime. In fact, as suggested by Houpt and McDonnell [28], it is likely that

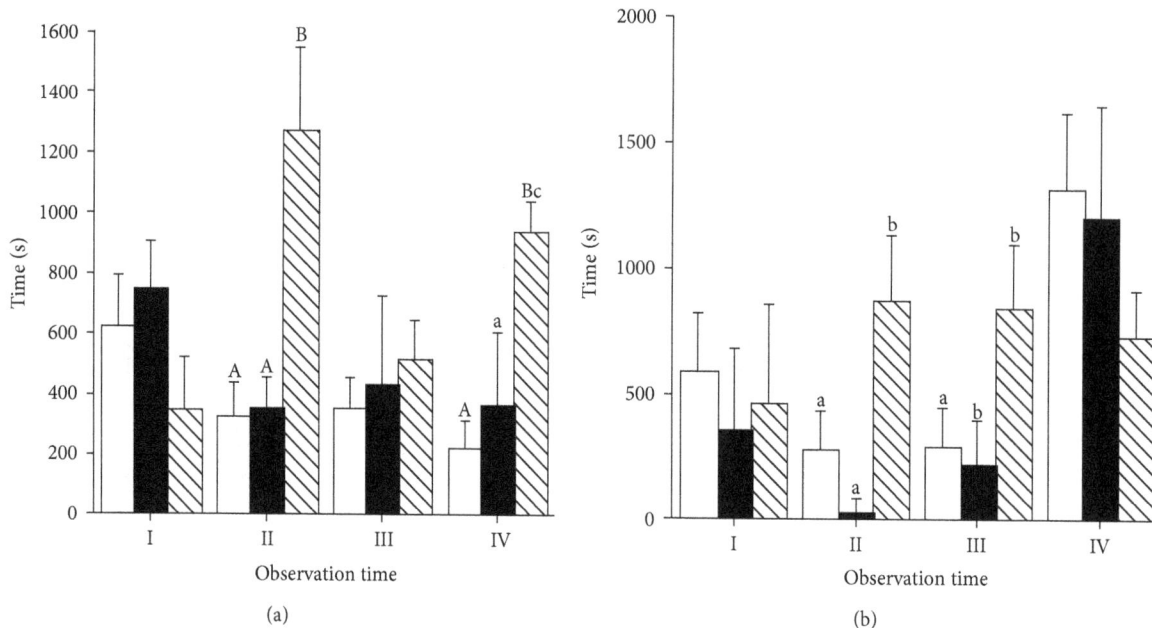

FIGURE 2: Effect of different types of physical exercise (race blank; maximal exercise shaded; daily exercise lined) on standing up activity (a) and resting behaviour (b) of Standardbred horses housed in single stalls. Mares were examined at rest in their stalls (Time I), immediately after exercise (Time II), one (Time III), and two hours (Time V) after the completion of exercise. Values are expressed as means ± SE. For parameters where a significant effect of type of exercise × time interaction was noted, means with different capital and low letters indicate significant difference ($P < 0.01$ and $P < 0.05$, resp.) between types of exercises.

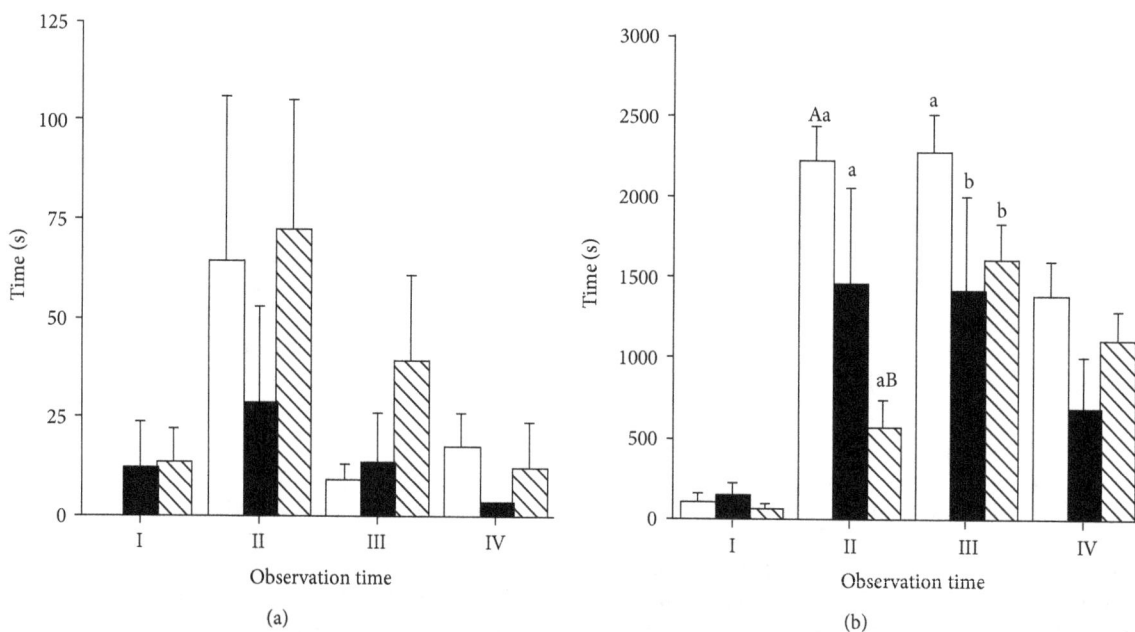

FIGURE 3: Effect of different types of physical exercise (race blank; maximal exercise shaded; daily exercise lined) on drinking (a) and eating activity (b) of Standardbred horses housed in single stalls. Mares were examined at rest in their stalls (Time I), immediately after exercise (Time II), one (Time III), and two hours (Time V) after the completion of exercise. Values are expressed as means ± SE. For parameters where a significant effect of type of exercise × time interaction was noted, means with different capital and low letters indicate significant difference ($P < 0.01$ and $P < 0.05$, resp.) between types of exercises.

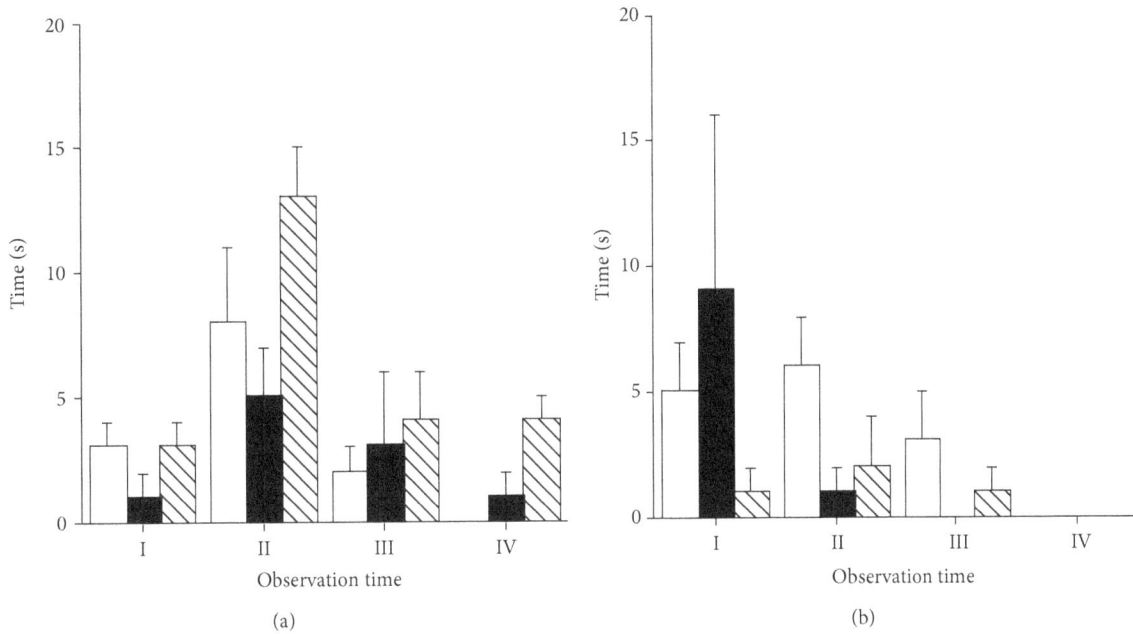

FIGURE 4: Effect of different types of physical exercise (race blank; maximal exercise shaded; daily exercise lined) on urinating (a) and defecating activity (b) of Standardbred horses housed in single stalls. Mares were examined at rest in their stalls (Time I), immediately after exercise (Time II), one (Time III), and two hours (Time V) after the completion of exercise. Values are expressed as means ± SE.

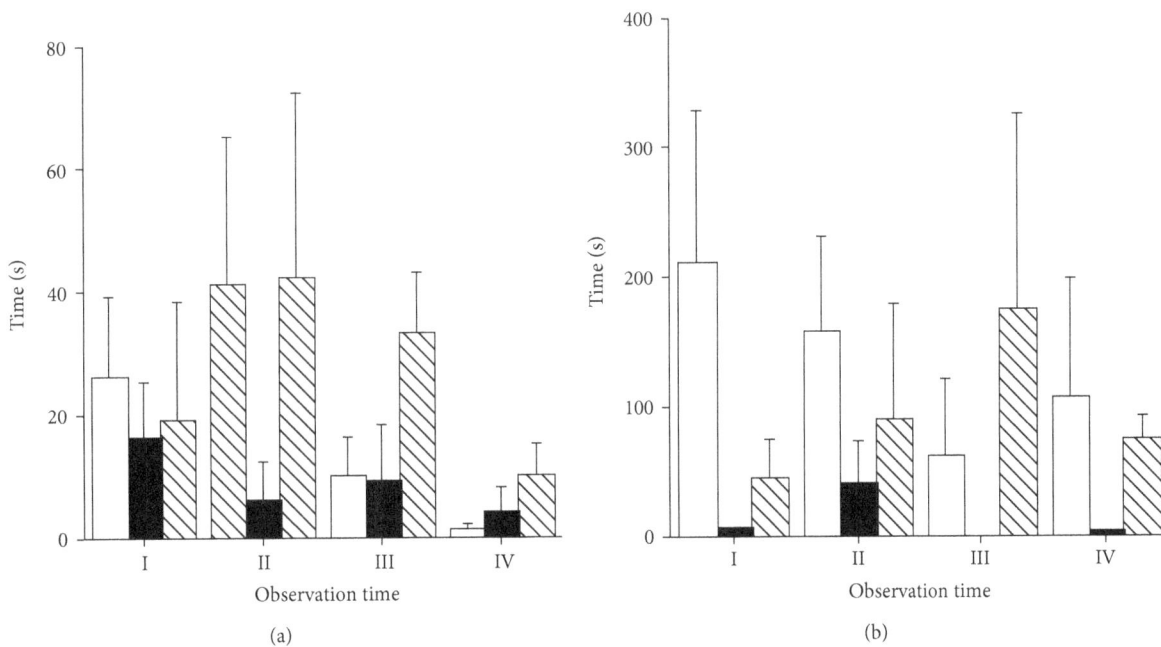

FIGURE 5: Effect of different types of physical exercise (race blank; maximal exercise shaded; daily exercise lined) on stereotypic behaviour (a) and exploitive activity (b) of Standardbred horses housed in single stalls. Mares were examined at rest in their stalls (Time I), immediately after exercise (Time II), one (Time III), and two hours (Time V) after the completion of exercise. Values are expressed as means ± SE.

good management also contributed to the low incidence of stereotypies. Although housing in single stalls and a stimuli poor environment is usually positively correlated with the development of abnormal behaviours [7], our data indicated that the horses were well adapted to their routinely management as they were trained on a daily basis, fed

thrice, and handled many times a day. In addition, human activities (feeding, grooming, and cleaning) were conducted daily for 10 hours in the stable, suggesting that the horses were well accustomed to human presence and that they were handled and looked after properly. Finally, the presence of few crib-biting events could be more closely correlated with the feeding other than the training [7]. Therefore, in agreement with Werhahn et al. [11], our data suggest that a regular training regime does not increase the occurrence of stereotypies in Standardbred confined in single stalls.

5. Conclusion

In conclusion, after all physical exercises tested in this study, horses increased eating and drinking behaviour, whereas they decreased resting. In consequence, to guarantee a favourable physiological and behavioural restore, we would recommend that horses are offered food and fresh water in their boxes after cooling down. Overall, the assessment of horse behaviour after physical exercise by means of a focal ethogram represents a useful tool to monitor equine welfare. This could easily be adopted by the horse industry with the use of CCTV technology.

Conflict of Interests

The authors declare that there is no conflict of interests regarding the publication of this paper. None of the authors of this paper has a financial or personal relationship with other people or organizations that could inappropriately influence or bias the content of the paper.

References

[1] H. Werhahn, E. F. Hessel, and H. F. A. van den Weghe, "Competition horses housed in single stalls (I): behavior and activity patterns during free exercise according to its configuration," *Journal of Equine Veterinary Science*, vol. 32, no. 1, pp. 45–52, 2012.

[2] B. Padalino, P. de Palo, A. Tateo, and P. Centoducati, "La gestione del cavallo trottatore: indagine in Puglia," *Ippologia*, vol. 16, no. 4, pp. 15–18, 2005.

[3] R. Freire, P. Buckley, and J. J. Cooper, "Effects of different forms of exercise on post inhibitory rebound and unwanted behaviour in stabled horses," *Equine Veterinary Journal*, vol. 41, no. 5, pp. 487–492, 2009.

[4] J. Ladewing, "The other 23 hours of the day," in *Proceedings of the 9th ISES Conference*, July 2013.

[5] M. VanDiereholock and T. Vogel-vanVreeswijk, "Revolutionary equine group housing system with automatic roughage feeding system moving in between a group: the effect of increasing from 3 to 6 feeding runs," in *Proceedings of the 9th ISES Conference*, July 2013.

[6] J. J. Cooper and M. J. Albentosa, "Behavioural adaptation in the domestic horse: potential role of apparently abnormal responses including stereotypic behaviour," *Livestock Production Science*, vol. 92, no. 2, pp. 177–182, 2005.

[7] P. D. McGreevy, P. J. Cripps, N. P. French, L. E. Green, and C. J. Nicol, "Management factors associated with stereotypic and redirected behaviour in the thoroughbred horse," *Equine Veterinary Journal*, vol. 27, no. 2, pp. 86–91, 1995.

[8] J. J. Cooper and G. J. Mason, "The identification of abnormal behaviour and behavioural problems in stabled horses and their relationship to horse welfare: a comparative review," *Equine Veterinary Journal Supplements*, no. 27, pp. 5–9, 1998.

[9] C. Nicol, "Understanding equine stereotypies," *Equine Veterinary Journal Supplements*, no. 28, pp. 20–25, 1999.

[10] S. M. Pell and P. D. McGreevy, "A study of cortisol and beta-endorphin levels in stereotypic and normal Thoroughbreds," *Applied Animal Behaviour Science*, vol. 64, no. 2, pp. 81–90, 1999.

[11] H. Werhahn, E. F. Hessel, and H. F. A. van den Weghe, "Competition horses housed in single stalls (II): effects of free exercise on the behavior in the stable, the behavior during training, and the degree of stress," *Journal of Equine Veterinary Science*, vol. 32, no. 1, pp. 22–31, 2012.

[12] W. Martin-Rosset, *L'alimentazione del cavallo*, Edagricole, Bologna, Italy, 1990.

[13] A. Tateo, M. Siniscalchi, B. Padalino, S. Dimatteo, P. Centoducati, and A. Quaranta, "Parametri ematochimici e fisiologici in cavalli trottatori sottoposti ad esercizio su bagnasciuga e in pista," *Ippologia*, vol. 1, pp. 21–25, 2008.

[14] T. R. Rietmann, A. E. A. Stuart, P. Bernasconi, M. Stauffacher, J. A. Auer, and M. A. Weishaupt, "Assessment of mental stress in warmblood horses: heart rate variability in comparison to heart rate and selected behavioural parameters," *Applied Animal Behaviour Science*, vol. 88, no. 1-2, pp. 121–136, 2004.

[15] M. Becker-Birck, S. Biau, N. Ill, J. Aurich, E. Mostl, and C. Aurich, "Heart rate, heart rate variability and cortisol release in the horse and its rider: different response to training and a public equestrian performance," in *Proceedings of the 8th ISES*, Edinburgh, July 2012.

[16] D. Marlin and K. Nankervis, *Equine Exercise Physiology*, Backwell Publishing, Malden, Mass, USA, 2002.

[17] D. R. Hodgson, R. E. Davis, and F. F. McConaghy, "Thermoregulation in the horse in response to exercise," *The British Veterinary Journal*, vol. 150, no. 3, pp. 219–235, 1994.

[18] N. Miraglia, D. Bergero, and D. Gagliardi, *Il cavallo atleta*, Edagricole, Bologna, Italy, 2000.

[19] K. Carson and D. G. M. Wood-Gush, "Equine behaviour: II. A review of the literature on feeding, eliminative and resting behaviour," *Applied Animal Ethology*, vol. 10, no. 3, pp. 179–190, 1983.

[20] H. Caanitz, L. O'Leary, K. Houpt, K. Petersson, and H. Hintz, "Effect of exercise on equine behavior," *Applied Animal Behaviour Science*, vol. 31, no. 1-2, pp. 1–12, 1991.

[21] A. Tateo, B. Padalino, M. Boccaccio, A. Maggiolino, and P. Centoducati, "Transport stress in horses: effects of two different distances," *Journal of Veterinary Behavior*, vol. 7, no. 1, pp. 33–42, 2012.

[22] M. Kiley-Worthington, "The behavior of horses in relation to management and training—towards ethologically sound environments," *Journal of Equine Veterinary Science*, vol. 10, no. 1, pp. 62–75, 1990.

[23] J. J. Hagan and B. Bohus, "The effects of endorphins on cardiac responses during an emotional stress," *Physiology and Behavior*, vol. 31, no. 5, pp. 607–614, 1983.

[24] P. McGreevy, *Equine Behaviour: A Guide for Veterinarians and Equine Scientists*, Sydney, Australia, Saunders, 2008.

[25] J. A. Mench and G. J. Mason, *Animal Welfare*, CAB International, Wallingford, UK, 1997.

[26] C. Fureix, P. Jego, S. Henry, L. Lansade, and M. Hausberger, "Toward an ethological animal model of depression? A study on horses," *PLoS ONE*, vol. 7, no. 6, Article ID e39280, 2012.

[27] I. Bachmann, L. Audigé, and M. Stauffacher, "Risk factors associated with behavioural disorders of crib-biting, weaving and box-walking in Swiss horses," *Equine Veterinary Journal*, vol. 35, no. 2, pp. 158–163, 2003.

[28] K. A. Houpt and S. M. McDonnell, "Equine stereotypes," *Compendium on Continuing Education for the Practising Veterinarian*, vol. 15, pp. 1265–1271, 1993.

15

Effect of Moxidectin Treatment at Peripartum on Gastrointestinal Parasite Infections in Ewes Raised under Tropical Andes High Altitude Conditions

J. J. Vargas-Duarte,[1,2] H. Lozano-Márquez,[2,3]
H. A. Grajales-Lombana,[3] C. Manrique-Perdomo,[3] D. A. Martínez-Bello,[4]
C. Saegerman,[5] M. Raes,[2] and N. Kirschvink[2]

[1]Genetic Institute, National University of Colombia, Carrera 30 No. 45-03, Edificio 426, Bogotá D.C., Colombia
[2]Unit of Integrated Veterinary Research, Department of Veterinary Medicine, University of Namur, rue de Bruxelles 61,
  5000 Namur, Belgium
[3]Faculty of Veterinary Medicine and Animal Science, National University of Colombia, Carrera 30 No. 45-03,
  Edificio 481, Bogotá D.C., Colombia
[4]Faculty of Veterinary Medicine, Cooperative University of Colombia, Calle 30 No. 33-51, Bucaramanga, Colombia
[5]Research Unit of Epidemiology and Risk Analysis Applied to Veterinary Sciences (UREAR),
  Fundamental and Applied Research for Animal and Health (FARAH), University of Liège, boulevard de Colonster 20,
  4000 Liège, Belgium

Correspondence should be addressed to J. J. Vargas-Duarte; jjvargasd@unal.edu.co

Academic Editor: Guillermo Virkel

This study tested the impact of moxidectin at peripartum on nematode fecal egg count (FEC) and clinical parameters on ewes in the high altitude tropical Andes of Colombia. FEC and clinical evaluations were performed on 9 occasions in 43 naturally infected ewes before and during gestation and after lambing. Moxidectin (Mox, $200\,\mu g\,kg^{-1}$) was applied at late pregnancy (T_1, $n = 15$) or 48 hours after parturition (T_2, $n = 14$). 14 untreated ewes served as controls (C). Suckling lambs ($n = 58$) remained untreated and underwent four clinical and parasitological evaluations until 8 weeks after birth. Mox efficacy equaled 99.3% (T_1) and 96.9% (T_2). Highest mean FEC value reflecting periparturient nematode egg rise (PPER) was recorded in C ewes at 4–6 weeks after lambing. Significant FEC reductions were found in T_1 (94.8%) and T_2 (96.7%) ewes ($p < 0.05$). All lambs showed a significant and ewes-group independent increase in FEC before weaning ($p < 0.05$). Clinical parameters (anemia and diarrhea) showed time- and treatment-related differences ($p < 0.05$). Monitoring of FEC and clinical parameters linked to gastrointestinal parasite infections allowed demonstrating that postpartum or preweaning are two critical periods to nematode infection for sheep raised under tropical Andes high altitude conditions. Use of Mox as anthelmintic treatment prevented PPER.

1. Introduction

Sheep parasites belong to the main constraints that reduce sustainability of wool, milk, and meat production worldwide [1–3]. To prevent parasite dissemination in small ruminant flocks, assessment of the magnitude of gastrointestinal parasite burdens in different productive categories is required [4, 5]. Indeed, lambs have been described as the most susceptible

category to gastrointestinal parasites and it is assumed that adult animals can deal with parasite infection and minimize its pathogenic activity [5, 6]. However, it has been shown that periparturient ewes are highly susceptible to gastrointestinal nematode infections and are the largest contributors to pasture contamination with nematode eggs [7, 8].

In mature ewes, a transient loss of immunity to gastrointestinal nematodes begins around lambing time and continues for several weeks after parturition. This impaired resistance is associated with an increase in strongylid fecal egg count (FEC) commonly referred to as the periparturient nematode egg rise (PPER) [5, 9–14]. PPER has been described mainly in sheep breeds exploited in temperate regions. Indeed, the flocks' seasonal management allows the spring contamination of pasture with nematode eggs shed by lactating ewes and the concomitant infection of lambs with the infective larvae hatched from those eggs [15, 16]. Although well known, the exact cause of PPER remains poorly understood. Increased FEC has been also associated with variations in hormonal profiles at peripartum (prolactin and cortisol levels) and low levels of metabolisable protein intake during late pregnancy and lactation [13, 17–21].

In tropical regions of South America, sheep production is based on extensive grazing with limited management and sanitary practices, which leads to increased mortality rates and reduced productivity due to gastrointestinal nematodes [22–24]. Under these conditions, the importance of a PPER and its epidemiological consequences in small ruminants remain to be established [7, 25–28]. On the one hand, infective larvae may be continuously available in the tropics and reproductive cycles and lambing are not strictly seasonal events as in temperate countries. Indeed, in Colombian flocks, lambing might occur during the entire year, but two main annual periods of births during April–June and November-December at the end of rainy periods are described [29]. On the other hand, physiopathological consequences of PPER in lactating ewes and their offspring are believed to be important in the tropics because the infectious pressure persists at a high level and because nutritional management is often heterogeneous [24, 26, 30, 31]. Consequently, environmental parameters, reproductive cycle features, and feeding management practices are fundamental tools for rational anthelmintic treatment [3, 4, 32]. In order to minimize nematode egg outputs and to regulate pasture contamination with infective third larval stages in tropical sheep production systems, strategic treatment of highly infected animal groups, as periparturient ewes, is recommended [2, 8, 33, 34].

Among the available chemical groups used to control gastrointestinal nematodes in sheep, macrocyclic lactones represent the cornerstone of current anthelmintic drug control [35]. Moxidectin (Mox), a macrocyclic lactone of the chemical family of milbemycins, has been widely used during the last 30 years [36]. However, the intensive use of this broad-spectrum antiparasitic compound could lead to the emergence of resistance in gastrointestinal nematodes [35, 36]. This situation has encouraged the search for treatment strategies to optimize Mox potential, avoiding unnecessary treatments, particularly in geographic areas where Mox use is not a frequent practice and resistance is not yet fully present [36, 37].

The present study hypothesized (1) that PPER occurs in Colombian sheep raised under Andean high altitude tropical conditions during the period of the highest lambing rate (April–June), (2) that Mox is still an effective anthelmintic molecule at tropical Andes, and (3) that Mox strategic treatment of ewes administered either at late pregnancy or early peripartum period would prevent PPER.

2. Materials and Methods

The study was conducted at the Center for Sheep Research, Technological Development and Extension of the National University of Colombia, located in Mosquera-Cundinamarca ($4°40'57''N, 74°12'50''W$) at 2510 m above sea level. The mean temperature during the study period was $13.5°C$ and the monthly average rainfall 86 mm. The protocols employed followed the national guidelines for care and use of animals (Colombian Law 89/1989) and were approved by the Ethical Committee of the Faculty of Veterinary Medicine and Animal Science of National University of Colombia (CB-035-2013).

2.1. Animals. This study enrolled 43 healthy wool ewes of four breeds (Colombian creole, Romney Marsh, Hampshire, and Corriedale). Ewes were grazing together in *Lolium perenne* and *Pennisetum clandestinum* pastures and were supplemented with concentrate feed, hay, and mineralized salt according to physiological requirements. Fresh drinking water was available *ad libitum*. Ewes' clinical and parasitological follow-up was performed during one complete reproductive cycle (dry period, mating period, pregnancy period, and postpartum period). Since birth, lambs ($n = 58$) were kept with their dams and underwent the same follow-up.

2.2. Experimental Design. A longitudinal study was conducted during 40 weeks and included nine sampling periods where parasitological and clinical evaluations were performed in relation to ewe's reproductive state (Figure 1). The last anthelmintic treatment was applied more than four weeks before the beginning of the follow-up (fenbendazole; $10 \, mg \cdot kg^{-1}$ once daily during three days). Ewes were investigated before breeding, around mating (natural reproduction with a mating period of 34 days), at midpregnancy ($\sim$80 days of pregnancy), at late pregnancy (7–29 days before lambing), at immediate peripartum (6 days before until 2 days after lambing), at early postpartum (2–15 days after lambing), at intermediate postpartum (15–30 days after lambing), at late postpartum (30–45 days after lambing), and at preweaning (46–60 days after lambing). Lambs were investigated since birth at the same time points as their dams. At late pregnancy, ewes were ranked on the basis of body weight, body score, and parasite infection burden and allocated into three groups. Ewes of group T_1 ($n = 15$) received a single Mox (Cydectin, Fort Dodge Animal Health) subcutaneous injection of $200 \, \mu g \, kg^{-1}$ of body weight at late pregnancy ($\sim$135 days of gestation). Ewes of group T_2 ($n = 14$) received a single Mox subcutaneous injection of $200 \, \mu g \, kg^{-1}$ body weight 2 days after lambing. Control ewes (C group, $n = 14$) remained untreated throughout the whole study. Five further fortnightly samplings were performed after lambing.

2.3. Clinical and Zootechnical Parameters. The animals were monitored daily during the entire course of the experiment. Development of clinical signs related to parasite

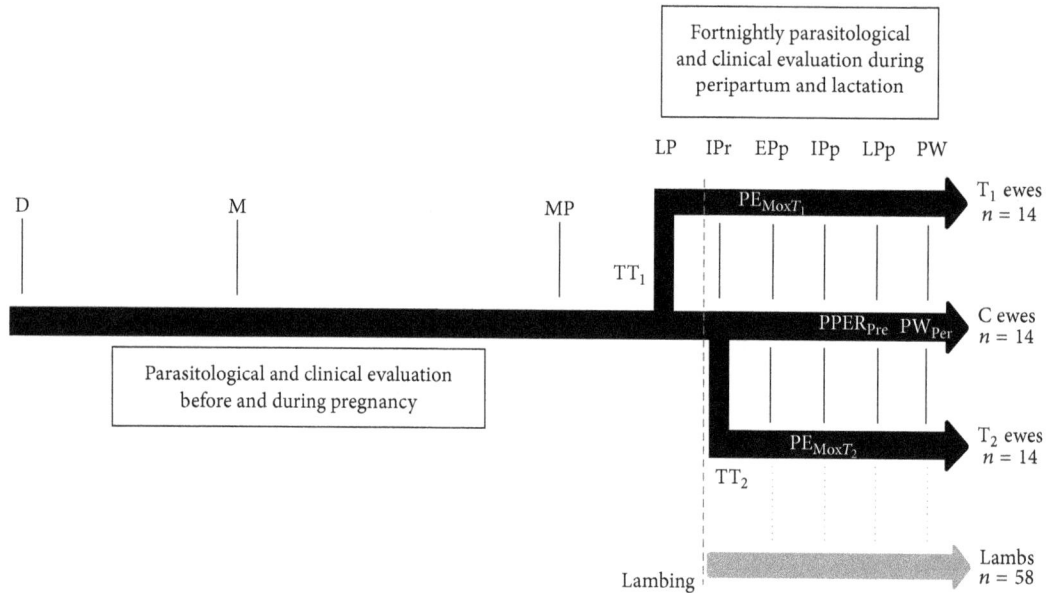

FIGURE 1: Experimental design to describe periparturient nematode egg rise (PPER) of ewes naturally infected with gastrointestinal nematodes and to measure the efficacy and persistency of peripartum strategic treatment with moxidectin (Mox) either at the onset of late pregnancy (TT_1) or at the end of immediate peripartum (TT_2) period under tropical Andes high altitude conditions. Parasitological and clinical evaluations included FEC by McMaster test, anemia detection by FAMACHA© system, diarrhea assessment by Dag scoring, body weight, and body condition assessment. Fecal egg count reduction (FECR) was employed to test posttreatment moxidectin efficacy 15 days after treatment (PE_{MoxT_1} and PE_{MoxT_2}), the prevention of PPER at late postpartum ($PPER_{Pre}$) period, and preweaning persistency (PW_{Per}). Ewes in control group (C) and offspring of all ewes were untreated against gastrointestinal nematodes. D: dry ewes; M: mating; MP: midpregnancy; LP: late pregnancy; Ipr: immediate postpartum; Epp: early postpartum; Ipp: intermediate postpartum; LPp: late postpartum; and PW: preweaning.

infections (depression, ataxia, and/or submandibular edema) was monitored. Body weight and body condition were recorded monthly. Except for dry period, scores of anemia (FAMACHA©) and diarrhea (Dag score) were measured at each sampling period according to Broughan and Wall [38], Di Loria et al. [39], and Macarthur et al. [21] recommendations.

2.4. Parasitological Follow-Up. Parasite burden determination was performed by fecal sampling in all ewes at the 9 established periods and in lambs at four occasions. FEC were obtained by the modified McMaster test according to the methodology described by Henriksen and Christensen [40] with a minimum detection level of 50 eggs per gram of feces. In cases of parasite burdens higher than 4000 strongylid eggs per gram and associated clinical signs of nematode infection (FAMACHA© level ≥4 or elevated Dag score), C ewes and/or the untreated lambs were selectively treated and withdrawn. Additionally, lambs whose fecal oocyst count was higher than 4000 *Eimeria* oocysts per gram of feces, received an oral toltrazuril anticoccidial treatment (Coccicalf, California Company S.A., 20 mg kg^{-1} of body weight).

2.5. Statistical Analysis. To estimate FEC reduction (FECR) induced by treatments, the equations recommended by Dobson et al. [41] were employed to calculate the following.

(1) Mox Posttreatment Efficacies. Consider $PE_{Mox} = 100 \times [1 - (T_{i15}/T_{i0}) \times (C_0/C_{15})]$, where T_{i0} and T_{i15} are the arithmetic

means of pretreatment and 15-day posttreatment FEC of treated groups (T_1 or T_2) and C_0 and C_{15} are the arithmetic means of C group at the corresponding sampling times. Mox resistance was suspected when posttreatment FECR was less than 95% and resistance was declared when the upper 95% confidence interval of the percentage reduction was less than 95% [42].

(2) PPER Prevention Induced by Mox Treatments. Consider $PPER_{Pre} = 100 \times [1 - (T_{iLPp}/C_{LPp})]$, where T_{iLPp} and C_{LPp} are late postpartum arithmetic means of FEC in treated (T_1 and T_2) and C groups, respectively.

(3) Preweaning Mox Treatments Persistency. Consider $PW_{Per} = 100 \times [1 - (T_{iPW}/C_{PW})]$, where T_{iPW} and C_{PW} are preweaning arithmetic means of FEC in treated (T_1 and T_2) and C groups, respectively.

Resampling-bootstrap method was employed to provide 95% confidence intervals for anthelmintic efficacies [41]. The package "eggCounts" in R software version 3.1.0 was employed [43].

Statistical analysis of data was conducted employing a two-factor ANOVA with repeated measures on one factor in order to evaluate the effect of both treatment and sampling time on FEC and clinical parameters. If necessary, logarithmic transformation was performed in order to achieve a normal data distribution. Clinical variables as FAMACHA©, Dag score, and body condition were discriminated into categories and presented as median (minimum and maximum

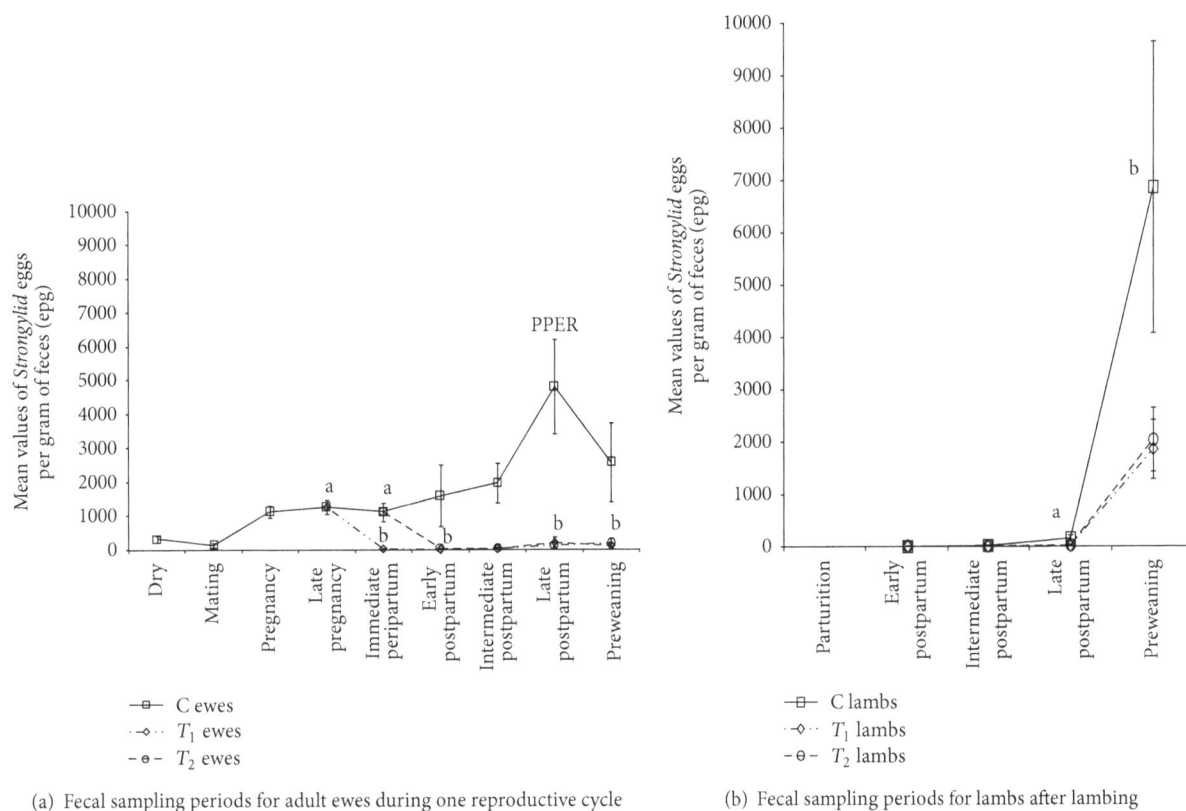

(a) Fecal sampling periods for adult ewes during one reproductive cycle

(b) Fecal sampling periods for lambs after lambing

FIGURE 2: Mean gastrointestinal parasite burdens (± standard error of mean) registered during one complete reproductive cycle in ewes and their offspring. (a) shows the peak in FEC at late pregnancy in C ewes (PPER) and the significant ([b]) and sustained FECR induced by T_1 and T_2 peripartum strategic treatment with moxidectin (two-factor ANOVA, $p < 0.05$) preventing the PPER ($PPER_{Pre}$). (b) shows the significant increase in FEC at preweaning ([b]) in ewes' offspring (two-factor ANOVA, $p < 0.05$). Adult ewes $n = 43$ (14 C, 15 T_1, and 14 T_2). Suckling lambs $n = 58$ lambs (18 born from C ewes, 20 from T_1 ewes, and 20 from T_2 ewes).

values). A ratio change for each clinical and zootechnical variable was calculated by dividing the median values before treatment (dry, mating, midpregnancy, and late pregnancy) over the median after treatment (early, intermediate, late, and preweaning period). Group effect on ratio changes was assessed by one-factor ANOVA and Tukey tests. p values less than 0.05 ($p < 0.05$) were considered significant. Statistical analysis was performed using the software SPSS Statistics 21.0.

3. Results

An effect of treatment and sampling time on FEC was established ($p < 0.05$). Mean FEC from ewes before and during mating period were significantly lower than those registered during pregnancy and lactation in C ewes. PPER occurred in C ewes at late postpartum period, 4–6 weeks after lambing, and induced a significant increase in FEC ($p < 0.05$) (Figure 2(a)).

Peripartum Mox treatment in T_1 and T_2 ewes significantly reduced FEC 15 days after treatment and efficiently prevented PPER ($p < 0.05$). No differences between T_1 and T_2 mean for FEC after treatment were observed; FEC remained low until preweaning period in both groups.

Significant differences by treatment and sampling time were recorded for clinical parameters ($p < 0.05$). Mox treatment applied to group T_1 prevented increase in FAMACHA values after lambing as observed in C and T_2 groups (Table 2). No major changes were found for body weight and body condition scores.

A significant increase in FEC occurred to lambs at preweaning period (Figure 2(b)), two weeks after FEC peak in control ewes ($p < 0.05$). Although no significant differences among preweaning FEC were observed between lambs born to C, T_1, or T_2 ewes ($p < 0.05$), untreated control ewes offspring showed a sharper increase in FEC (Figure 2(b)) and required treatment. Lambs' clinical parameters did not show significant differences over time or in function of ewes' treatment group (data not shown).

4. Discussion

The present study evaluated under field conditions the magnitude of PPER of gastrointestinal nematodes in Colombian wool sheep and tested the efficacy of Mox and its impact on two periparturient treatment schemes in ewes at lambing at the period of the highest birth rate in Andean flocks. PPER and treatment efficiency and persistency were evaluated in

TABLE 1: FECR induced by moxidectin strategic treatment of periparturient ewes during the same reproductive cycle.

Time of treatment	Evaluated period	Mean FEC ± SEM		Efficacy of treatment	
		Untreated control ewes $n = 11^*$	Treated ewes $n_{T_1} = 15$ and $n_{T_2} = 14$	% FECR	95% CI
Before lambing (T_1)	Before treatment	1705 ± 537	1060 ± 314	—	—
	15 days after treatment (PE_{Mox})**	745 ± 351	3 ± 3	99.3	97–100
	Late postpartum ($PPER_{Pre}$)**	4168 ± 1417	217 ± 172	94.8	66.2–99.6
	Preweaning (PW_{Per})**	2582 ± 1205	123 ± 59	95.2	79.4–98.9
48 h after lambing (T_2)	Before treatment	1277 ± 491	1043 ± 358	—	—
	15 days after treatment (PE_{Mox})**	1205 ± 316	27 ± 18	96.1	89.1–100
	Late postpartum (PPR_{Pre})**	4168 ± 1417	136 ± 64	96.7	85.9–99.5
	Preweaning (PW_{Per})**	2582 ± 1205	193 ± 140	92.5	53–98.8

T_1: late pregnancy treated group; T_2: 48 hours postlambing treated group; PE_{Mox}: posttreatment efficacy induced by moxidectin; $PPER_{Pre}$: PPER prevention induced by moxidectin; PW_{Per}: preweaning moxidectin persistency; FEC: fecal egg count; SEM: standard error of mean; FECR: fecal egg count reduction; 95% CI: 95% confidence intervals. *Three C ewes with high FEC and associated clinical signs were excluded after intermediate postpartum period due to Mox treatment by ethical considerations and their data were not included in the analysis. **Significant effect of treatments (one-way ANOVA and Tukey tests, $p < 0.05$) in FEC by evaluated period.

TABLE 2: Treatment-induced differences in the median of ratio change of clinical (FAMACHA© and Dag score) and zootechnical (body weight and body condition) parameters.

Measured parameters	Median (min–max)		
	Untreated control group $n = 11^*$	Late pregnancy Mox injection $n = 15$	48 hours postlambing Mox injection $n = 14$
Change ratio			
FAMACHA**	0.73 (0.5–1)[a]	1 (0.67–1.25)[b]	0.67 (0.67–1)[a]
Dag score**	1.75 (0.5–2)[a]	1 (0.67–3)[b]	1.16 (0.67–2)[ab]
Body weight	1.19 (1.06–1.28)	1.16 (1.02–1.4)	1.19 (1.05–1.42)
Body condition	1.04 (0.82–1.03)	1 (0.7–1.2)	1 (0.67–1.3)

Data were calculated by dividing the median of the parameter values before treatment (dry, mating, midpregnancy, and late pregnancy) over its median after treatment (early, intermediate, late, and preweaning period). Min: minimum value; max: maximum value; FAMACHA© values (1–5); Dag score values (0–5); body condition values (1–5). *Three C ewes with high FEC and associated clinical signs were excluded after intermediate postpartum period due to Mox treatment. **Significant differences between treatments (one-way ANOVA, $p > 0.05$). Treatment differences (Tukey test, $p > 0.05$) are denoted by superscripts.

terms of FEC as well as in terms of clinical (anemia and diarrhea score) and zootechnical (weight, body condition) performances.

The study was conducted under field conditions with naturally infected ewes. As the animals belonged to the Sheep Research Center of National University in Bogota, they had been selected among a larger group in order to allow an optimal standardization of the study conditions and the investigation of a reduced number of animals (14-15 ewes per group). Local (Creole) or well adapted breeds (Romney Marsh, Hampshire, and Corriedale) were kept on typical Colombian altitude pastures. If keeping all animal groups (T_1, T_2, and C) on the same pasture allowed an optimal standardization of the infectious third larvae pressure, it also diminished the effect of the treatments that were tested. Indeed, in spite of the high efficacy and persistence of Mox strategic treatment, it is likely that FECR observed in ewes would have been even better if separated pastures would have been used after treatment. It might also be assumed that the

lack of zootechnical impact (body weight and body condition score) of the treatments was at least partially due to standardization of the infectious pressure. Keeping the animals on separated pastures would have increased group-related differences among ewes and particularly among lambs. However, our study aimed to simulate local breeding conditions, that is, extensive grazing and no separation of treated from untreated animals. Untreated animals favor the "refugia" population of parasites by inducing a dilution effect on eggs shed by treated animals, although most treatment practices still rely on systematic treatment of animal groups [44].

The fluctuation in FEC observed throughout ewe's reproductive cycle might have been linked to ewe's productivity stage and the endocrine, immunological, and metabolic changes [6, 13, 16]. Low mean FEC in mature ewes at dry and mating periods could be related to minimum maintenance nutritional requirements and to the active immunological response described against gastrointestinal nematodes in empty adult ewes that limit the establishment of consumed infective larvae and the development and reproduction of parasitic stages [13, 18].

In contrast, nutritional requirements are increased during pregnancy and late pregnancy; hence, it is possible that the increased mean FEC recorded during pregnancy but especially at late pregnancy could be related to higher nutritional demands leading to augmented intake of contaminated herbage with infective larval stages but also to the onset of immunity breakdown towards gastrointestinal nematodes. In this study, the highest percentage of ewes with body condition values ≥3 was recorded at late pregnancy period (88.4%). Macarthur et al. [14] have described that ewe's body condition values ≥3 at late pregnancy improve the productive performance of lactating ewes and suckling lambs and reduce the risk of immune relaxation to gastrointestinal nematodes during peripartum period. This suggests that an adequate nutrient supply by pasturing and supplementation in the flock could reduce the impact on the severity of gastrointestinal infections during lactation. It has been also established that immunological deficiencies against gastrointestinal nematodes start at late pregnancy and they were related to low levels of both circulating eosinophils and total antibodies directed against nematodes 23 days before lambing [45]. The FEC values observed in this study at late pregnancy (Table 1) suggest the need to establish strategic treatment protocols at this critical period, reducing pasture contamination and offspring infection after lambing.

At immediate peripartum period, there was a slight reduction in FEC in control ewes, followed by a significant increase during lactation (Figure 2(a)). On the contrary, ewes of groups T_1 and T_2 displayed a significant and sustained decrease in FEC after periparturient treatment. Although T_1 ewes maintained a slightly lower gastrointestinal nematode burden during all lactation, no differences in terms of FEC or zootechnical parameters were observed between groups T_1 and T_2.

At intermediate and late postpartum period a continuous and drastic increase in mean FEC was observed in control ewes. At this time ewes should increase their catabolism of fat tissue in order to ensure the production of milk to support their lambs [21]. Late postpartum FEC peak reached in control ewes coincides with the systemic and local relaxation of the immunological response against nematodes reported by Beasley et al. [45] six weeks after lambing. It has been described that during these periods the rate of establishment of adult parasites is increased and the ewes lost their ability to suppress nematodes fecundity allowing a further significant increase in FEC [21, 45]. The stress caused by birth process, nursing, and maternal behavior could favor the already depressed systemic immunity and promote the PPER [14]. Indeed, relaxation of immunity against gastrointestinal nematodes was observed in control ewes, in which 35.7% ($n = 5$) had FEC higher than 4000 eggs per gram at late postpartum period and 21.4% ($n = 3$) registered FAMACHA© values ≥4. Only one anemic ewe was recorded in T_2 group.

The significance of PPER observed at late postpartum period in this trial contributes to high larvae pasture contamination especially when susceptible lambs are grazing alongside the ewes, thereby increasing their chances of becoming heavily infected. Our results showed that after the late postpartum peak in C ewes there was a significant increase in lambs' FEC at preweaning period, due to the ingestion of pasture contaminated with nematode infective larvae. An effective acquired immunological response in lambs is only gradually developed during the first year of life [6]. Strategic treatment of ewes seemed to somewhat protect their lambs delaying nematode infection (Figure 2(b)). It is possible that delayed egg excretion in lambs born from treated ewes was due to prolonged Mox secretion by milk suckling. Imperiale et al. [46] showed that residual concentrations of Mox were recovered in milk up to 35 days after treatment (between 17.8 and 183.5 ng mL^{-1} daily). Considering that daily milk intake ranges from 1000 to 2000 mL in lambs, milk secretion of 100 ng mL^{-1} Mox per day would lead to ingestion of 100–200 μg Mox per lamb per day. Although this temporal excretion of Mox could reduce FEC, it also exposes lambs' nematodes to subtherapeutic doses reducing "*refugia*" population of parasites and predisposing to resistance processes [47]. Recently Dever and Kahn [48] have demonstrated that anthelmintics extremely lipophilic as Mox administered at the rate of 1 mg kg^{-1} of body weight to lactating ewes could reduce significantly FEC in suckling offspring and expose lambs to subtherapeutic doses of the drug, a risk factor for the development of anthelmintic resistance. Our study employed only 200 mg mL^{-1} and due to differences in treatment period application (late pregnancy or immediate peripartum), T_1 offspring received lower Mox by milk than T_2. In order to reduce the risk of milk Mox residues, late pregnancy treatment 35 days before lambing could be recommended.

As mentioned earlier, all animals enrolled in this study were kept together in order to standardize infectious larvae pressure and to favor "*refugia*" gastrointestinal nematode population. Despite the high estimated PE$_{Mox}$ and PW$_{Per}$, it would however be interesting to assess the protective effect of ewes' peripartum treatment in animals housed on separate pastures in order to evaluate the impact of treatment on FEC and clinical parameters in ewes and lambs whose infectious larvae pressure would be lower than in the present study where untreated control ewes continued to contaminate the environment of treated ewes and their untreated offspring.

5. Conclusions

This study describes the FEC changes throughout ewes' reproductive stages and confirmed that PPER exists under tropical Andes high altitude conditions in Colombia. Mox treatment applied prior to or shortly after lambing efficiently prevented PPER and reduced changes of FAMACHA and Dag scores over time. FEC increase occurring in suckling lambs at preweaning period tended to be delayed by treating ewes at peripartum period. Although larger animal groups are needed to characterize the impact of PPER on zootechnical parameters, this study suggests that ewes raised under tropical Andes high altitude conditions are prone to undergo changes of pathophysiological indicators in response to increased gastrointestinal nematode burdens that could be useful in targeted treatment strategies.

Disclosure

Preliminary results were presented as an abstract at the 2nd Benelux Congress on Physiology and Pharmacology, Maastricht, 4th-5th April 2014.

Conflict of Interests

None of the authors of this paper has a financial or personal relationship with other people or organizations that could inappropriately influence or bias the content of the paper.

Acknowledgment

The authors thank "Coopération Universitaire Belge," ARES, Belgium, for financial support.

References

[1] S. Gaba, J. Cabaret, C. Chylinski, C. Sauvé, J. Cortet, and A. Silvestre, "Can efficient management of sheep gastro-intestinal nematodes be based on random treatment?" *Veterinary Parasitology*, vol. 190, no. 1-2, pp. 178–184, 2012.

[2] M. R. Knox, R. B. Besier, L. F. Le Jambre et al., "Novel approaches for the control of helminth parasites of livestock VI: summary of discussions and conclusions," *Veterinary Parasitology*, vol. 186, no. 1-2, pp. 143–149, 2012.

[3] D. M. Leathwick and R. B. Besier, "The management of anthelmintic resistance in grazing ruminants in Australasia—strategies and experiences," *Veterinary Parasitology*, vol. 204, no. 1-2, pp. 44–54, 2014.

[4] J. B. da Silva, C. P. Rangel, B. de Azevedo Baêta, and A. H. da Fonseca, "Risk factors relating to helminth infections in cows during the peripartum," *Revista Brasileira de Parasitologia Veterinaria*, vol. 21, no. 2, pp. 92–96, 2012.

[5] V. Goldberg, G. Ciappesoni, and I. Aguilar, "Modelling the faecal worm egg count curve during the periparturient period in uruguayan merino sheep," *Spanish Journal of Agricultural Research*, vol. 10, no. 4, pp. 986–992, 2012.

[6] I. G. Colditz, D. L. Watson, G. D. Gray, and S. J. Eady, "Some relationships between age, immune responsiveness and resistance to parasites in ruminants," *International Journal for Parasitology*, vol. 26, no. 8-9, pp. 869–877, 1996.

[7] S. Tembely, A. Lahlou-Kassi, J. E. O. Rege et al., "Breed and season effects on the peri-parturient rise in nematode egg output in indigenous ewes in a cool tropical environment," *Veterinary Parasitology*, vol. 77, no. 2-3, pp. 123–132, 1998.

[8] N. D. Sargison, "Pharmaceutical treatments of gastrointestinal nematode infections of sheep—future of anthelmintic drugs," *Veterinary Parasitology*, vol. 189, no. 1, pp. 79–84, 2012.

[9] L. P. Kahn, M. R. Knox, and G. D. Gray, "Enhancing immunity to nematode parasites in pregnant and lactating sheep through nutrition and genetic selection," in *Recent Advances in Animal Nutrition in Australia*, J. L. Corbett, Ed., vol. 12, pp. 15–22, University of New England, Armidale, Australia, 1999.

[10] P. Sakkas, J. G. M. Houdijk, S. Athanasiadou, and I. Kyriazakis, "Sensitivity of periparturient breakdown of immunity to parasites to dietary protein source," *Journal of Animal Science*, vol. 90, no. 11, pp. 3954–3962, 2012.

[11] A. M. Beasley, L. P. Kahn, and R. G. Windon, "The periparturient relaxation of immunity in Merino ewes infected with *Trichostrongylus colubriformis*: endocrine and body compositional responses," *Veterinary Parasitology*, vol. 168, no. 1-2, pp. 51–59, 2010.

[12] A. C. Kotze, B. M. Hines, and A. P. Ruffell, "A reappraisal of the relative sensitivity of nematode pharyngeal and somatic musculature to macrocyclic lactone drugs," *International Journal for Parasitology: Drugs and Drug Resistance*, vol. 2, pp. 29–35, 2012.

[13] A. R. Sykes, "Environmental effects on animal production: the nutritional demands of nematode parasite exposure in sheep," *Asian-Australasian Journal of Animal Sciences*, vol. 13, pp. 343–350, 2000.

[14] F. A. Macarthur, L. P. Kahn, and R. G. Windon, "Immune response of twin-bearing Merino ewes when infected with *Haemonchus contortus*: effects of fat score and prepartum supplementation," *Livestock Science*, vol. 157, no. 2-3, pp. 568–576, 2013.

[15] A. R. Williams, J. C. Greeff, P. E. Vercoe, R. J. Dobson, and L. J. E. Karlsson, "Merino ewes bred for parasite resistance reduce larval contamination onto pasture during the peri-parturient period," *Animal*, vol. 4, no. 1, pp. 122–127, 2010.

[16] N. D. Sargison, D. J. Bartram, and D. J. Wilson, "Use of a long acting injectable formulation of moxidectin to control the periparturient rise in faecal Teladorsagia circumcincta egg output of ewes," *Veterinary Parasitology*, vol. 189, no. 2–4, pp. 274–283, 2012.

[17] L. P. Kahn, M. R. Knox, G. D. Gray, J. M. Lea, and S. W. Walkden-Brown, "Enhancing immunity to nematode parasites in single-bearing Merino ewes through nutrition and genetic selection," *Veterinary Parasitology*, vol. 112, no. 3, pp. 211–225, 2003.

[18] A. M. Beasley, L. P. Kahn, and R. G. Windon, "The influence of reproductive physiology and nutrient supply on the periparturient relaxation of immunity to the gastrointestinal nematode *Trichostrongylus colubriformis* in Merino ewes," *Veterinary Parasitology*, vol. 188, no. 3-4, pp. 306–324, 2012.

[19] L. A. Jones, P. Sakkas, J. G. M. Houdijk, D. P. Knox, and I. Kyriazakis, "Amelioration of the periparturient relaxation of immunity to parasites through a reduction in mammalian reproductive effort," *International Journal for Parasitology*, vol. 42, no. 13-14, pp. 1127–1134, 2012.

[20] F. J. McPherson, S. Shini, A. W. Gibbon, and M. J. D'Occhio, "Protein supplementation in the first 100 days of gestation fails to enhance resistance of weaned Merino lambs against *Haemonchus contortus*," *Livestock Science*, vol. 150, no. 1–3, pp. 11–21, 2012.

[21] F. A. Macarthur, L. P. Kahn, and R. G. Windon, "Regulating maternal production of twin-bearing Merino ewes through fat score and prepartum supplementation when infected with Haemonchus contortus," *Livestock Science*, vol. 157, no. 2-3, pp. 442–451, 2013.

[22] V. H. Suarez, "Helminthic control on grazing ruminants and environmental risks in South America," *Veterinary Research*, vol. 33, no. 5, pp. 563–573, 2002.

[23] M. B. Molento, F. S. Fortes, D. A. S. Pondelek et al., "Challenges of nematode control in ruminants: focus on Latin America," *Veterinary Parasitology*, vol. 180, no. 1-2, pp. 126–132, 2011.

[24] A. N. Henrioud, "Towards sustainable parasite control practices in livestock production with emphasis in Latin America," *Veterinary Parasitology*, vol. 180, no. 1-2, pp. 2–11, 2011.

[25] J. F. Torres-acosta, R. I. Rodríguez-Vivas, and R. Cámara-Sarmiento, "Efecto del parto sobre la eliminación de huevecillos

de nemátodos y ooquistes de Eimeria en cabras criollas," *Revista Biomédica*, vol. 6, no. 4, pp. 208–215, 1995.

[26] E. Romjali, A. Batubara, V. S. Pandey, and R. M. Gatenby, "Short communication Peri-parturient rise in faecal strongyle egg counts of different genotypes of sheep in North Sumatra, Indonesia," *Veterinary Parasitology*, vol. 68, no. 1997, pp. 191–196, 2000.

[27] N. Mandonnet, M. Bachand, M. Mahieu et al., "Impact on productivity of peri-parturient rise in fecal egg counts in Creole goats in the humid tropics," *Veterinary Parasitology*, vol. 134, no. 3-4, pp. 249–259, 2005.

[28] M. Mahieu and G. Aumont, "Periparturient rise in Martinik Hair Sheep and perspectives for gastrointestinal nematode control," *Tropical Animal Health and Production*, vol. 39, no. 6, pp. 387–390, 2007.

[29] D. C. Moreno-Vargas and H. A. Grajales-Lombana, "Caracterización del proceso administrativo y de mercado en los sistemas ovinos del trópico alto colombiano," *Revista Cienci Animal*, no. 7, pp. 85–98, 2014.

[30] M. Knox and J. Steel, "Nutritional enhancement of parasite control in small ruminant production systems in developing countries of south-east Asia and the Pacific," *International Journal for Parasitology*, vol. 26, no. 8-9, pp. 963–970, 1996.

[31] R. A. Rocha, A. F. T. Amarante, and P. A. Bricarello, "Comparison of the susceptibility of Santa Inês and Ile de France ewes to nematode parasitism around parturition and during lactation," *Small Ruminant Research*, vol. 55, no. 1–3, pp. 65–75, 2004.

[32] G. Morales, E. Sandoval, L. A. Pino, and Z. Rondón, "Evaluación de dos criterios de utilidad en un programa de control de la infección por nematodos gastrointestinales en ovinos mediante tratamiento antihelmíntico selectivo," *Zootecnia Tropical*, vol. 26, no. 2, pp. 141–150, 2008.

[33] M. Tibbo, K. Aragaw, J. Philipsson et al., "A field trial of production and financial consequences of helminthosis control in sheep production in Ethiopia," *Preventive Veterinary Medicine*, vol. 84, no. 1-2, pp. 152–160, 2008.

[34] G. Cringoli, L. Rinaldi, V. Veneziano, L. Mezzino, J. Vercruysse, and F. Jackson, "Evaluation of targeted selective treatments in sheep in Italy: effects on faecal worm egg count and milk production in four case studies," *Veterinary Parasitology*, vol. 164, no. 1, pp. 36–43, 2009.

[35] P. Godoy, J. Lian, R. N. Beech, and R. K. Prichard, "Haemonchus contortus P-glycoprotein-2: in situ localisation and characterisation of macrocyclic lactone transport," *International Journal for Parasitology*, vol. 45, no. 1, pp. 85–93, 2015.

[36] M. Lloberas, L. Alvarez, C. Entrocasso et al., "Comparative tissue pharmacokinetics and efficacy of moxidectin, abamectin and ivermectin in lambs infected with resistant nematodes: impact of drug treatments on parasite P-glycoprotein expression," *International Journal for Parasitology: Drugs and Drug Resistance*, vol. 3, pp. 20–27, 2013.

[37] D. Márquez, G. Jiménez, F. García, and C. Garzón, "Resistencia a los antihelmínticos en nemátodos gastrointestinales de bovinos en municipios de Cundinamarca y Boyacá," *Corpoica Ciencia y Tecnología Agropecuaria*, vol. 9, no. 1, pp. 113–123, 2008.

[38] J. M. Broughan and R. Wall, "Faecal soiling and gastrointestinal helminth infection in lambs," *International Journal for Parasitology*, vol. 37, no. 11, pp. 1255–1268, 2007.

[39] A. Di Loria, V. Veneziano, D. Piantedosi et al., "Evaluation of the FAMACHA system for detecting the severity of anaemia in sheep from southern Italy," *Veterinary Parasitology*, vol. 161, no. 1-2, pp. 53–59, 2009.

[40] S. A. Henriksen and J. P. Christensen, "Demonstration of Isospora suis oocysts in faecal samples," *Veterinary Record*, vol. 131, no. 19, pp. 443–444, 1992.

[41] R. J. Dobson, B. C. Hosking, C. L. Jacobson et al., "Preserving new anthelmintics: a simple method for estimating faecal egg count reduction test (FECRT) confidence limits when efficacy and/or nematode aggregation is high," *Veterinary Parasitology*, vol. 186, no. 1-2, pp. 79–92, 2012.

[42] G. C. Coles, C. Bauer, F. H. M. Borgsteede et al., "World Association for the Advancement of Veterinary Parasitology (W.A.A.V.P.) methods for the detection of anthelmintic resistance in nematodes of veterinary importance," *Veterinary Parasitology*, vol. 44, no. 1-2, pp. 35–44, 1992.

[43] P. R. Torgerson, M. Paul, and R. Furrer, "Evaluating faecal egg count reduction using a specifically designed package 'eggCounts' in R and a user friendly web interface," *International Journal for Parasitology*, vol. 44, no. 5, pp. 299–303, 2014.

[44] F. Kenyon, A. W. Greer, G. C. Coles et al., "The role of targeted selective treatments in the development of refugia-based approaches to the control of gastrointestinal nematodes of small ruminants," *Veterinary Parasitology*, vol. 164, no. 1, pp. 3–11, 2009.

[45] A. M. Beasley, L. P. Kahn, and R. G. Windon, "The periparturient relaxation of immunity in Merino ewes infected with Trichostrongylus colubriformis: parasitological and immunological responses," *Veterinary Parasitology*, vol. 168, no. 1-2, pp. 60–70, 2010.

[46] F. A. Imperiale, M. R. Busetti, V. H. Suárez, and C. E. Lanusse, "Milk excretion of ivermectin and moxidectin in dairy sheep: assessment of drug residues during cheese elaboration and ripening period," *Journal of Agricultural and Food Chemistry*, vol. 52, no. 20, pp. 6205–6211, 2004.

[47] J. A. van Wyk, "Refugia—overlooked as perhaps the most potent factor concerning the development of anthelmintic resistance," *Onderstepoort Journal of Veterinary Research*, vol. 68, no. 1, pp. 55–67, 2001.

[48] M. Dever and L. Kahn, "Decline in faecal worm egg counts in lambs suckling ewes treated with lipophilic anthelmintics: Implications for hastening development of anthelmintic resistance," *Veterinary Parasitology*, vol. 209, no. 3-4, pp. 229–234, 2015.

16

Detection of *Babesia caballi* and *Theileria equi* in Blood from Equines from Four Indigenous Communities in Costa Rica

María Fernanda Posada-Guzmán,[1] **Gaby Dolz,**[1,2]
Juan José Romero-Zúñiga,[2] **and Ana Eugenia Jiménez-Rocha**[3]

[1]*Maestría en Enfermedades Tropicales, Posgrado Regional en Ciencias Veterinarias Tropicales, Universidad Nacional, Campus Presbítero Benjamín Nuñez, P.O. Box 86, 3000 Heredia, Costa Rica*
[2]*Programa de Investigación en Medicina Poblacional, Escuela de Medicina Veterinaria, Universidad Nacional, Campus Presbítero Benjamín Nuñez, P.O. Box 86, 3000 Heredia, Costa Rica*
[3]*Laboratorio de Parasitología, Escuela de Medicina Veterinaria, Universidad Nacional, Campus Presbítero Benjamín Nuñez, P.O. Box 86, 3000 Heredia, Costa Rica*

Correspondence should be addressed to Gaby Dolz; gaby.dolz.wiedner@una.cr

Academic Editor: Remo Lobetti

A cross-sectional study was carried out in four indigenous communities of Costa Rica to detect presence and prevalence of *Babesia caballi* and *Theileria equi* and to investigate factors associated with presence of these hemoparasites. General condition of horses (n = 285) was evaluated, and hematocrits and hemoglobin were determined from blood samples of 130 horses, which were also analyzed using blood smears, nested polymerase chain reaction (PCR), and immunosorbent assay (c-ELISA). The general condition of the horses (n = 285) in terms of their body and coat was between regular and poor, and hematocrit and hemoglobin average values were low (19% and 10.65 g/dL, resp.). Erythrocyte inclusions were observed in 32 (24.6%) of the samples. Twenty-six samples (20.0%) gave positive results for *B. caballi* and 60 (46.2%) for *T. equi*; 10 horses (7.7%) showed mixed infection, when analyzed by PCR. Using c-ELISA, it was found that 90 (69.2%) horses had antibodies against *B. caballi* and 115 (88.5%) against *T. equi*, while 81 (62.3%) showed mixed reactions. There were no factors associated with the presence of *B. caballi* and *T. equi*. These results contrast with results previously obtained in equines in the Central Valley of Costa Rica.

1. Introduction

Equine piroplasmosis is a horse infection produced by *Babesia caballi* and *Theileria equi* protozoan that belong, respectively, to the Babesiidae and Theileriidae families of the order Piroplasmida. The two agents may infest an animal at the same time and they are transmitted by ticks [1, 2].

The parasites that cause equine piroplasmosis are endemic in most parts of the world, including America. Seroprevalence between 20% and 90% is reported in Latin America, where the prevalence of *T. equi* is greater than that of *B. caballi*, while in regions of the Northern Hemisphere a greater prevalence of *B. caballi* than of *T. equi* has been observed; in addition, mixed infections were reported close to 30% [3–6].

Piroplasmosis is difficult to diagnose in endemic regions where clinical signs are variable rather than specific [7, 8]. *T. equi* is considered to be the most pathogenic, able to generate fevers of up to 40°C, lymphadenopathy, hepatomegaly, and bilirubinuria [9, 10].

Causative agents of equine piroplasmosis can be observed under a microscope through Giemsa-stained blood smears; however, this technique has the disadvantage of being subjective and having low sensitivity, mostly in horses with low parasitemia ($<10^4$ infected erythrocytes/μL) [6, 11, 12]. Indirect immunofluorescence assay (IFA) and immunosorbent assays (ELISA) are the serological tests required by the World Organization on Animal Health (OIE) for horses that have to be transported from one country to another [2]. Animals that are persistently infected or with an active infection will show high antibody titers, while, in horses that eliminate the agent, antibodies will decrease to the point where they cannot be detected in a period of six to ten months [13].

The polymerase chain reaction (PCR) technique for *B. caballi* and *T. equi* is highly efficient, since it can detect low levels of parasitemia, determines the infecting species, and also allows the detection of persistently infected animals and chronic carriers [14–17]. However, time and cost of implementation are two inconvenient aspects of this technique.

The different species of tick genera involved in the transmission of equine piroplasmosis, *Amblyomma, Dermacentor*, and *Rhipicephalus*, have been reported in the country by Álvarez et al. [18]. Until now, four serologic studies have been carried out in Costa Rica, detecting the presence of antibodies against *B. caballi* and *T. equi* in equines participating in a rally ($n = 41$) [19], for exportation purposes ($n = 21$) [20], from slaughterhouses ($n = 51$) [21], and also from thoroughbred stabled equines ($n = 181$) from the Central Valley [22], where the prevalence of 44.3% to 59.0% for *B. caballi* and of 34.0% to 47.0% for *T. equi* was determined.

The situation of piroplasmosis in indigenous horses in these communities has not been studied, even though these animals provide source of subsistence to their owners, and effective parasite control is lacking [3]. In contrast, most horses of the rest of the country are tested and dewormed regularly by their owners, especially when they are housed in stables or to participate in competitions. The objective of the present study was to determine the presence of current and past infections of *B. caballi* and *T. equi* in blood samples in horses of indigenous communities and determine risk factors associated with the presence of these agents.

2. Materials and Methods

2.1. Study Type and Reference Population. A descriptive cross-sectional observational study was carried out between March and October 2011 in the communities of Vereh, Paso Marcos, Alto Pacuare, and Amubre (Figure 1). The first three communities are in the Cabecar reserve, in Chirripó, Turrialba (9°41′45.81 to 9°48′46.12 North and 83°25′51.90 to 83°29′21.50 West), while the Amubre community is in Talamanca and belongs to the Bribri group (9°30′ North and 83°40′ West). Each community was visited once.

2.2. Data and Sample Collection. A survey with closed answers was conducted with each owner of an animal regarding the origin and general health care of the horse. Then a general clinical exam was carried out, and blood samples were taken. On an individual clinical record the presence of clinical signs was recorded (anemia, weakness, anorexia, cachexia, and hemoglobinuria), as well as the horse's body condition [23], coat condition, and tick presence.

Blood samples from all horses in work places were collected. The samples were transported under refrigeration to the laboratory, where clinical analysis and blood smear were carried out; samples were finally stored at −20°C for their molecular analysis. Blood samples without EDTA were

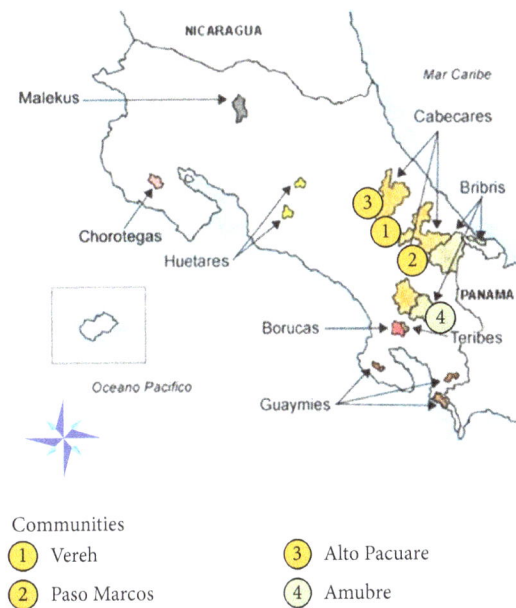

FIGURE 1: Location of indigenous communities in Costa Rica, showing the four sites sampled (taken from http://costarica1.bligoo.com .mx/?page=2 and modified).

centrifuged for 10 minutes at 10000 g and stored at −20°C for serological analysis.

The total number of samples collected in each community is shown in Table 1. Of the 285 samples taken in the field, 45% were selected from each community (for a total of 130 horses). The samples were selected on the basis of convenience, that is, the most affected were chosen over the least affected (horses presenting clinical signs or having ticks on them), and tested for erythrocyte inclusions and by PCR and ELISA.

2.3. Clinical Analyses and Blood Smears. Hematocrit values were determined for 130 samples in a HETTICH microcentrifuge (18600 g, 5 minutes); value was determined with a DAMON/IEC hematocrit reader. A densitometer was used to measure hemoglobin. Reported normal value for hematocrit was 37.9% ± 3.4% and for hemoglobin 14.9 g/dL ± 1.3 g/dL [4]. The Giemsa staining described by Akkan et al. [9] was used for these 130 samples for blood smears; samples in which there was at least one intraerythrocyte hemoparasite were considered positive.

2.4. Extraction, Polymerase Chain Reaction (PCR), and Sequencing. The Promega Wizard Genomic DNA Purification Kit (Madison, Wisconsin, USA) was used to extract the DNA from the 130 blood samples. Nested PCR as described by Battsetseg et al. [14] was carried out. Primers BC48F1 and BC48R3 were used for *B. caballi* for the first PCR and BC48F11 and BC48R31 for the second PCR. The mix for the first reaction was 12.5 μL and contained 6.5 μL of Dream Taq PCR Master Mix 2X (Fermentas), 0.5 μL of each primer (100 pmol/μL), 1 μL of DNA (1.9–2.6 μg), and 4.5 μL of nuclease-free water (Fermentas), and the amplification conditions were

TABLE 1: Results of the clinical exam of equines ($n = 285$) in four indigenous communities in Costa Rica.

Variable	Variable level	n	%	CI 95% LL	CI 95% UL
Community	Vereh	66	23.2	18.3	28.1
	Paso Marcos	80	28.1	22.9	33.4
	Alto Pacuare	72	25.3	20.3	30.3
	Amubre	67	23.5	18.6	24.3
Age	Young	110	38.6	32.9	44.3
	Adult	145	50.9	45.1	56.7
	ND	30	10.5	7.0	14.1
Body condition	Poor-regular	196	68.8	63.4	74.2
	Good	77	27.0	21.9	32.2
	ND	12	4.2	1.9	6.5
Fur condition	Poor-regular	218	76.5	71.6	81.4
	Good	61	21.4	16.6	26.2
	ND	6	2.1	0.4	3.8
Mucous membranes	Pale-jaundiced	54	18.9	14.4	23.5
	Pink	212	74.4	69.3	79.5
	ND	19	6.7	3.8	9.6
Number of ticks	≥50	149	52.3	46.5	58.1
	<50	134	47.0	41.2	52.8
	ND	2	0.7	−0.3	1.7

ND: no data available; CI 95%: confidence interval 95%; LL: lower limit; UL: upper limit.

4 minutes of initial denaturalization at 96°C, 40 repeated denaturing cycles (94°C for 1 minute), aligning (56°C for 2 minutes), extension (72°C for 2 minutes), and 5 minutes of final extension at 72°C. For the second PCR the conditions were the same, except that the aligning temperature was 50°C for 2 minutes, and 1 µL of the first PCR was used for the reaction. DNA extracted from a positive horse, donated by the University of Veterinary Medicine Hannover, Germany, was used as a positive control. Nuclease-free water (Fermentas) was used as a negative control.

Primers EMA-5 and EMA-6 (first PCR) and EMA-7 and EMA-8 (second PCR) were used for *T. equi*. The mix for the first PCR reaction was the same as the one for the PCR of *B. caballi*. The conditions were 10 minutes of initial denaturalization at 95°C, 40 repeated denaturing cycles (94°C for 1 minute), aligning (60°C for 1 minute), extension (72°C for 1 minute), and 5 minutes of final extension at 72°C. For the second PCR the conditions were the same as those described. For the reaction, 1 µL of product from the first PCR was used. DNA extracted from a positive horse, donated by the School of Veterinary Medicine and Zootechnics of the University of Sao Paulo, Brazil, was used as a positive control. Nuclease-free water (Fermentas) was used as a negative control.

The products obtained were subjected to electrophoresis (100 volts, 45 minutes) in agarose gels at 2% in TBE with GelRed. Samples that showed products with a size of 430 bp (*B. caballi*) and 218 bb (*T. equi*) were considered positive.

An amplified product of a blood sample that gave positive results for *B. caballi* and another one that tested positive for *T. equi* were sent to Macrogen, Korea, to be sequenced. Sequences were compared with others reported in GenBank, using MEGA 5.05 software and the BLAST program (National Center for Biotechnology Information, Bethesda, Maryland, USA).

2.5. Competitive Immunoassays (c-ELISA). The 130 selected sera were analyzed with competitive ELISA (VMRD Inc., Pullman, Washington, United States) to detect antibodies against *B. caballi* and *T. equi*, following recommended protocols. Sera that showed percentages of inhibition greater than or equal to 40% were considered positive.

2.6. Statistical Analysis. Absolute and relative frequency analyses were carried out on the characteristics of the 285 horses present in the four communities. In addition, the global percentage of positive samples was calculated for both PCR and c-ELISA, as well as the specific percentage per indigenous community studied. Finally the factors associated with the presence of each protozoan were determined (positive samples to PCR) using Poisson regression. The statistical analysis was carried out using the program STATA I/C 13 (StataCorp, USA).

3. Results

A total of 240 indigenous individuals came to the four locations, with 285 horses. Body condition was found to be poor in 84 (29.5%) and regular in 112 (39.3%) horses; likewise, coat condition was poor (39, 13.7%) or regular (179, 62.8%). No significant differences were determined between communities (Table 1).

TABLE 2: Absolute frequency and percentage of horses testing positive for B. caballi and T. equi using nested PCR and c-ELISA in four indigenous communities of Costa Rica (n = 285).

Community (N)	n	B. caballi n+ (%)		T. equi n+ (%)		B. caballi and T. equi n+ (%)	
		PCR	ELISA	PCR	ELISA	PCR	ELISA
Vereh (66)	30	8 (26.7)	20 (66.7)	12 (40.0)[a]	26 (86.7)	2 (6.7)	17 (56.7)
Amubre (66)	30	10 (33.3)	20 (66.7)	10 (33.3)[a]	28 (93.3)	4 (13.3)	20 (66.7)
Paso Marcos (80)	37	6 (16.2)	22 (59.5)	9 (24.3)[a]	35 (94.6)	2 (5.4)	22 (59.5)
Alto Pacuare (73)	33	2 (6.1)	28 (84.8)	29 (87.9)[b]	26 (78.8)	2 (6.1)	22 (66.7)
Total	130	26 (20.0)	90 (69.2)	60 (46.2)	115 (88.5)	10 (7.7)	81 (62.3)

N = total horses sampled; n = total horses analyzed; n+ = total positive by test.
The percentage (%) is calculated with respect to the total of animals analyzed by community. Superscripts indicate a statistical difference at the 0.05 significance level within the column, between rows.

Hematocrit and hemoglobin average values were 19.0% and 10.65 g/dL, respectively. A total of 26 (20.0%) and 60 (46.2%) horses were positive in PCR for B. caballi and T. equi, respectively; 10 (7.7%) showed mixed infections. Positive blood samples for B. caballi and T. equi showed 98.6% (355/360 bp) homology with B. caballi (JN217099) and 99.1% (231/233 bp) with T. equi (AF261824), respectively. Erythrocyte inclusions were observed in a total of 32 (24.6%) horses. From these positive results, the PCR only confirmed 19 (59.3%) as positive. In 98 (75.4%) samples, inclusions were not found, but 57 (43.8%) were positive in PCR analysis for one of the two agents.

A total of 124 (95.4%) of the 130 horses analyzed with c-ELISA were found to have antibodies against one of the two agents: 90 (69.2%) against B. caballi and 115 (88.5%) against T. equi; of these, 81 (62.3%) had antibodies against the two agents. For B. caballi, 25 (19.2%) samples were positive using c-ELISA and PCR and 39 (30.0%) negative in both tests. In 50.0% (65) of samples identified as seropositive, the presence of B. caballi was not confirmed through PCR, while only one seronegative sample yielded positive results using PCR. For T. equi, 53 (40.8%) samples were positive and 8 (6.2%) negative using the two techniques. In 47.7% (62) of seropositive samples presence of T. equi was not confirmed using PCR, while seven (5.4%) seronegative samples reacted PCR positive. Table 2 shows the distribution of horses found positive using PCR; significant differences were observed only in the PCR for T. equi between Alto Pacuare and the other communities.

In the Poisson regression analysis, as well as in logistic regression analysis, to determine epidemiological association with results of c-ELISA and PCR, respectively, factors associated with any of the conditions studied were not identified.

4. Discussion

The clinical exam and survey showed that most horses (196/285, 68.8%) had a body condition between regular and poor, which may be due to the low quality of the food they consume or the lack of programs to treat them for parasites. Owners indicated that they fed their horses with grass. Only 12.3% treated them for parasites a year ago, while the remaining (87.7%) did not treat them for parasites. Therefore it cannot be ruled out that gastrointestinal parasitism could have contributed to the anorexia and emaciation that were determined [3]. In addition, a high level of tick infestation was observed (99.3%) in the horses from all locations. Since ticks are not just vectors for piroplasmosis but also consume blood, this may have affected the low hematocrit and hemoglobin values found in the present study [8].

Although seroprevalence from B. caballi and T. equi was determined only from 130 horses in indigenous communities, selected from the most affected to least affected, it was much higher (69.2% and 88.5%, resp.) than that reported in thoroughbred stabled equines in Costa Rica (19% and 38%, resp.) [22]. Additionally, these agents had not been detected before through molecular techniques in our country. PCR determined the presence of these agents in 66.2% (B. caballi 20.0%, T. equi 46.2%) of the horses analyzed, findings that were confirmed with sequencing. The high presence of hemoparasites detected in the horses through PCR analysis is consistent with data reported in other Latin American countries [3, 4, 24], although it must be taken into consideration that the most affected horses were chosen and analyzed in the present study.

Some studies suggest a higher infection rate of B. caballi than with T. equi [5, 25] while others [26] found greater seroprevalence of T. equi than of B. equi, which is consistent with previous findings of Jiménez et al. [22] in thoroughbred stabled equines of the Central Valley of our country and with our findings. The laboratory results suggest that the two agents are endemic in the zones where indigenous communities are located, indicating piroplasm presence without causing serious diseases in the horses. In this respect, 7.7% of animals detected with mixed infections did not present clinical characteristics different than those of animals with simple infections [1]. Endemicity in indigenous communities is probably due to the presence of a great amount of ticks, which were found on the horses and which constantly transmit piroplasms from infected to susceptible animals. This may also represent a potential risk for indigenous individuals, because most of them live in close proximity to their animals and may acquire babesial agents through ticks [1, 27, 28].

Horses with positive PCR and ELISA results represent animals with chronic infections. A greater percentage of horses persistently infected with *T. equi* than with *B. caballi* were observed, which is in agreement with other reports [6, 17, 29]. Horses with positive PCR and negative ELISA results represent animals with recent infections. In addition, in this study, more animals were detected with early *T. equi* than with *B. caballi* infections. Finally, only approximately 50% of the animals had antibodies, implying that these horses recently overcame the infection [29]; this however should be further investigated [6]. Special attention should be given to the fact that a greater presence of *T. equi* was detected in indigenous communities, because this agent is considered more pathogenic and has been related to babesial infections in humans due to its taxonomic closeness to *Theileria microti* (formerly *Babesia microti*), which causes most clinical cases in humans. Although *B. caballi* and *T. equi* (named as *B. equi*) serologically positive human cases have been reported [1, 27, 28], the OIE concludes that human babesiosis is a disease that has not been sufficiently studied, and a risk for human populations cannot be ruled out [2].

Blood smears were shown to have a low sensitivity (24.6%) to detect hemoparasites, although they are a simple, inexpensive, and useful tool to diagnose the disease in the field [2, 6].

The results obtained in the different communities did not show significant differences, which is probably due to similarities of climate and ecological factors, as well as in the ways in which indigenous individuals handle their animals, which were very similar in the four communities [30], and the fact that most affected horses were chosen. Differences in sex, race, or ages of the horses did not appear to influence the chances for infection with *B. caballi* and *T. equi*, which is consistent with findings by Kakoma and Mehlhorn [31] but contrasts with findings of Jiménez et al. [22], who reported that thoroughbred stabled equines in the Central Valley with access to pastures and older than three years were more likely to be seropositive to *B. caballi* and *T. equi*, respectively. Significant effects of the variables analyzed in the present study between groups of horses with positive and negative results to *B. caballi* and *T. equi* were not observed.Body and coat condition were not good in most horses; it was also found that they showed low hematocrit and hemoglobin values, and all animals had ticks. Although not treating the horses for parasites is considered to be an important factor in determining the occurrence of equine piroplasmosis, since it favors the presence of ticks that act as vectors of the disease, this did not turn out to be statistically significant either, given that most animals had not been dewormed [2, 12].

5. Conclusions

The ability to diagnose infected animals with certainty is important to be able to provide correct treatment and to prevent further hemoparasite transmission to susceptible animals. The present study proved that using two diagnostic techniques, one direct (PCR) and the other indirect (c-ELISA), is advisable to discern between animals pursuing

an active or persistent infection. It is recommended that indigenous communities be informed of the risk to horses and inhabitants of contracting an infection with babesial agents from the ticks that infest their animals, and integral tick control should be promoted in the locations studied, seeking to prevent the spread of disease between horses and its transmission to indigenous individuals.

Disclosure

Preliminary results were presented as a Poster at the XXI National Congress of Veterinary Medicine, San José, Costa Rica, 11–13 November 2014.

Conflict of Interests

No conflict of interests is declared.

Acknowledgment

The authors would like to thank Vicerrectoría de Investigación, Universidad Nacional, Heredia, Costa Rica.

References

[1] J. Maslin, F. Beugnet, B. Davoust, and F. Klotz, "Babésioses," *EMC—Maladies Infectieuses*, vol. 1, no. 4, pp. 281–292, 2004.

[2] World Organization for Animal Health (OIE), Equine Piroplasmosis. Aetiology, Epidemiology, Diagnosis, Prevention and Control References, http://www.oie.int/fileadmin/Home/eng/Animal_Health_in_the_World/docs/pdf/Disease_cards/EQUINE_PRIOPLASMOSIS.pdf.

[3] M. Teglas, E. Matern, S. Lein, P. Foley, S. M. Mahan, and J. Foley, "Ticks and tick-borne disease in Guatemalan cattle and horses," *Veterinary Parasitology*, vol. 131, no. 1-2, pp. 119–127, 2005.

[4] R. Castellanos, J. L. Canelón, V. Calzolaio, F. Aguinaco, Á. López, and R. Montesinos, "Estudio hematológico y detección de hemoparásitos en caballos criollos venezolanos de dos hatos del estado de Apure, Venezuela (Hematologic study in Venezuelan Creole horses from two herds of the state of Apure, Venezuela)," *Revista Científica de la Facultad de Ciencias Veterinarias de la Universidad del Zulia*, vol. 20, no. 2, pp. 153–160, 2010.

[5] R. Rosales, A. Rangel-Rivas, A. Escalona et al., "Detection of *Theileria equi* and *Babesia caballi* infections in Venezuelan horses using Competitive-Inhibition ELISA and PCR," *Veterinary Parasitology*, vol. 196, no. 1-2, pp. 37–43, 2013.

[6] L. N. Wise, L. S. Kappmeyer, R. H. Mealey, and D. P. Knowles, "Review of equine piroplasmosis," *Journal of Veterinary Internal Medicine*, vol. 27, no. 6, pp. 1334–1346, 2013.

[7] M. T. E. P. Allsopp, B. D. Lewis, and B. L. Penzhorn, "Molecular evidence for transplacental transmission of *Theileria equi* from carrier mares to their apparently healthy foals," *Veterinary Parasitology*, vol. 148, no. 2, pp. 130–136, 2007.

[8] R. Zobba, M. Ardu, S. Niccolini et al., "Clinical and laboratory findings in equine piroplasmosis," *Journal of Equine Veterinary Science*, vol. 28, no. 5, pp. 301–308, 2008.

[9] H. A. Akkan, M. Karaca, M. Tutuncu, S. Deger, I. Keles, and Z. Agaoglu, "Serologic and microscopic studies on Babesiosis

in horses in the Eastern border of Turkey," *Journal of Equine Veterinary Science*, vol. 23, no. 5, pp. 181–183, 2003.

[10] M. F. B. Ribeiro, J. A. G. da Silveira, and C. V. Bastos, "Failure of the *Amblyomma cajennense* nymph to become infected by *Theileria equi* after feeding on acute or chronically infected horses," *Experimental Parasitology*, vol. 128, no. 4, pp. 324–327, 2011.

[11] D. Lewis, E. R. Young, D. G. Baggott, and G. D. Osborn, "*Babesia divergens* infection of the Mongolian gerbil: titration of infective dose and preliminary observations on the disease produced," *Journal of Comparative Pathology*, vol. 91, no. 4, pp. 565–572, 1981.

[12] F. Mujica, C. Massard, M. P. Franque, A. Coronado, M. Forlano, and C. Suarez, "Grado de infección y mortalidad en la garrapata del caballo *Anocentor nitens* (Acari: Ixodidae) naturalmente infectada por el protozoa *Babesia caballi* (Apicomplexa: Babesiidae)," *Revista Científica*, vol. 14, pp. 440–443, 2004.

[13] A. Morilla, "Inmunología de la babesiosis (Babesiosis immunology)," http://www.fmvz.unam.mx/fmvz/cienciavet/revistas/C-Vvol3/CVv3c09.pdf.

[14] B. Battsetseg, S. Lucero, X. Xuan et al., "Detection of natural infection of *Boophilus microplus* with *Babesia equi* and *Babesia caballi* in Brazilian horses using nested polymerase chain reaction," *Veterinary Parasitology*, vol. 107, no. 4, pp. 351–357, 2002.

[15] J. Rampersad, E. Cesar, M. D. Campbell, M. Samlal, and D. Ammons, "A field evaluation of PCR for the routine detection of *Babesia equi* in horses," *Veterinary Parasitology*, vol. 114, no. 2, pp. 81–87, 2003.

[16] D. Vargas, R. Bonet, P. Oliva, and S. Campano, "Implementación de la técnica de PCR en la identificación de *Babesia* spp. en equinos," *Parasitología Latinoamericana*, vol. 59, no. 3-4, pp. 179–182, 2004.

[17] D. Boldbaatar, X. Xuan, B. Battsetseg et al., "Epidemiological study of equine piroplasmosis in Mongolia," *Veterinary Parasitology*, vol. 127, no. 1, pp. 29–32, 2005.

[18] V. Álvarez, V. Hernández, and J. Gamboa, "Catálogo de garrapatas suaves (Acari: Argasidae) y duras (Acari: Ixodidae) de Costa Rica," *Revista Brenesia, Costa Rica*, vol. 63-64, pp. 81–88, 2005.

[19] R. Pineda, *Influence of equine infectious anemia (EIA) and babesiosis in endurance horses in Costa Rica [Bachelor thesis]*, Veterinary Medicine, Universidad Nacional de Costa Rica, Heredia, Costa Rica, 1998.

[20] A. Gómez, *Equine ambulatory medicine [Bachelor thesis]*, Veterinary Medicine, Universidad Nacional de Costa Rica, Heredia, Costa Rica, 2007.

[21] C. Vega, *Seroprevalencia de piroplasmosis equina en caballos mantenidos en cuadra y caballos destinados a matadero en Costa Rica [Bachelor thesis]*, Universidad Nacional de Costa Rica, Heredia, Costa Rica, 2011.

[22] D. Jiménez, J. J. Romero-Zuñiga, and G. Dolz, "Serosurveillance of infectious agents in equines of the Central Valley of Costa Rica," *Open Veterinary Journal*, vol. 4, no. 2, pp. 107–112, 2014.

[23] D. R. Henneke, G. D. Potter, J. L. Kreider, and B. F. Yeates, "Relationship between condition score, physical measurements and body fat percentage in mares," *Equine Veterinary Journal*, vol. 15, no. 4, pp. 371–372, 1983.

[24] Z. Asgarali, D. K. Coombs, F. Mohammed, M. D. Campbell, and E. Caesar, "A serological study of *Babesia caballi* and *Theileria equi* in Thoroughbreds in Trinidad," *Veterinary Parasitology*, vol. 144, no. 1-2, pp. 167–171, 2007.

[25] D. Aguirre, M. Carfune, M. Rada, and S. Torioni de Echade, "Babesiosis clínica en equinos de Cerrillos, Salta, Argentina," *Revista de Investigaciones Agropecuarias*, vol. 33, no. 3, pp. 123–133, 2004.

[26] A. Heim, L. M. Passos, M. F. Ribeiro et al., "Detection and molecular characterization of *Babesia caballi* and *Theileria equi* isolates from endemic areas of Brazil," *Parasitology Research*, vol. 102, no. 1, pp. 63–68, 2007.

[27] R. Melendez, "Babesiosis: una zoonosis emergente en regiones templadas y tropicales. Una revisión," *Revista Científica*, vol. 10, no. 1, pp. 13–18, 2000.

[28] A. M. Kjemtrup and P. A. Conrad, "Human babesiosis: an emerging tick-borne disease," *International Journal for Parasitology*, vol. 30, no. 12-13, pp. 1323–1337, 2000.

[29] A. Moretti, V. Mangili, R. Salvatori et al., "Prevalence and diagnosis of *Babesia* and *Theileria* infections in horses in Italy: a preliminary study," *Veterinary Journal*, vol. 184, no. 3, pp. 346–350, 2010.

[30] L. Camacho and H. Watson, "La educación tradicional de la comunidad cabecar de Chirripó: algunas consideraciones," *InterSedes, Costa Rica*, vol. 11, no. 20, pp. 137–153, 2010.

[31] I. Kakoma and H. Mehlhorn, "Babesia of domestic animals," in *Parasitic Protozoa*, pp. 141–216, Academic Press, Millbrae, Calif, USA, 1994.

17

Testicular and Related Size Evaluations in Nigerian Sahel Goats with Optimal Cauda Epididymal Sperm Reserve

Y. Abba[1,2] and I. O. Igbokwe[1]

[1]Department of Veterinary Pathology, Faculty of Veterinary Medicine, University of Maiduguri, PMB 1069, Maiduguri 600233, Borno State, Nigeria
[2]Department of Veterinary Pathology and Microbiology, Faculty of Veterinary Medicine, Universiti Putra Malaysia, 43400 Serdang, Selangor, Malaysia

Correspondence should be addressed to I. O. Igbokwe; ikeigbokwe@gmail.com

Academic Editor: Maria Laura Bacci

Testicular sizes of animals are important for identification of those with adequate sperm production. The aim of this study was to define the testicular and related size estimates that would be associated with optimal cauda epididymal sperm counts (ESC) in Sahel goats based on postmortem evaluations. A stratified quota sample population of 125 male goats inclusive of all testicular sizes was taken at a slaughterhouse in Maiduguri, Nigeria. The bucks were aged 18–30 months and weighed 17.04 ± 2.99 (12–25) kg. Body, testicular, and epididymal weights of each goat with other related size measurements were estimated. ESC was determined from homogenized tissue using a manual cytometer. At the cut-off ESC of $>1.1 \times 10^9$ sperm heads, 66 (52.80%) of the goats had optimal ESC which was associated with testicular weight of 59.90 ± 16.10 (31.40–86.20) g, gonadosomatic index of 3.51 ± 0.69 (2.00–4.50) g/kg, and scrotal circumference of 19.07 ± 1.29 (17.00–21.80) cm. The size variables of the scrotum and testis correlated with one another and with the ESC. These findings provide data that may be used to anticipate adequate antemortem sperm reserve based on testicular size during preliminary selection of sires for breeding from a sexually mature Sahel buck population.

1. Introduction

The breeds of goats in Nigeria are either dwarf (West African Dwarf type, WAD) or long-legged (Sahel type). The ecotypes of Sahel goats in northern Nigeria are Borno White (BW), Kano or Savannah Brown (KB), and Red Sokoto (RS), with no morphological features for external differentiation apart from coat color [1–5]. Investigations of Sahel bucks to establish baseline data required for evaluation of their reproductive health are scanty, but reports are available on their potential for sperm production [6–16].

Normospermia could be anticipated when cauda epididymal sperm reserve is adequate, since the sperm output in the semen depends on the quantity of sperm stored in the cauda epididymides [17]. Reference values of testicular size and sperm cell counts in cauda epididymides of Nigerian goats at postmortem or after castration, based on adequate

number of reference individuals, were not accessible, but such values ought to be available to indicate normal variations observed in healthy populations so that it would be possible to identify individuals having abnormal values in unhealthy conditions [18]. Four postpubertal WAD goats at 5 months of age weighing 8.90–11.00 kg in the early dry season had cauda epididymal sperm reserve of 1.57 ± 0.32 (1.20–1.90) $\times 10^9$ [9]. At the age of 12–14 months and weighing 19.52 ± 1.25 kg, 15 WAD goats were reported to have cauda epididymal sperm reserve of 1.46 ± 0.26 (1.20–1.70) $\times 10^9$ [15]. The WAD goats, in these reports, were intensively managed and fed adequately with supplements to obviate the effect of undernutrition on reproductive capacity [9, 15] and could be presumed to represent reproductively sound animals in the population. There is no evidence that the potential for sperm production differed between WAD and Sahel breeds [19]. Increasing age and body weight positively correlated with testicular sizes of goats [20–23]. Larger testes correlated with their scrotal circumferences [19, 24–26]. Testicular and cauda epididymal sperm reserves positively correlated with testicular weights and scrotal circumferences in RS goats [8].

The Sahel goat has adequate sperm production at 3 months of age with sperm cell concentration increasing with age [11]. The quality of sperm was reported to improve with age and later diminish with ageing of the buck beyond 30 months, but sperm quality was better in the dry than wet season [12, 16]. Bilateral testicular hypoplasia [27, 28] and atrophy [28, 29] associated with small-sized testes and aspermatogenesis occur among Sahel bucks [30]. Unilateral cryptorchid Sahel bucks had similar sperm concentration with normal bucks, but the percentage of sperm cell abnormalities was higher than normal [31]. Breeding programmes require assurance of the reproductive capacity of sires, but in areas with low technical and laboratory support for semen evaluation, farmers may need a reference range of testicular sizes, without extraneous mitigating conditions, which may be associated with adequate sperm reserve for reproductive efficiency.

In this study, the testicular sizes of sexually mature Nigerian Sahel goats were evaluated with their scrotal and epididymal sizes and testicular and cauda epididymal sperm counts with the aim of identifying goats with optimal sperm output from testicular and related size variables.

2. Materials and Methods

One hundred and twenty-five apparently healthy male Sahel goats in good body condition aged 18–30 months and weighing 10–25 kg, presented for slaughter at the metropolitan abattoir, Maiduguri, Nigeria, were selected by stratified quota sampling to capture those with various testicular sizes from small to large sizes with bilateral symmetry and the right-sided testis was consistently used for the study. They were aged by dental examination and weighed. The scrotal length (SL) and circumference (SC) were estimated with measuring tape. The testes (with their epididymides), with bilateral symmetry and without apparent lesions other than varying size, were collected and transported in an ice pack to the laboratory where the testes and epididymides were separated by dissection and weighed. The gonadosomatic index (GSI, g/kg) was estimated as the ratio of each testicular weight to body weight. The epididymosomatic index (ESI, g/kg) was also estimated as a ratio of each epididymal weight to body weight. Testicular longitudinal length (TLL) and mid-circumference (TMC) were estimated with a measuring tape. Sperm heads in homogenized testicular and cauda epididymal tissues were counted with a manual cytometer (haemocytometer) as earlier described by Amann and Lambiase [32] and Igbokwe et al. [33] with dilution of homogenates to facilitate counts and dilution factor used in the final calculation of counts. Optimal cauda epididymal sperm reserve was adjudged as $\geq 1.10 \times 10^9$ sperm cells [9, 15].

The data obtained were summarized as means ± standard deviations, means were compared by two-way analysis of variance with Tukey post hoc test, and coefficients

(r) of correlation were determined using computer software (GraphPad Instat, 1993 version, http://www.graphpad .com/scientific-software/instat/). Correlation coefficients were significant ($p < 0.05$) at >0.30 [34].

3. Results

Sixty-six (52.80%) out of 125 bucks had normal cauda epididymal sperm cell count of >1.10×10^9, and the data on their ages, BW, testicular (TSC) and cauda epididymal (ESC) sperm counts, and scrotal, testicular, and epididymal size variables are summarized in Table 1. The correlation coefficients in the relationships among the variables are presented in Table 2. The BW of the bucks increased ($p < 0.05$) with age and the sperm counts from the testes and cauda epididymides were higher ($p < 0.05$) at 30 months than 18 and 24 months of age. BW correlated ($r = 0.49$–0.70) with testicular and epididymal size variables (SC, SL, TW, TLL, and TMC) but did not correlate ($r = 0.15$–0.27) significantly ($p > 0.05$) with GSI and sperm counts (TSC, ESC). GSI correlated with TW ($r = 0.80$) and EW ($r = 0.77$) as well as SC, SL, TLL, and TMC ($r = 0.58$–0.80) but failed to correlate significantly ($p > 0.05$) with TSC ($r = 0.22$) and ESC ($r = 0.25$). ESC correlated significantly ($p < 0.05$) with scrotal size variables (SC, SL), some testicular size variables (TW, TLL, and TMC), and EW, whereas TSC did not have significant ($p > 0.05$) correlation with these variables. However, ESC correlated ($r = 0.55$; $p < 0.05$) with TSC as EW also correlated ($r = 0.92$; $p < 0.05$) with TW. The size variables of the scrotum and testis correlated ($r = 0.70$–0.77; $p < 0.05$) with one another.

4. Discussion

Majority of the bucks surveyed had optimal ESC and those with lower ESC than the cut-off sperm count were excluded from this report, having been evaluated for hypospermatogenesis and aspermatogenesis as earlier reported [30]. The bucks with optimal and suboptimal ESC had similar age range; the later had lower testicular weights (3.50–54.10 g) and gonadosomatic index values (0.40–2.80 g/kg) than the former [30, 35]. The incidence of testicular hypoplasia and atrophy had been reported recently among our Sahel goat populations [27–29], suggesting the need to determine the appropriate testicular sizes with optimal sperm output. This report provides such data on Sahel bucks with optimal ESC in the semiarid Sahel region and agrees with some limited data earlier reported of some testicular size parameters of mature RS and BW bucks [21]. RS bucks, aged 24–30 months, had mean testicular weight of 83.70 g at mean body weight of 17.80 kg [8]; and the GSI was 4.70 g/kg [35]. At 12–36 months, RS bucks weighed 22.50–30.00 kg with testicular weights of 55.00–103.00 g [21] and GSI of 2.40–3.40 g/kg [35], whereas BW bucks weighed 18.60–28.90 kg with testicular weights of 50.00–100.50 g [21] and GSI of 2.60–3.50 g/kg [35]. In the present study, the testicular weights of Sahel bucks were 31.40–86.20 g where body weights were 12.00–25.00 kg giving the GSI as 2.00–4.50 g/kg.

TABLE 1: Age-related variations in body weights, testicular and epididymal size estimates, and sperm counts in Nigerian Sahel goats.

| Parameters | Age (months) | | | All goats ($n = 66$) | Range (Min.–Max.) |
	18 ($n = 14$)	24 ($n = 25$)	30 ($n = 27$)		
Body weight (kg)	14.00 ± 1.13^a	16.67 ± 2.82^b	18.74 ± 2.29^c	17.04 ± 2.99	12.00–25.00
Sperm cell count ($\times 10^9$)					
Cauda epididymal	1.68 ± 0.31^a	1.68 ± 0.38^a	2.34 ± 0.80^b	1.94 ± 0.67	1.12–4.66
Testicular	0.14 ± 0.10^a	0.15 ± 0.01^a	0.27 ± 0.20^b	0.23 ± 0.30	0.03–1.88
Scrotal size					
Length (cm)	8.39 ± 0.68^a	9.66 ± 2.32^b	9.89 ± 0.61^b	9.29 ± 0.91	7.50–11.00
Circumference (cm)	17.82 ± 0.67^a	18.87 ± 1.22^b	19.91 ± 1.01^c	19.07 ± 1.29	17.00–21.80
Testicular size					
Gonadosomatic index (g/kg)	2.85 ± 0.38^a	3.43 ± 0.67^b	3.98 ± 0.41^c	3.51 ± 0.69	2.00–4.50
Weight (g)	39.58 ± 5.73^a	56.30 ± 11.26^b	74.34 ± 7.65^c	59.90 ± 16.10	31.40–86.20
Longitudinal length (cm)	8.94 ± 0.68^a	10.02 ± 1.07^b	11.13 ± 0.79^c	10.23 ± 1.20	7.80–12.90
Mid-circumference (cm)	10.23 ± 0.65^a	11.36 ± 0.87^b	12.71 ± 0.62^c	11.57 ± 1.30	9.10–13.70
Epididymal size					
Weight (g)	6.46 ± 1.17^a	8.15 ± 1.53^b	10.11 ± 0.69^c	8.57 ± 1.82	4.60–11.70
Epididymal-testicular weight ratio (g/g)	0.16 ± 0.02^a	0.15 ± 0.02^a	0.13 ± 0.01^b	0.15 ± 0.02	0.11–0.19
Epididymosomatic index (g/kg)	0.46 ± 0.08^a	0.49 ± 0.10^{ab}	0.54 ± 0.05^b	0.51 ± 0.08	0.28–0.64

[a,b,c]Means ± standard deviation with different superscripts are significantly different ($p < 0.05$).

TABLE 2: Correlation coefficients* (r) in matrix of relationships among testicular and related variables and associated sperm counts.

Variables	GSI	SC	SL	TW	TLL	TMC	EW	ESC	TSC	BW
Gonadosomatic index (GSI)	1									
Scrotal circumference (SC)	0.58	1								
Scrotal length (SL)	0.59	0.84	1							
Testicular weight (TW)	0.80	0.77	0.72	1						
Testicular longitudinal length (TLL)	0.60	0.74	0.70	0.89	1					
Testicular mid-circumference (TMC)	0.76	0.77	0.76	0.96	0.89	1				
Epididymal weight (EW)	0.77	0.68	0.64	0.92	0.83	0.89	1			
Cauda epididymal sperm count (ESC)	0.25	0.34	0.30	0.36	0.35	0.37	0.39	1		
Testicular sperm count (TSC)	0.22	0.15	0.20	0.16	0.12	0.17	0.21	0.55	1	
Body weight (BW)	0.15	0.60	0.49	0.70	0.76	0.69	0.60	0.27	0.04	1

*$r \geq 0.3$ is significant ($p < 0.05$).

The age for sexual maturity for Sahel bucks is 3–12 months [11]. The earliest age reported for adequate sperm production was 5 months in WAD bucks [9] and 5.70 months in British bucks [36]. Tropical male goats were reported to reach puberty and sexual maturity at 3.20 and 4.40 months of age, respectively [37], but male Nubian goats reached puberty at 8 months of age [38]. The Sahel bucks, in this study, were expected to have adequate sperm output at >18 months, if the testicular sizes were appropriate and testicular hypoplasia was precluded. As the bucks got older up to 30 months of age, the sperm output was increased because the bucks had increasing BW and testicular size. The testes of Sahel goats grow until mature body weight is attained at ≥30 months of age [39]. Previous reports indicated that testicular size positively correlated with sperm production in bulls, rams, boars, stallions [40, 41], and WAD and cashmere goats [15, 42]. Therefore, the TW and related size parameters would be imperative in selecting sire that is reproductively

sound as proposed by Ott and Memon [43]. Scrotal size parameters (SC, SL) correlated with BW, TW, and sperm output in this study, similar to earlier reports [23, 25, 26, 43–48]. The testicular size parameters (TW, GSI, TLL, and TMC) increased with age, indicating that testicular growth was sustained within the period because of expansion of the seminiferous tubular epithelium and associated increase in sperm output, indicating that more mature bucks will have better sperm ejaculation to enhance siring capacity. While BW of the bucks increased with age, BW had low insignificant correlation with TSC and ESC, suggesting that BW variation may not be an absolutely efficient predictor of sperm output in the bucks, in spite of the finding that BW had strong correlation with testicular size (TW, TLL, and TMC) and moderate correlation with scrotal size (SC, SL). The strong correlation between TSC and ESC justifies the dependence of semen sperm count on testicular sperm production and cauda epididymal sperm reserves. However, there was lack of remarkable dependence of testicular sperm count on testicular and related size variables among the goats. Biometric evaluations may establish assumptions of testicular sperm production, but assessment of quality of sperm ejaculates will still be necessary to have enhanced assurance of reproductive soundness of siring Sahel bucks.

In conclusion, the data in this report highlighted a relationship between morphometric parameters associated with size of testis and the sperm reserve that could influence semen quality in terms of sperm output. The impact is anchored on the provision of reference data for the locality on the testicular size measurements which may be useful in prediction of adequate sperm production and normospermia during preliminary selection of sires for breeding purposes.

Conflict of Interests

None is declared.

Acknowledgments

Ismaila Gadaka, HND, provided technical assistance during the research. Abba was on study fellowship at the University of Maiduguri and received partial financial support for this research.

References

[1] D. Bourn, W. Wint, R. Blench, and E. Woolley, "Nigerian livestock resources survey," *World Animal Review*, vol. 78, pp. 49–58, 1994.

[2] I. O. Igbokwe, A. Y. Ribadu, and M. M. Bukar, "Erythrocyte glutathione concentrations in Nigerian Sahel goats," *Small Ruminant Research*, vol. 30, no. 1, pp. 1–6, 1998.

[3] I. S. R. Butswat and D. T. RZaharadden, "Comparisms of some reproductive parameters in Red Sokoto and Kano brown breeds of goats," *Nigerian Journal of Animal Production*, vol. 25, pp. 1–5, 1998.

[4] R. Blench, "Traditional livestock breeds: geographical distribution and dynamics in relation to the ecology of West Africa," Working Paper 122, Overseas Development Institute, London, UK, 1999.

[5] H. D. Kwari, M. N. Sivachelvan, and A. G. Chibuzo, "Characterization of Sahel goat in Borno state, Nigeria, for certain qualitative traits," *Nigerian Journal of Experimental and Applied Biology*, vol. 5, no. 2, pp. 151–154, 2004.

[6] S. O. Ogwuegbu, B. O. Oko, M. O. Akusu, and T. A. Aire, "Gonadal and extragonadal sperm reserves of the maradi (Red Sokoto) goat," *Bulletin of Animal Health Production in Africa*, vol. 33, pp. 139–141, 1985.

[7] H. D. Kwari and S. O. Ogwuegbu, "Morphometric studies of the reproductive organs, Gonadal and extra-Gonadal sperm reserves of the Kuri Bull and Borno white buck of the Sahelian zone of North-Eastern part of Nigeria," *Tropical Veterinarian*, vol. 10, pp. 83–87, 1992.

[8] C. S. Daudu, "Spermatozoa output, testicular sperm reserve and epididymal storage capacity of the Red Sokoto goats indigenous to northern Nigeria," *Theriogenology*, vol. 21, no. 2, pp. 317–324, 1984.

[9] I. I. Bitto and G. N. Egbunike, "Seasonal variations in sperm production, gonadal and extragonadal sperm reserves in pubertal West African dwarf bucks in their native tropical environment," Livestock Research for Rural Development, Volume 18, Article #134, 2006, http://www.lrrd.org/lrrd18/9/bitt18134.htm.

[10] I. I. Bitto and G. N. Egbunike, "Seasonal variations in the morphometric characteristics of the pubertal West African Dwarf buck in its native tropical environment," *International Journal of Morphology*, vol. 24, no. 4, pp. 637–642, 2006.

[11] V. A. Maina, S. U. R. Chaudhari, and G. D. Mshelia, "Spermiogram of the white ecotype of Sahel bucks in Maiduguri Metropolis," *Pakistan Journal of Biological Sciences*, vol. 9, no. 2, pp. 307–309, 2006.

[12] V. A. Maina, S. U. R. Chaudhari, G. D. Mshelia, and A. Williams, "Influence of season on semen characteristics of Sahel bucks in Borno state," *Journal of Applied Sciences*, vol. 6, no. 2, pp. 353–356, 2006.

[13] V. A. Maina, S. U. R. Chaudhari, and A. Y. Ribadu, "Effect of ecotype on semen characteristics of Sahel goats in Borno State," *Journal of Applied Sciences*, vol. 6, no. 5, pp. 1220–1224, 2006.

[14] I. I. Bitto, G. N. Egbunike, and M. O. Akusu, "Seasonal variation in the histometric characteristic of the reproductive organs of pubertal West African Dwarf goats in their native tropical environment," *International Journal of Morphology*, vol. 26, no. 2, pp. 397–401, 2008.

[15] S. O. C. Ugwu, "Relationship between scrotal circumference, in situ testicular measurements and sperm reserves in the West African Dwarf Goats," *African Journal of Biotechnology*, vol. 8, no. 7, pp. 1354–1357, 2009.

[16] M. O. Oyeyemi, A. P. Fayomi, D. A. Adeniji, and O. M. Ojo, "Gonadal and extragonadal spermiogram of Sahel buck in the humid zone of Nigeria," *Current Research Journal of Biological Sciences*, vol. 3, no. 5, pp. 468–471, 2011.

[17] W. E. Berndtson, "Methods for quantifying mammalian spermatogenesis: a review," *Journal of Animal Science*, vol. 44, no. 5, pp. 818–833, 1977.

[18] A. Geffré, K. Friedrichs, K. Harr, D. Concordet, C. Trumel, and J.-P. Braun, "Reference values: a review," *Veterinary Clinical Pathology*, vol. 38, no. 3, pp. 288–298, 2009.

[19] N. K. Alade, A. A. Shettima, and I. B. Watirahyel, "Differences between the testicular and semen quality characteristics of three breeds of goats in a semi arid environment," *Journal of Arid Agriculture*, vol. 16, pp. 145–149, 2006.

[20] Y. Mekasha, A. Tegegne, A. Abera, and H. Rodriguez-Martinez, "Body size and testicular traits of tropically-adapted bucks raised under extensive husbandry in Ethiopia," *Reproduction in Domestic Animals*, vol. 43, no. 2, pp. 196–206, 2008.

[21] A. O. Raji, J. U. Igwebuike, and J. Aliyu, "Testicular biometry and its relationship with body weight of indigenous goats in a semi arid region of Nigeria," *Journal of Agricultural and Biological Sciences*, vol. 3, no. 4, pp. 6–9, 2008.

[22] K. S. Kabiraj, M. S. A. Hoque, M. A. M. Khandoker, and S. S. Husain, "Testicular biometry and its relationship with body weight and semen output of Black Bengel bucks in Bangladesh," *Journal of Cell and Animal Biology*, vol. 5, no. 2, pp. 27–32, 2011.

[23] A. Shoyombo, O. Fasanya, U. Bunjah, and H. Yakubu, "On-farm prediction of testicular characteristics in bucks at specific ages," *World Journal of Life Sciences and Medical Research*, vol. 2, no. 3, pp. 114–117, 2012.

[24] N. K. Alade, A. Abdulkareem, and S. B. Adamu, "Breed differences in body weight, body and testicular measurements and

their relationship in Red Sokoto and Sahel goats at weaning," *Sahel Journal of Veterinary Science*, vol. 6, no. 1, pp. 13–17, 2007.

[25] N. K. Alade, C. L. Ezeokoli, and I. D. Mohammed, "The relationships between body weight, testicular weight, age and the scrotal circumference of goats in the semi-arid Maiduguri, Nigeria," *Animal Production Research Advances*, vol. 5, no. 1, 2009.

[26] N. K. Alade, S. Mbap, and I. D. Muhammed, "Testicular characteristics: gonadal and extra gonadal sperm reserves and their relationship with body weight in Sahel goats," *African Journal of Agricultural Research and Development*, vol. 2, no. 2, pp. 91–94, 2009.

[27] I. O. Igbokwe, A. E. Ikpo, H. A. Grema, F. M. Mshelbwala, and N. A. Igbokwe, "Bilateral testicular hypoplasia among mature Sahel bucks in Nigeria," *Turkish Journal of Veterinary and Animal Sciences*, vol. 35, no. 2, pp. 111–115, 2011.

[28] Y. Abba, S. Simon, H. I. Gambo, I. O. Igbokwe, and Y. Iliyasu, "Pathological conditions associated with the male reproductive tract of the sahel bucks," *Veterinary Medicine International*, vol. 2014, Article ID 406431, 5 pages, 2014.

[29] F. M. Mshelbwala and I. O. Igbokwe, "Severe bilateral testicular atrophy among Sahel goats in Maiduguri, Nigeria," *Sahel Journal of Veterinary Science*, vol. 9, pp. 17–20, 2010.

[30] Y. Abba and I. O. Igbokwe, "Aspermatogenesis and hypospermatogenesis in culled Sahel goats in Nigeria," *Reproduction in Domestic Animals*, vol. 47, supplement 4, pp. 416–613, 2012, Proceedings of the International Conference on Animal Reproduction in Vancouver, Canada, Abstract #1007, p. 468.

[31] I. O. Igbokwe, Y. Abba, S. U. Geidam, and N. A. Igbokwe, "Sperm output from unilateral cryptorchid Sahel goats," *Comparative Clinical Pathology*, vol. 23, no. 4, pp. 819–822, 2014.

[32] R. P. Amann and J. Y. Lambiase, "The male rabbit III: determination of daily sperm production by means of testicular homogenates," *Journal of Animal Science*, vol. 28, pp. 369–374, 1969.

[33] N. A. Igbokwe, U. K. Sandabe, S. Sanni, B. Wampana, I. M. Wiam, and I. O. Igbokwe, "Aqueous stem-bark extract of *Ficus sycomorus* increases sperm production and pH of sperm microenvironment in growing albino rat," *Animal Reproduction*, vol. 6, no. 4, pp. 509–515, 2009.

[34] P. Singha, *An Introductory Text on Biostatistics*, Ahmadu Bello University Press, Zaria, Nigeria, 1992.

[35] Y. Abba, *Quantitative and histopathological assessment of aspermatogenesis and hypospermatogenesis in Sahel goats with bilateral testicular hypoplasia [MVSc Dissertation]*, Department of Veterinary Pathology, University of Maiduguri, Maiduguri, Nigeria, 2011.

[36] N. Ahmad and D. E. Noakes, "Sexual maturity in British breeds of goat kids," *British Veterinary Journal*, vol. 152, no. 1, pp. 93–103, 1996.

[37] W. J. A. Payne and R. Wilson, *An Introduction to Animal Husbandry in the Tropics*, Blackwell Science, London, UK, 1999.

[38] P. K. Chakraborty, L. D. Stuart, and J. L. Brown, "Puberty in the male Nubian Goat: serum concentrations of LH, FSH and testosterone from birth through puberty and semen characteristics at sexual maturity," *Animal Reproduction Science*, vol. 20, no. 2, pp. 91–101, 1989.

[39] F. M. Mshelbwala, *Prevalence and pathology of retained (cryptorchid) and descended testes in Nigerian Sahel goats [MVSc dissertation]*, Department of Veterinary Pathology, University of Maiduguri, Maiduguri, Nigeria, 2010.

[40] R. H. Foote, "Factors influencing the quantity and quality of semen harvested from bulls, rams, boars and stallions," *Journal of Animal Science*, vol. 47, no. 2, pp. 1–11, 1978.

[41] R. P. Amann, "A critical review of methods for evaluation of spermatogenesis from seminal characteristics," *Journal of Andrology*, vol. 2, no. 1, pp. 37–58, 1981.

[42] S. W. Walkden-Brown, B. J. Restall, and W. A. Taylor, "Testicular and epididymal sperm content in grazing Cashmere bucks: seasonal variation and prediction from measurements in vivo," *Reproduction, Fertility and Development*, vol. 6, no. 6, pp. 727–736, 1994.

[43] R. S. Ott and M. A. Memon, "Breeding soundness examinations of rams and bucks, a review," *Theriogenology*, vol. 13, no. 2, pp. 155–164, 1980.

[44] T. A. Bongso, M. R. Jainudeen, and A. S. Zahrah, "Relationship of scrotal circumference to age, body weight and onset of spermatogenesis in goats," *Theriogenology*, vol. 18, no. 5, pp. 513–524, 1982.

[45] G. S. Bilaspuri and K. Singh, "Developmental changes in body weight and testicular characteristics in Malabari goat kids," *Theriogenology*, vol. 37, no. 2, pp. 507–520, 1992.

[46] G. S. Bilaspuri and K. Singh, "Distinction between Malabari and Beetal goat breeds," *Small Ruminant Research*, vol. 10, no. 3, pp. 201–208, 1993.

[47] A. M. Al-Ghalban, M. J. Tabbaa, and R. T. Kridli, "Factors affecting semen characteristics and scrotal circumference in Damascus bucks," *Small Ruminant Research*, vol. 53, no. 1-2, pp. 141–149, 2004.

[48] M. O. Oyeyemi, A. P. Fayomi, D. A. Adeniji, and O. M. Ojo, "Testicular and epididymal parameters of sahel buck in the humid zone of Nigeria," *International Journal of Morphology*, vol. 30, no. 2, pp. 489–492, 2012.

18

Systemic *Candida parapsilosis* Infection Model in Immunosuppressed ICR Mice and Assessing the Antifungal Efficiency of Fluconazole

Yu'e Wu,[1] Fangui Min,[1] Jinchun Pan,[1] Jing Wang,[1] Wen Yuan,[1] Yu Zhang,[1] Ren Huang,[1] and Lixin Zhang[2]

[1]*Guangdong Laboratory Animals Monitoring Institute, Guangdong Provincial Key Laboratory of Laboratory Animals, Guangzhou 510663, China*
[2]*Institute of Microbiology, Chinese Academy of Sciences, Beijing 100080, China*

Correspondence should be addressed to Yu Zhang; zhangyugzh@hotmail.com, Ren Huang; labking@sohu.com, and Lixin Zhang; lzhang03@gmail.com

Academic Editor: William Ravis

This study was to establish a systemic *C. parapsilosis* infection model in immunosuppressed ICR mice induced by cyclophosphamide and evaluate the antifungal efficiency of fluconazole. Three experiments were set to confirm the optimal infectious dose of *C. parapsilosis*, outcomes of infectious model, and antifungal efficiency of fluconazole in vivo, respectively. In the first experiment, comparisons of survival proportions between different infectious doses treated groups showed that the optimal inoculum for *C. parapsilosis* was 0.9×10^5 CFU per mouse. The following experiment was set to observe the outcomes of infection at a dose of 0.9×10^5 CFU *C. parapsilosis*. Postmortem and histopathological examinations presented fugal-specific lesions in multiorgans, especially in kidneys, characterized by inflammation, numerous microabscesses, and fungal infiltration. The CFU counts were consistent with the histopathological changes in tissues. Th1/Th2 cytokine imbalance was observed with increases of proinflammatory cytokines and no responses of anti-inflammatory cytokines in sera and kidneys. In the last experiment, model based evaluation of fluconazole indicated that there were ideal antifungal activities for fluconazole at dosages of 10–50 mg/kg/d. Data demonstrates that the research team has established a systemic *C. parapsilosis* infection model in immunosuppressed ICR mice, affording opportunities for increasing our understanding of fungal pathogenesis and treatment.

1. Introduction

Candida, usually kept as harmless commensals in healthy individuals, may become opportunistic pathogens in susceptible hosts, especially in severely drug-immunosuppressed or immunodeficient patients [1–3]. During the past two decades, the candidemia causative agent has changed from *C. albicans* to non-*C. albicans*, and the patients infected with the non-*C. albicans* were gradually increased. *Candida* infections have accounted for about 8 to 9 percent of hospital-acquired infections and become the fourth most common cause of such infections [4, 5]. *C. parapsilosis,* a typical commensal of human skin, has emerged notoriously for its capacity to grow in total parenteral nutrition and to form biofilms on catheters and other implanted devices [6, 7]. During the last decade, the incidence of *C. parapsilosis* has dramatically increased and become the second most commonly isolated *Candida* species from blood cultures.

Given the incidence of disease and the unacceptably high mortality associated with *C. parapsilosis*, there is an urgent need of more effective preventive, diagnostic, and therapeutic strategies. Experimental animal models are a critical component of understanding the pathogenesis and host resistance to infection and to development of more efficacious antifungal therapies. Previously, an immunocompromised mouse model of *C. parapsilosis* established by us has been used to evaluate microbial metabolites as combination agents for the treatment of fungal infections [8]. After further optimization for establishment procedures, the animal model was more stable and presented outcomes of systemic infection. The present paper will describe in detail the outcomes of the systemic mouse *C. parapsilosis* model, including mortality, tissues fungal burdens, histopathology, serum and renal cytokines, and the usage of the model for evaluation of fluconazole.

2. Materials and Methods

2.1. Animals and Ethics Statement. SPF female ICR mice aged from 4 to 6 weeks and weighed 20 to 22 g were used in this study. Animals were purchased from SLAC Laboratory Animal Centre Co., Shanghai, and had never been used for any experimental procedures previously. After arrival, animals were acclimated for 3 days before the experiments.

Animal use protocols were reviewed and approved by IACUC of Guangdong Laboratory Animal Monitoring Institute in accordance with the *Guide for the Care and Use of Laboratory Animals* [9]. Animals were bred in negative pressure isolation cages in an animal negative pressure facility with an approval of and oversight by the Local Provincial Institutional Environmental Health and Safety Office.

2.2. Fungal Strain and Inoculum Preparation. *C. parapsilosis* ATCC22019 normally stored at −86°C was used in this study. Stock inoculum suspensions of *C. parapsilosis* were obtained from >20 h cultures in RPMI medium 1640 incubated at 30°C with shaking at 150 rpm. And >95% of *C. parapsilosis* cells should be blastoconidia by microscopic examination.

2.3. Cyclophosphamide Induced Immunosuppression. Ten mice were intraperitoneally injected with cyclophosphamide (CY) (100 mg/kg weight/d) for continuous 3 days. Blood samples (0.20 mL) were collected via fossa orbitalis vein daily from 0 to 6 days after the injection of CY. Then, total leukocyte counts were performed by the *Sysmex XT-2000iv* automatic hematology analyzer. Another 10 mice receiving normal saline were set as controls.

2.4. Study Design. The first experiment was set to confirm the infectious dose. The immunosuppressed mice receiving CY were inoculated with 0.1 mL *C. parapsilosis* suspension via tail vein at doses of 1×10^2 CFU, 0.9×10^5 CFU, 5.0×10^5 CFU, and 8×10^5 CFU, respectively. The control mice receiving normal saline were inoculated with 0.1 mL normal saline via tail vein. According to the results of survival curves, the optimal infectious dose would be confirmed.

In the second experiment, another immunosuppressed group inoculated with optimal infectious dose of *C. parapsilosis* was set to observe the outcomes of infection. At days 1, 4, and 6 postinfection, 3 mice were euthanized, sera were collected, and target organs (heart, liver, spleen, lung, kidney, and brain) were excised for tissue fungal burdens, pathological examination, and cytokine measurement.

The third experiment was designed to evaluate fluconazole (Sigma). Four groups of infected mice were treated intraperitoneally with fluconazole at the dosages of 0, 0.5, 10, and 50 mg/kg/d of body weight 1 h postinfection for 7

consecutive days. Survival rates and tissue fungal burdens were used to evaluate the antifungal efficacy of fluconazole.

2.5. Clinical Assessment. Animals were observed daily throughout the study for alterations in behavior, appetite, and mortality.

2.6. Postmortem and Histopathological Examinations. The mice were sacrificed by CO_2 inhalation. Heart, liver, spleen, lung, kidney, brain, stomach, and bladder were removed immediately and preserved in 10% formalin. After paraffin embedding and sectioning, standard 5 μm sections were cut and stained with hematoxylin and eosin (H&E) and periodic acid-Schiff (PAS).

2.7. Tissue Fungal Burdens. Half of the target organs were homogenized in 1.0 mL of sterile normal saline. Tissue homogenates from individual mice were serially diluted on SDA plates and incubated for 48 h at 35°C. Results are expressed as CFU log_{10} per organ.

2.8. Cytokine Measurement. IL-1α, IL-1β, IL-2, IL-4, IL-5, IL-6, IL-10, IL-17, IL-23, GM-CSF, IFN-γ, and TNF-α in serial sera and renal samples of control and infected mice were measured by cytometric bead array.

2.9. Data Analysis. All data was expressed as mean ± SD. Between-group differences of quantitative data were analyzed by *t*-tests. While the between-group differences of survival cures were performed by *Log-rank (Mantel-Cox) Test*. Significance was judged at the 0.05 level.

3. Results

3.1. CY Induced Immunosuppression. No significant changes were found in total leukocyte counts for the control mice injected with saline. However, the mice receiving CY showed a time corresponding decrease from days 1 to 4. At day 4, the total leukocyte counts of mice receiving CY reached the lowest levels followed by a gradual increase to basal levels till day 14 (Figure 1). The results indicate that the optimal infection time points are days 3 to 6 after CY administration.

3.2. Confirmation of Infectious Dose by Survival Proportions. In the first study, every immunosuppressed group presented death of animals postinfection. All except 1×10^2 CFU group died out from days 1 to 15 postinfection. For 1×10^2 CFU group, 92% of animals survived until 12 days postinfection for necropsy.

The survival curves were shown in Figure 2. 0.9×10^5 CFU group showed significant differences with the other groups (*Log-rank Test*, $P < 0.05$). The median survival times of 0.9×10^5 CFU, 5.0×10^5 CFU, and 8.0×10^5 CFU groups are 5.5 days, 2 days, and 2.5 days, respectively. These data indicated that the optimal inoculum for *C. parapsilosis* was 0.9×10^5 CFU per mouse in immunosuppressed mice.

3.3. Clinical Signs of the Model. The clinical symptoms of distress, such as that decreased movement, decreased food

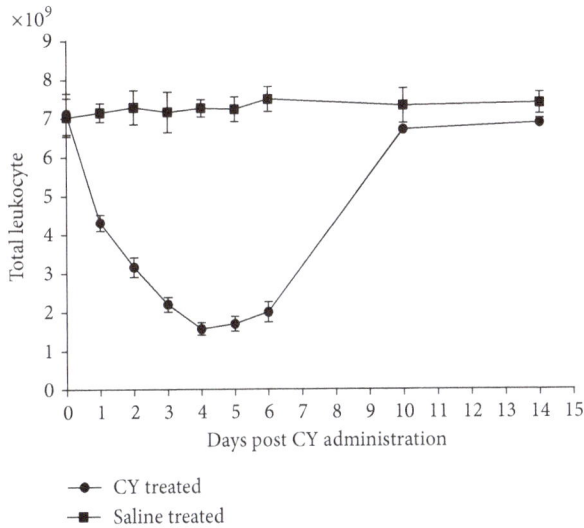

FIGURE 1: Total leukocyte counts. A time corresponding decrease was found in CY treated mice from days 1 to 4. The lowest data emerged at day 4 ($n = 10$).

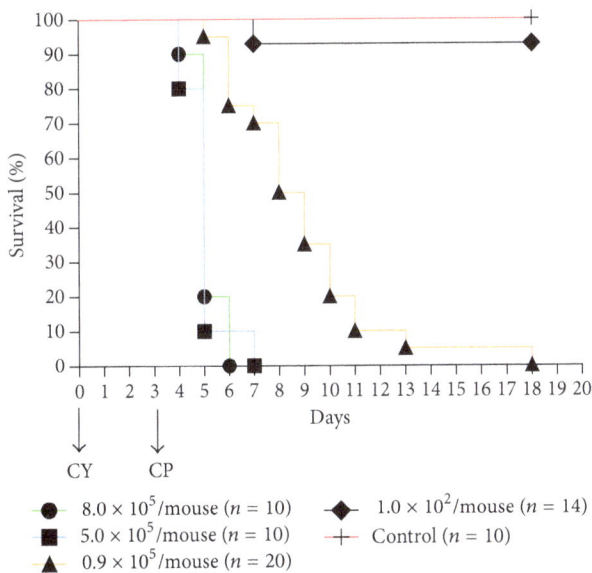

FIGURE 2: Survival curves. The mortality showed positive associations with infectious dose. And the optimal inoculum for *C. parapsilosis* was 0.9×10^5 CFU per immunosuppressed mouse.

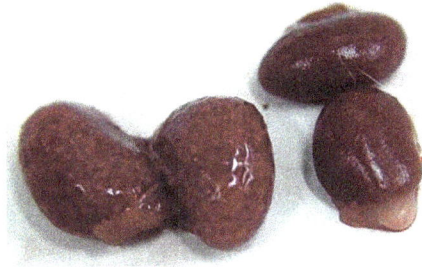

FIGURE 3: Gross observation of kidneys. The right two kidneys were the normal controls and the left swollen kidneys covered with petechiae were from infected mice.

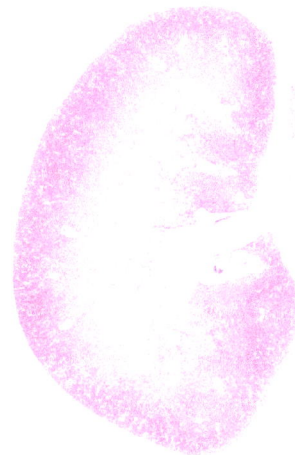

(a)

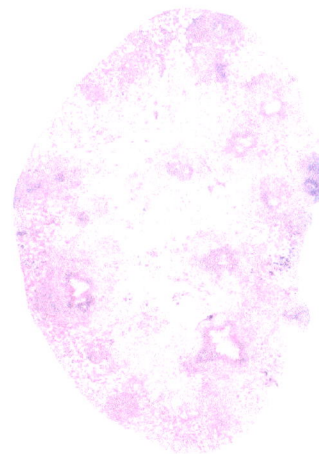

(b)

FIGURE 4: Histopathological changes in kidneys. Figure 4(a) was the control mouse showing no observed lesions. Figure 4(b) was the infected mouse presenting numerous granulomas in tissue section of the kidney.

and water consumption, weight loss, self-imposed isolation, and difficult breathing, were conspicuous in most infected animals 2 days postinfection. Each infected group presented death of animals during the infection period. Before death, most of them exhibited severe neurologic disorders, including opisthotonus, torticollis, and ataxia.

3.4. Gross Observation of the Model. At necropsy, swollen kidneys covered with white foci were observed in all infected mice (Figure 3). Some cases showed petechiae and petechial bleeding on the surface of the lung lobes and brains. Besides, moderate enlargements of the spleens were observed in most animals. No specific gross lesions were found in other organs.

3.5. Histological Analysis of the Model. At day 1, the lesions in all organs were relatively temperate, characterized by inflammation and slightly fungal infiltration of kidney tissues.

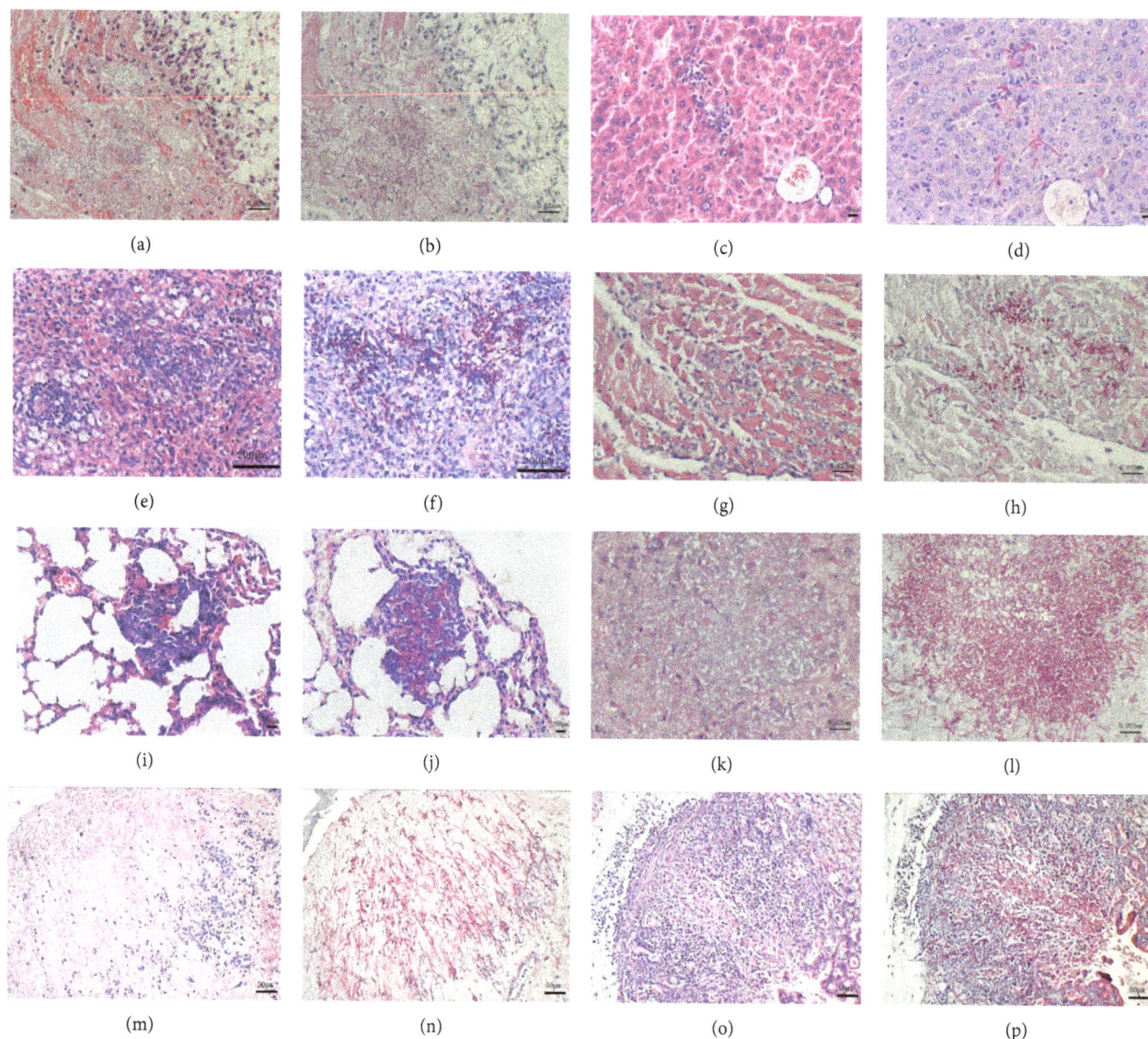

FIGURE 5: Histological findings of infected immunosuppressed mice. Figures 5(a), (c), (e), (g), (i), (k), (m), and (o) were H&E stained sections displaying the representative lesions in kidney, liver, spleen, heart, lung, brain, stomach, and bladder walls, respectively. Figures 5(b), (d), (f), (h), (j), (l), (n), and (p) stained by PAS showed fungal mycelia infiltration in kidney, liver, spleen, heart, lung, brain, stomach, and bladder walls, respectively.

At s 4 and 6, representative lesions could be observed in most organs. The kidney suffered the most severe lesions compared to the other organs or tissues. Numerous granulomas were diffused in renal cortex and medulla (Figure 4). Microscopic examination revealed that all granulomas contained fungal mycelia, blastospores, and chlamydospore-like structures (Figures 5(a) and 5(b)). The liver only experienced minor lesions, presenting periportal infiltration with a few polymorphonuclear leukocytes and fungal elements (Figures 5(c) and 5(d)). The spleen demonstrated the nonspecific lesion of the decrease of lymphocytes in white pulp and infiltration of a few PAS-positive fungal elements (Figures 5(e) and 5(f)). A certain number of granulomas or focal necrosis could be observed in the cardiac muscles, which were always composed by a necrotic center, infiltration of leukocytes,

mycelia, blastospores, and PAS-positive components (Figures 5(g) and 5(h)). Some certain focal necroses infiltrated by erythrocytes, lymphocyte-like cells, PAS-positive mycelia, blastospores, and chlamydospore-like structures were found in lung interstitium (Figures 5(i) and 5(j)). The lesions in brains were relatively more severe than the other organs, except kidneys. Focal liquefactive necrosis with abundant invading fungal pseudohyphae disrupted much of the forebrain (Figures 5(k) and 5(l)). Multifocal to coalescent necrosis and fungal invasions were observed in the gastric wall, which destroyed the deep structures of gastric wall including lamina propria, lamina muscularis, and stratum subvascular (Figures 5(m) and 5(n)). Similar lesions and extensive fungal invasion to gastric wall were also present within the bladder wall (Figures 5(o) and 5(p)).

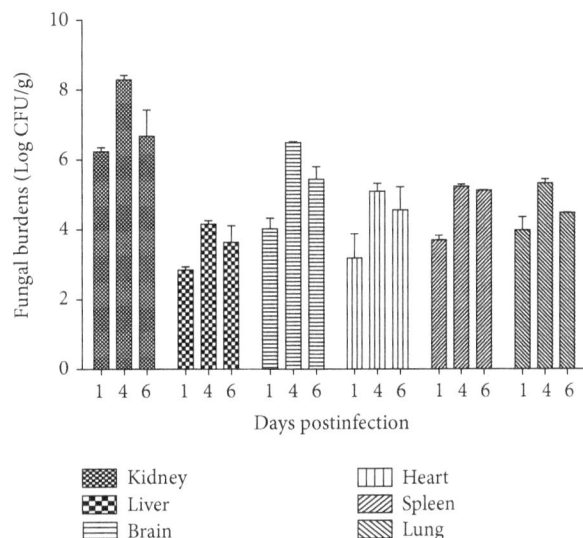

FIGURE 6: Dynamic changes of tissue fungal burdens. Tissue fungal burdens showed a transient increase during the infection period. And the kidney suffered the highest CFU scores.

3.6. Tissue Fungal Burdens of the Model. *C. parapsilosis* could be detected out from the kidney, liver, brain, heart, spleen, and lung tissue suspension from day 1 postinfection. The dynamic changes of fungal burdens were the same in these organs, showing a transient increase with a brief peak at day 4 postinfection (Figure 6). The kidneys presented with much higher CFU scores compared with the other organs of the same time (t-test, $P < 0.05$).

3.7. Cytokine Levels of the Model. For the CY group, all the detected serum and renal cytokines showed no significant changes all the time. Unlike the CY group, the *C. parapsilosis* infected mice presented different dynamic changes in serum and renal cytokines (Figure 7). Serum IL-6 and TNF-α showed a transient increase and reached the highest points at day 4, followed by the increase of serum IFN-γ. The other serum cytokines (IL-2, IL-4, IL-5, IL-10, IL-17, IL-23, GM-CSF, IL-1α, and IL-1β) showed no specific changes. Renal IL-6, TNF-α, IFN-γ, IL-1α, and IL-1β presented significant increases from days 4 to 6 postinfection. However, the other renal cytokines (IL-2, IL-4, IL-5, IL-10, IL-17, IL-23, and GM-CSF) presented no specific changes.

3.8. Model Based Evaluation of Antifungal Activity of Fluconazole. Four groups of infectious models were used to evaluate the antifungal efficiency of fluconazole by administrating different dosages of fluconazole. During the experiment period, all animals of 50 mg/kg/d group survived, while mortalities of 100%, 80%, and 40% were observed in 0, 0.5, and 10 mg/kg/d groups, respectively. Survival curves were generated and compared between each 2 groups (Figure 8). Significant differences were found between 50 mg/kg/d group and the other groups (*Log-rank Test*, $P < 0.05$). There were also significant differences between 10 mg/kg/d group and the others. No significant differences were shown between 0.5 mg/kg/d group and the control. After receiving

fluconazole, 50 mg/kg/d group showed a significant decline of renal fungal burdens (Figure 9). Though there were declines in mortalities of 0.5 and 10 mg/kg/d groups, the renal fungal burdens significantly increased at day 4 postinfection (t-test, $P < 0.05$) (Figure 9). When compared with the control, renal fungal burdens of both 50 and 10 mg/kg/d groups at days 4 and 6 were significantly lower than the control (t-test, $P < 0.05$). Results indicated that there were ideal antifungal activities for fluconazole at dosages of 10–50 mg/kg/d.

4. Discussion

C. albicans has been kept as the major species associated with human *Candida* infections for decades. And the majority of experimental animal models for *Candida* species have focused on *C. albicans* too. Though many kinds of animals have been used to study *Candida* infections, the rodent infection models occupied the majority for economic reasons, easy handling, and the availability of genetic modification [10]. In this paper, we will try to introduce an ideal *C. parapsilosis* infection model based on immunosuppressed ICR mice.

Many regents have been used to obtain the immunosuppressed mice, for example, cortisone acetate and hydrocortisone succinate [11]. Here, we used CY to induce immunosuppression in ICR mice. Mice presented a time transient decrease of the total leukocyte counts and reached the lowest point at day 4 after receiving CY for 3 consecutive days at a dosage of 100 mg/kg body weight. Result demonstrated that days 3 to 6 after CY administration were the optimal infection time points. And the day 4 was chosen to infect mice in this study.

To assure the infectious dose of *C. parapsilosis*, immunosuppressed mice were infected with 4 dosages, respectively. According to the results of survival curves, the dosage of 0.9×10^5 CFU *C. parapsilosis* was the optimal infectious dose in immunosuppressed ICR mice. The morphology

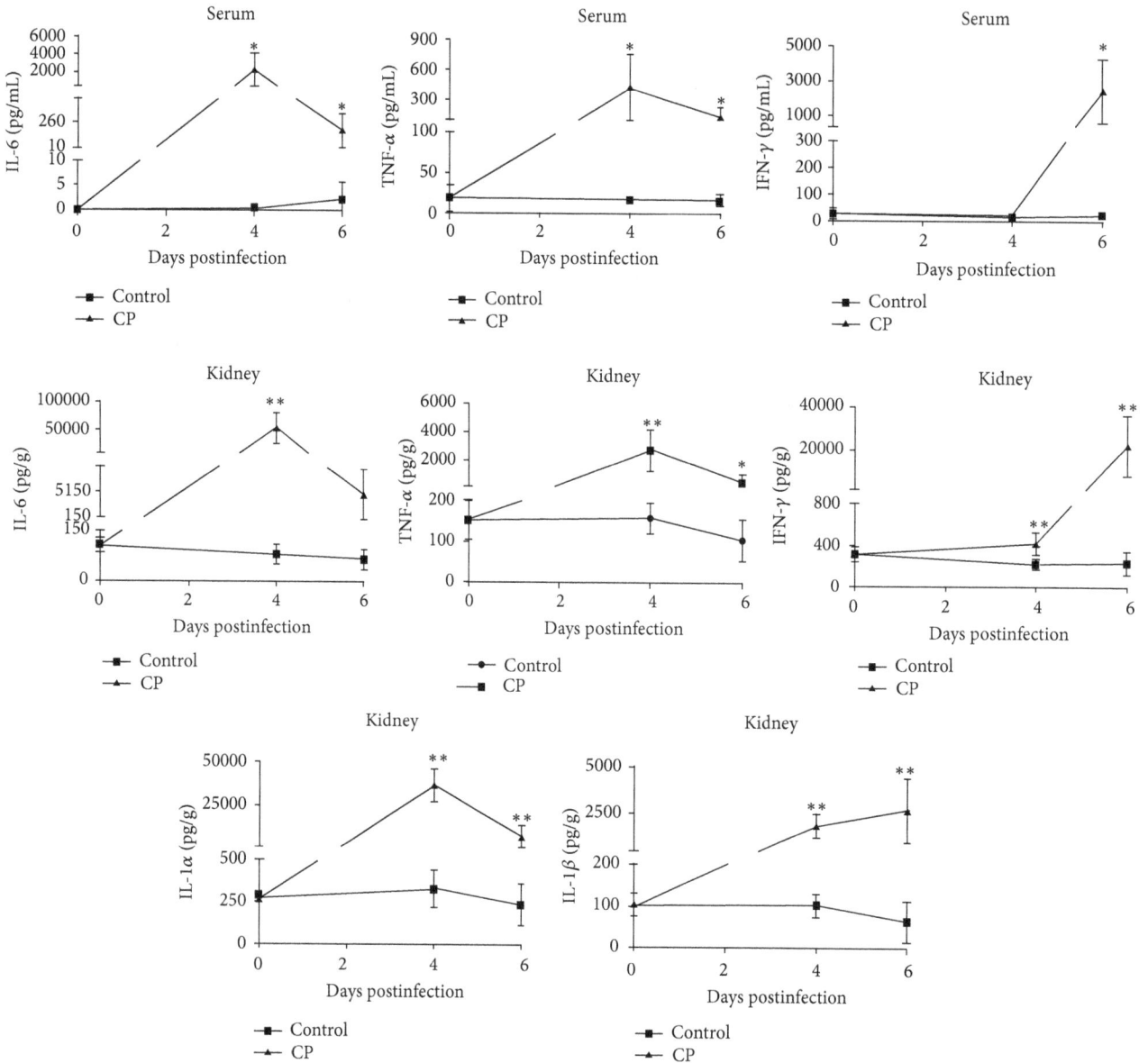

FIGURE 7: Dynamic changes of serum and renal cytokines. Serum IL-6, TNF-α, and IFN-γ and renal IL-6, TNF-α, IFN-γ, IL-1α, and IL-1β presented significant increases during the infection period.

of *Candida* species was important to animal models. Our previous experiments showed that mycelium *C. parapsilosis* has more virulence than fungal spores. And the inoculums containing >95% fungal spores were used in this study.

The infection model based on 0.9×10^5 CFU *C. parapsilosis* presented a median survival time of 5.5 days, which was long enough to satisfy researches on antifungal agents. Histopathology and tissues fungal burdens revealed the model to be a systemic infection one, and the kidneys suffered the most severe lesions, indicating that kidney could be a suitable target organ for screening antifungal agents. The fungal burdens showed a transient increase with a brief peak at day 4 postinfection in multiple organs, demonstrating that day 4 postinfection was an optimal time point to assess the fungal burdens for research or evaluation of antifungal

agents, which were further identified by using the infectious model in evaluation of antifungal activity of fluconazole. Some serum and renal proinflammatory cytokines were induced and consistent with the tissue fungal burdens, while anti-inflammatory cytokines showed no significant increase. Th1/Th2 cytokine imbalance might result in high mortality of infected mice.

This project established a systemic *C. parapsilosis* infection model in immunosuppressed ICR mice. In this model, multiorgans, including kidneys, liver, lungs, spleen, brains, and bladder wall, represented numerous microabscesses, which demonstrated congestion, hemorrhages, tubular degeneration, and heterophilic infiltration. This model affords opportunities for increasing our understanding of fungal pathogenesis and treatment.

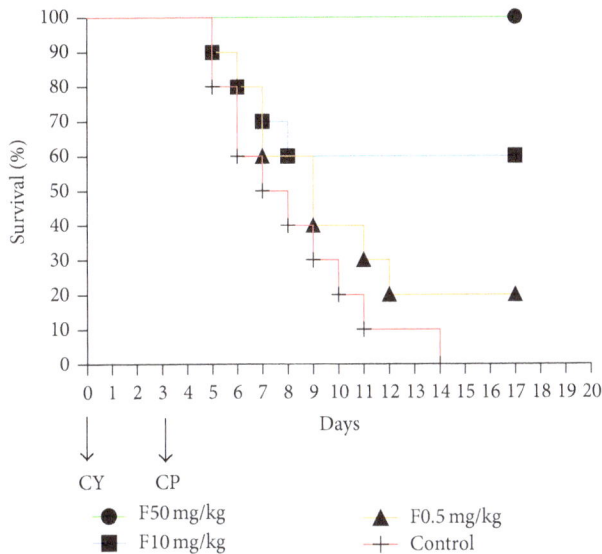

FIGURE 8: Survival curves of fluconazole treated mice ($n = 10$ per group). Comparisons between each two groups except 0.5 and 10 mg/kg/d groups that showed significant differences (*Log-rank Test*, $P < 0.05$).

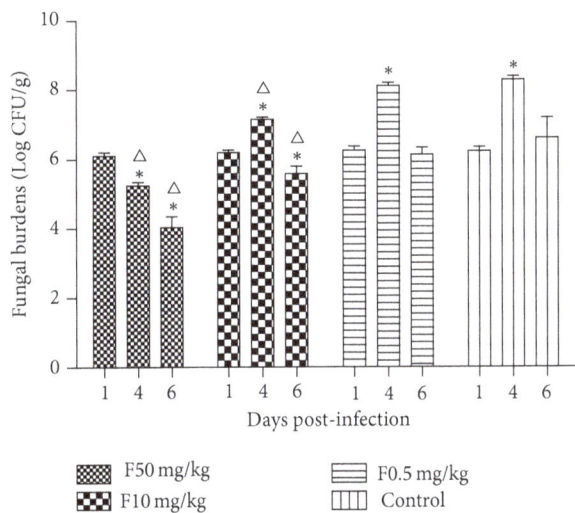

FIGURE 9: Renal fungal burdens of fluconazole treated mice ($n = 5$ per day). 50 mg/kg/d group showed a significant decline of renal fungal burdens, while, the other groups showed a transient increase during the experiment period. $^*P < 0.05$, t-test, versus that of day 1. $^\triangle P < 0.05$, t-test, versus that of control of the same time point.

Conflict of Interests

The authors declare that there is no conflict of interests regarding the publication of this paper.

Authors' Contribution

Yu'e Wu and Fangui Min are co-first authors. Yu'e Wu, Fangui Min, Yu Zhang, and Ren Huang conceived and designed the study. The first five coauthors performed the experiments.

Lixin Zhang provided the fungal strain and gave constructive advices. All coauthors read and approved the final paper.

Acknowledgment

This work was supported by Grants 2010B060500019 and 2014A010107018 of Guangdong Provincial Science and Technology Project.

References

[1] J. Marchena-Gomez, T. Saez-Guzman, M. Hemmersbach-Miller et al., "Candida isolation in patients hospitalized on a surgical ward: significance and mortality-related factors," *World Journal of Surgery*, vol. 33, no. 9, pp. 1822–1829, 2009.

[2] T. Nakamura and H. Takahashi, "Epidemiological study of *Candida* infections in blood: susceptibilities of *Candida* spp. to antifungal agents, and clinical features associated with the candidemia," *Journal of Infection and Chemotherapy*, vol. 12, no. 3, pp. 132–138, 2006.

[3] S.-Y. Ruan and P.-R. Hsueh, "Invasive candidiasis: an overview from Taiwan," *Journal of the Formosan Medical Association*, vol. 108, no. 6, pp. 443–451, 2009.

[4] A. M. Tortorano, G. Dho, A. Prigitano et al., "Invasive fungal infections in the intensive care unit: a multicentre, prospective, observational study in Italy (2006–2008)," *Mycoses*, vol. 55, no. 1, pp. 73–79, 2012.

[5] H. Wisplinghoff, H. Seifert, R. P. Wenzel, and M. B. Edmond, "Current trends in the epidemiology of nosocomial bloodstream infections in patients with hematological malignancies and solid neoplasms in hospitals in the United States," *Clinical Infectious Diseases*, vol. 36, no. 9, pp. 1103–1110, 2003.

[6] R. Saha, S. Das Das, A. Kumar, and I. R. Kaur, "Pattern of Candida isolates in hospitalized children," *Indian Journal of Pediatrics*, vol. 75, no. 8, pp. 858–860, 2008.

[7] Z. Y. Zhang, K. C. Qian, and S. L. Chen, "Distribution of Candidemia and antifungal drugs assay in our hospital from 2005–2008," *Modern Medicine & Health*, vol. 25, pp. 3411–3412, 2009.

[8] L. X. Zhang, K. Z. Yan, Y. Zhang et al., "High-throughput synergy screening identifies microbial metabolites as combination agents for the treatment of fungal infections," *Proceedings of the National Academy of Sciences of the United States of America*, vol. 104, no. 11, pp. 4606–4611, 2007.

[9] National Research Council, *Guide for the Care and Use of Laboratory Animals*, National Academy Press, Washington, DC, USA, 2011.

[10] F. de Bernardis, L. Morelli, T. Ceddia, R. Lorenzini, and A. Cassone, "Experimental pathogenicity and acid proteinase secretion of vaginal isolates of *Candida parapsilosis*," *Journal of Medical and Veterinary Mycology*, vol. 28, no. 2, pp. 125–137, 1990.

[11] G. M. Chaves, M. A. de Q Cavalcanti, A. M. A. Carneiro-Leão, and S. L. Lopes, "Model of experimental infection in healthy and immunosuppressed Swiss albino mice (*Mus musculus*) using *Candida albicans* strains with different patterns of enzymatic activity," *Brazilian Journal of Microbiology*, vol. 35, no. 4, pp. 324–329, 2004.

19

Elephant (*Elephas maximus*) Health and Management in Asia: Variations in Veterinary Perspectives

David Miller,[1] **Bradford Jackson,**[2] **Heidi S. Riddle,**[3] **Christopher Stremme,**[4] **Dennis Schmitt,**[5,6] **and Thaddeus Miller**[7]

[1]*P.O. Box 2786, Loveland, CO 80539-2786, USA*
[2]*University of Alabama at Birmingham, Birmingham, AL, USA*
[3]*Riddle's Elephant and Wildlife Sanctuary, AR, USA*
[4]*Elephant Health Care Program (EHCP) of the Veterinary Society for Sumatran Wildlife Conservation (Vesswic), Sumatra, Indonesia*
[5]*William H. Darr School of Agriculture, Missouri State University, Springfield, MO, USA*
[6]*Ringling Bros. Center for Elephant Conservation, Polk City, FL, USA*
[7]*University of North Texas Health Science Center, Fort Worth, TX, USA*

Correspondence should be addressed to David Miller; dsmdaczm@gmail.com

Academic Editor: Lorraine M. Sordillo

There is a need to identify strategic investments in Asian elephant (*Elephas maximus*) health that will yield maximal benefits for overall elephant health and conservation. As an exploratory first step, a survey was administered to veterinarians from Asian elephant range countries at a workshop and via email to help prioritize health-related concerns that will mostly benefit elephants. Responses were received from 45 veterinarians from eight countries that had a range of experience with captive and wild elephants. The occurrence of medical conditions and responses to treatment varied among responses. However, injuries, parasitism, and gastrointestinal disease were reported as the most common syndromes responsible for elephant morbidity, whereas injury and infectious disease not due to parasitism were the most commonly reported sources of elephant mortality. Substandard nutrition, water quality and quantity deficiencies, and inadequate or absent shelter were among the factors listed as barriers to optimal elephant health. While this survey's results do not support definitive conclusions, they can be used to identify where and how subsequent investigations should be directed. Rigorous assessment of the relative costs and benefits of available options is required to ensure that investments in individual and population health yield the maximal benefits for elephants.

1. Introduction

Wildlife conservation, veterinary and public health, and other organizations allocate human, physical, and economic resources according to perceived needs and available resources [1–3]. The allocation decision process can be complicated, such as where investment in animal health does not complement conservation objectives and vice versa. Baseline information on where and how to direct and integrate efforts for animal health and conservation is generally incomplete and sometimes absent when organizations make resource allocation decisions. Consequently, exploratory work needs

to be conducted to clarify the primary issues of concern. This approach is not unlike traditional public health and veterinary population health programs where problems are identified, and the costs and benefits of interventional strategies are established, as a part of overall program development and prioritization of resource allocations [3, 4].

Asian elephants (*Elephas maximus*) are an endangered species that illustrate the challenges of optimizing and integrating resource allocations for animal health and conservation [5]. Across their range, Asian elephants face conflict with humans, habitat destruction and fragmentation, diseases, and other challenges [6]. Wild elephant populations may be adversely or positively affected by captive populations, which have limited fecundity and undocumented levels of compromised health. Addressing these and other challenges with a unified and appropriate policy or practice is complicated because there are many differences in the culture, attitudes, and infrastructure experienced by elephant personnel located in different Asian elephant range countries. Consequently, what should take priority in efforts to sustain wild and captive elephant populations is unclear. To catalog the collective experience and skills among elephant veterinarians in Asia is a necessary early step to more clearly understand existing challenges and more effectively design strategies that will reverse or slow trends that threaten elephant health and population viability.

We report findings from a review of the published literature to document the types of studies and topics relevant to elephant health and conservation in Asian elephant range countries. This is followed by the results of an initial survey of veterinarians across Asian elephant range countries. Our survey was by necessity conducted in a nonrandom, semiformal fashion and cannot be interpreted as fully representative. It can, however, begin to lay the foundations for more comprehensive work by both using a new approach and identifying knowledge gaps critical to the appropriate design and successful conduct of subsequent work. Because management practices and their effects may ripple between wild and captive elephant populations, we considered the overall conservation of Asian elephants by systematically collecting data related to common elephant health concerns from veterinarians with elephant expertise working in Asia. We used a survey instrument that included questions concerned with background information, basic veterinary concerns, laboratory facilities, elephant handler (mahout) health, perceived needs for improved elephant health, and common diseases or conditions. This provides preliminary information that supports methods development and hypothesis generation for subsequent work to improve elephant health and conservation programs in Asia.

2. Methods

2.1. Literature Review. We conducted a search of the PubMed database (http://www.ncbi.nlm.nih.gov/pubmed) using the terms "elephant" and "Asia" (26 August, 2014). Titles, author address, and abstracts (where available) were reviewed to establish whether the research was conducted in Asian elephant range countries; references that clearly were not from these countries were excluded. Studies were characterized, where possible, by study design (laboratory, controlled trials, hybrid, case report or series, cross-sectional surveys, case-control, cohort study, policy, review, hybrid, and unable to determine) and topic categories (basic veterinary concerns, laboratory capacity, needs assessments, common disease conditions, and treatment).

2.2. Survey Development. We developed and administered a 13-page, 21-field survey instrument to explore the veterinary knowledge and practices of a convenience sample

of veterinarians from Asian elephant range countries (see the Appendix). The English language instrument included closed- and open-ended questions to collect data in 6 areas: (1) basic background information (country, employment, elephant caseload, and the elephant population's characteristics); (2) basic veterinary concerns (prevalence of various clinical conditions); (3) laboratory facilities (availability of various laboratory services); (4) informal impressions of mahout health (clinical conditions observed and knowledge of routine screening); (5) needs assessment (clinician's needs for medicine, treatment, diagnostics, basic husbandry, and mahout training that could improve elephant health); and (6) common disease conditions (ranked medical conditions, treatment, and outcomes). Questions were developed to gain insights into broad, coarse-scale trends in elephant health and serve as a starting point for where to direct subsequent, more focused investigations. The survey was drafted in consultation with veterinarians with expertise in elephant health and others, including a biostatistician and a biomedical systems researcher, in order to provide the most comprehensive, relevant, and valid information available given the constraints of circumstance, language, and practice. The survey was pilot tested for ease of readability and completion.

2.3. Study Population. Data was collected from two populations: a convenience sample of veterinarians participating in an elephant health workshop (Regional Asian Elephant Veterinary Workshop held in Banda Aceh, Sumatra, Indonesia from March 27–30, 2012) and a convenience sample of veterinarians that were subsequently contacted via networking and responded via email. Potential participants were excluded if they had insufficient written English language proficiency to consent to participate in or complete the survey. All respondents were offered the opportunity to respond anonymously. The study population represented a broad spectrum of involvement in elephant health and varying levels of experience.

All veterinarians attending the workshop who consented to participate were administered the survey during the first morning's session, prior to any presentations that could influence responses. Surveys were collected immediately after completion and subsequently scanned to create permanent electronic records. Emailed survey responses were solicited from veterinarians that were known but unable to attend the workshop.

Prudent and conservative research practice requires that when planning studies and recruiting study participants, the potential harm to participants must be minimal and fully disclosed. In keeping with these standards, our methods and survey instruments were reviewed and approved as appropriate by the University of North Texas Health Science Center (Fort Worth, Texas, USA), Office for the Protection of Human Subjects, Institutional Review Board.

2.4. Data Analysis. Data from surveys was entered into electronic format by one investigator (B.J.) and verified by a second investigator (D.M.). In an attempt to compensate for uneven English language skills, we used a web-based program (Google Translate; https://translate.google.com/) or a native translator. Where this strategy allowed survey completion by workers with otherwise insufficient English language proficiency, those responses were included; where language barriers precluded interviewees from giving consent or substantially completing the survey in spite of translation attempts, the responses were not included.

Except where marked differences were noted, data from responses obtained from workshop and email responses and data from respondents working with captive and wild elephants were combined for analysis. This was done for the purpose of obtaining sufficiently large sample sizes to gain insights into the broad issues of interest to this study, rather than focus on precision or outliers. In addition, responses from those that worked with both captive and wild populations often did not distinguish between the two populations. The appropriateness of this approach was qualitatively confirmed by examining the data for substantial differences between the sample populations. Descriptive analyses were conducted; categorical responses are presented as absolute numbers and percentages and continuous responses are presented as means ± standard deviations (SD). As a means of accounting for the diversity of responses and limited diagnostic capacity available to clinicians, observed medical conditions were qualitatively grouped into syndromes and reported by rank; syndrome scores were not reported to avoid inferences that were not appropriate based on the convenience sampling scheme.

3. Results

3.1. Literature Review. The literature search identified 202 references from 1963 to present. Many references had limited information available, but 70 were identified as relevant. The most common study designs were ecological/natural history, case reports or series, and laboratory-based investigations that documented physiological or biomedical reference ranges and measurements (Table 1). The most common study topics were descriptions of common disease conditions. Of 44 reports that could be identified as being conducted in a single country, over half were conducted in India ($n = 15$) and Sri Lanka ($n = 10$).

3.2. Survey Overview. Responses were obtained from 45 individuals from a total of 8 Asian elephant range countries for a total of 8595 data points; 15 of these data points were not legible or could not be translated and were excluded (Table 2). Most ($n = 27$, 60%) respondents were government employees. Over half of the respondents worked with elephants full-time ($n = 24$, 53%), with the remainder having part-time ($n = 11$, 24%) or exclusively academic responsibilities. The duration of relevant experience among respondents ranged from 0.5–30 years (mean 10.7, SD ± 6.8 years).

TABLE 1: Study designs and topic categories that characterize elephant studies conducted in Asia that were identified in a PubMed search.

	Number
Study design	
Ecological or natural history	21
Case report or series	18
Laboratory-based investigation	17
Cross-sectional survey	8
Policy	3
Review	3
Study topic category*	
Common disease conditions	31
Basic veterinary concerns	15
Treatment	2
Needs assessment	1

*Twenty-one studies could not be categorized by these topics.

The mean number of elephants checked per month by government (23.1 SD ± 27.4) and nongovernment (26.6 SD ± 30.5) veterinarians was similar but varied widely by individual respondent (occasional to 100 elephants examined per month) as did the reported number of elephants seen at least twice per year (occasional to 3000 elephants). Fewer (11% versus 42%) respondents reported their primary work (80–100% of contacts) to be with wild rather than captive elephants.

None of the respondents indicated that all of the elephants in their area were reproducing, but 71% indicated that at least some elephants had successfully reproduced. Seven respondents did not provide responses regarding elephant reproduction. A variety of primary uses for elephants were indicated by respondents; responses of "all" or "most" indicated their use in: zoos ($n = 7$), tourism ($n = 13$), logging ($n = 6$), forest patrol ($n = 7$), conflict management ($n = 2$), or education ($n = 3$).

3.3. Basic Veterinary Concerns. Most elephants that were regularly examined had some medical abnormalities; few respondents (14%) indicated that 80–100% of elephants that were regularly checked had no visible signs of disease. Reported conditions that together comprised a small percentage of the total "abnormal" report included evidence of systemic illness, upper or lower respiratory disease, weight loss, diarrhea or other gastrointestinal problems; ectoparasites; nonectoparasitic skin disease; endoparasites observed in feces; eye disease; oral disease, tusk or molar disease; trunk disease; foot disease or other sources of lameness; wounds other than skin lesions; infant mortality; reproductive problems; reduced work endurance; and anorexia. Responses were not uniform within or between countries. Gastrointestinal

TABLE 2: Characteristics of elephant health survey respondents.

Row labels	Number of respondents	Mean number of years of elephant care	Percentage of work with captive elephants (number of respondents)		Percentage of work with wild elephants (number of respondents)	
			0–19%	80–100%	0–19%	80–100%
India	8	9.9	1	3	4	2
Indonesia	21	10.0	1	9	9	1
Laos	2	2.8		1	1	
Malaysia	1	9.0				1
Myanmar	1	10.0				
Nepal	2	13.0		1	1	
Sri Lanka	7	16.4	4	3	2	1
Thailand	3	8.3		2	3	
Grand total (mean ± SD)	45	(10.7 ± 6.8)	6	19	20	5

disease was not confined to captive animals, as two respondents with a focus on wild populations indicated that 40–59% of their elephants had colic and/or diarrhea. Regional differences were reported for nonparasitic skin diseases; half of Indian respondents indicated that 40–59% of elephants had nonparasitic skin diseases, whereas most (86%) respondents from Sri Lanka reported that nonparasitic skin diseases were uncommon (0–19% of regularly inspected elephants). Respondents from five countries reported that <40% of their elephants were shedding endoparasite ova or larvae (the number of responses from each country varied from 1 to 15). The highest prevalence (60–79%) of eye disease was reported for Indian elephants (38% of respondents). Oral, tusk, and molar disease was reported sporadically, with two respondents indicating that these conditions were observed in 40–59% of elephants, and one respondent indicating a prevalence of 60–79%. These oral conditions were not coreported with responses from three countries where anorexia was reported for 60–79% of elephants; most responses indicated that 0–19% of elephants had anorexia. Stereotypic behavior as common as 60–100% in some populations was reported, and stereotypies were not restricted to captivity, as three respondents reported 20–80% of free-ranging elephants with stereotypic behavior. Two workshop participants from Indonesia reported a prevalence of 20–39% for trunk disease, whereas the remaining responses indicated a prevalence of < 20%. The prevalence of simple foot disease was reported to be 20–60% by half of the respondents. Complicated foot disease was reported to be < 40% by 62% of the respondents, and three respondents indicated that > 20% of the free-ranging elephants had complicated foot disease. Only 13% of respondents reported that > 20% of elephants had infant mortality or reproductive problems.

Most (84%) of the respondents had conducted necropsies, at a mean of 5.37/year (SD ± 12.05) (range < 1 to 40/year). A variety of pathologic findings, including specific etiologies and specific organ lesions, were reported for necropsies (Table 3). However, no single condition exceeded 11% of the total. Trauma from all causes (human elephant conflict, intraspecific aggression, traumatic injuries, and lightening) comprised 18% of the reported findings, which exceeded the sum of infectious diseases (16%) due to parasitism, and infectious bacterial and viral diseases.

3.4. Laboratory Facilities Questionnaire. Hematology (56%), laboratory analyses for routine organ function (e.g., AST, alkaline phosphatase, BUN, creatinine, etc.) (51%), and light microscopy for fecal parasite testing (78%) were always or mostly available to over half of respondents (Table 4). Light microscopy for blood parasite testing was always or mostly available to 44% of respondents. Approximately one quarter of respondents had access to other diagnostic modalities, with 53–84% having no access to nutrition-related, virology, or imaging diagnostics. With the exception of blood mineral, blood nutrition, virology, and toxicology, respondents working primarily with captive animals had greater access to diagnostics.

3.5. Mahout Health Questionnaire. Only 29% of the respondents indicated that the health of mahouts was routinely screened, although another 20% were unsure of whether mahout health screens were conducted. Respondents mostly indicated that few (0–19%) mahouts had frequent sneezing or coughing, sudden weight loss, eye disease, abnormal joints or limbs, skin abnormalities, or lethargy. One respondent reported that 60–79% of mahouts had abnormal limbs, joints, or skin, and this individual also reported 40–59% had lethargy, eye disease, frequent coughing, and frequent sneezing.

3.6. Needs Assessment. Most respondents indicated that an important need is improvement in basic husbandry. More than 2/3rds of respondents indicated a need for improved

TABLE 3: Major postmortem pathologic findings reported by survey respondents. Respondents were able to report more than one finding per necropsy.

Reported postmortem pathologic findings	%
Human elephant conflict (electrocution, poisoning, poaching, train collision, gunshot, wells, pit traps, snares, etc.)	10.4
Hemorrhage	10.2
Endoparasites	7.5
Gastrointestinal stasis or torsion	6.7
Lung lesions	6.5
Liver lesions	4.3
Old age	4.1
Undetermined	4.1
Injuries from intraspecific aggression	3.9
Toxin	3.5
Splenic lesions	3.5
Tetanus	3.5
Cardiac lesions	3.3
Renal lesions	3.3
Enteritis	3.1
Traumatic injuries	3.1
Sepsis	2.7
Emaciation	2.4
Skin lesions	2.2
Rabies	1.4
Tuberculosis	1.4
Elephant endotheliotropic herpes virus	1.4
Autolysis	1.2
Cyanosis	1.0
Peritonitis	1.0
Lightning	0.8
Salmonellosis	0.8
Arthritis	0.8
Anemia	0.6
Nasal and oral mucosa ulceration	0.6
Abscess	0.4
Eye conditions	0.4
Grand total	100

supplements, and narrative responses indicated great interest (n = 32 responses, 71%) in improving the nutritional offerings provided to elephants. Most (64%) respondents indicated a need for improved elephant shelters, although some captive elephants resided in "deep forest" and were not considered in need of shelter. Many respondents listed a need for facilities for conducting treatments (56%) and managing adult bulls in musth (51%). Half (51%) of respondents had concerns for

water quality and/or quantity. Narrative responses indicated concern for safe drinking and bathing water and a need for filtration and water quality testing. Most respondents indicated a need for improved mahout training in the areas of daily routine health (80%), elephant biology and behavior (64%), elephant restraint and handling tools (62%), and drug use and administration methods for elephants (60%).

Overall drug availability limitations (64%) were considered the greatest constraint for addressing elephant health needs (Table 5). The most common preventive medications administered included anthelmintics (n = 28), vaccination (n = 11), vitamins (n = 9), and minerals (n = 6). Antibiotics were also listed as preventive medications by a few respondents (n = 5). Respondents described multiple anthelmintics and regular rotations of drugs, and practical concerns such as short expiration times were reported. Routinely administered vaccinations included tetanus toxoid (n = 21), rabies (n = 14), hemorrhagic septicemia (Pasteurella multocida) (n = 6), foot-and-mouth disease (n = 6), anthrax (n = 4), blackleg/black quarter disease (Clostridium chauvoei) (n = 3), and tuberculosis (mycobacterial species and vaccine type not specified) (n = 1). Narrative responses indicated that vaccine availability and cost concerns limit the number of elephants that are vaccinated, and there was concern for the absence of elephant-specific vaccines. Narrative responses also elaborated on owner financial limitations and the inability of mahouts to continue drug and other treatments. Untrained or uncooperative elephants (36%) were commonly reported constraints for administration of medications and performing diagnostics. Additional recommendations for improved preventive health programs included a need to increase the number of knowledgeable veterinarians and mahouts.

The scarcity of diagnostics that could be the basis for optimizing treatments (67%) was listed as a common obstacle. Limited test availability (64%) and a shortage of trained personnel (51%) represented the greatest obstacles for performing diagnostic procedures. Narrative responses noted the absence of elephant-specific assays, limitations of existing technologies for such a large species, problems with storage of samples, levels of professionalism, and slow laboratory turnaround times.

3.7. Common Disease Conditions. The most common syndromes reported as causes of morbidity in range country Asian elephants were injuries, endo- and ectoparasitism, and gastrointestinal disease (Table 6). While many of the syndromes were reported by respondents that had either predominantly captive or wild responsibilities, injuries due to human-elephant conflict, as well as poisoning, were reported exclusively for wild populations, with one exception. Abscesses, cancer, nonparasitic infectious diseases (rabies, tetanus, anthrax, herpes, and tuberculosis), overwork, renal disease, reproductive problems, skin disease, stereotypical behavior, tusk pathology, and ventral edema were reported exclusively for captive elephants, although none of these were common. Lameness was also exclusively reported for

TABLE 4: Availability of laboratory facilities reported by survey respondents ($n = 45$).

Diagnostic modality	Always available (number)	Mostly available (number)	Sometimes available (number)	Never available (number)	No response (number)
Hematology	7	17	17	3	1
Organ indices	8	15	16	6	
Blood mineral	4	6	13	22	
Blood nutrition	2		19	24	
Hair nutrition		1	6	38	
Toxin detection		6	17	22	
Hormone analysis	3	1	17	22	2
Fecal parasite microscopy	22	13	9	1	
Blood parasite microscopy	12	8	21	4	
Microbiology culture and antibiotic sensitivity	4	8	26	7	
Methods for identifying viral pathogens	1		14	30	
Histopathology	4	6	26	8	1
Ultrasound	2	4	11	28	
Radiology	1	1	11	32	

TABLE 5: Survey respondents' ($n = 45$) perceptions of needed improvements in the diagnosis, treatment, and preventive medicine for elephants in Asian range countries.

Category of concerns	Specific concerns for each category	Number of respondents indicating a need (%)
Obstacles that prevent obtaining needed medications	Financial constraints	15 (33.3)
	Limited drug availability	29 (64.4)
	Import restrictions for drugs	18 (40)
Obstacles that prevent conducting needed treatments	Limited access to elephants (roads, etc.)	11 (24.4)
	Treatment not permitted by owner	4 (8.89)
	Absence of mahout cooperation	2 (4.44)
	Untrained/uncooperative elephants	16 (35.6)
	Limited diagnostics that could serve to direct appropriate treatments	30 (66.7)
Obstacles to performing diagnostic procedures	Financial constraints	15 (33.3)
	Limited diagnostic test availability	29 (64.4)
	Import restrictions for diagnostic tests	11 (24.4)
	Broken equipment	6 (13.3)
	Lack of personnel training	19 (42.2)
	Shortage of trained personnel	23 (51.1)
Preventive medicine needs: food	Vitamin supplements	33 (73.3)
	Mineral supplements	34 (75.6)
	High nutrient supplements	31 (68.9)
Preventive medicine needs: shelter	Clinic for conducting treatments	25 (55.6)
	Nursery and/or sick elephant facilities	21 (46.7)
	Isolation facility	18 (40)
	Facility for musth bulls	23 (51.1)
Preventive medicine needs: water	Control of H_2O quality	13 (28.9)
	Control of H_2O quantity	13 (28.9)
Preventive medicine needs: mahout training topics	Daily routine health	36 (80)
	Elephant restraint and handling tools	28 (62.2)
	Elephant biology and behavior	29 (64.4)
	Drug use and administration	27 (60)

TABLE 6: Major syndromes reported for morbidity and mortality in Asian elephants in range countries, listed in order of most common to least common. Items in ( ) are subcategories of the immediately preceding topic.

Syndromes: morbidity	Syndromes: mortality
Injury	Injury
(Gunshot wounds)	(Gunshot)
Parasitism	Infectious disease not due to parasitism
Gastrointestinal disease	Gastrointestinal disease
(Diarrhea)	(Diarrhea)
Ocular disease	Poisoning
Foot pathology	Old-age related
Malnutrition	Nonspecific
Abscess	Parasitism
Infectious disease not due to parasitism	Malnutrition
Lameness	Renal disease
Skin disease	Cardiac disease
Stereotypical behavior	Hemorrhagic disease
Overwork	Lack of veterinary care
Poisoning	Lameness
Renal disease	Musth
Cancer	Respiratory disease
Ventral edema	Dehydration
Drug reaction	Prolonged recumbency
Reproductive problem	Seizure
Tusk pathology	Congenital disease
	Neurologic disease
	Reproductive problem
	Chemical immobilization

captive elephants, although foot pathology was reported for both captive and wild populations. Infectious disease due to parasitic and nonparasitic causes had a cumulative percentage score (21%) that was less for injuries due to all causes (27%), although causes of gastrointestinal disease, ocular disease, skin disease, abscesses, foot pathology, and lameness could have had infectious disease or injury components that could not be established with this study. Of 14 respondents reporting bacterial or viral infections by name (elephant endotheliotropic herpes virus or EEHV, tuberculosis, anthrax, foot and mouth disease, tetanus, elephant pox, *Salmonella, Clostridium,* or rabies), only 3 mostly or always had access to either microbiology or virology laboratory facilities.

Injuries (35%) were ranked as the leading cause of mortality, followed by infectious disease not due to parasitism (14%). Gastrointestinal disease, poisoning, geriatric, nonspecific, and parasitic etiologies were ranked similarly as causes of

mortality. Respondents from four different countries (India, Indonesia, Malaysia, and Sri Lanka) reported mortality due to poisoning, with similar numbers of reports from captive and wild populations. Organ-based disease (renal and cardiac) and malnutrition were similarly ranked less than 5% as a cause of mortality, followed by a number of miscellaneous causes. Gunshot, explosives, railway accidents, poaching, human-elephant conflict, and snares were reported primarily from Sri Lanka (71%) and wild populations. Poaching was also reported for respondents from India, Malaysia, and Indonesia. Traumatic causes of mortality reported for captive populations included intra-specific fighting, work accidents, lightning, and other injuries.

Nine syndromes (injuries, gastrointestinal disease, malnutrition, lameness, foot disease, infectious disease, parasitic disease, ocular disease, and miscellaneous) were subjectively identified among respondent's lists of standard treatments, success rates, and treatment needs, with recognition that these categories were not strictly distinct and did not represent formal diagnoses (Table 7). Subcategories for each syndrome were identified where treatment, and/or success rates, and treatment needs were distinct. A range of treatments, success rates with and without treatment, mortality, and clinician needs were reported, with variable numbers of reports for each category. Respondents also identified basic medical (e.g., suture), husbandry (e.g., elephant training for routine preventive care and improved housing), and diagnostic (e.g., clinical laboratory, diagnostic imaging) needs.

4. Discussion

This study represents the key first step of ensuring that the most important needs for elephant health and conservation in Asia receive the highest priorities [3]. Our literature review indicated that elephant health and conservation reports are predominantly descriptive with few efforts to address population-level concerns. Our interest in conducting the survey was in developing a new approach and identifying broad trends to serve as a starting point for identifying where more focused efforts are needed. By necessity, a convenience sampling scheme was used. Consequently, as with all observational studies, limited inferences are possible from this data. However, a broad overview of the data suggests that the health and conservation needs of elephants vary regionally. Even if this is not true, the differences among responses suggest regional variation in perspectives that must be considered when addressing elephant health and conservation needs. Differing perceptions of the questions and categories, the survey administration methods used, and other biases may limit confidence in the absolute numbers or relative ranks of syndromes and other observations. Thus, while this study could not resolve all questions, gaps in clarity and other sources of uncertainty can direct future efforts. This will increase the odds that strategic investments yield the maximal benefits for elephant conservation.

4.1. Literature Review. Our literature review indicated that published research on elephants in Asian range countries

TABLE 7: Syndromes and treatments that are available or are needed and currently unavailable, as well as outcomes with and without treatment.

	Injury	Gastrointestinal disease	Malnutrition	Lameness	Foot diseases	Infectious disease	Parasitic disease	Ocular disease
Standard treatment	Abscesses and myiasis, general and unspecified wounds: flush with saline, H₂O₂, iodine, chlorhexidine; surgical drainage; topical and systemic antibiotics 7–15 d (oxytetracycline and penicillin); local betamethasone and unspecified anti-inflammatories; conservative compress; vitamins; analgesics; tetanus toxoid; fly repellants; fluid therapy; rest. Gunshot: anesthesia; wound dressing; broad spectrum antibiotic	General: antibiotics; fluids; oral electrolytes; antibiotics (ampicillin, gentamycin); ranitidine; tolterodine; budesonide; metaclopromide; nonsteroidal anti-inflammatories; antispasmotics; vitamins; minerals. Colic: enema; fluids and electrolytes; exercise; nonsteroidal agents; bath in pool; antibiotics; anthelmintics; liver extract. Constipation/impaction: fluids; rectal palpation; supportive therapy; enemas; purgatives; rest; parasympathomimetics; spasmolytics. Bloat: supportive therapy; per rectum neurostimulation; antibloat agents; rectal enemas; exercise; flunixin meglumine. Diarrhea: antibiotics; fluids; diet correction; astringents; antiparasitics; fecal culture. Malabsorption: vitamin and mineral levels in blood; nutritional supplements	Improved food quality; vitamins, minerals, and other food supplements; antiparasitic agents; regular monitoring of serum levels	Nonsteroidal anti-inflammatories; steroids; herbal drugs; hot massage; cool compresses; antibiotics; supportive treatment; rest. Fractures: bandage; rest/restriction of movement; plaster cast	Routine foot care; dry location tethering; isolation. Cleaning or bath with H₂O₂, iodine or formalin. Local, topical, or systemic antibiotics (tetracycline, broad-spectrum, or based on culture and sensitivity.) Local steroids; supportive therapy	General: antibiotics. Tuberculosis: antibiotics (rifampin, ethambutol, or isoniazide) or no treatment. EEHV: famcyclovir, acyclovir. Tetanus: antispasmodic drugs; antibiotics; hydration; tetanus toxoid. Elephant pox: antibiotics; fluids; vitamins; local therapy	General: topical and systemic antiparasitic agents (fenbendazol, albendazol, mebendazol, ivermectin, oxyclozanide); supportive therapy; routine fecal examination. Balantidia: no response. Trypanosomiasis: Berenil. Cobboldia spp. and filarial: ivermectin	Ophthalmic topicals: gentamycin, chloramphenicol, nonsteroidal anti-inflammatories, doxycycline, and tetracycline. Systemic drugs: nonsteroidal anti-inflammatories. Not specified: antibiotics, herbal medications, antifungals, analgesics, glaucoma drugs. Surgery
Percentage resolved without treatment (range/number of respondents)†	General: 0–80% Gunshot: 50%	General: 1–60% Colic: 0–10% Constipation/impaction: 0–30% Bloat: 0–100% Diarrhea: 0–30% Malabsorption: 0%	0–20%	General: 0–20% (70% for arthritis) Fractures: 0–20%	0–70%	Tuberculosis: 0–30% EEHV: 0–20% Tetanus: no responses Elephant pox: 1%	General: 0–30% Balantidia: 0% Trypanosomiasis: 20% Cobboldia spp. and filarial: 10–20%	Conjunctivitis/keratitis: 0–50% Nonspecific ocular disease: 1–40%

TABLE 7: Continued.

	Injury	Gastrointestinal disease	Malnutrition	Lameness	Foot diseases	Infectious disease	Parasitic disease	Ocular disease
Percentage that die without treatment†	General: 0–70% Gunshot: 50%	General: 0–70% Colic: 0–80% Constipation/impaction: 0–50% Bloat: 1–1005 Diarrhea: 0–100% Malabsorption: 100%	0–20%	General: 0–5% (40% degenerative joint disease) Fractures: 20–100%	0–50%	Tuberculosis: 0–60% EEHV: 0–80% Tetanus: 100% Elephant pox: 90%	General: 0–50% Balantidia: 0% Trypanosomiasis: 80% Cobboldia spp. and filarial: 50–60%	Conjunctivitis/keratitis: Conjunctivitis/keratitis: 0–10% Nonspecific ocular disease: 0–5%
Percentage cured with standard treatment†	General: 25–100% Gunshot: 90%	General: 90–100% Colic: 70–100% Constipation/impaction: 60–100% Bloat: 80–100% Diarrhea: 60–90% Malabsorption: no response	100%	General: 70–80% (40% degenerative joint disease) Fractures: 15–60%	30–90%	Tuberculosis: 20–80% EEHV: 25–40% Tetanus: 30% Elephant pox: 100%	General: 80–100% Balantidia: 1000% Trypanosomiasis: 50% Cobboldia spp. and filarial: 90–100%	Conjunctivitis/keratitis: 50–100% Nonspecific ocular disease: 40–100%
Percentage mortality with standard treatment†	General: 0–10% Gunshot: 10%	General: 0–5% Colic 0–20%: Constipation/impaction: 0–20% Bloat: 0–1% Diarrhea: 0–40% Malabsorption: no response	0%	General: 0% (50% degenerative joint disease) Fractures: 10–85%	0–40%	Tuberculosis: 0–20% EEHV: 25–60% Tetanus: 70% Elephant pox: 10%	General: 0–10% Balantidia: 0% Trypanosomiasis: 50% Cobboldia spp. and filarial: 5–10%	Conjunctivitis/keratitis: 0–10% Nonspecific ocular disease: 0%
Treatments that are wished for	General: Suture; minor surgical instruments; antibiotics; drugs that enhance granulation or destroy pyrogenic membranes; hoisting facility; topical cream; radiology access	General: routine anthelmintics; probiotics Colic: improved diagnostics, drug efficacy, husbandry records, trochars, diet, and routine anthelmintics; Constipation/impaction: endoscopic surgery Bloat: no responses Diarrhea: improved diagnostics; uncertain Malabsorption: no response	Improved food and supplement resources; reduced corruption of government funds; standardized nutritional guidelines	Improved drugs; improved diagnostic tools; acupuncture; hoisting facility	Elephant training for routine, hygienic foot care and foot care tools; improved staff training; increased enclosure size; cryosurgery; radiology capacity; shoes to prevent wound contamination	General: emphasis on prevention; medications specific for organism Tuberculosis: cheaper drugs with less toxicity and shorter treatment protocols; testing options; EEHV: early diagnostic tools; famcyclovir Tetanus: uncertain Elephant pox: clinical laboratory facility	General: preventive therapy; improved diagnostics and drug efficacy; therapeutic baths Balantidia: no response Trypanosomiasis: less toxic drug Cobboldia spp. and filarial: improved laboratory diagnostics and improved mobility to improve response time	Increased variety of drugs available (concerns for antibiotic resistance and efficacy); improved housing (preventive); clinic for morbid animals; ophthalmoscopes and improved diagnostics; improved drug application methods; improved surgical options

Miscellaneous conditions included urinary tract infections, heat stroke, snake bite, photosensitivity, poisoning, ventral edema, septicemia, and pneumonia.

†Inconsistencies in numbers (percentages that exceed or are less than 100%) are due to subjectivity and recall bias or language barriers.

was primarily descriptive and was concentrated in a few countries. There have been efforts to survey elephant health in Asia [7]. However, there is a dearth of broad-scale studies that can guide researchers and funders by identifying prioritized needs that are most likely to have a beneficial impact on captive and free-ranging elephant health and conservation. While case reports and other descriptive studies can be useful for sharing valuable information, they reflect the interests and support for publication of the authors and are difficult to place in context per the impact of these conditions on elephant populations. Consequently, available literature is not sufficient for guiding strategic approaches for the use of limited resources to benefit elephant health and conservation in Asia.

4.2. Survey Overview. As with all questionnaires, recall and other biases, the format of closed questions, and other concerns are limitations [8]. As is common for conservation-related questionnaires, formal validation of the questionnaire, opportunistic sampling from a limited sampling frame, respondents' source of employment, and other concerns exist. Also, exclusion of non-English speaking veterinarians and those without access to the Web, as well as culturally-based misinterpretation of the questions, are among potential limitations of this study. In particular, biases are possible due to representation from only 8 of 13 Asian elephant range countries and overrepresentation of respondents from one country (Indonesia, where the workshop was held). In retrospect, inclusion of 0% and 100% categories may have eliminated some of the ambiguity associated with the ranges that the questionnaire provided. Efforts to improve the study's relevancy and scope included external review of the questionnaire's format by multiple professionals prior to distribution, increasing the sample size and the range of countries by distributing the questionnaire in person at a workshop and via electronic networking, offering the option of anonymous responses, and inclusion of respondents with primarily captive, primarily free-ranging, and mixed-setting elephant experience. Ultimately, while this study is the first effort to objectively investigate the health-related syndromes and needs of elephants in Asia, it serves as a coarse-scale starting point for optimizing resource allocation for this region's elephants.

4.3. Basic Survey Information. The small number of responses from some countries and for some categories, as well as incomplete responses that further limited the dataset, precluded formal statistical comparisons. The full sampling frame of English and non-English speaking elephant veterinarians in all 13 Asian elephant range countries could not be established. Qualitatively similar results for respondents that received the questionnaire via in-person and electronic networking resulted in joint summary of the results, except where noted. As many respondents did not strictly work with captive or free-ranging elephant populations, distinctions among captive and free-ranging elephants are limited. Although respondents could respond anonymously, 60% of respondents were government employees, the majority of

elephants were owned by the government, and the degree to which government policy influenced responses is unclear.

4.4. Basic Veterinary Concerns. While most elephants were classified as having few visible signs of disease, substantial variation was observed among the responses and a number of different conditions were responsible for the total number of abnormalities reported. There is a need to establish whether differences in veterinary knowledge and/or training, elephants trained for examinations, support for diagnostic facilities, regional differences in disease, husbandry, individuals' perceptions, or other reasons can account for differences in reported conditions between and within countries. In particular, the cost effectiveness for improved husbandry and preventive care should be explored further. Each of the respondents ($n = 9$) indicating that >40% of regularly checked elephants had colic or constipation also indicated a need for improved food quality, access to medications, and the presence of endoparasites in >20% of elephants, and most also indicated a need for improved water quality. This data suggests that improved basic husbandry and routine prophylaxis may reduce the prevalence of these conditions and possibly others related to work endurance, fecundity, anorexia, and oral health. Alternatively, some interventions may be uncertain. For instance, only 54% of respondents reported routine use of anthelmintics in countries where fecal shedding of parasites was classified as uncommon, although limited diagnostic availability may be responsible for under-diagnosis of fecal shedding. Limited diagnostic availability also raises uncertainty as to whether agents, such as the parasite *Cobboldia elephantis* [9], are focally or widely distributed. Responses indicating foot disease and stereotypic behavior in free-ranging populations are of uncertain significance and may warrant further investigation for perspective on management of captive populations. Low fecundity reported in the Basic Information section of the questionnaire and few respondents reporting low infant mortality or reproductive problems warrant clarification of whether the reported infrequency of reproductive problems is real or the consequence of reproduction being a low management priority for these populations. An understanding of where clusters for some conditions truly exist, where diagnostic facilities or clinician training are limited, and how to facilitate increased training of mahouts and elephants for preventive medicine, diagnostics, and treatment is needed.

Most respondents conducted necropsies, although the need for improved equipment and the physical challenges were noted and might affect the accuracy of necropsy results. In addition, the likelihood that not all elephants are necropsied (for a variety of reasons) is a bias that limits population-level inferences. Trauma-related necropsy findings were marginally more common than the sum of mortalities due to all infectious causes. However, improved diagnostic capacity might result in different proportions of pathologic findings. The diversity of conditions noted by respondents indicates the need to identify the medical conditions that can be most cost-effectively managed to improve animal welfare and/or population stability or growth; focusing on one or a few diseases that are not strategically selected to ensure that resource investments have a substantive impact may not result in improved individual or population-level health and welfare.

4.5. Laboratory Facilities. Basic hematology and blood chemistries were always available to only 9% of the respondents. This is consistent with the absence of studies in our literature review that document the laboratory capacity for diagnosing elephant medical conditions in Asian elephant range countries. While light microscopy was available for fecal parasitology for most respondents, there is uncertainty why only 44% always or mostly also have access to light microscopy for identifying blood parasites. This could be because light microscope optics for evaluation of fecal ova are less (10–40X) than needed to evaluate the presence of blood parasites (100X oil immersion). Alternatively, this discrepancy may be linked to responses elsewhere in the questionnaire indicating a need for improved personnel training. Few respondents had access to histopathology all or most of the time. In light of this, the dearth of testing available for nutritional concerns, toxins, microbes, or diagnostic imaging is not surprising. These diagnostic limitations affect both antemortem and postmortem diagnoses. Consequently, many of the diagnoses listed in the questionnaire are likely based on clinical signs or gross pathology only. This limits inferences possible from this and other elephant health studies that are conducted in Asia, and therefore increases uncertainty about the prevalence and impact of various disease conditions on elephant health, welfare, and population viability. Better confidence in the diagnoses would require investment in improved laboratory facilities and trained personnel. This would likely improve antemortem diagnoses and clinical case management, as well as assessments of population health and disease.

4.6. Mahout Health Questionnaire. Mahout and elephant health may be closely linked by the mahouts' ability to care for their elephants, the elephants' ability to work, and other factors [10], and this potential link was not discussed in studies identified in our literature review. The informal observations of the veterinarians responding to this survey serve as a starting point for investigating this concept from the perspective of trained medical professionals.

Only six individuals from six countries reported that >19% of mahouts had any of the listed medical conditions. Possible reasons for these discrepancies include clusters of disease occurrence, a majority of respondents focusing their attention on elephants rather than mahouts, or other reasons. Addressing mahout health could result in improved elephant health by improving the mahouts' ability to provide care to their elephants or as part of a strategy to gain support for elephant-oriented health and welfare programs. Further investigations in this area are warranted to clarify this survey's findings.

4.7. Needs Assessment. Responses to both open and closed format questions indicated notable needs on several levels. Basic elephant husbandry needs reported by respondents included improved nutrition; elephant shelters and musth bull facilities; water quality and/or quantity; and mahout training. Respondents indicated that improved elephant care required better diagnostic capacity; facilities to perform treatments; trained personnel; trained and cooperative elephants; and improved drug and vaccine availability. The absence of reliable diagnostics limits the therapeutic value of many drugs due to uncertain diagnoses and also curbs confidence in the results of many studies of elephant disease.

Based on other species, the most cost-effective priorities for improving elephant health and welfare in Asia may be addressed via preventive medicine programs, basic husbandry, diagnostic capacity, prophylactic medications, and training of veterinarians and mahouts. As more than two thirds of all respondents indicated a need for improved nutrition, provision of an appropriate diet is a strategy that will theoretically support all other health objectives. Similarly, provisions of appropriate shelter and water are fundamental husbandry concepts that should be considered for programs intended to improve elephant health and welfare. Vaccines for rabies, *Clostridium chauvoei*, hemorrhagic septicemia (*Pasteurella multocida*), and tetanus could be cost-effective preventive measures, although efficacy and the relative cost-effectiveness of all vaccination options warrant further investigation. Also worthy of further investigation is the degree to which elephant health could be improved by increased use or appropriate rotation of anthelmintics and development of effective education programs for veterinarians and mahouts. Owner financial constraints or perceptions of the benefits of health measures may limit the potential to enact preventive and medical treatment programs. Conventional medical strategies are largely relevant to captive elephants. Broader scale studies that incorporate ecological and sociological factors are likely more relevant to improving the health of free-ranging elephants.

4.8. Common Disease Conditions. Injuries and parasitism were the most common medical conditions seen in captive and free-ranging elephants, with injuries due to human-elephant conflict restricted to free-ranging populations (Table 6). These medical conditions are candidates for preventive management in captive populations via administration of antiparasitic agents and husbandry modifications for minimizing intra-elephant conflict. Strategies for mitigating human-elephant conflict may reduce mortality in wild populations [11, 12]. Ocular disease due to eye worms and other causes was a comparatively common condition, although the response to treatment was often successful for captive elephants. While lameness was reported exclusively for captive elephants, recognition of foot pathology in free-ranging elephants warrants further investigation, as it has relevance to concerns for captive elephant management and welfare [13–15]. Gastrointestinal disease, including colic, bloat, and constipation, was common in captive animals and was also reported for wild populations. Although gastrointestinal disease represents a broad range of etiologies, the degree to which improved nutrition and access to safe water can reduce the prevalence of gastrointestinal disease and malnutrition for elephants is worth exploring further, especially in calves. Infectious disease was uncommonly reported, although the degree to which this represents deficiencies in access to diagnostic laboratories versus a legitimately low concern is uncertain. In particular, diseases such as EEHV and TB that garner much attention in nonrange, for example, North America and Europe, captive elephant populations are difficult to consider when many Asian countries do not appear to have mycobacterial and virologic veterinary testing capabilities sufficient for providing accurate diagnoses. Similarly, assessing many of the less common diseases is difficult in the absence of reliable diagnostic support. Nevertheless, questionnaire responses suggest that injuries may cause over one-third of mortalities, and this estimate may be low if abscesses or other conditions are secondary to injuries.

A range of responses to treatment was evident (Table 7). This could be because combining narrative reports into consolidated categories such as injuries, gastrointestinal disease, lameness, and foot disease represent combining multiple etiologies with differing prognoses. Alternatively, the variation in outcomes may represent variation in clinician training and expertise or differing levels of access to medications and other resources. If this is the case, investments in training and medical resources could improve treatment outcomes. Even where treatment appears to generally be successful, such as for ecto- and endoparasites, improved access to antiparasitic drugs and research demonstrating drug efficacy may improve outcomes.

Causes of morbidity and mortality may adversely affect individual animal health and welfare or have population-level impacts on fecundity and/or mortality rates. Syndromes with mortality rates that exceed morbidity rates may disproportionately affect population dynamics, and thus may warrant greater support for research and interventions. Injuries and infectious disease not due to parasitism may represent a greater impact on elephant mortality than expected (Table 6). However, this study's design precludes definitive conclusions for such comparisons.

5. Conclusions

Objective data can assist with prioritizing goals and improving the decision process for maximizing the benefits of health and conservation programs [3, 16]. Results from this questionnaire serve as a starting point for determining how to allocate resources to best benefit elephant health and welfare in Asia, as existing literature is insufficient to support such efforts. While the medical concerns listed by respondents have varying degrees of overlap and should be considered on a coarse scale, trauma was consistently listed as the most common cause of elephant morbidity and mortality. In addition, deficiencies in basic husbandry and diagnostics for elephants were commonly listed. Consequently, captive elephants may benefit most by addressing basic concerns such as nutrition, water availability and quality, and housing. Similarly, minimizing human-elephant conflict for wild populations is a substantial challenge. However, addressing these challenges may yield the greatest health benefits because prevention is often the most cost-effective approach [17].

A focus on one or a few diseases that are not strategically selected risks wasting limited resources by investing in programs that have little or no impact on overall elephant conservation efforts. There is a need to clarify the tradeoffs that exist and establish the outcomes that will likely result from investments in elephant health. Consequently, elephant health programs should be well-supported as a part of overall elephant conservation efforts in Asia.

Appendix

Survey of Elephant Health and Management in Asia

A. Basic Information

Survey of Elephant Health and Management in Asia. This is the first form for the respondents to fill out. The purpose of this form is to obtain basic information about the extent to which the respondent works with elephants. See Table 8.

B. Basic Veterinary Concerns

Survey of Elephant Health and Management in Asia. This questionnaire is a self-report form. The purpose of this form is to obtain percentages of elephants seen by the respondent with select health conditions. See Table 9.

C. Laboratory Facilities Questionnaire

Survey of Elephant Health and Management in Asia. The purpose of this form is to determine the capability of laboratory facilities available for diagnostics. See Table 10.

D. Mahout Health Questionnaire

Survey of Elephant Health and Management in Asia. The purpose of this form is to determine whether the mahouts have any observable health conditions. See Table 11.

E. Needs Assessment

Survey of Elephant Health and Management in Asia. The purpose of this form is to identify common needs and/or barriers to optimal elephant health. See Table 12.

F. Common Disease Conditions

Survey of Elephant Health and Management in Asia. The purpose of this form is to obtain information on common disease conditions encountered and how these diseases are handled by the respondent. See Table 13.

TABLE 8

Date: ————————————

(1) Which Asian range country do you work in? ——

     (a) What region within that country? ——

(2a) Do you work for a government agency?

     □ No   □ Yes   If yes, what type?

                           □ Forestry

                           □ Wildlife

                           □ Livestock

                           □ Other ————————

(2b) Do you work for a nongovernment agency (NGO)?

     □ No   □ Yes   If yes, what type? ————————————————————————————————

(2c) If you responded "no" to both (2a) and (2b) please indicate your employment type   ————————————————————

(3) How often do you work with elephant health care?   □ Full time   □ Part time   □ Occasionally

(4) Approximately how many years have you worked with elephant health care? ————————————————————years

(5) How many elephants do you check and/or treat on average **each month**? ———————————————————Elephants

(6) In the area where you are working, how many individual elephants do you see for treatment and/or health check on **a regular basis (minimum 2 times per year)?** ————————————————————Elephants

(7) In the area where you are working, how many of the captive elephants (males and females) have successfully reproduced? □ All   □ Some   □ None

What is the percentage of your work with captive or wild elephants:	0–19%	20–39%	40–59%	60–79%	80–100%
(8a) With captive elephants?	□	□	□	□	□
(8b) With wild elephants?	□	□	□	□	□

In the area where you are working, what is the percentage of the captive elephants owned:	0–19%	20–39%	40–59%	60–79%	80–100%
(9a) By the government?	□	□	□	□	□
(9b) By private owners/institutions?	□	□	□	□	□

(10) **For which type of activities are the elephants utilized?**	All of them	Most of them	Some of them	A few of them	None of them
Zoo exhibition	□	□	□	□	□
Tourism	□	□	□	□	□
Logging	□	□	□	□	□
Forest and habitat patrols	□	□	□	□	□
Human elephant conflict management	□	□	□	□	□
Education awareness programs	□	□	□	□	□
Not utilized	□	□	□	□	□

TABLE 9

Date: ————————————————

(11) On average, how many elephants that you checked regularly (at least 2 times a year) had evidence of the following:	0–19%	20–39%	40–59%	60–79%	80–100%
No visible signs of diseases or disorders	☐	☐	☐	☐	☐
Systemic illness	☐	☐	☐	☐	☐
Upper respiratory disease	☐	☐	☐	☐	☐
Lower respiratory disease	☐	☐	☐	☐	☐
Weight loss	☐	☐	☐	☐	☐
Diarrhea	☐	☐	☐	☐	☐
Other intestinal problems such as colic or constipation	☐	☐	☐	☐	☐
Ectoparasites, such as lice, mites, and ticks	☐	☐	☐	☐	☐
Skin disease caused by reasons other than ectoparasites	☐	☐	☐	☐	☐
Microscopic detection of infestation with endoparasites	☐	☐	☐	☐	☐
Shedding endoparasites with feces	☐	☐	☐	☐	☐
Eye disease	☐	☐	☐	☐	☐
Oral disease	☐	☐	☐	☐	☐
Tusk or molar problems	☐	☐	☐	☐	☐
Trunk disease	☐	☐	☐	☐	☐
Simple foot problems (overgrown toenails or foot pads, simple cracks or splits in nails and pad without infection and lameness)	☐	☐	☐	☐	☐
Complicated foot problems (pad and nail infections, serious injuries, pain, swelling, and lameness)	☐	☐	☐	☐	☐
Non-foot lameness	☐	☐	☐	☐	☐
Wounds other than skin lesions	☐	☐	☐	☐	☐
Infant mortality	☐	☐	☐	☐	☐
Reproductive problems	☐	☐	☐	☐	☐
Reduced endurance for work	☐	☐	☐	☐	☐
Reduced appetite	☐	☐	☐	☐	☐
Stereotypical behavior	☐	☐	☐	☐	☐

(11b) **Have you conducted any postmortem examinations (necropsies) or witnessed the conduction of these examinations in elephants?**

☐ No   ☐ Yes

(11c) **If yes, how many cases per year?**   ————————————————

What were the major pathological findings in these examinations?

("undetermined" can be listed as a finding)

(1) ————————————

(2) ————————————

(3) ————————————

(4) ————————————

(5) ————————————

(6) ————————————

TABLE 10

Date: —————————————————

(12a) **How often are the following labs and diagnostic facilities available?**	Never	Sometimes	Mostly	Always
Laboratory for conducting **routine hematology**	☐	☐	☐	☐
Laboratory for **analyzing blood for routine organ function indices** (e.g., AST, Alk Phos, BUN, Creat, protein, glucose, etc.)	☐	☐	☐	☐
Laboratory **for conducting routine blood mineral analyses** (e.g., Na, CL, Ca, P, etc.)	☐	☐	☐	☐
Laboratory for **analyzing blood for nutritional indices** (e.g., vitamins, fatty acids, micronutrients, etc.)	☐	☐	☐	☐
Laboratory for **analyzing hair for nutritional indices** (e.g., vitamins, micronutrients, etc.)	☐	☐	☐	☐
Laboratory for **detection of toxins**	☐	☐	☐	☐
Laboratory for conducting **hormone analysis**	☐	☐	☐	☐

(12b) **How often are the following labs and diagnostic facilities available?**	Never	Sometimes	Mostly	Always
Light microscopy for **fecal parasite testing**	☐	☐	☐	☐
Light microscopy for **blood parasite testing**	☐	☐	☐	☐
Microbiology lab for **determination of bacterial pathogens and antibiotic sensitivity**	☐	☐	☐	☐
Microbiology lab for **determination of viral pathogens**	☐	☐	☐	☐
Histopathology	☐	☐	☐	☐
Ultrasonography	☐	☐	☐	☐
Radiology (or X-rays)	☐	☐	☐	☐

TABLE 11

Date: —————————————————

(13) **Are mahouts regularly screened for any diseases?**		☐ Yes	☐ No	☐ Unsure	
(13a) **Approximately what is the percentage of mahouts you have seen with the following conditions?**	0–19%	20–39%	40–59%	60–79%	80–100%
Frequent sneezing	☐	☐	☐	☐	☐
Frequent coughing	☐	☐	☐	☐	☐
Sudden weight loss	☐	☐	☐	☐	☐
Eye disease	☐	☐	☐	☐	☐
Abnormal joints or limbs	☐	☐	☐	☐	☐
Abnormal skin conditions	☐	☐	☐	☐	☐
Lethargy (loss of energy)	☐	☐	☐	☐	☐

TABLE 12

Date: —————————————

(14) What are the obstacles that **prevent you from** obtaining **needed medicines** (check all that apply)?

    ☐ Costs for medicines/financial limitations of elephant owner

    ☐ Limited availability of medicines on the local market

    ☐ Import restriction for medicines not available on the local market

    ☐ Other   If "other", please specify———————

(15) What are the obstacles that **prevent you from** conducting **needed treatments** (check all that apply)?

    ☐ Limited access to the area where the elephant is located (road conditions, no transportation, etc.)

    ☐ Treatment not permitted by elephant owner

    ☐ Mahouts that do not cooperate

    ☐ Elephants that are not trained/do not tolerate needed treatment procedures

    ☐ Limited diagnostic techniques to sufficiently diagnose diseases and identify ideal treatment schemes

    ☐ Other   If "other", please specify———————

(16) What are the obstacles that **prevent you from** performing **needed diagnostic procedures** (check all that apply)?

    ☐ Costs for tests/financial limitations of elephant owner

    ☐ Limited availability of diagnostic tests

    ☐ Import restriction for diagnostic tests or supplies that limit availability

    ☐ Inability to keep equipment in working order

    ☐ Lack of training

    ☐ Insufficient availability of trained personnel to conduct tests

    ☐ Other   If "other", please specify———————

(17) What are the **preventive medicine program needs** that exist (check all that apply)?

Elephant food:

    ☐ Vitamin supplements

    ☐ Mineral supplements

    ☐ Specific food supplements with high nutrients

    ☐ Other; please specify——————

Shelter:

    ☐ Special location and facilities for the conduction of treatments (a clinic)

    ☐ Shelter for sick elephants and/or mothers with calf

    ☐ Isolation facility

    ☐ Specific facility/restraint for musth bulls

    ☐ Others; please specify—————

Water:

    ☐ Control of water quality

        If yes, please describe techniques/measurements used to control water quality

        ————————————————

        ————————————————

    ☐ Control of water quantity provided/made available

Table 12: Continued.

Medications:

What kind of preventive medications are administered?

(Please list as many as you are aware of)

————————————————

————————————————

————————————————

Vaccinations:

What are the vaccinations administered? (Please list as many as you are aware of)

————————————————

————————————————

————————————————

Mahout training:

□ Training about daily routine health care procedures

□ Training about different restraint and handling tools

□ Training about elephant biology and behavior

□ Appropriate use of basic drugs and administering basic medications

□ Other (if "other," please specify)

————————————————

————————————————

————————————————

(18) What kind of preventive programs would you suggest as useful to be conducted in your area, and which currently cannot be conducted? (Please provide details where possible)

(A) **Elephant food**————————————————————————————————

(B) **Shelter**————————————————————————————————

(C) **Water**————————————————————————————————

(D) **Medications**————————————————————————————————

(E) **Vaccinations**————————————————————————————————

(F) **Mahout management training**————————————————————————

(G) **Veterinary training**————————————————————————————

(H) **Other**————————————————————————————————

TABLE 13

Date: ——————————————

(19) What are the six main medical issues you find with elephants in your care (i.e., injuries, disease, parasitism, malnutrition, etc.) ranked in order, **from most common to least common?**

    (1) Most common——————————————

    (2) ——————————————

    (3) ——————————————

    (4) ——————————————

    (5) ——————————————

    (6) Least common——————————————

(20) What are the six main causes of elephant mortality that you see ranked in order, **from most common to least common?** ("undetermined" can be listed as a cause)

    (1) Most common cause ——————————

    (2) ——————————————

    (3) ——————————————

    (4) ——————————————

    (5) ——————————————

    (6) Least common cause ——————————

The following question requests information on the most common disease conditions that you encounter, treatment option used, the treatment results, and ideal future treatment options. Please list the diseases in order from the most common to the least common.

Disease:	(Most Common Disease)		
	(1) ————————	(2) ————————	(3) ————————
Standard treatment:			
Percentage that resolved without treatment:	————%	————%	————%
Percentage that died without treatment:	————%	————%	————%
Percentage cured with standard treatment:	————%	————%	————%
Percentage of mortality with standard treatment:	————%	————%	————%
Treatment option(s) that you would like to have available for the future:			

Disease:			(Least Common Disease)
	(4) ————————	(5) ————————	(6) ————————
Standard treatment:			
Percentage that resolved without treatment:	————%	————%	————%
Percentage that died without treatment:	————%	————%	————%
Percentage cured with standard treatment:	————%	————%	————%
Percentage of mortality with standard treatment:	————%	————%	————%
Treatment option(s) that you would like to have available for the future:			

Conflict of Interests

The authors declare that there is no conflict of interests regarding the publication of this paper.

Acknowledgments

Partial support was provided by Asian Elephant Support and a U.S. Fish and Wildlife Service Grant (no. 96200-1-G019) that funded the Regional Asian Elephant Veterinary Workshop in Aceh, Indonesia, March 27–30, 2012. The following individuals are thanked for contributing information to this study: Drs. D. E. Anggraini, T. Angkwanish, A. R. Arasyi, P. Basumatary, Budianto, I. Budiana, A. Chandy, V. Chanthavong, B. Choudhury, A. Dangolla, R. Deswita, K. Gairhe, Husnurrizal, P. Homkong, S. Ilayaraja, Y. Khadpekar, J. Melia, O. Perera, V. Perera, A. Ponnusamy, W. Pramesywari, T. Prasad, S. Raharjo, C. Rajapaksa, D. Ramirez, N. Rickyawan, K. K. Sarma, C. Stremme, R. Suharta, E. Suyanti, J. Thapa, M. Wahyu, R. R. Wahyuni, W. Wardana, C. G. Wijesinghe, A. Zachariah, and several anonymous respondents. The authors thank Koko Sasongko for translations.

References

[1] K. A. Wilson, M. F. McBride, M. Bode, and H. P. Possingham, "Prioritizing global conservation efforts," *Nature*, vol. 440, no. 7082, pp. 337–340, 2006.

[2] B. S. Halpern, C. R. Pyke, H. E. Fox, J. C. Haney, M. A. Schlaepfer, and P. Zaradic, "Gaps and mismatches between global conservation priorities and spending," *Conservation Biology*, vol. 20, no. 1, pp. 56–64, 2006.

[3] M. V. Maciosek, A. B. Coffield, N. M. Edwards, T. J. Flottemesch, and L. I. Solberg, "Prioritizing clinical preventive services: a review and framework with implications for community preventive services," *Annual Review of Public Health*, vol. 30, pp. 341–355, 2009.

[4] M. W. Sanderson and D. P. Gnad, "Biosecurity for reproductive diseases," *Veterinary Clinics of North America: Food Animal Practice*, vol. 18, no. 1, pp. 79–98, 2002.

[5] Convention on International Trade in Endangered Species of Wild Fauna and Flora (CITES), *Appendices I, II and III*, Convention on International Trade in Endangered Species of Wild Fauna and Flora, Geneva, Switzerland, 2013.

[6] R. Sukumar, "A brief review of the status, distribution and biology of wild Asian elephants," *Internationl Zoo Yearbook*, vol. 40, no. 1, pp. 1–8, 2006.

[7] A. Ramanathan and A. Mallapur, "A visual health assessment of captive Asian elephants (Elephas maximus) housed in India," *Journal of Zoo and Wildlife Medicine*, vol. 39, no. 2, pp. 148–154, 2008.

[8] I. Dohoo, W. Martin, and H. Stryhn, *Veterinary Epidemiologic Research*, AVC, Charlottetown, Canada, 2003.

[9] R. Venu, T. Thoiba Singh, R. Veeraharin, D. Rajesh, and C. Srilatha, "First report of Cobboldia elephantis (Cobbold, 1866) larvae in a free ranging wild elephant from Andhra Pradesh, India," *Journal of Parasitic Diseases*, pp. 1–3, 2013.

[10] S. Boonmee, K. Chanawongse, M. Uttisaen, and K. Rewdang, "Taboo and health behavior of mahout in elephant biosphere of Thailand and Lao People's Democratic Republic," *Mediterranean Journal of Social Sciences*, vol. 3, no. 11, pp. 369–374, 2012.

[11] P. Bal, C. D. Nath, K. M. Nanaya, C. G. Kushalappa, and C. Garcia, "Erratum to: elephants also like coffee: trends and drivers of human-elephant conflicts in coffee agroforestry landscapes of Kodagu, Western Ghats, India," *Environmental Management*, vol. 48, no. 2, pp. 263–275, 2011.

[12] J. G. Estes, N. Othman, S. Ismail et al., "Quantity and configuration of available elephant habitat and related conservation concerns in the Lower Kinabatangan floodplain of Sabah, Malaysia," *PLoS ONE*, vol. 7, no. 10, Article ID e44601, 2012.

[13] C. Stremme, A. Lubis, and M. Wahyu, "Implementation of regular veterinary care for captive Sumatran elephants," *Gajah*, vol. 27, pp. 6–14, 2007.

[14] K. Rajankutty, "Foot disorders and their care in elephants," in *Healthcare Management of Captive Asian Elephants*, G. Ajitkumar, K. Anil, and P. Alex, Eds., pp. 111–113, Kerala Agricultural University Press, Mannuthy, India, 2009.

[15] K. Sarma, *Elephant Care*, Directorate of Project Elephant, Ministry of Environment & Forests, Government of India, New Delhi, India, 2011.

[16] A. S. Pullin, T. M. Knight, D. A. Stone, and K. Charman, "Do conservation managers use scientific evidence to support their decision-making?" *Biological Conservation*, vol. 119, no. 2, pp. 245–252, 2004.

[17] U. E. Bauer, P. A. Briss, R. A. Goodman, and B. A. Bowman, "Prevention of chronic disease in the 21st century: elimination of the leading preventable causes of premature death and disability in the USA," *The Lancet*, vol. 384, no. 9937, pp. 45–52, 2014.

20

Inhibition of *Pasteurella multocida* Adhesion to Rabbit Respiratory Epithelium Using Lectins

Magda Patricia Carrillo, Nhora María Martinez, María del Pilar Patiño, and Carlos Arturo Iregui

Pathobiology Group, Laboratory of Veterinary Pathology, Faculty of Veterinary Medicine and Zootechnics, National University of Colombia, Bogotá D.C., Colombia

Correspondence should be addressed to Carlos Arturo Iregui; caireguic@unal.edu.co

Academic Editor: Philip H. Kass

This study aimed to evaluate the ability of a panel of lectins to inhibit the ability of *Pasteurella multocida* to adhere to and affect the rabbit respiratory epithelium. Nasal septa from rabbit fetuses were cultured with various lectins before the addition of *P. multocida*. The percentage of bacteria adhering to the epithelium was evaluated semiquantitatively by indirect immunoperoxidase (IIP) staining. The goblet cells (GCs) were counted in semithin sections stained with toluidine blue and served as the main morphological criterion to evaluate the inhibitory effect of the lectins. The lectins PNA, WGA, RCA_{120}, and DBA significantly inhibited the adhesion of *P. multocida* to the ciliated epithelium ($P < 0.05$) and prevented the pathogen-induced increase in the number of GCs ($P < 0.05$) compared with those of positive control tissues. In addition, VVA, SJA, UEA I, DSL, SBA, and ECL significantly inhibited the increase in GCs compared with that of the control tissues. The results suggest that less aggressive therapeutic strategies, such as treatment with lectins, may represent alternative approaches to control bacterial respiratory infections.

1. Introduction

Adhesion of pathogenic microorganisms to epithelial surfaces is an important step in the infection and colonization of a susceptible host [1–4]. Infection by pathogens is generally initiated by the specific recognition of host epithelial surfaces. Receptors present in the mucin layer can act as binding sites during microbial adhesion. Lectin/glycoconjugate interactions are known for their high specificity and play a significant role in the adhesion of bacteria and other microorganisms to the epithelial surfaces of their hosts. In their infection strategy, bacteria often use sugar-binding proteins, such as lectins and the adhesins pili or fimbriae, to recognize and bind to host glycoconjugates [5–7]. In gram-negative bacteria, the lipopolysaccharide (LPS) on the outer membrane has also been reported as an important structure involved in carbohydrate-lectin interactions [8–10].

Bacterial resistance to antibiotics is an ever-increasing concern. An alternative disease intervention strategy is to target important steps in disease pathogenesis rather than targeting the pathogen directly; in this case, we would seek to mitigate disease by limiting pathogen attachment to host cells and thereby reduce colonization using substances that, in contrast to antibacterial agents, do not destroy the pathogens but rather interfere with their first pathogenic step, namely, their attachment to host cells. Accordingly, antiadhesion therapies have been documented for the enteropathogen *E. coli* K99 in swine and calves; adhesion and infection of this bacterium can be prevented using carbohydrates (CHOs) [11–13]. In the same manner, the specific sialic acid adhesion of *Helicobacter pylori* to human gastric mucus and erythrocytes was inhibited by high molecular mass constituents derived from cranberries [14].

Pasteurella multocida, which is considered a normal component of the upper respiratory tract flora in a variety of animal species, is a well-known pathogen responsible for a range of diseases and economic losses in bovines, swine, canines, laboratory animals, rabbits, and birds [15–19]. This pathogen has also been associated with respiratory tract infections in humans [20]. Although the pathogenic process

Table 1: Lectins and their characteristics [34, 35, 37]. Man, mannose; Glc, glucose; GalNAc, N-acetylgalactosamine; GlcNAc, N-acetylglucosamine; Gal, galactose; Fuc, fucose; Neu5Ac, N-acetylneuraminic acid.

Abbreviation	Latin name	Common name	Carbohydrate specificity
		Source of lectin	
Con A	*Canavalia ensiformis*	Jack bean	Man/Glc
DBA	*Dolichos biflorus*	Horse gram	GalNAc(α1-3)/GalNAc
DSL	*Datura stramonium*	Jimson weed or thorn apple	(GlcNAc)2-4
ECL	*Erythrina cristagalli*	Coral tree	Gal/GalNAc
GSL I	*Griffonia simplicifolia I*	Unknown	Gal/GalNAc
GSL II	*Griffonia simplicifolia II*	Unknown	GlcNAc
Jacalin	*Artocarpus integrifolia*	Jackfruit	Gal/GalNAc
LCA	*Lens culinaris*	Lentil	Man/Glc
LEL	*Lycopersicon esculentum*	Tomato	(GlcNAc)2-4
PNA	*Arachis hypogaea*	Peanut	Gal β1-3/GalNAc
PSA	*Pisum sativum*	Garden pea	Man/Glc
RCA$_{120}$	*Ricinus communis*	Castor oil bean	Galβ1-4/GalNAc
SBA	*Glycine max*	Soybean	Gal/GalNAc
SJA	*Sophora japonica*	Japanese pagoda tree	Gal/GalNAc
STL	*Solanum tuberosum*	Potato	(GlcNAc)2-4
UEA I	*Ulex europaeus I*	Gorse or furze	Fuc
VVA	*Vicia villosa*	Hair vetch	GalNAc
WGA	*Triticum vulgaris*	Wheat germ	GlcNAc/Neu5Ac

is not completely understood, *P. multocida* can transition from being a normal inhabitant of the host to a pathogen capable of causing disease and death. Strategies to control *P. multocida* disease include vaccines and antibiotics, which can have limited efficacy [21, 22].

A major capsular component of all *P. multocida* serogroup A strains is hyaluronic acid [23, 24], the adherent properties of which have been described [25, 26]; additionally, the LPS of *P. multocida* A serovar 3 strain Pm70 possesses CHO sequences similar to those found on several host epithelial surfaces [27, 28]. These findings suggest that both structures might be susceptible targets for antiadhesive therapy by their corresponding lectins or CHOs.

In a search for alternative strategies to control *P. multocida* infections with fewer side effects, this *ex vivo* study explored the possibility of inhibiting *P. multocida* adhesion to the respiratory epithelium (nasal septum) of fetal rabbits using lectins. The results showed that lectin pretreatment reduced the number of bacteria adhering to the apical surface of the epithelium and blocked the pathogen-induced increase in the number of GCs in respiratory tissues, thus raising the possibility of an alternative control strategy for bacterial infection.

2. Materials and Methods

2.1. P. multocida Strains. *P. multocida* isolates from Pm147/08 to Pm160/08 were obtained from the turbinates, trachea, or lungs of diseased rabbits with rhinitis and bronchopneumonia [29]. Routine microbiology tests and PCR amplification and sequencing of the hyaD gene in the cap locus, which encodes proteins involved in the synthesis and assembly of

the type A capsule (GenBank accession number AF067175) [30, 31], confirmed the identity of *P. multocida* type A.

P. multocida isolates were passed through mice by intraperitoneal inoculation. Mice were euthanized after the first signs of disease, and the bacterium was recovered from the heart, liver, lung, and trachea and cultured on BHI agar at 37°C for 24 h before use. The bacterial mass was collected and diluted in glucose-enriched essential medium (MEM), achieving a final concentration of 10^7 CFU/mL via counting and plating.

2.2. Lectins. A total of 18 distinct lectins from three commercial kits (Vector Laboratories) were used (Table 1). These lectins are extracted from various plants and included Con A, DBA, DSL, ECL, GSL I, GSL II, Jacalin, LCA, LEL, PNA, PSA, RCA$_{120}$, SBA, SJA, STL, UEA I, VVA, and WGA. They were selected based on a range of specificities for multiple sugars [32–37].

2.3. Ex Vivo Culture of Rabbit Fetal Nasal Septa. This study was conducted with the approval of the Bioethics Committee of the Faculty of Veterinary Medicine of the National University of Colombia.

Eight pregnant female rabbits at their 26th gestational day were anesthetized with xylazine (5 mg kg^{-1}) and ketamine (35 mg kg^{-1}). The fetuses were delivered by caesarean and immediately euthanized by medullar sectioning; the females were also euthanized with an overdose of anesthetics immediately after the surgery. The skin, mandible, muscle, and palate of the fetuses were removed, and the nasal cavity was cross-sectioned with a sterile blade to obtain three slices, each

0.3 cm thick, from each animal. Sections were washed three times in MEM before tissue culture.

2.4. Inhibitory Effect of Natural Lectins on P. multocida Adherence to the Rabbit Respiratory Epithelium.

To evaluate the potential inhibitory effects of lectins on *P. multocida* adhesion, an experiment was designed to block potential receptors for the bacterium on the apical membrane of epithelial cells. Six cross sections of nasal septa and bacteria were separately evaluated using each lectin (applied at $0.2\,\mu g\,mL^{-1}$); six additional sections cultured without *P. multocida* or lectin and three sections incubated with each lectin alone were used as negative controls; six additional explants were incubated only with the bacterium and were used as positive controls. Tissue sections were immersed in 10 mL MEM supplemented with lectin in a 5 cm diameter Petri dish and incubated in a humid chamber with 5% CO_2 and 95% O_2 for 1 h. The samples were then washed three times with MEM to eliminate the nonadherent lectin. Next, 10^7 CFU of *P. multocida* was added to the samples, and they were incubated for 2 h. Three explants of each lectin treatment were fixed with 3.7% buffered formalin and three with Trump fixative (40% formalin, 25% glutaraldehyde) for 24 h. Control tissues were fixed in a similar manner [29, 38, 39].

2.5. Tissue Processing

2.5.1. Immunohistochemistry.
A polyclonal antiserum raised in an adult female sheep was used. Briefly, as a first dose, $250\,\mu g/mL$ of *P. multocida* was injected with complete Freund adjuvant (CFA); 7 days later, a booster dose with incomplete Freund adjuvant was applied. Finally, two doses of the antigen without adjuvant were inoculated one week apart. Animals were bled at 35 days p.i.; serum collected before inoculation served as a negative control. To eliminate cross-reactions, the serum was immunoadsorbed with normal nasal tissues of other fetuses. The serum was diluted 1 : 25 in sterile Tris-buffered saline (pH 7.6); 5 mL of the antiserum was then diluted in 1 mL of macerated sterile tissues previously washed with physiological salt solution. The mixture was centrifuged at 1000 rpm for 1 h at room temperature, and the supernatant was collected and frozen at −20°C until use. The working dilution of the primary antiserum was determined by indirect immunodot; a similar procedure was followed for the second antibody.

The number of bacteria adhered to the ciliated border of the respiratory epithelial cells was assessed by an indirect immunoperoxidase (IIP) technique [40, 41]. The tissues were embedded in paraffin and cut into 3 μm thick sections. The polyclonal antiserum raised in sheep was used as the specific primary antibody, and a commercial antiserum against ovine IgG produced in donkey was used as a secondary antibody (Sigma, Aldrich) [42]. Nasal septa of rabbits affected by the rhinitic and pneumonic forms of the disease were used as positive controls for the IIP technique.

The level of *P. multocida* adherence to the epithelium was assessed by a semiquantitative procedure as follows: both epithelial surfaces of the nasal septa were considered the full area (100%) to which the bacteria could adhere, and a mean adherence level was determined; no bacteria adhering to the surface were scored as 0%; bacteria attached to >0–30% of the epithelial surface were considered to be of focal adhesion; bacteria adhered to >30–60% of the surface were considered to be multifocal; and bacteria adhered to >60% of the surface were interpreted to be of diffuse adherence.

2.6. Semithin Sections.
Tissue sections fixed for 24 h in Trump solution were decalcified in 10% EDTA for seven days, washed with 0.1 mmol phosphate-buffered saline (pH 7.3), postfixed in 1% osmium tetroxide, dehydrated in an ascending alcohol gradient, and finally embedded in Epon 812 (Polysciences). Sections (0.5 μm thick) were cut with a microtome (Microm) and stained with toluidine blue for approximately 30 s.

Tissue sections were evaluated by light microscopy using 100x objective. The number of cells (with cell nuclei used as the counting unit) in eight continuous fields of respiratory epithelium was analyzed in each of 3 replicates. The protective role of lectins was determined by calculating the percentage of GCs relative to those of other respiratory epithelial cells [29, 43]. In addition, increased GC activity was considered when cells showed an enlarged size, increased mucin release, and apical cytoplasm that protruded over their neighbor cells [44].

2.7. Statistical Analysis.
The mean proportions of ciliated respiratory epithelium covered by adhered and nonadhered *P. multocida* were compared among the various lectin treatments and positive control tissues by ANOVA in a completely random model. To determine differences between treatments, a Dunnett test was performed, with $P < 0.05$ accepted as significant. To analyze the GC activity when the hypothesis was significant ($P < 0.05$), a Dunnett test was performed to compare each lectin treatment with the positive control [45].

3. Results

3.1. Inhibition of P. multocida Adhesion to the Respiratory Epithelium of Nasal Septa: IIP Staining.
Immunostaining of *P. multocida* on the apical surface of the respiratory epithelium in lectin-treated tissues ranged from localized (>0–30%) (Figure 1(b)) to multifocal (>30–60%) (Figure 1(c)); by contrast, in positive control tissues (tissues exposed only to the bacterium), the immunostaining was similar in all replicates, with a generalized granular appearance covering almost 90% of the epithelial surface (Figure 1(d)).

The lectins LCA (*Lens culinaris*), PNA (*Arachis hypogaea*), WGA (*Triticum vulgaris*), RCA$_{120}$ (*Ricinus communis*), and DBA (*Dolichos biflorus*) significantly ($P < 0.05$) inhibited *P. multocida* adherence to the ciliated border of respiratory epithelial cells compared with that of the positive control tissues (Figure 2).

3.2. Semithin Sections.
The respiratory epithelia of nasal septa exposed only to *P. multocida* showed an increase in the

(a)

(b)

(c)

(d)

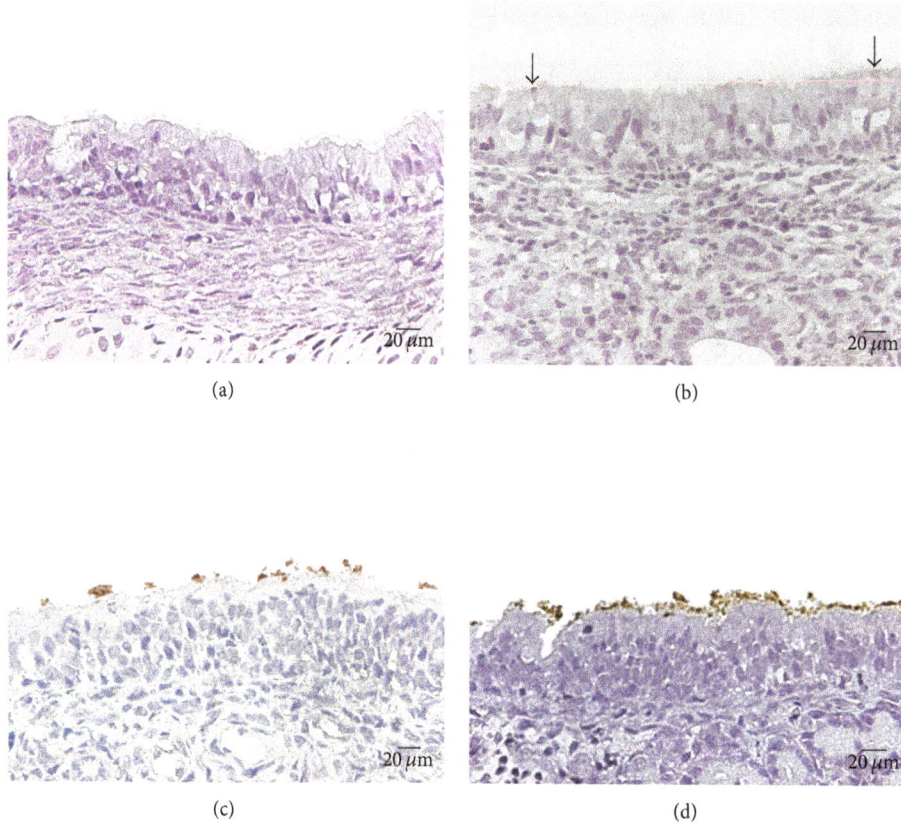

FIGURE 1: IIP technique for determining the percentage of the epithelial surface covered by adherent *P. multocida*. (a) Normal fetal rabbit respiratory nasal epithelium of IIP, negative control; light microscopy (LM), scale bar = 20 μm. (b) Respiratory epithelium of the nasal septa of rabbit fetus preincubated with PNA plus *P. multocida* (sparse focal immunostaining (arrows); >0–30% of the epithelial surface); LM, scale bar = 20 μm. (c) Tissue preincubated with VVA and *P. multocida* showing multifocal immunostaining (>30–60% of the surface covered with bacteria); LM, scale bar = 20 μm. (d) Tissue incubated with *P. multocida* without lectins (positive control) showing generalized immunostaining (>60% of the epithelial surface covered by bacteria); LM, scale bar = 20 μm.

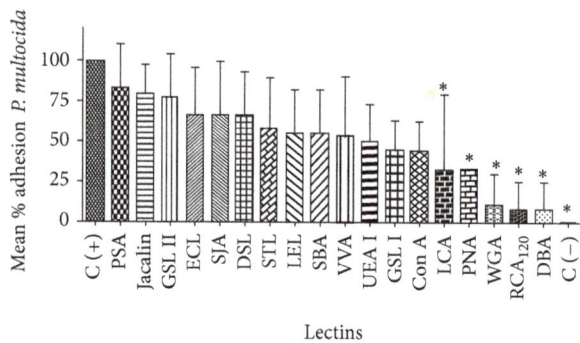

FIGURE 2: Inhibition of *P. multocida* adhesion to the ciliated respiratory epithelium of rabbit fetuses exposed to various lectins. Adhesion is expressed as mean percentage of the ciliated border epithelium coated by adhered bacteria. *Significant inhibition ($P <$ 0.05) compared with the positive control tissues. C (−): negative control.

number of GCs compared with that of the control specimens (Figures 3(a) and 4). This increased number of GCs (Figure 3(c)) was accompanied by an enhanced production

and release of mucus, such that the apical surface of these cells protruded above their neighboring ciliated cells, with their contents liberated into the lumen (Figure 3(c)). No increase in the number or activity of GCs was observed when nasal septa were incubated separately with each lectin.

The lectins VVA (*Vicia villosa*), DBA (*Dolichos biflorus*), RCA$_{120}$ (*Ricinus communis*), SJA (*Sophora japonica*), UEA I (*Ulex europaeus I*), WGA (*Triticum vulgaris*), DSL (*Datura stramonium*), SBA (*Glycine max*), ECL (*Erythrina cristagalli*), and PNA (*Arachis hypogaea*) also showed significant inhibitions ($P <$ 0.05) of the GC number and activity (Figure 4).

4. Discussion

The current strategies for preventing *P. multocida* infection in susceptible species, including rabbits, are limited to a few vaccines and antibiotics, but these approaches have shown inconsistent results [46–49]. In this study, we have explored a novel strategy to impede the adherence of this microorganism to the respiratory epithelia of rabbits using lectins while simultaneously investigating which molecules could protect the epithelium without having to kill the bacteria. Implementing an *ex vivo* experimental protocol, our data

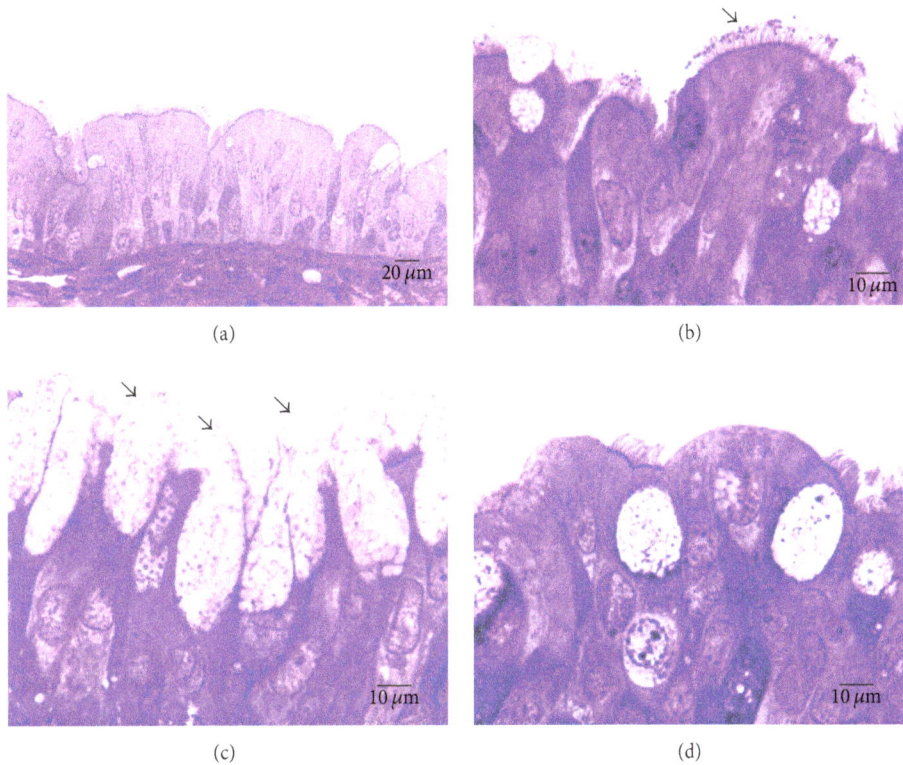

FIGURE 3: Toluidine blue staining of respiratory nasal epithelia of rabbit fetuses exposed to *P. multocida*. (a) Normal epithelium not exposed to bacteria or lectins; LM, scale bar = 20 μm. (b-c) Nasal septa of positive control tissues exposed only to *P. multocida*. (b) *P. multocida* adhering to cilia (arrow); LM, scale bar = 10 μm. (c) GCs showing increased numbers and excretory activity. All of the GCs are protruding above the apical limit of their neighboring cells and liberating their contents (arrows); LM, scale bar = 10 μm. (d) Nasal epithelium exposed to both bacteria and PNA. The lectin inhibited the increase in the number of GCs, though some loss of cilia can still be observed; LM, scale bar = 10 μm.

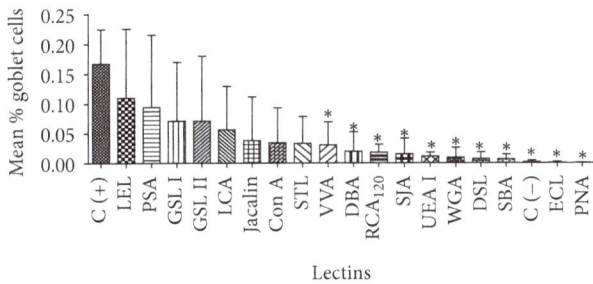

FIGURE 4: Inhibition of the increase in the percentage of GCs in the respiratory epithelia of nasal septa treated with various lectins. *Significant inhibition ($P < 0.05$) by lectins compared with positive control tissues. C (−): negative control.

demonstrate that certain lectins inhibited the attachment of *P. multocida* to the respiratory epithelia of fetal rabbit nasal septa and also prevented the pathogen-induced increase in the number of GCs.

In this study, treatment with the lectins PNA (Gal β1–3/GalNAc), WGA (GlcNAc/Neu5Ac), RCA$_{120}$ (Galβ1–4/ GalNAc), DBA (GalNAc (α1–3)/GalNAc), and LCA (Man/ Glc) significantly inhibited *P. multocida* adhesion to rabbit nasal respiratory epithelia and, in the cases of PNA, WGA, RCA$_{120}$, and DBA also prevented an increase in the number and activity of GCs. These results suggest three possible explanations for the inhibitory activity of these lectins: (1) LCA, PNA, WGA, RCA$_{120}$, and DBA bind to their specific CHO moieties present on the apical surface of the respiratory epithelium, thereby masking putative CHO receptors for corresponding lectins on the bacterial surface similar to those targeted in this work; (2) these lectins, on their side, recognize CHOs on the bacterial capsule and/or its LPS that serve as ligands for the corresponding lectin receptors on the apical membrane of the respiratory epithelium; and (3) both events occur simultaneously. Mason et al. [50] demonstrated that the PNA, LCA, RCA$_{120}$, and WGA lectins recognize CHOs on the upper respiratory epithelium of laboratory rodents, partially confirming our results. In addition, Perfumo et al. [51] reported that lectins similar to those tested in this study (DBA, SBA, PNA, and RCA$_{120}$) bind to receptors on the respiratory epithelial cells of the nasal cavity of healthy swine, as well as those suffering from atrophic rhinitis caused by *P. multocida* and *B. bronchiseptica*. Taken together, these findings indicate that CHOs and lectins with corresponding specificities are present on the apical surfaces of the respiratory epithelia of various animal species and most likely also on the surfaces of *P. multocida* and *B. bronchiseptica*, serving as receptors and ligands, respectively.

WGA recognizes GlcNAc (β1) and D-glucuronic acid residues, which are constituents of hyaluronan, a major nonsulfated glycosaminoglycan ubiquitous in all connective tissues; hyaluronan has also been described on both the apical and basal surfaces of the airway epithelium [52–55] and in tracheal secretions [56]. Hyaluronic acid is also a major capsular component of all *P. multocida* serogroup A strains [23, 24]. *P. multocida* serogroup A has been shown to adhere strongly to HeLa cells, turkey air sac macrophages, and alveolar macrophages; bacterial adhesion was reduced by treatment of the bacteria with hyaluronidase (to reduce the amount of capsule) or the addition of hyaluronic acid [25, 26]. Similarly, a spontaneous acapsular variant of *P. multocida* serogroup A did not adhere to turkey air sac macrophages [26]. Glorioso et al. [57] studied the adhesion of *P. multocida* isolated from rabbits to monolayers of HeLa cell cultures and to parakeratotic pharyngeal cells. Their most significant finding was that GlcNAc treatment inhibited bacterial adhesion to both cell lines. These results suggest that lectin-like molecules that serve as receptors for the microorganism are present on both epithelial surfaces. The main adherent role was attributed to *P. multocida* fimbriae [58]. These findings were complemented by those of Al-Haddawi et al. [59], who demonstrated that *P. multocida* A3 fimbriae isolated from rabbits recognize GlcNAc on the cilia of the respiratory epithelium; they were also able to competitively block this binding using the same CHO. Conversely, Jacques et al. [60] and Hatfaludi et al. [8] state that, despite the fact that *P. multocida* possesses various structures able to contribute to its binding of the respiratory epithelial cells of swine and rabbits *in vitro*, the LPS and type IV fimbria are likely the main mediators of the adhesion, acting as the CHO and lectin ligands, respectively. It is conceivable that, in our studies, WGA simultaneously bound hyaluronan residues on the apical surface of the respiratory epithelium and on the capsule of *P. multocida*, thereby exerting a double inhibitory effect.

However, the protective effect of WGA in this research could also be attributed to the inhibition of adherence of *P. multocida* LPS to hyaluronan on the apical membrane of the nasal respiratory epithelial cells. Protective activity against LPS-induced septic shock, acute lung injury, and airway hyperreactivity has been demonstrated by pretreatment with high molecular weight hyaluronan ($<5 \times 10^5$), indicating that soluble hyaluronan can prevent the adherence of LPS to membrane-bound hyaluronan [61, 62].

The increase in the number and activity of GCs observed in this study could be due to the stimulation of the bacterium itself but is more likely related to the presence of substances liberated by *P. multocida*, mainly its LPS. Using the same *ex vivo* model as in this study, a previous study from our group exposed nasal cultures to *P. multocida* or its LPS separately; in both cases, the main response of the respiratory epithelium was a statistically significant increase in the number and activity of GCs compared with those of controls [29]. Previous studies have also reported hyperplasia and increased activity in the GCs of the respiratory epithelium following exposure to LPS [63–65]. Intranasal instillation of endotoxin

in rats induces an inflammatory response characterized by an increase in the quantity or secretion of mucosubstances, as well as the infiltration of inflammatory cells into the epithelium, mainly PMNs [63]. Several mechanisms have been proposed to explain the positive effect of LPS on mucus production. Aside from the activity of various components of the PMNs, the expression of mucin genes, without the need for other secondary mediators, has been induced in cell cultures and nasal explants exposed only to endotoxin [66, 67]. Recent *in vivo* and *in vitro* work on the LPS of *Pseudomonas aeruginosa* reinforced these observations, as the expression of the mucin MUC5AC in mucin-producing cells of the airways was stimulated by treatment with this molecule [68]. Additional experiments by our group, in which the nasal septa of rabbit fetuses were only exposed to *P. multocida*, showed that the LPS was spontaneously released by the bacterium on the apical surface of the epithelial cells, where it entered the ciliated cells. This event was accompanied by increases in the number and activity of GCs, without any evidence of inflammatory cells [69]. These results reinforce the hypothesis that the LPS of *P. multocida* was one of the main targets of the inhibitory effect of the lectin WGA observed in this work.

Except for LCA, all lectins that prevented *P. multocida* adherence to the epithelium (PNA, WGA, RCA$_{120}$, and DBA) also inhibited the increase in the number of GCs. It is not clear why LCA did not also have an inhibitory effect on these cells.

A different effect was found for VVA, SJA, UEA, DSL, SBA, and ECL, which significantly prevented the elevation in the number of GCs but did not significantly inhibit *P. multocida* adherence to the respiratory epithelium. Although we do not have a convincing explanation for the lack of inhibitory effect on *P. multocida* adhesion, part of the inhibitory effect of VVA, SJA, SBA, and ECL on GC number could be attributable to their specificity for CHOs residues containing Gal/GalNAc (and of DSL for GlcNAc), as these are important constituents of the LPS of *P. multocida* serovar 3, Pm70 [27].

Analysis of the *P. multocida* 3 Pm70 genome sequence identified two predicted filamentous hemagglutinin genes (fhaB1 and fhaB2) that might have similar adherent activities as that of the filamentous hemagglutinin protein of *Bordetella pertussis*, FhaB-FhaB1 FhaB2, for the adhesion to host cells [8, 70, 71]. This protein has at least three separate binding activities: a glycosaminoglycan binding site [72–74], an integrin-binding arginine-glycine-aspartate (RGD) sequence [75, 76], and a CHO recognition domain that mediates attachment to ciliated respiratory epithelial cells and macrophages [77–80]. The FhaB1 and FhaB2 proteins of *P. multocida* could have similar ligand affinity for CHO receptors on the airway epithelia of rabbits.

The results of this study indicate that *P. multocida* type A binds to the apical surface of rabbit nasal respiratory epithelia through several CHO-containing receptors, likely via bacterial surface structures, such as the capsule, LPS, type IV fimbriae, or lectin-like structures that may specifically bind to those glycosidic receptors, all of which would be potential targets for the inhibitory effect of the lectins observed in this work. We propose that, in addition to the potential use of lectins to inhibit the deleterious effects of *P. multocida* adhesion and colonization, it could also be more effective to employ the corresponding sugars, that is, D-Man, D-Glc, and GlcNAc, the effects of which have recently been demonstrated [81]. This approach would allow the key receptors on the respiratory epithelial cells to be occupied by the sugars or endocytosed upon sugar binding, reducing their numbers and leaving no binding sites for the microorganisms' sugar molecules [9, 13, 82]. The use of natural substances to inhibit pathogen adhesion to host cells might be an advantageous strategy that does not exert evolutionary pressure to generate more pathogenic forms of the microorganisms [6, 9].

5. Conclusions

A number of lectins were found to impede the attachment of *P. multocida* to the respiratory epithelia of fetal rabbit nasal septa *ex vivo*. The inhibition of *P. multocida* adhesion protected the respiratory cells from the lesions caused by the pathogen, and it is therefore highly probable that the undamaged mucosa would be able to clear the pathogen by innate protective mechanisms, such as mucociliary clearance. Preventing *P. multocida* colonization and cell damage in the upper respiratory tract may impede the bacteria from reaching deeper regions of the lungs. Our results support future investigations into whether the CHOs identified herein can also inhibit *P. multocida* adhesion in rabbits *in vivo*.

Conflict of Interests

The authors declare that there is no conflict of interests regarding the publication of this paper.

Acknowledgments

Special thanks are given to Dr. Noel Verjan from Tolima University, Colombia, and to Dr. Ben Adler from Monash University for their critical review of the paper. The authors are also thankful to Dr. Cristobal Corredor for his invaluable advice on lectins.

References

[1] W. P. Reed and R. C. Williams Jr., "Bacterial adherence: first step in pathogenesis of certain infections," *Journal of Chronic Diseases*, vol. 31, no. 2, pp. 67–72, 1978.

[2] M. S. Neiderman, "The pathogenesis of airway colonization: lessons learned from the study of bacterial adherence," *European Respiratory Journal*, vol. 7, no. 10, pp. 1737–1740, 1994.

[3] L. Lu and W. A. Walker, "Pathologic and physiologic interactions of bacteria with the gastrointestinal epithelium," *The American Journal of Clinical Nutrition*, vol. 73, no. 6, pp. 1124S–1130S, 2001.

[4] T. J. Foster, "Colonization and infection of the human host by staphylococci: adhesion, survival and immune evasion," *Veterinary Dermatology*, vol. 20, no. 5-6, pp. 456–470, 2009.

[5] A. Imberty and A. Varrot, "Microbial recognition of human cell surface glycoconjugates," *Current Opinion in Structural Biology*, vol. 18, no. 5, pp. 567–576, 2008.

[6] M. Hartmann and T. K. Lindhorst, "The bacterial lectin FimH, a target for drug discovery—carbohydrate inhibitors of type 1 fimbriae-mediated bacterial adhesion," *European Journal of Organic Chemistry*, vol. 2011, no. 20-21, pp. 3583–3609, 2011.

[7] H. Connell, W. Agace, P. Klemm, M. Schembri, S. Mårild, and C. Svanborg, "Type 1 fimbrial expression enhances *Escherichia coli* virulence for the urinary tract," *Proceedings of the National Academy of Sciences of the United States of America*, vol. 93, no. 18, pp. 9827–9832, 1996.

[8] T. Hatfaludi, K. Al-Hasani, J. D. Boyce, and B. Adler, "Outer membrane proteins of *Pasteurella multocida*," *Veterinary Microbiology*, vol. 144, no. 1-2, pp. 1–17, 2010.

[9] I. Ofek and N. Sharon, "Visions & reflections: a bright future for anti-adhesion therapy of infectious diseases," *Cellular and Molecular Life Sciences*, vol. 59, no. 10, pp. 1666–1667, 2002.

[10] D. Bravo, A. Hoare, A. Silipo et al., "Different sugar residues of the lipopolysaccharide outer core are required for early interactions of *Salmonella enterica* serovars Typhi and Typhimurium with epithelial cells," *Microbial Pathogenesis*, vol. 50, no. 2, pp. 70–80, 2011.

[11] M. Mouricout, J. M. Petit, J. R. Carias, and R. Julien, "Glycoprotein glycans that inhibit adhesion of *Escherichia coli* mediated by K99 fimbriae: treatment of experimental colibacillosis," *Infection and Immunity*, vol. 58, no. 1, pp. 98–106, 1990.

[12] M. Mouricout, "Swine and cattle enterotoxigenic *Escherichia coli*-mediated diarrhea. Development of therapies based on inhibition of bacteria-host interactions," *European Journal of Epidemiology*, vol. 7, no. 6, pp. 588–604, 1991.

[13] N. Sharon, "Atomic basis of protein-carbohydrate interactions: an overview," in *Protein-Carbohydrate Interactions in Infectious Diseases*, C. Bewley, Ed., Royal Society of Chemistry, London, UK, 2006.

[14] O. Burger, I. Ofek, M. Tabak, E. I. Weiss, and N. Sharon, "A high molecular mass constituent of cranberry juice inhibits helicobacter pylori adhesion to human gastric mucus," *FEMS Immunology Medical Microbiology*, vol. 29, no. 4, pp. 295–301, 2000.

[15] M. Harper, J. D. Boyce, and B. Adler, "*Pasteurella multocida* pathogenesis: 125 years after pasteur," *FEMS Microbiology Letters*, vol. 265, no. 1, pp. 1–10, 2006.

[16] N. García, *Caracterización fenotípica y genética de aislados de Pasteurella multocida obtenidos de ganado porcino [Ph.D. thesis]*, Universidad Complutense de Madrid, Madrid, Spain, 2010.

[17] E. J. Hotchkiss, J. C. Hodgson, E. Schmitt-van de Leemput, M. P. Dagleish, and R. N. Zadoks, "Molecular epidemiology of *Pasteurella multocida* in dairy and beef calves," *Veterinary Microbiology*, vol. 151, no. 3-4, pp. 329–335, 2011.

[18] N. Sthitmatee, Y. Kataoka, and T. T. Sawada, "Molecular epidemiology of Japanese avian *Pasteurella multocida* strains by the single-enzyme amplified fragment length polymorphism and pulsed-field gel electrophoresis," *The Journal of Veterinary Medical Science*, vol. 72, no. 11, pp. 1465–1470, 2010.

[19] I. I. A. Suelam and L. K. Samie, "Molecular diversity of *Pasteurella multocida* isolated from different rabbit outbreaks at Zagazig suburbs, Egypt," *Global Veterinaria*, vol. 6, no. 2, pp. 208–212, 2011.

[20] S. Miyoshi, H. Hamada, A. Miyoshi et al., "*Pasteurella multocida* pneumonia: zoonotic transmission confirmed by molecular epidemiological analysis," *Geriatrics and Gerontology International*, vol. 12, no. 1, pp. 159–163, 2012.

[21] C. Kehrenberg, N. T. Thu Tham, and S. Schwarz, "New plasmid-borne antibiotic resistance gene cluster in *Pasteurella multocida*," *Antimicrobial Agents and Chemotherapy*, vol. 47, no. 9, pp. 2978–2980, 2003.

[22] K. K. Kumarasamy, M. A. Toleman, T. R. Walsh et al., "Emergence of a new antibiotic resistance mechanism in India, Pakistan, and the UK: a molecular, biological, and epidemiological study," *The Lancet Infectious Diseases*, vol. 10, no. 9, pp. 597–602, 2010.

[23] K. K. Pandit and J. E. Smith, "Capsular hyaluronic acid in *Pasteurella multocida* type A and its counterpart in type D," *Research in Veterinary Science*, vol. 54, no. 1, pp. 20–24, 1993.

[24] H. Rosner, H.-D. Grimmecke, Y. A. Knirel, and A. S. Shashkov, "Hyaluronic acid and a $(1 \rightarrow 4]$-β-D-xylan, extracellular polysaccharides of *Pasteurella multocida* (Carter type A) strain 880," *Carbohydrate Research*, vol. 223, pp. 329–333, 1992.

[25] J. Esslinger, R. S. Seleim, G. Hermann, and H. Blobel, "Adhesion of *Pasteurella multocida* to Hela cells and macrophages of different animal species," *Revue de Medecine Veterinaire*, vol. 145, no. 1, pp. 49–53, 1994.

[26] I. M. Pruimboom, R. B. Rimler, M. R. Ackermann, and K. A. Brogden, "Capsular hyaluronic acid-mediated adhesion of *Pasteurella multocida* to turkey air sac macrophages," *Avian Diseases*, vol. 40, no. 4, pp. 887–893, 1996.

[27] F. St. Michael, E. Vinogradov, J. Li, and A. D. Cox, "Structural analysis of the lipopolysaccharide from *Pasteurella multocida* genome strain Pm70 and identification of the putative lipopolysaccharide glycosyltransferases," *Glycobiology*, vol. 15, no. 4, pp. 323–333, 2005.

[28] R. S. Houliston, S. Bernatchez, M.-F. Karwaski et al., "Complete chemoenzymatic synthesis of the Forssman antigen using novel glycosyltransferases identified in *Campylobacter jejuni* and *Pasteurella multocida*," *Glycobiology*, vol. 19, no. 2, pp. 153–159, 2009.

[29] P. Esquinas, *Interacción in vitro entre la Pasteurella multocida y/o su lipopolisacárido con epitelio de septo nasal de conejo [M.S. dissertation]*, Universidad Nacional de Colombia, Bogotá, Colombia, 2007.

[30] K. M. Townsend, J. D. Boyce, J. Y. Chung, A. J. Frost, and B. Adler, "Genetic organization of *Pasteurella multocida* cap loci and development of a multiplex capsular PCR typing system," *Journal of Clinical Microbiology*, vol. 39, no. 3, pp. 924–929, 2001.

[31] J. A. Steen, P. Harrison, T. Seemann et al., "Fis is essential for capsule production in *Pasteurella multocida* and regulates expression of other important virulence factors," *PLoS Pathogens*, vol. 6, no. 2, Article ID e1000750, 2010.

[32] C. Barbeito, A. Massone, and M. Quiroga, *Aplicación de Las Técnicas de Lectinhistoquimica. Aplicaciones en Patología Veterinaria*, Universidad Nacional de La Plata, La Plata, Argentina, 1990.

[33] M. Slifkin and R. J. Doyle, "Lectins and their application to clinical microbiology," *Clinical Microbiology Reviews*, vol. 3, no. 3, pp. 197–218, 1990.

[34] S. A. Brooks, U. Schumacher, and A. J. C. Leathem, "Sources of lectins and other reagents for histochemistry," in *Lectin Histochemistry*, Royal Microscopical Society, Oxford, UK, 1997.

[35] J. Rhodes and J. Milton, "Lectin-binding specifications," in *Lectins Methods and Protocols*, J. Rhodes and J. Milton, Eds., Humana Press, Totowa, NJ, USA, 1998.

[36] N. Sharon and H. Lis, "Plant lectins," in *Lectins*, N. Sharon and H. Lis, Eds., Springer, Dordrecht, The Netherlands, 2007.

[37] K. Turton, R. Natesh, N. Thiyagarajan, J. A. Chaddock, and K. R. Acharya, "Crystal structures of Erythrina cristagalli lectin with bound N-linked oligosaccharide and lactose," *Glycobiology*, vol. 14, no. 10, pp. 923–929, 2004.

[38] M. Stinson and J. Wang, "Lectin inhibition of bacterial adhesion to animal cells. Part XII: use of lectins in the investigation in pathogen-host interaction," in *Lectins Methods and Protocols*, J. Rhodes and J. Milton, Eds., Humana Press, New York, NY, USA, 1998.

[39] H. Al-Haj Alia, T. Sawadaa, H. Hatakeyamab, Y. Katayamac, N. Ohtsukid, and O. Itohd, "Invasion of chicken embryo fibroblast cells by avian *Pasteurella multocida*," *Veterinary Microbiology*, vol. 104, no. 1-2, pp. 55–62, 2004.

[40] E. Heyderman, "Immunoperoxidase technique in histopathology: applications, methods, and controls," *Journal of Clinical Pathology*, vol. 32, no. 10, pp. 971–978, 1979.

[41] T. Ogawa, K. Gamoh, K. Aoki et al., "Validation and standardization of virus neutralizing test using indirect immunoperoxidase technique for the quantification of antibodies to rabies virus," *Zoonoses and Public Health*, vol. 55, no. 6, pp. 323–327, 2008.

[42] J. Kenny, "Immunochemical methods in cell and molecular biology: R. J. Mayer and J. H. Walker. pp 325. Academic Press, London. 1987," *Biochemical Education*, vol. 17, no. 3, p. 164, 1989.

[43] C. Gallego, A. M. Middleton, N. Martínez, S. Romero, and C. Iregui, "Interaction of *Bordetella bronchiseptica* and its lipopolysaccharide with *in vitro* culture of respiratory nasal epithelium," *Veterinary Medicine International*, vol. 2013, Article ID 347086, 9 pages, 2013.

[44] P. Esquinas, L. Botero, M. D. P. Patiño, C. Gallego, and C. Iregui, "Ultrastructural comparison of the nasal epithelia of healthy and naturally affected rabbits with *Pasteurella multocida* A," *Veterinary Medicine International*, vol. 2013, Article ID 321390, 8 pages, 2013.

[45] R. Martínez and N. Martínez, *Diseño de Experimentos Análisis de Datos Estándar y no Estándar*, Guadalupe ltda, Bogotá, Colombia, 1997.

[46] R. B. Rimler, P. A. Rebers, and K. R. Rhoades, "Fowl cholera: cross-protection induced by *Pasteurella multocida* separated from infected turkey blood," *Avian Diseases*, vol. 23, no. 3, pp. 730–741, 1979.

[47] M. A. Suckow, T. L. Bowersock, K. Nielsen, C. E. Chrisp, P. L. Frandsen, and E. B. Janovitz, "Protective immunity to *Pasteurella multocida* heat-labile toxin by intranasal immunization in rabbits," *Laboratory Animal Science*, vol. 45, no. 5, pp. 526–532, 1995.

[48] J. Boyce, C. Lo, I. Wilkie, and B. Adler, *Pasteurella in Pathogenesis of Bacterial Infections in Animals*, C. L. Gyles, J. F. Prescott, G. Songer, C. O. Thoen, Eds., Blackwell Publishing, Malden, Mass, USA, 2010.

[49] A. Dowling, J. C. Hodgson, M. P. Dagleish, P. D. Eckersall, and J. Sales, "Pathophysiological and immune cell responses in calves prior to and following lung challenge with formalin-killed *Pasteurella multocida* biotype A:3 and protection studies involving subsequent homologous live challenge," *Veterinary Immunology and Immunopathology*, vol. 100, no. 3-4, pp. 197–207, 2004.

[50] C. M. Mason, S. Q. Azizi, and A. R. dal Nogare, "Respiratory epithelial carbohydrate levels of rats with gram-negative bacillary colonization," *The Journal of Laboratory and Clinical Medicine*, vol. 120, no. 5, pp. 740–745, 1992.

[51] C. J. Perfumo, N. Mores, A. D. Armocida, I. A. Piffer, A. R. Massone, and S.-I. Itagaki, "Histochemical and lectinhistochemical studies on nasal mucosa of pigs with or without respiratory diseases," *Journal of Veterinary Medical Science*, vol. 60, no. 9, pp. 1021–1023, 1998.

[52] S. J. Green, G. Tarone, and C. B. Underhill, "Distribution of hyaluronate and hyaluronate receptors in the adult lung," *Journal of Cell Science*, vol. 90, no. 1, pp. 145–156, 1988.

[53] S. M. Casalino-Matsuda, M. E. Monzon, G. E. Conner, M. Salathe, and R. M. Forteza, "Role of hyaluronan and reactive oxygen species in tissue kallikrein-mediated epidermal growth factor receptor activation in human airways," *The Journal of Biological Chemistry*, vol. 279, no. 20, pp. 21606–21616, 2004.

[54] R. T. Pirinen, R. H. Tammi, M. I. Tammi et al., "Expression of hyaluronan in normal and dysplastic bronchial epithelium and in squamous cell carcinoma of the lung," *International Journal of Cancer*, vol. 79, no. 3, pp. 251–255, 1998.

[55] M. E. Lauer, S. C. Erzurum, D. Mukhopadhyay et al., "Differentiated murine airway epithelial cells synthesize a leukocyte-adhesive hyaluronan matrix in response to endoplasmic reticulum stress," *Journal of Biological Chemistry*, vol. 283, no. 38, pp. 26283–26296, 2008.

[56] M. E. Monzon, S. M. Casalino-Matsuda, and R. M. Forteza, "Identification of glycosaminoglycans in human airway secretions," *American Journal of Respiratory Cell and Molecular Biology*, vol. 34, no. 2, pp. 135–141, 2006.

[57] J. C. Glorioso, G. W. Jones, and H. G. Rush, "Adhesion of type A *Pasteurella multocida* to rabbit pharyngeal cells and its possible role in rabbit respiratory tract infections," *Infection and Immunity*, vol. 35, no. 3, pp. 1103–1109, 1982.

[58] C. G. Ruffolo, J. M. Tennent, W. P. Michalski, and B. Adler, "Identification,purification, and characterization of the type 4 fimbriae of *Pasteurella multocida*," *Infection and Immunity*, vol. 65, no. 1, pp. 339–343, 1997.

[59] M. H. Al-Haddawi, S. Jasni, M. Zamri-Saad et al., "In vitro study of *Pasteurella multocida* adhesion to trachea, lung and aorta of rabbits," *Veterinary Journal*, vol. 159, no. 3, pp. 274–281, 2000.

[60] M. Jacques, N. Parent, and B. Foiry, "Adherence of Bordetella bronchiseptica and *Pasteurella multocida* to porcine nasal and tracheal epithelial cells," *Canadian Journal of Veterinary Research*, vol. 52, no. 2, pp. 283–285, 1988.

[61] J. Muto, K. Yamasaki, K. R. Taylor, and R. L. Gallo, "Engagement of CD44 by hyaluronan suppresses TLR4 signaling and the septic response to LPS," *Molecular Immunology*, vol. 47, no. 2-3, pp. 449–456, 2009.

[62] F. E. Lennon and P. A. Singleton, "Role of hyaluronan and hyaluronan-binding proteins in lung pathobiology," *The American Journal of Physiology—Lung Cellular and Molecular Physiology*, vol. 301, no. 2, pp. L137–L147, 2011.

[63] J. R. Harkema and J. A. Hotchkiss, "*In vivo* effects of endotoxin on nasal epithelial mucosubstances: ouantitative histochemistry," *Experimental Lung Research*, vol. 17, no. 4, pp. 743–761, 1991.

[64] T. Shimizu, Y. Takahashi, S. Kawaguchi, and Y. Sakakura, "Hypertrophic and metaplastic changes of goblet cells in rat nasal epithelium induced by endotoxin," *American Journal of Respiratory and Critical Care Medicine*, vol. 153, no. 4, pp. 1412–1418, 1996.

[65] J. Tamaoki, K. Takeyama, I. Yamawaki, M. Kondo, and K. Konno, "Lipopolysaccharide-induced goblet cell hypersecretion in the guinea pig trachea: inhibition by macrolides," *The American Journal of Physiology*, vol. 272, no. 1, pp. L15–L19, 1997.

[66] N. Beckmann, B. Tigani, R. Sugar et al., "Noninvasive detection of endotoxin-induced mucus hypersecretion in rat lung by MRI," *The American Journal of Physiology—Lung Cellular and Molecular Physiology*, vol. 283, no. 1, pp. L22–L30, 2002.

[67] J. G. Wagner, S. J. van Dyken, J. R. Wierenga, J. A. Hotchkiss, and J. R. Harkema, "Ozone exposure enhances endotoxin-induced mucous cell metaplasia in rat pulmonary airways," *Toxicological Sciences*, vol. 74, no. 2, pp. 437–446, 2003.

[68] W. Li, F. Yan, H. Zhou et al., "*P. aeruginosa* lipopolysaccharide-induced MUC5AC and CLCA3 expression is partly through Duox1 *in vitro* and *in vivo*," *PLoS ONE*, vol. 8, no. 5, Article ID e63945, 2013.

[69] C. Gallego, S. Romero, P. Esquinas, and C. Iregui, "Proposed pathogenic roles of the lipopolysaccharide of *Pasteurella multocida* A during the first steps of the infection in rabbits," in *Proceedings of the International Pasteurellaceae Conference*, Prato, Italy, 2014.

[70] C. Locht, R. Antoine, and F. Jacob-Dubuisson, "*Bordetella pertussis*, molecular pathogenesis under multiple aspects," *Current Opinion in Microbiology*, vol. 4, no. 1, pp. 82–89, 2001.

[71] B. J. May, Q. Zhang, L. L. Li, M. L. Paustian, T. S. Whittam, and V. Kapur, "Complete genomic sequence of *Pasteurella multocida*, Pm70," *Proceedings of the National Academy of Sciences of the United States of America*, vol. 98, no. 6, pp. 3460–3465, 2001.

[72] J. H. Hannah, F. D. Menozzi, G. Renauld, C. Locht, and M. J. Brennan, "Sulfated glycoconjugate receptors for the *Bordetella pertussis* adhesin filamentous hemagglutinin (FHA) and mapping of the heparin-binding domain on FHA," *Infection and Immunity*, vol. 62, no. 11, pp. 5010–5019, 1994.

[73] F. D. Menozzi, R. Mutombo, G. Renauld et al., "Heparin-inhibitable lectin activity of the filamentous hemagglutinin adhesin of *Bordetella pertussis*," *Infection and Immunity*, vol. 62, no. 3, pp. 769–778, 1994.

[74] S. Mattoo and J. D. Cherry, "Molecular pathogenesis, epidemiology, and clinical manifestations of respiratory infections due to *Bordetella pertussis* and other *Bordetella* subspecies," *Clinical Microbiology Reviews*, vol. 18, no. 2, pp. 326–382, 2005.

[75] D. A. Relman, M. Domenighini, E. Toumanen, R. Rappuoli, and S. Falkow, "Filamentous hemagglutinin of *Bordetella pertussis*: nucleotide sequence and crucial role in adherence," *Proceedings of the National Academy of Sciences of the United States of America*, vol. 86, no. 8, pp. 2637–2641, 1989.

[76] D. A. Relman, E. T. Tuomanen, S. Falkow, D. T. Golenbock, K. Saukkonen, and S. D. Wright, "Recognition of a bacterial adhesin by an integrin: macrophage CR3 (αMβ2, CD11b/CD18) binds filamentous hemagglutinin of *Bordetella pertussis*," *Cell*, vol. 61, no. 7, pp. 1375–1382, 1990.

[77] E. Tuomanen, H. Towbin, G. Rosenfelder et al., "Receptor analogs and monoclonal antibodies that inhibit adherence of *Bordetella pertussis* to human ciliated respiratory epithelial cells," *The Journal of Experimental Medicine*, vol. 168, no. 1, pp. 267–277, 1988.

[78] K. Saukkonen, C. Cabellos, M. Burroughs, S. Prasad, and E. Tuomanen, "Integrin-mediated localization of *Bordetella pertussis* within macrophages: role in pulmonary colonization," *Journal of Experimental Medicine*, vol. 173, no. 5, pp. 1143–1149, 1991.

[79] S. M. Prasad, Y. Yin, E. Rodzinski, E. I. Tuomanen, and H. R. Masure, "Identification of a carbohydrate recognition domain in filamentous hemagglutinin from *Bordetella pertussis*," *Infection and Immunity*, vol. 61, no. 7, pp. 2780–2785, 1993.

[80] P. A. Cotter, M. H. Yuk, S. Mattoo et al., "Filamentous hemag-glutinin of *Bordetella bronchiseptica* is required for efficient establishment of tracheal colonization," *Infection and Immunity*, vol. 66, no. 12, pp. 5921–5929, 1998.

[81] C. Gallego, M. P. Patiño, N. Martínez, and C. A. Iregui, *Prevention of Disease and Lesions Caused by P. multocida in Rabbits by Using Carbohydrates*, European Society of Clinical Microbiology and Infectious Diseases, Barcelona, Spain, 2014.

[82] N. Sharon, "Lectins: carbohydrate-specific reagents and biolog-ical recognition molecules," *The Journal of Biological Chemistry*, vol. 282, no. 5, pp. 2753–2764, 2007.

21

Environmental Attributes to Respiratory Diseases of Small Ruminants

Anu Rahal,[1] Abul Hasan Ahmad,[2] Atul Prakash,[1] Rajesh Mandil,[1] and Aruna T. Kumar[3]

[1] *Department of Veterinary Pharmacology and Toxicology, Uttar Pradesh Pandit Deen Dayal Upadhyaya Pashu Chikitsa Vigyan Vishwavidyalaya Evam Go-Anusandhan Sansthan (DUVASU), Mathura 281001, India*
[2] *Department of Veterinary Pharmacology and Toxicology, Govind Ballabh Pant University of Agriculture & Technology, Pantnagar 263145, India*
[3] *Directorate of Information and Publications of Agriculture, KAB-I, New Delhi 110012, India*

Correspondence should be addressed to Anu Rahal; rahalanu72@gmail.com

Academic Editor: Amit Kumar

Respiratory diseases are the major disease crisis in small ruminants. A number of pathogenic microorganisms have been implicated in the development of respiratory disease but the importance of environmental factors in the initiation and progress of disease can never be overemphasized. They irritate the respiratory tree producing stress in the microenvironment causing a decline in the immune status of the small ruminants and thereby assisting bacterial, viral, and parasitic infections to break down the tissue defense barriers. Environmental pollutants cause acute or chronic reactions as they deposit on the alveolar surface which are characterized by inflammation or fibrosis and the formation of transitory or persistent tissue manifestation. Some of the effects of exposures may be immediate, whereas others may not be evident for many decades. Although the disease development can be portrayed as three sets of two-way communications (pathogen-environment, host-environment, and host-pathogen), the interactions are highly variable. Moreover, the environmental scenario is never static; new compounds are introduced daily making a precise evaluation of the disease burden almost impossible. The present review presents a detailed overview of these interactions and the ultimate effect on the respiratory health of sheep and goat.

1. Introduction

Indian livestock sector has emerged as one of the key components of national as well as agricultural growth with an annual contribution of 3.93% (2,41,177 crore) of national GDP and 22.14% share in the agricultural GDP. Today, India ranks first with respect to buffalo, second in cattle and goats, and third in sheep population in comparison to the world livestock population [1]. It also provides self-employment opportunities to almost 6.7% of rural work force. Presently, livestock sector holds a substantial share in fulfillment of human food demand and this share is expected to further get doubled by 2030 [2]. To discharge this increasing demand of livestock products, it is essential that India increases the animal population, improves feed conversion efficiency, implements better reproductive policy, and overall improves the livestock health and productivity, that is, excess use of drugs as food additives, fattening agents, prophylactic antipathogenic drugs, boosters of reproductivity, and so forth. The attempt to increase livestock products (meat, eggs, and milk) production has also resulted in the production, accumulation, and dumping of large amounts of different kinds of wastes or pollutants in the environment all over the world. Aerosolization of microbial pathogens, endotoxins, drug residues, pesticides, offensive odour, and dust particles are all inevitable consequences of the generation and handling of waste material of the food production process, originating from animals. For optimizing livestock productivity, it is mandatory that small ruminant rearers realize that they form the front for identification and prophylaxis of entry of disease-causing agents (pathogens) into production systems [3–5] for a reduction in current on-farm vulnerabilities, upgrading food safety and food security, and enhancing their competence for production of a safer and wholesome product [6].

Broadly, the term "environmental pollution" refers to presence of any agent or a chemical in the environment of an individual which is potentially hazardous to either the environmental or individual's health. As such, environmental pollutants may take many forms: chemicals, organisms, and biological materials, as well as energy in its various forms (e.g., noise, radiation, and heat). The actual number of potential pollutants is therefore incalculable. Less than 1% of these pollutants have been subjected to a detailed appraisal in terms of their toxicity and health risks [7]. Furthermore, environmental conditions are never static; they undergo change over time and rare events may occur which may produce long-term health consequences in the exposed living populations. Such interactions between pathogens, their hosts, and novel environments may alleviate or compound the individual pathological responses, ultimately affecting its viability and contributing to insidious persistence or ultimate destruction of life. A suitable example may be the effect of abiotic factors which include insularity, climate, and volcanism on the prevalence and severity of disease in free-ranging sheep on Hawaii's Island [8].

Respiratory diseases are the major disease crisis in small ruminants [9, 10]. A number of epidemiological surveys have established the presence of the principal respiratory viruses and bacteria in majority of respiratory outbreaks. Repeated attempts have been made to tackle these outbreaks by prior vaccination but only limited success has been achieved. The present review discusses the contributions of environmental factors to initiation and progression of respiratory diseases in small ruminants.

2. Respiratory System of Small Ruminants

The respiratory tract of an adult goat comes into contact with approximately 7-8 liters of air per minute, that is, 11,000 liters of air in a day. Thus, the quality of inhaled air has major implications on the respiratory health of the animals. The respiratory system of sheep and goats is quite adaptable against a plethora of air contaminants [11] but disruption of defensive mechanisms to get rid of inhaled material may occur if an individual is exposed to highly concentrated particles in certain situations or if an exposure occurs during strenuous labour. Airborne contaminants may then serve as a primary cause of respiratory disease or can exacerbate a preexisting respiratory conditions or pulmonary disease. Depending on the inhaled substance, acute or chronic reactions occur as particles are deposited on the alveolar surface. Acute reactions are characterized by swelling (oedema) and inflammation [12], while chronic reactions are characterized by connective tissue scarring (fibrosis) and the formation of specific aggregates of immune cells (granulomas) [13]. Some of the effects of exposures may be immediate, whereas others such as lung disease related to asbestos deposits may not present for many decades [14].

3. Factors Affecting Development of Diseases

The production of disease in an animal is determined by three basic factors: the host, the pathogen, and the environment

[15]. The relationship between these three factors can best be represented in the form of a triangle. It is the balance between these three components that decides the initiation and progress of disease. For initiating disease development, an interaction between a highly virulent pathogen and a susceptible host in a disease favourable environment is required. The environment plays a major role in modulating the virulence of the pathogen [16–18] as well as reducing the host defence [19] and thus increasing the susceptibility of the host. A pathogenic agent can certainly gain entry into the animal body and initiate disease development process but the immune system of host can phagocytise the pathogen (e.g., by secreting chemical factors) and thus check the disease progress. On contrary to this, the host can also influence the environment by alterations in the microclimate requirements for disease production for example, abrasions, wound, malnutrition, path physiological conditions, and immunocompromised status [20]. A thorough consideration of interactions amongst these factors allows assessment of risk for disease outbreaks and intervention to reduce the amount of disease.

The severity of onset of clinical disease in the host is decided chiefly by the pathogenicity of the prevalent population of the pathogen. The term pathogenicity includes both virulence and aggressiveness. The adaptation mechanisms of the pathogen to the altered environmental factors play an important role in determining its survival in the host and the environment as a whole. The reduction in heterozygosity in disease resistance genes of bighorn sheep (*O. canadensis*) populations has been associated with highest lungworm parasite loads [21] as compared to domestic sheep which with a lengthier period of local adaptation and enhanced vigor might have also conferred resistance to common parasitic diseases. *Muellerius* spp. infections also typically do not produce clinical disease in domestic sheep [22] but may be more pathogenic in nonadapted hosts such as bighorn [23, 24] and possibly mouflon [25].

The foremost host factor affecting disease development is the presence of susceptible animals in the population. If the host population is largely susceptible to the pathogen in the vicinity, the disease may have the privilege to get transformed into an epidemic. The key player in determining the susceptibility to any pathogen is the immune status of the animal which, in turn, relies on number of environmental variables for its fluctuations. The preceding immune status of the host is frequently critical in determining the occurrence of disease; for example, low virulence pathogens usually produce clinical disease only in immunocompromised hosts while highly virulent pathogens may show morbidity even in healthy host. Animals whose lungs are already compromised from previous diseases usually fall prey to toxicity by leukotoxins and lipopolysaccharides, both potent toxins that, in high levels, act as chemotactic factors for inflammatory cells and promote inflammation and severe lung damage [26]. In kids, such acute outbreaks can occur with low morbidity rates but high mortality rates.

While lungworm infestations in sheep are quite common, the severity of lung lesions was observed only in sheep regularly exposed to high concentrations of volcanic gases after the eruption of Kīlauea in 2008 which may have contributed to immunocompromised lung health, reduced resistance to parasitic infections, and increased susceptibility for severe inflammatory reactions [8]. Such severity of disease is also observed in conjunction with bacterial and/or viral infections or other stress factors characteristic of bighorn sheep pneumonia complex [27–29].

4. Environmental Variables

Environmental variables have conventionally been accepted as the major determinants for disease development (Figure 1). Even the traditional and chemical disease prophylactic and therapeutic control measures employ this concept for manoeuvring the environment to make it less congenial for disease progress. The prevalence of lung disease is unevenly distributed over the world [30] and can be traced down to regional environmental challenges along with other factors such as nutrition. As it is difficult to assess the prevalence, duration, and amount of exposure, the precise risk each environment factor poses is hard to define. Wildlife species of European mouflon sheep (*Ovis gmelini musimon*) translocated to Hawaiian Islands for sport hunting provided a unique opportunity to understand how disease processes may be affected by environmental conditions [8].

5. Aerographic Conditions

The aerographic conditions commonly include the state of atmospheric air in terms of temperature, wind velocity, clouds, precipitation, and volcanic eruptions. The prevailing climatic conditions have a major impact on the survival of the pathogens [31]. An alteration in weather conditions of a geographical area has always witnessed an outburst of infectious diseases and has been labelled as predisposer of disease epidemics. Small ruminants are well adapted to extreme temperatures, with their body hair coats providing insulation against cold and heat [32]. Sheep, in general, are more susceptible than goats to high temperatures and humidity [33]. Any alteration in the environmental temperature affects the incubation period, the life cycle (the time between infection and sporulation), and the contagious period (the time during which the pathogen continues to propagate the infection amongst the population). At higher temperatures the life cycle of the pathogen usually gets speeded up with the result that epidemics develop at a faster rate. Under cooler conditions, the pathogens develop dormancy and the progress of epidemic is slower leading to a decline in incidence as well as severity of disease.

High humidity increases the risk of heat stress at any air temperature. The heat index (temperature + humidity) is considered as a more accurate measure of heat stress (hyperthermia) by veterinarians than temperature alone [34]. Heat stress lowers the natural immune defense of animals, thus, making them more susceptible to disease. An increase in the incidence of pneumonia is a common observation in extremely hot weather [35]. The resistance to parasitic and other opportunistic diseases is also reduced. *P. multocida* often exists as a commensal in the upper respiratory tracts of majority of livestock species and has also been identified as the most frequently isolated bacteria from pneumonic lung [36] but the importance of predisposing factors in the development of pneumonia can never be overestimated.

Moisture also influences outbreak of respiratory diseases caused by microorganisms like bacteria and fungi and nematodes [37]. The influence of rain splash and running water on dispersal of pathogen is also important for explosive nature of the disease [38]. Free water or the collision of raindrops facilitates the dissemination of many fungi and nearly all bacteria. It is a useful adaptation for a pathogen that facilitates dispersal and germination as well as establishment of infection in the host. Pathogens like fungi and nematodes require a latent period for germination of spores and setting up of infection in the host animal. As both these processes are time taking as well as unavoidable for disease initiation, the duration of persistence of favourable climatic conditions has an important influence on infection.

In addition, the dissemination and resulting concentration of the pollutant may vary significantly depending on the prevailing (e.g., meteorological) conditions at that time. Patterns of atmospheric dispersion, for example, change not only in relation to wind speed and direction but also temperature inversion effect and atmospheric stability [39]. Statistically significant relationship was found between incidence of pneumonia as a cause of lamb death and climatic factors such as rainfall, humidity, and intensity and direction of wind [40].

Animal housing is also an important consideration in evaluating the impact of outdoor aerographic conditions on the health of the animals. Animals living indoors are less likely to be affected by rain and thunderstorms but poor ventilation and unhygienic barns are usually associated with severe outbreaks of respiratory diseases. The grazing goats have been reported to show about 2-3-fold higher morbidity as compared to the stall-fed animals [41]. Amongst the indoor factors responsible for microbial pollution the most important is the animal itself and its bedding material. Confinement of circulating air also prevents dissemination of the microbial load and hence facilitates the disease initiation. The moisture content of the bedding material may further assist in production of spores and metabolites of different bacterial and fungal strains resulting in a chronic inflammatory and immunosuppressive response.

6. Climate

Climate is the statistical information that expresses the variation of weather at a given place for a specified interval of time. Climate change is likely to directly affect the physiological profile of animal by altering the homeostasis and other thermoregulatory functions and hence its health and productivity. Climate may also influence health of animals indirectly by disturbing the nutritional supply thus, decreasing resistance to diseases and pests.

Impact of Climate Change. Inter-Governmental Panel on Climate Change has projected that global earth temperature will increase by 1.8–4.0°C by the end of this century [42].

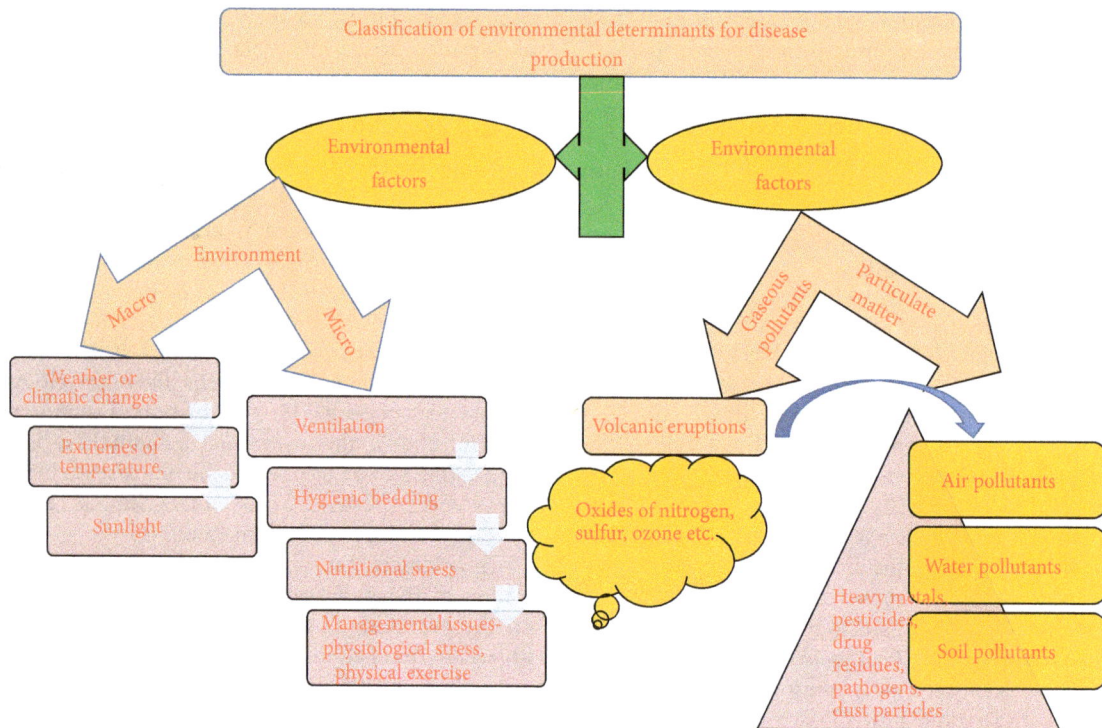

FIGURE 1: Classification of environmental determinants for disease production.

This increase in global temperature could potentially cause scarcity of water and food resources and dissemination of infectious diseases and heat-related deaths. The significance of temperature is further promoted in context of temperate regions as compared to the tropics, where temperatures are relatively uniform throughout the year [43]. Further, the subsequent climatic changes are expected to increase the possibility of vector-borne and other diseases and transformation in pattern of disease transmission. The maximum effect of climatic variation on transmission of disease is likely to occur at the lower and upper limits (14–18 and 35–40°C, resp.) of the range of temperature at which the transmission of infection takes place [44]. Rise in temperature and alterations in rainfall pattern will favor the disbursal of vector populations to unforeseen areas (higher altitude or temperate zones) [45]. In the tropics, diurnal oscillations in temperature are greater than the seasonal fluctuations, inducing many pathogens to sporulate by the combination of the decrease in temperature and the increase in humidity at night. The occurrence of Bluetongue in Europe and Rift Valley Fever in goats in East Africa are two well-documented examples of increased vector-borne disease risk in goats associated with climate change [46]. Further, microbial pathogens as well as their vectors may also show sensitivity to factors such as temperature, humidity, rainfall, ground water, wind velocity, and changes in vegetation and are bound to have an impact on emerging and reemerging infections of livestock. In a study conducted in Avikanagar (Rajasthan, India), cold stress along with frost and poor ventilation has been found to predispose lambs to E. coli-borne septicemia with major involvement of upper respiratory tract and lungs [47].

7. Atmospheric Pollution

Atmospheric pollution remains a major health hazard to all the living species throughout the world and shares about 8-9% of the total disease burden [7], but the risk is higher in developing countries, where poverty, lack of modern technology, and weak environmental legislation further substantiate the risk. The lungs serve as common interface between the animal body and the air environment in its close vicinity. Consequently, the lungs become a frequent dumping site for airborne pollutants. Thousands of environmental toxins and commercial chemicals such as heavy metals and pesticides are now in use, the particles of which may persist in the atmosphere as aerosol, fibres, fumes, mists, or dust. The effects of polluted air on domestic animals principally can either be caused by the indoor environment and by outdoor air pollution. Goats and, to a lesser extent, sheep are reared indoors but their indoor environment is quite comparable with the outdoor air conditions. Therefore, outdoor pollution is considered more important than the indoor pollution. Indoor pollution gains further significance in case of animals kept in overcrowded premises or in poor hygiene or ventilation.

7.1. Epidemiology of Atmospheric Pollution. Exposures to pollutants may occur through a number of pathways and exposure processes. Inhalation of environmental pollutants is generally over a considerable period of time and thus usually elicits health issues on chronic basis, but occasional inhalation of solid particles deposited from industrial exhaust on pasture land may directly cause an acute response. The increased incidence of pasture originated disease can be attributed to their short stature due to which they breathe closer to the ground as compared to cattle and hence are more likely to inhale the solid particulates deposited on the pasture. The lesions produced in small ruminants such as sheep and goat due to air pollution are chiefly inflammatory in nature as was observed in 1952 smog disaster (London, UK) that increased respiratory tract hyperresponsiveness and ultimately resulted in respiratory distress (and right-sided heart failure) of cattle that were housed in the city [48] owing to high level of sulphur dioxide. Owing to high solubility sulphur dioxide mainly irritates the anterior air passage characterised by acute bronchiolitis and the accompanying emphysema.

7.2. Interplay between Atmospheric Pollution and Health. The relationship between pollution and health is both a multifaceted and conditional process. For pollutants to have an adverse effect on health, susceptible individuals must receive a minimal dose of the pollutant, or its metabolite, over a period sufficient to trigger detectable symptoms. Pollutants rarely occur in isolation; typically they exist in combination [7]. Exposures are therefore not singular rather a mixture of pollutants, often with varied origins, some of which may have additive or synergistic effects [49, 50]. Unravelling the effects of individual pollutants is a herculean challenge that has yet to be adequately resolved in many areas of environmental toxicology. Individual pollutants may be implicated in a wide range of health effects, whereas few diseases can directly be attributed to a single pollutant. Long latent intervals, cumulative exposures, and multiple exposures to different pollutants which might act synergistically all create difficulties in unravelling associations between environmental pollution and health. Health consequences of environmental pollution are thus unpredictable, even for pollutants that are inherently lethal; the ultimate outcome will depend on the coincidence of both the discharge and dispersion processes that determine the rate of appearance and dilution of the pollutant in the environment.

7.3. Mechanism of Atmospheric Pollutants. Irrespective of the origin, the ultimate health hazard imposed by all pollutants depends upon their persistence, mobility, biotransformation, and their toxicity profile. The problems associated with the release of persistent pollutants like chlorinated pesticide, DDT (Dichlorodiphenyltrichloroethane), into the environment were highlighted with recognition of the global extent of contamination and a wide-range of environmental and health effects [51]. The signature movement in this regard took long back in 1962 when an American biologist, Rachel Carson, published a book, Silent Spring, and resulted in a large public protest that eventually led to a ban on agricultural use of DDT in the USA in 1972. This book detailed the environmental impacts of the indiscriminate spraying of DDT in the USA and questioned the logic of releasing large amounts of chemicals into the environment without fully understanding their effects on ecology or human health. Similar stories are now around the world in respect to chlorofluorocarbons and other atmospheric pollutants that are accepted as greenhouse gases or scavengers of stratospheric ozone [52] and perhaps also endocrine disruptors [53].

7.4. Factors Affecting Pollutants Severity. Mere persistent nature of a pollutant does not endorse the health risk; its presence in a form that is accessible to the lungs is also important to produce respiratory disease. The development of environmentally induced lung disease is a function of the intensity and duration of the exposure as well as the inherent toxicity of the inhaled substance and susceptibility of the host. The physical status of the inhaled substance (solid, fume, or mixture), the particle size, and other physicochemical characteristics (like solubility) principally determine the initial location of disease development. Smaller particles (0.1 to 1.0 μ) are more likely to reach the lung alveoli, but airborne particles up to 5 microns in size may also do so. In general, larger particles (10 μ or greater) are trapped and removed by the mucus and cilia of the upper respiratory tract. Inorganic mercury is persistent but less toxic and less readily bioavailable than methyl mercury, which gets converted naturally through chemical reactions by microorganisms [54, 55]. Conversely, many solid wastes pose little risk as long as they remain in their original form. The problem arises when their decomposition takes place, either because the decomposition products are inherently more toxic or because they show an increased accessibility to the respiratory system.

Ventilation is often a managemental problem for indoor sheep and goat farming. High level of ammonia is a common finding in the indoor atmosphere of small ruminants. Ammonia is a highly hydrosoluble respiratory toxicant which causes chronic dyspnea and clinical pictures consistent with restrictive lung dysfunction, obstructive lung disease, and bronchial hyperreactivity [56].

7.5. Types of Atmospheric Pollutants. Dumping of waste materials of either chemical or biological origin represents a major source of air pollution, though final release into the wider environment may only occur when these materials decompose or break up.

7.5.1. Particulate Matter. Respirable particles of air pollutants and gaseous agents affect different parts of the respiratory tree depending upon their inherent characteristics [57]. For particulate pollutants, particle size is more important while for gasses, relative solubility is important. In a study conducted on Hawaii Island, higher incidence of pathological lesions has been documented in lungworm infested sheep that were exposed to gaseous emissions from Kīlauea Volcano in contrast to lungworm infested sheep not in vicinity of volcanic discharges though latter had significantly more upper respiratory tract inflammation and hyperplasia suggestive of chronic antigenic stimulation, possibly associated with exposure to fine airborne particulates owing to reduced plant ground cover during extended drought conditions [8].

7.5.2. Gaseous Pollutants. Probably, gasses from Kīlauea Volcano such as sulfur dioxide contributed to severity of respiratory disease principally associated with chronic lungworm infections at Mauna Loa. Sulphur dioxide, because it is highly water soluble, initially affects the upper airway, while ozone, with its medium solubility, initially affects the middle airways and nitrogen dioxide, with its low solubility, initially affects the lower airways.

To affect the respiratory tree, the gaseous pollutants must be inhaled in a sufficient volume so that a minimal alveolar concentration is reached. Thereafter, the toxic potency of the pollutant will decide the degree of damage. Different physiological and environmental factors will also exert an influence on the overall toxicity; for example, physiological stress, metabolic acidosis, hypoxia, hypotension, hyponatremia, or hypomagnesaemia will potentiate the toxicity while CNS excitation or hypernatremia will subdue the hazard.

7.5.3. Microbial Contaminants. Bacterial infections in a sheep and goat farm are a common clinical and subclinical finding [58–60]. Some common respiratory commensal bacteria include *Pasteurella* spp. [36], *Staphylococcus* spp., *Streptococcus pneumoniae* [61], *Arcanobacterium pyogenes*, *Haemophilus* spp., and *Klebsiella pneumonia* while the common mycoplasmas isolated from sheep and goats are *Mycoplasma capricolum* subsp. *capripneumoniae* (a causal agent of caprine contagious pleuropneumonia), *M. mycoides* subsp. *capri* (involved in contagious agalactia syndrome), *M. bovis* [62], and *M. ovipneumoniae* [63]. Out of these, *M. ovipneumoniae* is one of the most important mycoplasmas involved in the respiratory diseases of sheep. Combined effects of ammonia and bacterial endotoxins predispose the animals to respiratory infections with viruses and bacteria, both primary pathogenic as well as opportunistic species. Although food producing animals appear to be capable of maintaining a high level of efficient growth in spite of marked degrees of respiratory disease [64], at a certain level of respiratory insufficiency rapid growth can no longer be attained. In that case the production results will be uneconomically. The viral infections also predispose the host to bacterial infection by a direct damage to respiratory clearance mechanisms and lung parenchyma, facilitating translocation of bacteria from the upper respiratory tract and establishment of infection in compromised lung and secondly, by interfering with the immune system's ability to respond to bacterial infection [65, 66].

8. Oxidative Stress as Predisposer

Respiratory diseases in sheep and goats are generally an outcome from physiological stress with viral and bacterial infections and adverse weather exposure [67]. Predisposing causes [68] are generally synergistic and include age, stress (comingling, weather, nutritional changes, etc.), and immunological background. Environmental risk factors include climate, ambient temperature, dust particles, stocking density, humidity, ventilation, and shipping distance.

Oxidative stress is a normal physiological phenomenon [69]. Under normal conditions, the physiologically important intracellular levels of reactive oxygen species (ROS) are maintained at a minimal requisite level by various enzyme systems participating in the *in vivo* redox homeostasis. Stress

is one of the basic requirements for disease development (Figure 2) [69, 70].

It can have several origins like environmental extremes for example, cold, heat, hypoxia, physical exercise, or malnutrition. Stress can also be categorized on the basis of duration and onset as acute and chronic stress. The stress due to exposure of cold or heat is generally acute and temporary and is released with the removal of cause. Similarly stress due to physical exercises or complete immobilization [71] is also acute in nature but nutritional and environmental stresses usually persist for a longer period of time. Dust, transporting, weaning, handling, mingling with infected animals, overcrowding, dehorning, and castration all add to the onset of disease. Decreasing the number of stress factors associated with a disease is also an important step in prevention. The less an animal is exposed to the stress factors, the more likely it will maintain an integral immune system to defend itself against infectious organisms [72]. Oxidative stress resulting from persistent inflammation due to an inhaled irritant can be the major factor involved in the change of the dynamics of immune responses of the respiratory system. These alterations can create an immunological chaos that could lead to loss of architectural integrity of cells and tissues ultimately leading to chronic conditions or cancers [73, 74].

The significant contribution of predisposing factors in the development of pneumonic lung owing to commensal pasteurella infection is well known [36]. A primary infection with *Mycoplasma ovipneumoniae* is frequently isolated from pneumonic sheep, but it can also be found in the respiratory tracts of healthy animals [75]. Nevertheless, it may predispose sheep to invasion of the lower respiratory tract by other organisms such as the parainfluenza-3 virus and *Mannheimia haemolytica* [76, 77]. Few reports also implicate *Mycoplasma ovipneumoniae* as a cause of severe respiratory disease in goats [78, 79]. Occurrence of clinical respiratory disease due to these pathogens is associated with poor management practices and occur as a consequence of severe stress for example, transportation stress, viral infections (e.g., parainfluenza-3 virus), lung parasites, prior bacterial infections, overcrowded pens, poor housing conditions, sudden environmental changes, and other stressful conditions.

9. Prophylactic and Therapeutic Management

The first step in preventing environmentally related lung disease is to recognize the exposure-disease relationship. Then, primary prevention may be accomplished with a reduction, modification, or elimination of the exposure or environment. Other interventions require global approach to prioritize and target environmental modifications with public health policy implications. Educating about the ill effects of air pollution is also an important aspect of prevention of environmentally induced lung disease.

Broad spectrum antibacterial agents may be effective in treating bacterial infections in sheep and goats and may include fluoroquinolones such as enrofloxacin, ciprofloxacin, florfenicol, and ceftiofur along with suitable anti-inflammatory agents [80–83]. While selecting the drug

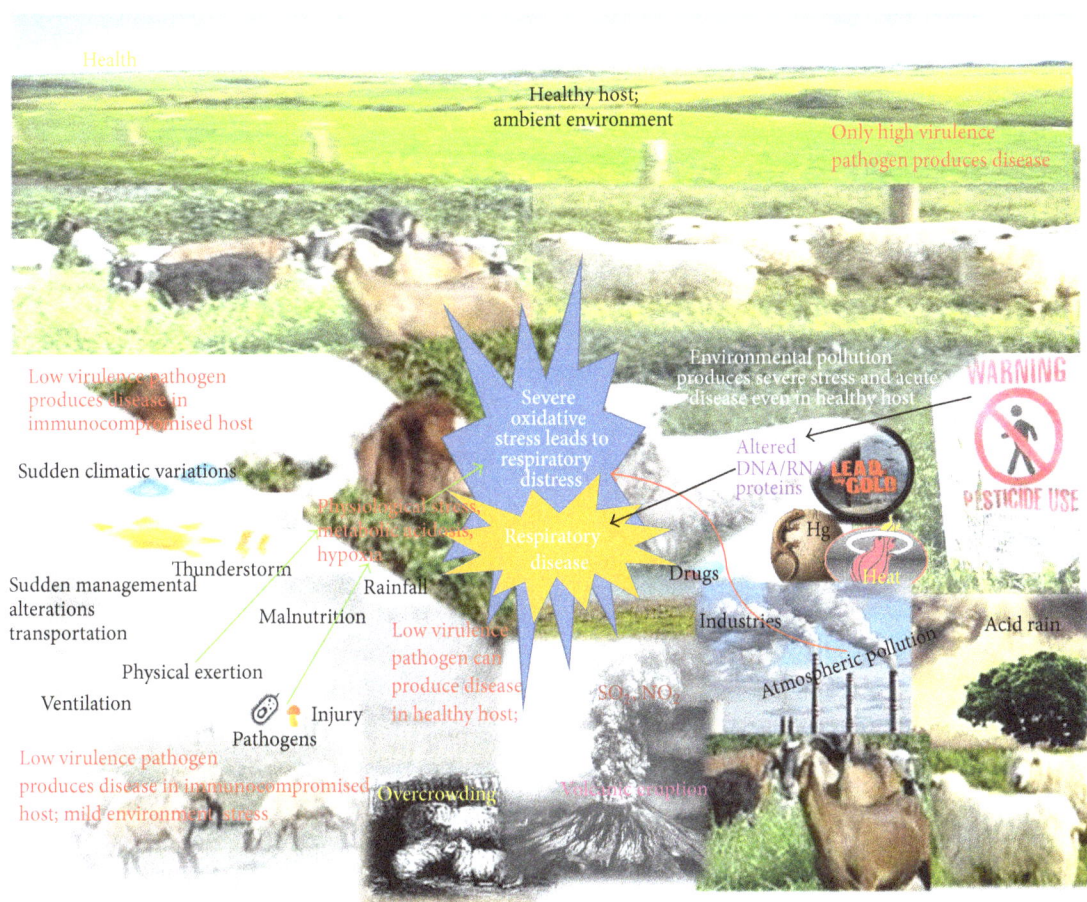

FIGURE 2: Environmental attributes to oxidative stress leading to initiation and progress of respiratory diseases.

combinations and their respective dosage regimen, drug interaction should to be considered in view of the pathophysiological status of the animal [84]. Several natural feed components have received great attention in the last two decades, and several biological activities showing promising anti-inflammatory, antioxidant, and antiapoptotic-modulatory potential have been identified [85–87]. Plants such as *Ocimum sanctum* have been used for ages to prevent and cure viral infection of man and animals [88].

Interleukin-1beta (IL-1beta) and tumor necrosis factor-alpha (TNF-alpha) have been proven to mediate the development of numerous inflammatory lung diseases [74]. A number of common indigenous plants such as *Cimicifuga racemosa*, *Mimosa pudica*, and so forth have shown excellent anti-inflammatory potential and can be added to regular feeding schedule of small ruminants for prophylaxis [86]. Zinc supplementation has been found to shorten duration of severe pneumonia in human infants. Perhaps, zinc as an adjuvant hastens recovery and reduces antimicrobial resistance [89]. Antioxidant supplements also seem to modulate the impact of ozone and particulates pollutants on lung function [90]. Vitamin C and E may blunt effect of ozone on lung function but do not seem to prevent symptoms.

10. Conclusions

Although the disease development can be described as three sets of two-way communications (pathogen-environment, host-environment, and host-pathogen), this is a generalization. All three groups of factors interact in a highly variable manner in any real life scenario, often in nonlinear ways that are difficult to compute and forecast.

Estimating the contribution of environmental pollution to the burden of disease is far from simple. The global atmospheric pollution scenario is too difficult to classify and define completely. Moreover, it is never static; new pollutants are being introduced to the air every day and too little is known about their interactions with respiratory health, or about their levels of exposure, to make reliable toxicity appraisal. These difficulties are more pronounced in developed countries, where disease surveillance, reporting of mortality, environmental monitoring, and population data systems are all relatively well approved. Still precise evaluation of the disease burden is yet worth the endeavour.

The animal biodiversity available in our country is a virtual goldmine of germplasm. Some of the indigenous breed of livestock like Jamunapari goat have unique characteristics of adaptability to adverse agroclimatic conditions, better disease tolerance, feed conversion efficiency, and zero managemental requirements. Therefore, maintain a livestock population that is sustainable in the present everday changing climatic scenario is a challenging task, which would require a change in breeding policy, perpetuating disease resistant and climate adaptable traits, capacity building, and regional and global cooperation.

Conflict of Interests

The authors declare that there is no conflict of interests in publication of this work.

References

[1] *19th Livestock Census Report*, The Hindu Business Line, 2012.

[2] WHO, "Global and regional food consumption patterns and trends," 2013, http://www.who.int/nutrition/topics/3_foodconsumption/en/index7.html.

[3] U. A. Madden, "Animal health challenges encountered resulting from disasters and emergencies," *Caprine Chronicle*, vol. 23, pp. 6–7, 2008.

[4] U. A. Madden, "Keys for small ruminant producers purchasing and raising goats and sheep," *The Journal of Extension*, vol. 48, Article ID 3TOT10, 2010, http://www.joe.org/2010june/tt10.php.

[5] J. Barnes, J. C. Meche, D. A. Hatch, and G. Dixon, "Strengthening agricultural entrepreneurship: a grant writing tool for agricultural producers," *Journal of Extension*, vol. 47, no. 1, Article ID 1TOT4, 2009.

[6] U. A. Madden, "Addressing food safety and security on farms," *Caprine Chronicle*, vol. 2, pp. 6–7, 2007.

[7] D. Briggs, "Environmental pollution and the global burden of disease," *British Medical Bulletin*, vol. 68, pp. 1–24, 2003.

[8] J. G. Powers, C. G. Duncan, T. R. Spraker et al., "Environmental conditions associated with lesions in introduced free-ranging sheep in Hawai," *Pacific Sciences*, vol. 68, pp. 65–74, 2013.

[9] A. Traore and R. T. Wilson, "Epidemiology and ecopathology of respiratory diseases of small ruminants in semi-arid West Africa," in *Proceedings of the International Livestock Research Institute Conference (ILRI '89)*, 1989, http://www.ilri.org/InfoServ/Webpub/fulldocs/X5489B/X5489B0Z.HTM.

[10] F. Vallerand and R. Branckaert, "La race ovine Djallonké au Cameroun: potentialités zootechniques, conditions d'élevage, avenir," *Revue d'élevage et de Médecine Vétérinaire des Pays Tropicaux*, vol. 28, pp. 423–518, 1975.

[11] http://www.fass.org/docs/agguide3rd/Chapter10.pdf.

[12] E. Ricciotti and G. A. Fitzgerald, "Prostaglandins and inflammation," *Arteriosclerosis, Thrombosis, and Vascular Biology*, vol. 31, no. 5, pp. 986–1000, 2011.

[13] T. A. Wynn, "Cellular and molecular mechanisms of fibrosis," *Journal of Pathology*, vol. 214, no. 2, pp. 199–210, 2008.

[14] L. Braun and S. Kisting, "Asbestos-related disease in South Africa: the social production of an invisible epidemic," *The American Journal of Public Health*, vol. 96, no. 8, pp. 1386–1396, 2006.

[15] A. Engering, L. Hogerwerfand, and J. Slingenbergh, "Pathogen-host-environment interplay and disease emergence," *Emerging Microbes Infections*, vol. 2, p. e5, 2013.

[16] M. J. Kuehn and N. C. Kesty, "Bacterial outer membrane vesicles and the host-pathogen interaction," *Genes & Development*, vol. 19, no. 22, pp. 2645–2655, 2005.

[17] L. Jelsbak, L. E. Thomsen, I. Wallrodt, P. R. Jensen, and J. E. Olsen, "Polyamines are required for virulence in *Salmonella enterica* serovar typhimurium," *PLoS ONE*, vol. 7, no. 4, Article ID e36149, 2012.

[18] J. L. Martínez and F. Baquero, "Interactions among strategies associated with bacterial infection: pathogenicity, epidemicity, and antibiotic resistance," *Clinical Microbiology Reviews*, vol. 15, no. 4, pp. 647–679, 2002.

[19] J. H. Madenspacher, K. M. Azzam, K. M. Gowdy et al., "p53 integrates host defense and cell fate during bacterial pneumonia," *Journal of Experimental Medicine*, vol. 210, pp. 891–904, 2013.

[20] C. G. Becker, D. Rodriguez, A. V. Longo, A. L. Talaba, and K. R. Zamudio, "Disease risk in temperate amphibian populations is higher at closed-canopy sites," *PLoS ONE*, vol. 7, Article ID e48205, 2012.

[21] G. Luikart, K. Pilgrim, J. Visty, V. O. Ezenwa, and M. K. Schwartz, "Candidate gene microsatellite variation is associated with parasitism in wild bighorn sheep," *Biology Letters*, vol. 4, no. 2, pp. 228–231, 2008.

[22] D. Pugh, *Sheep and Goat Medicine*, WB Saunders Company, Philadelphia, Pa, USA, 1st edition, 2002.

[23] M. J. Pybus and H. Shave, "*Muellerius capillaris* (Mueller, 1889) (Nematoda: Protostrongylidae): an unusual finding in Rocky Mountain bighorn sheep (*Ovis canadensis* canadensis Shaw) in South Dakota," *Journal of Wildlife Diseases*, vol. 20, no. 4, pp. 284–288, 1984.

[24] J. C. Demartini and R. B. Davies, "An epizootic of pneumonia in captive bighorn sheep infected with *Muellerius sp*," *Journal of Wildlife Diseases*, vol. 13, no. 2, pp. 117–124, 1977.

[25] M. S. Panayotova-Pencheva and M. T. Alexandrov, "Some pathological features of lungs from domestic and wild ruminants with single and mixed protostrongylid infections," *Veterinary Medicine International*, vol. 2010, Article ID 741062, 9 pages, 2010.

[26] L. Zecchinon, T. Fett, and D. Desmecht, "How *Mannheimia haemolytica* defeats host defence through a kiss of death mechanism," *Veterinary Research*, vol. 36, no. 2, pp. 133–156, 2005.

[27] D. J. Forrester, "Bighorn sheep lung worm pneumonia complex," in *Parasitic Diseases of Wild Mammals*, W. M. Samuel, M. J. Pybus, and A. A. Kocan, Eds., pp. 158–173, Iowa State University Press, Ames, Iowa, USA, 1971.

[28] R. J. Monello, D. L. Murray, and E. F. Cassirer, "Ecological correlates of pneumonia epizootics in bighorn sheep herds," *Canadian Journal of Zoology*, vol. 79, no. 8, pp. 1423–1432, 2001.

[29] T. R. Spraker, C. P. Hibler, G. G. Schoonveld, and W. S. Adney, "Pathologic changes and microorganisms found in bighorn sheep during a stress-related die-off," *Journal of Wildlife Diseases*, vol. 20, no. 4, pp. 319–327, 1984.

[30] http://extoxnet.orst.edu/tibs/epidemio.htm.

[31] S. V. Singh, A. V. Singh, A. Kumar et al., "Survival mechanisms of *Mycobacterium avium* subspecies paratuberculosis within host species and in the environment—a review," *Natural Sciences*, vol. 5, pp. 710–723, 2013.

[32] http://awionline.org/pubs/cq/sheep.htm.

[33] http://www.aces.edu/pubs/docs/A/ANR-1316/ANR-1316.pdf.

[34] M. Hale, L. Coffey, A. Bartlett, and C. Ahrens, "Sheep: Sustainable and Organic Production," 2010, https://attra.ncat.org/attra-pub/summaries/summary.php?pub=209.

[35] R. A. Mohamed and E. B. Abdelsalam, "A review on pneumonic pasteurellosis (respiratory mannheimiosis) with emphasis on pathogenesis, virulence mechanisms and predisposing factors," *Bulgarian Journal of Veterinary Medicine*, vol. 11, pp. 139–160, 2008.

[36] M. Yesuf, H. Mazengia, and M. Chanie, "Histopathological and bacteriological examination of pneumonic lungs of small ruminants slaughtered at Gondar, Ethiopia," *Am-Europian Journal of Scientific Research*, vol. 7, pp. 226–231, 2012.

[37] R. M. Maier, I. L. Pepper, and C. P. Gerb, *Environmental Microbiology*, Academic Press, 2009.

[38] K. C. Sahoo, A. J. Tamhankar, E. Johansson, and C. S. Lundborg, "Antibiotic use, resistance development and environmental factors: a qualitative study among healthcare professionals in Orissa, India," *BMC Public Health*, vol. 10, article 629, 2010.

[39] R. Colvile and D. J. Briggs, "Dispersion modelling," in *Spatial Epidemiology. Methods and Applications*, P. Elliott, J. C. Wakefield, N. G. Best, and D. J. Briggs, Eds., pp. 375–392, Oxford University Press, 2000.

[40] D. Lacasta, L. M. Ferrer, J. J. Ramos, J. M. González, and M. de las Heras, "Influence of climatic factors on the development of pneumonia in lambs," *Small Ruminant Research*, vol. 80, no. 1–3, pp. 28–32, 2008.

[41] A. Lago, S. M. McGuirk, T. B. Bennett, N. B. Cook, and K. V. Nordlund, "Calf respiratory disease and pen microenvironments in naturally ventilated calf barns in winter," *Journal of Dairy Science*, vol. 89, no. 10, pp. 4014–4025, 2006.

[42] Intergovernmental Panel on Climate Change (IPCC), "Climate change 2007: the physical science basis. Summary for policymakers," Fourth Assessment Report of the Intergovernmental Panel on Climate Change, http://www.ipcc.ch.

[43] K. Dhama, R. Tiwari, S. Chakraborty et al., "Global warming and emerging infectious diseases of animals and humans:current scenario, challenges, solutions and future perspectives—a review," *International Journal of Current Research*, vol. 5, pp. 1942–1958, 2013.

[44] A. K. Githeko, S. W. Lindsay, U. E. Confalonieri, and J. A. Patz, "Climate change and vector-borne diseases: a regional analysis," *Bulletin of the World Health Organization*, vol. 78, no. 9, pp. 1136–1147, 2000.

[45] R. W. Sutherst, "Global change and human vulnerability to vector-borne diseases," *Clinical Microbiology Reviews*, vol. 17, no. 1, pp. 136–173, 2004.

[46] E. A. Gould and S. Higgs, "Impact of climate change and other factors on emerging arbovirus diseases," *Transactions of the Royal Society of Tropical Medicine and Hygiene*, vol. 103, no. 2, pp. 109–121, 2009.

[47] G. G. Sonawane, F. Singh, B. N. Tripathi, S. K. Dixit, J. Kumar, and A. Khan, "Investigation of an outbreak in lambs associated with *Escherichia coli* O95 septicaemia," *Veterinary Practicenor*, vol. 13, pp. 72–75, 2012.

[48] E. J. Catcott, "Effects of air pollution on animals," *Monograph Series. World Health Organization*, vol. 46, pp. 221–231, 1961.

[49] J. P. Groten, F. R. Cassee, P. J. van blander, C. De-Rosa, and V. J. Feron, *Mixture in Toxicology*, Academic Press, New York, NY, USA, 1999, Edited by M. H. Schafer, S. G. Meclelan and F. Welsch.

[50] J. E. Simmons, "Chemical mixtures: challenge for toxicology and risk assessment," *Toxicology*, vol. 105, no. 2-3, pp. 111–119, 1995.

[51] F. Bro-Rasmussen, "Contamination by persistent chemicals in food chain and human health," *Science of the Total Environment*, vol. 188, no. 1, pp. S45–S60, 1996.

[52] M. McFarland and J. Kaye, "Chlorofluorocarbons and ozone," *Photochemistry and Photobiology*, vol. 55, no. 6, pp. 911–929, 1992.

[53] M. Joffe, "Infertility and environmental pollutants," *British Medical Bulletin*, vol. 68, pp. 47–70, 2003.

[54] WHO, *Mercury, Inorganic*, vol. 118, Environmental Health Criteria, Geneva, Switzerland, 1991.

[55] K. R. Smith, J. M. Samet, I. Romieu, and N. Bruce, "Indoor air pollution in developing countries and acute lower respiratory infections in children," *Thorax*, vol. 55, no. 6, pp. 518–532, 2000.

[56] R. E. de la Hoz, D. P. Schlueter, and W. N. Rom, "Chronic lung disease secondary to ammonia inhalation injury: a report on three cases," *The American Journal of Indian Medicine*, vol. 29, pp. 209–214, 1996.

[57] M. Georgiev, A. Afonso, H. Neubauer et al., "Q fever in humans and farm animals in four European countries, 1982–2010," *Euro Surveillance*, vol. 18, no. 8, 2013.

[58] W. van der Hoek, J. C. E. Meekelenkamp, F. Dijkstra et al., "Proximity to goat farms and *Coxiella burnetii* seroprevalence among pregnant women," *Emerging Infectious Diseases*, vol. 17, no. 12, pp. 2360–2363, 2011.

[59] L. Hogerwerf, A. Courcoul, D. Klinkenberg, F. Beaudeau, E. Vergu, and M. Nielen, "Dairy goat demography and Q fever infection dynamics," *Veterinary Research*, vol. 44, article 28, 2013.

[60] A. Kumar, A. K. Verma, A. K. Sharma, and A. Rahal, "Isolation and antibiotic sensitivity of *Streptococcus pneumoniae* infections with involvement of multiple organs in lambs," *Pakistan Journal of Biological Sciences*, vol. 16, pp. 2021–2025, 2013.

[61] A. Kumar, A. K. Verma, N. K. Gangwar, and A. Rahal, "Isolation, characterization and antibiogram of *Mycoplasma bovis* in sheep pneumonia," *Asian Journal of Animal and Veterinary Advances*, vol. 7, no. 2, pp. 149–157, 2012.

[62] A. Kumar, A. K. Verma, and A. Rahal, "*Mycoplasma bovis*, a multi disease producing pathogen: an overview," *Asian Journal of Animal and Veterinary Advances*, vol. 6, no. 6, pp. 537–546, 2011.

[63] R. Nicholas, R. Ayling, and L. McAuliffe, "Respiratory diseases of small ruminants," in *Mycoplasma Diseases of Ruminants*, R. Nicholas, R. Ayling, and L. Mcauliffe, Eds., pp. 171–179, CABI, Wallingford, UK, 2008.

[64] M. R. Wilson, R. Takov, R. M. Friendship et al., "Prevalence of respiratory diseases and their association with growth rate and space in randomly selected swine herds," *Canadian Journal of Veterinary Research*, vol. 50, no. 2, pp. 209–216, 1986.

[65] S. W. Martin and J. G. Bohac, "The association between serological titers in infectious bovine rhinotracheitis virus, bovine virus diarrhea virus, parainfluenza-3 virus, respiratory syncytial virus and treatment for respiratory disease in Ontario feedlot calves," *Canadian Journal of Veterinary Research*, vol. 50, no. 3, pp. 351–358, 1986.

[66] C. J. Czuprynski, F. Leite, M. Sylte et al., "Complexities of the pathogenesis of *Mannheimia haemolytica* and *Haemophilus somnus* infections: challenges and potential opportunities for prevention?" *Animal Health Research Reviews*, vol. 5, no. 2, pp. 277–282, 2004.

[67] P. R. Scott, "Treatment and control of respiratory disease in sheep," *Veterinary Clinics of North America—Food Animal Practice*, vol. 27, no. 1, pp. 175–186, 2011.

[68] R. J. Callan and F. B. Garry, "Biosecurity and bovine respiratory disease," *Veterinary Clinics of North America—Food Animal Practice*, vol. 18, no. 1, pp. 57–77, 2002.

[69] A. Rahal, A. Kumar, V. Singh et al., "Oxidative stress, prooxidants, and antioxidants: the interplay," *BioMed Research International*, vol. 2014, Article ID 761264, 19 pages, 2014.

[70] A. H. Ahmad, A. Rahal, and A. Tripathi, "Optimising drug potential of plants," in *Proceedings of the Symposium on Recent Trends in Development of Herbal Drugs: Challenges and Opportunities and 6th Annual Conference of ISVPT*, p. 9, Ranchi, India, November 2006.

[71] A. Rahal, V. Singh, D. Mehra, S. Rajesh, and A. H. Ahmad, "Prophylactic efficacy of *Podophyllum hexandrum* in alleviation of immobilization stress induced oxidative damage in rats," *Journal of Natural Products*, vol. 2, pp. 110–115, 2009.

[72] N. Valero, J. Mosquera, G. Añez, A. Levy, R. Marcucci, and M. A. de Mon, "Differential oxidative stress induced by dengue virus in monocytes from human neonates, adult and elderly individuals," *PLoS ONE*, vol. 8, Article ID e73221, 2013.

[73] M. Khatami, "Unresolved inflammation: "Immune tsunami" or erosion of integrity in immune-privileged and immune-responsive tissues and acute and chronic inflammatory diseases or cancer," *Expert Opinion on Biological Therapy*, vol. 11, no. 11, pp. 1419–1432, 2011.

[74] K. Dhama, S. K. Latheef, H. A. Samad et al., "Tumor necrosis factor as mediator of inflammatory diseases and its therapeutic targeting: a review," *Journal of Medical Sciences*, vol. 13, pp. 226–235, 2013.

[75] A. J. DaMassa, P. S. Wakenell, and D. L. Brooks, "Mycoplasmas of goats and sheep," *Journal of Veterinary Diagnostic Investigation*, vol. 4, no. 1, pp. 101–113, 1992.

[76] M. Giangaspero, R. A. Nicholas, M. Hlusek et al., "Seroepidemiological survey of sheep flocks from Northern Japan for Mycoplasma ovipneumoniae and Mycoplasma agalactiae," *Tropical Animal Health Production*, vol. 44, pp. 395–398, 2012.

[77] R. A. J. Nicholas, R. D. Ayling, and G. R. Loria, "Ovine mycoplasmal infections," *Small Ruminant Research*, vol. 76, no. 1-2, pp. 92–98, 2008.

[78] R. Gonçalves, I. Mariano, A. Núñez, S. Branco, G. Fairfoul, and R. Nicholas, "Atypical non-progressive pneumonia in goats," *Veterinary Journal*, vol. 183, no. 2, pp. 219–221, 2010.

[79] M. Rifatbegović, Z. Maksimović, and B. Hulaj, "*Mycoplasma ovipneumoniae* associated with severe respiratory disease in goats," *Veterinary Record*, vol. 168, no. 21, p. 565, 2011.

[80] A. Rahal, A. Kumar, A. H. Ahmad, and J. K. Malik, "Pharmacokinetics of diclofenac and its interaction with enrofloxacin in sheep," *Research in Veterinary Science*, vol. 84, no. 3, pp. 452–456, 2008.

[81] A. Rahal, A. Kumar, A. H. Ahmad, and J. K. Malik, "Pharmacokinetics of ciprofloxacin in sheep following intravenous and subcutaneous administration," *Small Ruminant Research*, vol. 73, no. 1–3, pp. 242–245, 2007.

[82] A. Rahal, A. Kumar, A. H. Ahmad, J. K. Malik, and V. Ahuja, "Pharmacokinetics of enrofloxacin in sheep following intravenous and subcutaneous administration," *Journal of Veterinary Pharmacology and Therapeutics*, vol. 29, no. 4, pp. 321–324, 2006.

[83] S. Verma, A. H. Ahmad, A. Rahal, and K. P. Singh, "Pharmacokinetics of florfenicol following single dose intravenous and intramuscular administration in goats," *Journal of Applied Animal Research*, vol. 36, no. 1, pp. 93–96, 2009.

[84] A. Rahal, A. H. Ahmed, A. Kumar et al., "Clinical drug interactions: a holistic view," *Pakistan Journal of Biological Sciences*, vol. 16, pp. 751–758, 2013.

[85] K. P. Singh, A. H. Ahmad, V. Singh, K. Pant, and A. Rahal, "Effect of *Emblica officinalis* fruit in combating mercury-induced hepatic oxidative stress in rats," *Indian Journal of Animal Sciences*, vol. 81, no. 3, pp. 260–262, 2011.

[86] R. Rathore, A. Rahal, R. Mandil, A. Prakash, and S. K. Garg, "Comparative anti-inflammatory activity of *Cimicifuga racemosa* and *Mimosa pudica*," *Australian Veterinary Practioner*, vol. 42, pp. 274–278, 2012.

[87] A. Rahal, A. Kumar, S. Chakraborty, R. Tiwari, S. K. Latheef, and K. Dhama, "Cimicifuga: a revisiting indigenous herb with multi-utility benefits for safeguarding human health—a review," *International Journal of Agronomy Plant Production*, vol. 4, pp. 1590–1601, 2013.

[88] Jayati, A. K. Bhatia, A. Kumar, A. Goel, S. Gupta, and A. Rahal, "*In vitro* antiviral potential of *Ocimum sanctum* leaves extract against New Castle disease virus of poultry," *International Journal of Microbiology and Immunology Research*, vol. 2, pp. 51–55, 2013.

[89] W. A. Brooks, M. Yunus, M. Santosham et al., "Zinc for severe pneumonia in very young children: double-blind placebo-controlled trial," *The Lancet*, vol. 363, no. 9422, pp. 1683–1688, 2004.

[90] I. Romieu, J. J. Sienra-Monge, M. Ramírez-Aguilar et al., "Antioxidant supplementation and lung functions among children with asthma exposed to high levels of air pollutants," *The American Journal of Respiratory and Critical Care Medicine*, vol. 166, no. 5, pp. 703–709, 2002.

22

Epidemiological Observations on Cryptosporidiosis in Diarrheic Goat Kids in Greece

Nektarios D. Giadinis,[1] Elias Papadopoulos,[2] Shawkat Q. Lafi,[3]
Vasiliki Papanikolopoulou,[1] Sofia Karanikola,[2] Anastasia Diakou,[2] Vergos Vergidis,[4]
Lihua Xiao,[5] Evi Ioannidou,[1] and Harilaos Karatzias[1]

[1]*Clinic of Farm Animals, Faculty of Veterinary Medicine, Aristotle University, 546 27 Thessaloniki, Greece*
[2]*Laboratory of Parasitology and Parasitic Diseases, Faculty of Veterinary Medicine, Aristotle University, 541 24 Thessaloniki, Greece*
[3]*Department of Pathology and Animal Health, Faculty of Veterinary Medicine, Jordan University of Science and Technology,*
 P.O. Box 3030, Irbid, Jordan
[4]*National Veterinary Laboratory, 69100 Komotini, Greece*
[5]*Division of Foodborne, Waterborne and Environmental Diseases, Centers for Disease Control and Prevention, Atlanta, GA, USA*

Correspondence should be addressed to Nektarios D. Giadinis; ngiadini@vet.auth.gr

Academic Editor: Yoshiaki Hikasa

This study aimed at investigating the occurrence of *Cryptosporidium* spp. in diarrheic goat kids in Greece and the risk factors associated with cryptosporidiosis. Altogether, 292 diarrheic 4–15-day-old goat kids from 54 dairy goat herds of Northern Greece were examined. Oocysts of *Cryptosporidium* spp. were detected in 223 of 292 (76.4%) goat kids and the intensity of infection was scored as "high" in 142 samples, "moderate" in 45 samples, and "low" in 36 samples. Larger herds (>200 animals) had higher infection rates than smaller ones, although this difference was not statistically significant. Significantly higher infection rates were observed in herds during late kidding season (1 January to 30 April) compared to the early one (1 September to 31 December). These results suggest that cryptosporidiosis is very common in diarrheic goat kids in Greece, especially in large herds during the late parturition season.

1. Introduction

Cryptosporidium spp. have a significant impact on health of neonatal 4–15-day-old goat kids, causing diarrhea, dehydration, and electrolyte imbalance. Cryptosporidiosis results in economic losses, because of the high morbidity and mortality rates, associated with the infection of this protozoan parasite. In addition, some of the *Cryptosporidium* isolates are zoonotic [1–4].

Cryptosporidium infection of diarrheic goat kids appears to be common in Southern Europe; many relative studies have been conducted in Turkey [5], Italy [6], Serbia [7], France [8, 9], Spain [10], and Cyprus [4]. Although cryptosporidiosis is an important cause of illness and mortality in goat kids, only one study has been conducted to date to investigate the risk factors involved in the acquisition of infections in this

animal species [8], while the rest are based on simple clinical observations [4, 5, 11].

In Greece, studies of neonatal cryptosporidiosis have been conducted to date in dairy calves [12] and lambs [13], but a similar study has not been conducted in goat kids. This study aimed at investigating the occurrence of *Cryptosporidium* spp. in diarrheic goat kids in Greece and at providing some epidemiological data that could contribute to the better understanding of cryptosporidiosis.

2. Materials and Methods

This study was conducted in Northern Greece from October 2011 to May 2013 in 54 goat herds (22,890 adult animals) with over 10% incidence of diarrhea in 4–15-day-old goat kids. Younger and older animals were not included in this study.

The herds included in this report consisted of local dairy crossbreeds maintained under the semi-intensive feeding system, which is the most common one in the country. They were regularly dewormed and vaccinated against clostridiosis. The selected herds had not received any anticryptosporidial medication prior to sampling. Each herd or animal was sampled only once.

The Ambulatory Clinic of the Faculty of Veterinary Medicine of Aristotle University visited the aforementioned goat herds. A complete history of the case was taken and rectal fecal samples were collected from at least 4 goat kids with diarrhea per herd. The samples were transferred to the Laboratory of Parasitology and Parasitic Diseases at the Faculty of Veterinary Medicine of Aristotle University and examined immediately.

The fecal samples were diluted with tap water and passed through a sieve (no. 150) in a centrifuge tube, centrifuged at $500\,g$ for 3 min and smears of $20\,\mu L$ of the sediment were dried, stained using the acid-fast Ziehl-Neelsen technique [14], and examined at 1000x magnification for *Cryptosporidium* spp. oocysts. The intensity of the infection was estimated semiquantitatively according to the average number of oocysts in 10 random fields. It was scored as light (<5 oocysts/10 fields), moderate (5–10 oocysts/10 fields), and high (>10 oocysts/10 fields). If no oocysts were detected, it was scored as negative.

Risk factors were also investigated and data on herd size ("large herds" ≥200 animals or "small herds" <200 animals) and kidding season were collected. Goat kids born from 1 September to 31 December were called "early," while those born from 1 January to 30 April were called "late."

Data were collected and entered in a data sheet and analysed using IBM SPSS 20.0 2011 software for Windows (IBM SPSS Corp., Armonk, NY, USA). Chi-square test (or Fisher's Exact Test) was used to determine the relationships between studied risk factors and sample positivity in goat herds. A P value ≤ 0.05 was considered statistically significant.

3. Results

Eight of the 54 goat herds had less than 200 adult animals, while the remaining 46 herds had ≥200 adult animals. Forty-five of the herds (83.3%) were found positive, with at least one animal infected with *Cryptosporidium* spp.: 5 in herds with <200 animals and 40 in herds with ≥200 animals. The herd size did not influence significantly ($P > 0.05$) the infection with *Cryptosporidium* spp. Most of the affected goat kids belonged to "late" kidding herds. In fact, 37 of the 45 positive herds (82.2%) were from "late" kidding and the remaining 8 (17.8%) were from "early" kidding. The difference between "early" and "late" herds was statistically significant ($P < 0.01$). All of the data in this paragraph are listed in Table 1.

On kid level, the occurrence rate of cryptosporidiosis was 76.4% (of the 292 goat kids that participated in the current study, 223 or 76.4% were infected with *Cryptosporidium* spp.). Regarding the intensity of the infection, 142 samples (48.63%) were scored as "high," 45 (15.41%) were scored as "moderate," and 36 (12.33%) were scored as "low," while the remaining 69 samples (23.63%) were "negative."

TABLE 1: Prevalence (%) of *Cryptosporidium* spp. infection in goat herds related to their size and time of kidding.

Goat herds	Herd size		Time of kidding		Total
	≥200 animals	<200 animals	Late	Early	
Infected	40	5	37	8	45 (83.3%)
Not infected	6	3	2	7	9 (16.7%)
Total	46	8	39	15	54

4. Discussion

Diarrhoea syndrome of neonatal goat kids causes significant losses worldwide and also in Greece [2, 15]. Cryptosporidiosis seems to be one of the most important causes of this syndrome in Greece and other countries [1, 16, 17].

In Greece, the contribution of *Cryptosporidium* spp. to neonatal goat kid diarrhoea and mortality has already been noticed in small number of goat herds [1, 18]. However, a systematic study has not been conducted to investigate its prevalence in goat herds with high neonatal goat kid diarrhoea incidence; the existing studies have investigated its prevalence in adult goats or herds with nonremarkable incidence of diarrhoea in neonatal goat kids [19–21].

The contribution of cryptosporidiosis in diarrhoea syndrome at the age of 4–15 days has been assessed to be 46% in Greek dairy calves [12] and 29% in lambs [13]. In the present study it was found that 76.4% of the diarrheic goat kids were positive for *Cryptosporidium* spp., as well as the 83.3% of the 54 examined goat herds. In fact, the data show that the problem of cryptosporidiosis seems to be much more common in the goat herds than in the sheep or dairy cattle in Greece [12, 13]. In a similar study in Cyprus the percentages were similarly high on both sheep and goat farms [4], although the percentage of positive goat herds was slightly higher than that in Greece (89.3% in Cyprus and 83.3% in Greece). Also, a high occurrence of *Cryptosporidium* infection has been found in diarrheic goat kids in a large French study by Delafosse and coworkers [8].

Herds with high animal stock were more likely to have *Cryptosporidium* spp. infection and cryptosporidiosis, although this difference was not statistically significant. In a similar study conducted in Cyprus the difference was found to be statistically significant [4], although the number of goat herds examined was lower. However, large herd size can be a risk factor for increased *Cryptosporidium* spp. infection, as it has been already shown in cattle [22] and sheep [4, 23, 24]. The increased herd size can affect the prevalence of *Cryptosporidium* spp. infection, because of inadequate management of these herds and close contact among susceptible animals [4].

"Late" kidding seems to be a factor that increases the possibility of clinical cryptosporidiosis. This finding confirms previous findings in goat kids [4, 8] and in lambs [4, 23]. The Greek goat-keepers usually clean animal premises once every year (in the summer); thus when the kidding season is extended the parasite contamination increases in the premises [4, 13]. This seems to be the most probable explanation for this condition, although a systematic research is necessary.

The majority of the examined diarrheic goat kids (48.63%) had a heavy *Cryptosporidium* spp. infection. In other studies in goats [8] and cattle [25], it was found that heavily infected goat kids and calves suffered from severe diarrhoea. It has also been previously reported that lambs or goat kids heavily infected with *Cryptosporidium* spp. can suffer from fatal diarrhoea with cryptosporidiosis being the sole cause or the predisposing factor for other pathological entities [1, 26, 27].

Furthermore, in neighbouring countries of Greece, the role of cryptosporidiosis in goat kids as well as in other animal species and human health has also been assessed [5, 7, 28–30]. Additionally, in Bulgaria, a study has been conducted for the presence of *Cryptosporidium* spp. in different water supplies [31]. Therefore, it seems that cryptosporidiosis is a common cause of diarrhoea in newborn goat kids in Greece and other countries of Balkan Peninsula. This could be due to the similar climatic and husbandry conditions, and definitely more extensive epidemiological studies in this area are necessary for the effective protection of animal and public health.

Conclusively, cryptosporidiosis is very common in diarrheic goat kids in Greece, especially for the large herds as well as for "late" kidding animals. This parasitic infection may pose a significant health and production issue in goat herds and a public health hazard.

Conflict of Interests

The authors declare that they have no conflict of interests regarding the publication of this paper.

References

[1] N. D. Giadinis, E. Papadopoulos, S. Q. Lafi, N. K. Panousis, M. Papazahariadou, and H. Karatzias, "Efficacy of halofuginone lactate for the treatment and prevention of cryptosporidiosis in goat kids: an extensive field trial," *Small Ruminant Research*, vol. 76, no. 3, pp. 195–200, 2008.

[2] M. C. Smith and D. M. Sherman, *Goat Medicine*, Wiley-Blackwell, New York, NY, USA, 2nd edition, 2009.

[3] S. M. Cacciò, A. R. Sannella, V. Mariano et al., "A rare *Cryptosporidium parvum* genotype associated with infection of lambs and zoonotic transmission in Italy," *Veterinary Parasitology*, vol. 191, no. 1-2, pp. 128–131, 2012.

[4] N. D. Giadinis, S. Symeoudakis, E. Papadopoulos, S. Q. Lafi, and H. Karatzias, "Comparison of two techniques for diagnosis of cryptosporidiosis in diarrhoeic goat kids and lambs in Cyprus," *Tropical Animal Health and Production*, vol. 44, no. 7, pp. 1561–1565, 2012.

[5] F. Sevinç, A. Şimşek, and U. Uslu, "Massive *Cryptosporidium parvum* infection associated with an outbreak of diarrhoea in neonatal goat kids," *Turkish Journal of Veterinary and Animal Sciences*, vol. 29, no. 6, pp. 1317–1320, 2005.

[6] S. Cacciò, F. Spano, and E. Pozio, "Large sequence variation at two microsatellite loci among zoonotic (genotype C) isolates of *Cryptosporidium parvum*," *International Journal for Parasitology*, vol. 31, no. 10, pp. 1082–1086, 2001.

[7] I. Pavlović, S. Ivanović, M. Žujović, and Z. Tomić, "Goat cryptosporidiosis and its importance at goat production pathology," *Biotechnology in Animal Husbandry*, vol. 26, no. 3-4, pp. 187–192, 2010.

[8] A. Delafosse, J. A. Castro-Hermida, C. Baudry, E. Ares-Mazás, and C. Chartier, "Herd-level risk factors for *Cryptosporidium* infection in dairy-goat kids in western France," *Preventive Veterinary Medicine*, vol. 77, no. 1-2, pp. 109–121, 2006.

[9] J. Petermann, C. Paraud, I. Pors, and C. Chartier, "Efficacy of halofuginone lactate against experimental cryptosporidiosis in goat neonates," *Veterinary Parasitology*, vol. 202, no. 3-4, pp. 326–329, 2014.

[10] J. Quílez, C. Vergara-Castiblanco, L. Monteagudo, E. D. Cacho, and C. Sánchez-Acedo, "Host association of *Cryptosporidium parvum* populations infecting domestic ruminants in Spain," *Applied and Environmental Microbiology*, vol. 79, no. 17, pp. 5363–5371, 2013.

[11] S. Tzipori, J. Larsen, M. Smith, and R. U. Luefl, "Diarrhoea in goat kids attributed to cryptosporidium infection," *Veterinary Record*, vol. 111, no. 2, pp. 35–36, 1982.

[12] N. Panousis, A. Diakou, E. Papadopoulos, N. Giadinis, H. Karatzias, and S. Haralampidis, "Prevalence of *Cryptosporidium* infection in dairy farms with a history of calves' diarrhoea," *Cattle Practice*, vol. 15, no. 1, pp. 89–92, 2007.

[13] N. Panousis, A. Diakou, N. Giadinis, E. Papadopoulos, H. Karatzias, and S. Haralampidis, "Prevalence of *Cryptosporidium* infection in sheep flocks with a history of lambs' diarrhoea," *Revue de Medecine Veterinaire*, vol. 159, no. 10, pp. 528–531, 2008.

[14] S. A. Henriksen and J. F. Pohlenz, "Staining of cryptosporidia by a modified Ziehl-Neelsen technique," *Acta veterinaria Scandinavica*, vol. 22, no. 3-4, pp. 594–596, 1981.

[15] V. Papanikolopoulou, A.-M. Pantikidou, and N. D. Giadinis, "Losses in lambs and goat kids up to 2 months old," in *Proceedings of the 12th Greek Veterinary Congress*, Athens, Greece, 2011.

[16] C. Paraud, I. Pors, and C. Chartier, "Evaluation of oral tilmicosin efficacy against severe cryptosporidiosis in neonatal kids under field conditions," *Veterinary Parasitology*, vol. 170, no. 1-2, pp. 149–152, 2010.

[17] J. A. Castro-Hermida, I. García-Presedo, A. Almeida, M. González-Warleta, J. M. C. Da Costa, and M. Mezo, "*Cryptosporidium* spp. And *Giardia duodenalis* in two areas of Galicia (NW Spain)," *Science of the Total Environment*, vol. 409, no. 13, pp. 2451–2459, 2011.

[18] A. Minas, E. Koutsoukou-Hartona, and M. Papasavvas, "Epidemiological survey for the detection of cryptosporidium oocysts in diarrheal lambs' and kids' faeces in the region of Larissa," *Bulletin of the Hellenic Veterinary Medical Society*, vol. 44, pp. 112–114, 1993.

[19] C. Papadopoulou, E. Xylouri, A. Mantzios, G. Spyropoulos, and S. Stoforos, "Cryptosporidiosis in farm animals in Greece," in *Proceedings of the 1st International Workshop on Cryptosporidiosis*, Edinburgh, UK, 1988.

[20] C. A. Himonas, K. S. Antoniadou-Sotiriadou, S. T. Sotiraki, and M. G. Papazahariadou, "Intestinal protozoa of animals in Macedonia," *Bulletin of the Hellenic Veterinary Medical Society*, vol. 49, pp. 300–306, 1998.

[21] N. Tzanidakis, S. Sotiraki, E. Claerebout et al., "Occurrence and molecular characterization of *Giardia duodenalis* and *Cryptosporidium* spp. in sheep and goats reared under dairy husbandry systems in Greece," *Parasite*, vol. 21, article 45, 2014.

[22] D. V. Nydam and H. O. Mohammed, "Quantitative risk assessment of *Cryptosporidium* species infection in dairy calves," *Journal of Dairy Science*, vol. 88, no. 11, pp. 3932–3943, 2005.

[23] A. C. Causapé, J. Quílez, C. Sánchez-Acedo, E. Del Cacho, and F. López-Bernad, "Prevalence and analysis of potential risk factors for *Cryptosporidium parvum* infection in lambs in Zaragoza (northeastern Spain)," *Veterinary Parasitology*, vol. 104, no. 4, pp. 287–298, 2002.

[24] B. Sari, M. Ö. Arslan, Y. Gicik, M. Kara, and G. T. Taşçi, "The prevalence of *Cryptosporidium* species in diarrhoeic lambs in Kars province and potential risk factors," *Tropical Animal Health and Production*, vol. 41, no. 5, pp. 819–826, 2009.

[25] M. Naciri, M. Paul Lefay, R. Mancassola, P. Poirier, and R. Chermette, "Role of *Cryptosporidium parvum* as a pathogen in neonatal diarrhoea complex in suckling and dairy calves in France," *Veterinary Parasitology*, vol. 85, no. 4, pp. 245–257, 1999.

[26] N. D. Giadinis, E. Papadopoulos, N. Panousis, M. Papazahariadou, S. Q. Lafi, and H. Karatzias, "Effect of halofuginone lactate on treatment and prevention of lamb cryptosporidiosis: an extensive field trial," *Journal of Veterinary Pharmacology and Therapeutics*, vol. 30, no. 6, pp. 578–582, 2007.

[27] N. D. Giadinis, E. Papadopoulos, P. Loukopoulos et al., "Illthrift in suckling lambs secondary to umbilical infections and possible implication of cryptosporidiosis as a risk factor," *Veterinary Medicine International*, vol. 2011, Article ID 382804, 3 pages, 2011.

[28] A. Bejan, V. Mircean, C. Radu, S. Sotiraki, and V. Cozma, "Epidemiology of *Cryptosporidium* pp. infection in goat kids in the central and the northwest part of Romania," *Scientia Parasitologica*, vol. 1, pp. 32–36, 2009.

[29] Z. Mišić, S. Katić-Radivojević, and Z. Kulišić, "*Cryptosporidium* infection in lambs and goat kids in Serbia," *Acta Veterinaria*, vol. 56, no. 1, pp. 49–54, 2006.

[30] A. Sejdini, R. Mahmud, Y. A. L. Lim et al., "Intestinal parasitic infections among children in central Albania," *Annals of Tropical Medicine and Parasitology*, vol. 105, no. 3, pp. 241–250, 2011.

[31] P. Karanis, I. Sotiriadou, V. Kartashev, C. Kourenti, N. Tsvetkova, and K. Stojanova, "Occurrence of *Giardia* and *Cryptosporidium* in water supplies of Russia and Bulgaria," *Environmental Research*, vol. 102, no. 3, pp. 260–271, 2006.

Dynamics of Progesterone, TNF-α, and a Metabolite of PGF2α in Blood Plasma of Beef Cows following Embryo Transfer

M. C. Mason,[1] J. Copeland,[1] E. J. Cuadra,[1] T. H. Elsasser,[2] Y. Jung,[3] and J. Larson[4]

[1] Department of Agriculture, Alcorn State University, 1000 ASU Drive No. 750, Alcorn State, Lorman, MS 39096, USA
[2] Bovine Functional Genomics Laboratory Beltsville Agricultural Center, USDA ARS, Beltsville, MD 20705, USA
[3] Cooperative Agricultural Research Center, Prairie View A&M University, P.O. Box 519, AGRL No. 112, Prairie View, TX, USA
[4] Department of Animal and Dairy Sciences, Mississippi State University, Mississippi State, MS 39762, USA

Correspondence should be addressed to E. J. Cuadra; cuadra@alcorn.edu

Academic Editor: Lorraine M. Sordillo

Lactating beef cows previously synchronized for estrus (d 0) were assigned to four treatments to assess their effectiveness in increasing blood progesterone (P4) and its effects on tumor necrosis factor-α (TNF-α) and prostaglandin F2α (PGF2α) after the transfer of embryos. At the time of transfer (d 7), cows received no treatment (control; $n = 16$), a controlled internal drug releasing device (CIDR; $n = 16$), human chorionic gonadotropin (hCG; $n = 15$), or gonadotropin releasing hormone (GnRH; $n = 15$). Blood samples were taken on d 7, 14, and 21 for analysis of P4 and tumor necrosis factor-α (TNF-α). Blood was collected (every 15 min for 2 h) in half the animals in each treatment group on d 14 and the remaining half on d 21 for analysis of prostaglandin F2α metabolite (PGFM). Retention rates were 56.2, 62.5, 46.7, and 13.3% for cows in the control, CIDR, hCG, and GnRH groups, respectively. Progesterone was greater ($P \leq 0.05$) in cows receiving hCG compared to others on d 14. Progesterone in all treatment groups increased from d 7 to d 14 and declined ($P \leq 0.05$) from d 14 to d 21. Contrary to pregnant cows, P4 and TNF-α declined from d 7 to d 21 in nonpregnant cows ($P \leq 0.05$). Although PGFM increased by d 21, there was no difference between pregnant and nonpregnant cows.

1. Introduction

Progesterone (P4) is abundantly reported in the literature as the primary and most intrinsic hormone associated with embryonic survival during early pregnancy [1, 2]. The emphasis in studying P4 is due to the ability exhibited by P4 in regulating uterine receptivity during implantation [3]. Moreover, low concentrations of P4 are associated with retention of pregnancy in beef cows [4]. Therefore, several studies have been recently designed to examine the effects of supplementing exogenous P4 on embryonic retention after the transfer of embryos. At present, this is commonly done by inserting a controlled internal drug releasing device (CIDR) at the time of breeding.

Our laboratory previously reported [5] that inserting a CIDR immediately after the transfer of embryos enhanced retention rates in recipient lactating and nonlactating beef cows. Similar results have been observed in cattle by other investigators [6, 7]. Conversely, Purcell et al. [5] did not detect beneficial effects on pregnancy rates by placing CIDR's immediately subsequent to embryo transfer in dairy cows.

Several factors might be responsible for the inconsistency in the research outcomes observed by supplementing exogenous P4 aimed to enhance embryonic retention of transferred embryos. In some cases, this may be attributed to the fact that a single CIDR may not deliver enough P4 to support pregnancy on recipients experiencing low circulating P4 [8] or perhaps failing to supplement adequate levels of P4 [6] at the time when majority of embryonic rejections have been suggested to occur after the transfer [7, 9, 10]. Furthermore, several trials have clearly demonstrated that exogenous supplementation of P4 impairs endogenous luteal production of P4 [10, 11] and caused marked regression of the corpus luteum (CL) during early pregnancy in cattle [12].

A more recent study conducted by our laboratory showed cows in the control group having increased pregnancy rates in parallel with increased concentrations of P4 during the first week after embryo transfer compared to a treated group with exogenous P4 via CIDR's [10]. Therefore, strategies to enhance endogenous production of P4 may be an alternative method to examine its role on key factors associated with embryonic retention of transferred embryos.

Some of the potential strategies to achieve this goal may be by either inducing the formation of an accessory CL or by boosting the synthesis of luteal tissue in the existing CL with the use of hormones. Hence, several hormonal treatments have been reported to manipulate secretion of endogenous P4 in cattle. Gonadotropin releasing hormone (GnRH) is reported to alter the synthesis of P4 [13] by manipulating growth of the follicle [14] and number of CL [15]. Consequently, administration of GnRH at the time of insemination results in increased conception rates in cattle [16–18]. In addition, human chorionic gonadotropin (hCG) has also commonly been used in cattle to boost endogenous concentrations of P4 in blood [19–21]. The increase in P4 may be a result of the formation of an accessory CL [22, 23] combined with promoting growth of the existing CL [22, 24]. Nevertheless, hCG inconsistently improves pregnancy rates [23–25]. Consequently, these hormones (GnRH and hCG) were used to boost endogenous P4 in the present study.

Prostaglandin F2α (PGF2α) and tumor necrosis factor-alpha (TNF-α) have been linked to retention of pregnancy by several investigators. Thus, it is well known that PGF2α is responsible for inducing regression of the CL [26], which is synthesized by the uterus and regulated by P4 [27]. In cyclic sheep, loss of P4 receptors allows for the uterine release of luteolytic pulses of PGF2α suggesting an inverse relationship. Tumor necrosis factor-alpha has both luteotropic and luteolytic functions [28]. Progesterone is considered to be a potent inhibitor of TNF-α messenger RNA (mRNA) and TNF-α protein production [29]. A decrease in TNF-α concentration on d 7 after the transfer of embryos may be associated with the decreased concentrations of P4 observed in the nonpregnant animals in a previous trial [10]. Therefore, the objective of this study was to assess the effectiveness of four treatments in increasing blood P4 and its effects on TNF-α and PGF2α. Our working hypothesis was that high concentrations of circulating P4 creates a window of time that facilitates synchrony between the embryo and the uterine environment by regulating concentrations of PGF2α and TNF-α in the uterine environment of the recipient.

2. Materials and Methods

2.1. Experimental Design and Hormonal Protocol. The study was approved by the Institutional Animal Care and Use Committee of Mississippi State University (11-023) and implemented at The Coastal Plain Branch Experiment Station of Mississippi State University in Newton, MS in the Spring of 2011. Lactating Angus crossbred cows were synchronized for estrous by receiving a CIDR (Eazi-Breed CIDR; Zoetis, Madison NJ) for 7 d. One d after removal, all cows

($n = 62$) received an injection of PGF2α (25 mg IM; Lutalyse; Zoetis). Cows were observed for estrus (d 0) four times per d (1 h at each time) during the 80 h post-PGF2α. Following manual evaluation of the CL via palpation per rectum, all cows exhibiting estrus with a CL received an embryo in the uterine horn ipsilateral to the CL on 7 d after estrus. At the time of transfer, cows were assigned to 1 of 4 treatments: no further treatment (Control, $n = 16$), a CIDR insert (CIDR, $n = 16$), an injection of hCG (1000 IU, IM; Sioux Biochemical, Inc, Sioux Center, IA; hCG, $n = 15$) or an injection of GnRH (100 μg, IM; Cystorelin; Merial, Duluth, GA; GnRH, $n = 15$).

2.2. Animals and Embryos. Animals were body condition scored (scale of 1 = emaciated; 9 = obese) by visual appraisal at the beginning of the project according to Whitman [30]. Embryos used in the study were donated by Mississippi State University. Flushing and freezing of the embryos were performed on d 7 after insemination. Embryos were a quality grade 1 [31] and developmental stages 4 and 5; the embryos were frozen in ethylene glycol and stored in liquid nitrogen until their use. The transfer of embryos was performed by an embryo transfer practitioner (Mid-South Reproductive Services, Baton Rouge, LA). Pregnancy diagnosis via palpation per rectum was determined at 60 d after transfer of the embryos.

2.3. Collection and Laboratory Analysis of Blood Samples. All samples were collected in 6.0 mL plastic vacutainers with no additives (Fisher Scientific, Pittsburg, PA) from the tail vein. Immediately after collection the samples were stored on ice until they could be centrifuged for 15 min at 1800 g, which was followed by long term storage at −20°C until later analysis. Blood samples for determination of 13, 14-dihydro-15-keto PGF2α metabolite (PGFM) were collected from half the animals within each treatment group on d 14 and the remaining half on d 21. On each of these two days, animals selected for collection of blood were additionally divided in two groups and collected every 15 min for 2 h in two individual restraining systems. Synthesis of PGF2α in each blood sample was inhibited as previously described by [32]. Blood samples were collected from all cows on d 7 (day of transfer), d 14, and d 21 for analysis of P4 and TNF-α.

The concentration of P4 in peripheral blood plasma was determined via radioimmunoassay that has been validated for use in bovine (Coat-a-Count Progesterone, Los Angeles, CA) and used according to the manufacturer's procedure. Plasma samples were assayed for concentrations of TNF-α via a double antibody radioimmunoassay as described by Kenison et al. [33], with the following changes. Antibody (rabbit anti-bovine TNF-α R7-93) generated against recombinant bovine TNF-α (kindly donated by Ciba-Geigy, Basel, Switzerland) was used as the primary antibody at a final tube dilution of 1 : 120,000 and recombinant bovine TNF-α (Kingfisher Biotech, St. Paul, MN) was radioiodinated and used as the assay tracer. Concentrations of PGFM were measured using an enzyme-linked immunosorbent assay (ELISA; Oxford Biomedical Research, Oxford, MI) and used according to the manufacturer's instructions. The intraassay and interassay coefficients of variation were 6.25 and 9.38%, respectively.

2.4. Statistical Analysis. Body condition scores of experimental animals were analyzed using the GLM procedure (SAS, Inst. Inc., Cary, NC). Data on conception rates (%) was also analyzed using the GLM procedure with a significance level of 5%; treatment means were compared using the Duncan multiple range test. Concentrations of P4, TNF-α, and PGFM in blood were analyzed using the MIXED procedure SAS (SAS Inst., Inc.) with repeated measures. The repeated measures model for the response plasma hormone concentrations on d 0, d 7, and d 14 contained the fixed effect of the treatments and the repeated factors of day and their corresponding interactions. Least squares means by the Bonferroni adjustment were analyzed and separated when a protected F test of $P \leq 0.05$ was detected. Correlation between P4 and PGFM concentrations were performed using the CORR procedure of SAS (SAS Inst., Inc.). All comparisons in the statistical analysis were established at a 5% level of significance. Throughout results, LSMeans ± standard errors are presented.

3. Results and Discussion

3.1. Progesterone. It is well documented in the literature that body condition of animals influences systemic P4 concentrations of cows [34, 35]. No significant differences were observed in body condition scores among cows in the hCG (5.76 ± 0.21), control (5.47 ± 0.18), GnRH (5.68 ± 0.11), and CIDR (5.67 ± 0.49) groups of this study. Pregnancy diagnosis via palpation per rectum at 60 d after transfer of the embryos revealed retention rates of 56.2% (9/16) for the control group, 62.5% (10/16) for the CIDR group, 13.3% (2/15) for the GnRH group, and 46.6% (7/15) for the hCG group. Pregnancy rates were not different between cows in the control, CIDR, and hCG groups ($P > 0.05$); however, percent pregnancy rate was lower ($P < 0.05$) in the GnRH group when compared to the control and CIDR groups. Other investigators have also observed a negative effect on conception rates in lactating dairy cows receiving treatment with GnRH right after artificial insemination [36]. Nevertheless, it has been shown to improve conception rate in repeat-breeder dairy cows when injected at the time of the fourth insemination [37].

An overall comparison between pregnant and nonpregnant animals (Figure 1) revealed that pregnant cows had increased ($P \leq 0.05$) concentrations of P4 on d 21 compared to nonpregnant cows in this study (Figure 1). These results are supported by previous reports revealing that majority of embryo losses occur between d 14 and d 21 of the gestation [7, 9, 10]. However, both nonpregnant and pregnant cows had an increase ($P \leq 0.05$) in concentration of P4 from d 7 to d 14, but a decrease ($P \leq 0.05$) from d 14 to d 21. However, regardless of the treatment only nonpregnant cows experienced a significant decrease in P4 ($P \leq 0.05$) from d 7 to d 21 of this study; this is attributed to the regression of the CL [38] due to factors impairing luteal activity taking

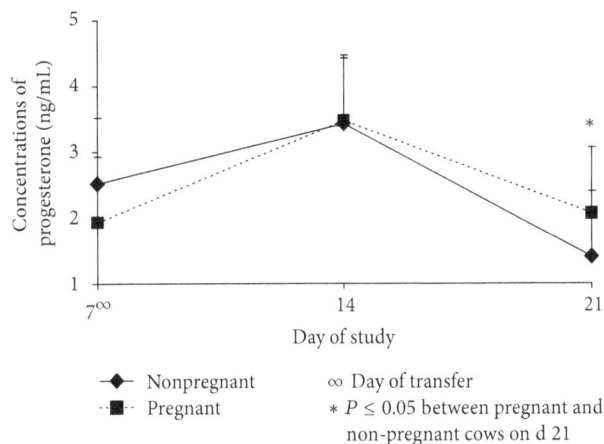

FIGURE 1: Concentrations (Mean ± SEM) of progesterone in pregnant and nonpregnant cows on d 7, d 14, and d 21.

place perhaps during the first days after the transfer [7]. Additionally, a previous study revealed that nonpregnant animals bearing a CIDR experienced an increase on P4 from d 7 to d 14 due to a P4 output by the regressing CL combined with the P4 released by the CIDR [10].

There was a significant treatment by pregnancy status interaction with cows failing to maintain pregnancy in the hCG group having significantly greater concentrations of P4 ($P \leq 0.05$) on d 14 (5.40 ± 0.58 ng/mL) and d 21 (2.91 ± 0.61 ng/mL) compared to nonpregnant cows in any other treatment groups on d 14 (2.27 ± 0.63, 2.32 ± 0.68, and 2.57 ± 0.44 ng/mL) and on d 21 (0.91 ± 0.63, 0.46 ± 0.44, and 1.24 ± 0.47 ng/mL) for the control, CIDR, and GnRH groups, respectively. Although nonpregnant cows in the control and CIDR groups had similar concentrations on d 7 and d 14, a decrease ($P \leq 0.05$) in the concentration of P4 occurred from d 14 (2.28 ± 0.56, 2.31 ± 0.68 ng/mL) to d 21 (0.90 ± 0.56, 0.46 ± 0.68 ng/mL; Table 1); Animals in these same two experimental groups are the only groups in the study experiencing a decrease in P4 from d 7 to d 21. Non-pregnant animals in the GnRH group also had a decline ($P \leq 0.05$) in P4 from d 14 (3.34 ± 0.44 ng/mL) to d 21 (1.24 ± 0.47 ng/mL); whereas, animals in the hCG group had an increase ($P \leq 0.05$) from d 7 (2.67 ± 0.59 ng/mL) to d 14 (5.4 ± 0.59 ng/mL); nevertheless, they similarly had a decrease ($P \leq 0.05$) in concentration of P4 from d 14 (5.4 ± 0.59 ng/mL) to d 21 (2.90 ± 0.62 ng/mL). Conversely, animals that maintained pregnancy in the control, CIDR and hCG group had an increase ($P \leq 0.05$; Table 1) in P4 from d 7 (2.27 ± 0.49, 1.54 ± 0.33, 2.17 ± 0.49 ng/mL) to d 14 (3.44 ± 0.49, 2.98 ± 0.36, 4.53 ± 0.78 ng/mL) along with a significant decline from d 14 to d 21.

It is believed that hCG may have increased overall secretion of P4 from the primary CL as well as from an induced secondary luteal structure during the first week of the study [39, 40]. Moreover, Mason et al. [10] also observed a significant increase in P4 7 d after the transfer in control and CIDR-treated cows retaining the embryos to completion of pregnancy.

TABLE 1: LSMeans and standard errors for concentrations of progesterone (ng/mL) in nonpregnant and pregnant cows within treatments.

Day	Control		CIDR[1]		GnRH[2]		hCG[3]	
	Nonpregnant	Pregnant	Nonpregnant	Pregnant	Nonpregnant	Pregnant	Nonpregnant	Pregnant
7[4]	2.22 ± 0.56^a	2.27 ± 0.49^a	2.54 ± 0.42^a	1.54 ± 0.33^a	$2.57 \pm 0.44^{a,b}$	1.07 ± 1.66^a	2.67 ± 0.46^a	2.17 ± 0.49^a
14	2.28 ± 0.56^a	3.44 ± 0.49^b	2.31 ± 0.47^a	2.98 ± 0.36^b	3.35 ± 0.44^a	1.16 ± 1.66^a	5.40 ± 0.73^b	4.53 ± 0.78^b
21	$0.90 \pm 0.56^{b,x}$	$2.54 \pm 0.49^{a,y}$	$0.46 \pm 0.33^{b,x}$	$1.73 \pm 0.25^{a,y}$	$1.25 \pm 0.47^{b,x}$	$0.85 \pm 1.66^{a,x}$	$2.94 \pm 0.94^{a,x}$	$2.11 \pm 0.95^{a,x}$

[a,b,c] Means within the same column lacking a common superscript are significantly different ($P \leq 0.05$).
[x,y] Means within row and within treatment group lacking a common superscript are significantly different ($P \leq 0.05$).
[1] Controlled internal drug release.
[2] Gonadotropin releasing hormone.
[3] Human chorionic gonadotropin.
[4] Day of embryo transfer.

TABLE 2: LSMeans and standard errors for concentrations of TNF-α (pg/mL) in nonpregnant and pregnant cows within treatments.

Day	Control		CIDR[1]		GnRH[2]		hCG[3]	
	Nonpregnant	Pregnant	Nonpregnant	Pregnant	Nonpregnant	Pregnant	Nonpregnant	Pregnant
7[4]	0.113 ± 0.02^a	0.124 ± 0.01^a	0.129 ± 0.03^a	0.112 ± 0.01^a	0.146 ± 0.01^a	0.095 ± 0.04^a	0.161 ± 0.02^a	0.160 ± 0.04^a
14	0.015 ± 0.02^a	0.119 ± 0.01^a	0.129 ± 0.01^a	0.124 ± 0.01^a	0.132 ± 0.01^a	0.102 ± 0.05^a	0.132 ± 0.02^{ab}	0.144 ± 0.02^a
21	0.116 ± 0.01^a	0.120 ± 0.01^a	0.126 ± 0.01^a	0.122 ± 0.01^a	0.122 ± 0.01^a	0.14 ± 0.02^a	$0.115 \pm 0.01^{b,x}$	$0.148 \pm 0.01^{a,y}$

[a,b,c] Means within the same column lacking a common superscript are significantly different ($P \leq 0.05$).
[x,y] Means within row and within treatment group lacking a common superscript are significantly different ($P \leq 0.05$).
[1] Controlled internal drug release.
[2] Gonadotropin releasing hormone.
[3] Human chorionic gonadotropin.
[4] Day of embryo transfer.

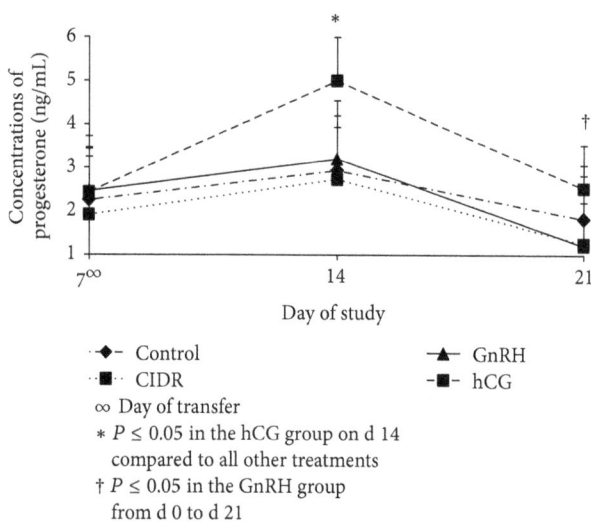

FIGURE 2: Concentrations (Mean ± SEM) of progesterone among treatment groups on d 7, d 14, and d 21. Treatment by day, concentration of progesterone decreased in cows from all treatments from d 14 to d 21 ($P \leq 0.05$); CIDR = controlled drug release; GnRH = gonadotropin releasing hormone; hCG = human chorionic gonadotropin.

Concentrations of P4 between treatment groups were not different at the time of transfer of the embryos (Figure 2) as a result of the previously synchronized estrus and the examination of the viability and presence of a well-developed CL in all animals on that day. Concentrations of P4 decreased ($P \leq 0.05$) from d 14 to d 21 in cows from all treatment groups; however, only cows within the GnRH group experienced decline in P4 concentrations ($P \leq 0.05$) from d 7 to d 21. This is in line with previous reports indicating that GnRH directly downregulates P4 release [41, 42]. On d 14, cows in the hCG group had increased concentrations of P4 compared to animals in all other treatment groups. On d 21, concentrations of P4 in cows in the hCG group were only greater ($P \leq 0.05$) than those in the GnRH group on that same day. Also, cows in the hCG group were the only ones with an increase ($P \leq 0.05$) in P4 from d 7 to d 14.

3.2. Tumor Necrosis Factor-α. Concentrations of TNF-α declined ($P \leq 0.05$) in animals in the hCG group from d 7 to d 21 (Figure 3). This same figure also shows a greater ($P \leq 0.05$) concentration of TNF-α in the hCG group compared to the GnRH group on d 7. The decrease ($P \leq 0.05$) in TNF-α between d 14 and d 21 also follows the decrease ($P \leq 0.05$) in concentrations of P4 within the hCG group.

The similar pattern of concentration between P4 and TNF-α suggests some type of link that allows this hormone and protein to act congruently [43]. When the treatment groups were looked at individually between the pregnant and nonpregnant cows (Table 2), decreased ($P \leq 0.05$) concentrations of TNF-α from d 7 to d 21 were observed in the nonpregnant cows of the hCG group; additionally, an increased ($P \leq 0.05$) concentration of TNF-α in the pregnant

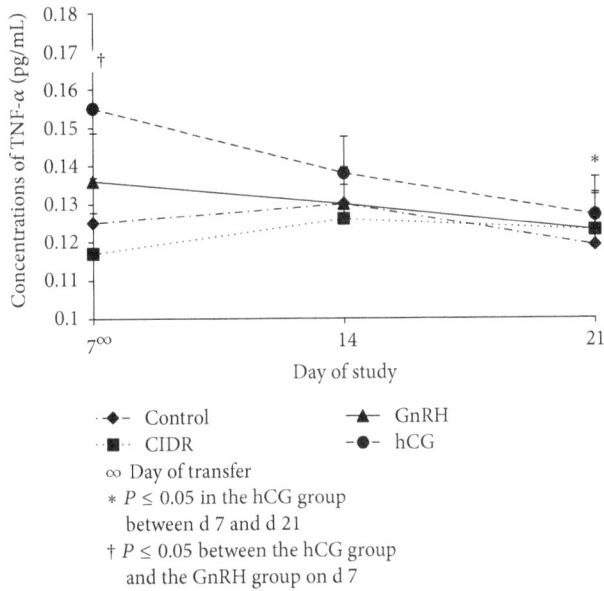

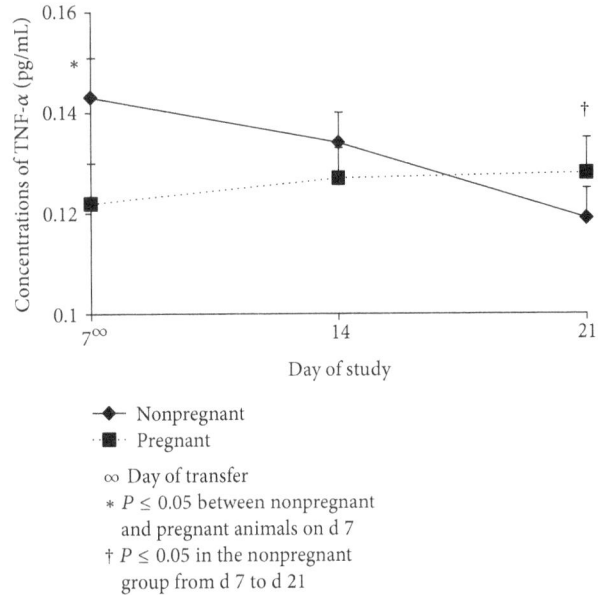

FIGURE 3: Concentrations (Mean ± SEM) of TNF-α among treatment groups on d 7, d 14, and d 21. Treatment x day interaction ($P \leq 0.05$); CIDR = controlled internal drug release; GnRH = gonadotropin releasing hormone; hCG = human chorionic gonadotropin.

FIGURE 4: Concentrations (Mean ± SEM) of TNF-α in pregnant and nonpregnant cows on d 7, d 14, and d 21. Pregnancy status x day interaction ($P \leq 0.05$); CIDR = controlled internal drug release; GnRH = gonadotropin releasing hormone; hCG = human chorionic gonadotropin.

cows was observed when compared to the nonpregnant cows on d 21 on that same group. Similar results were observed in a previous study where concentrations of TNF-α increased after hCG administration, suggesting a relationship between hCG and TNF-α via the Interleukin-6 receptor system [44, 45].

An overall comparison between pregnant and nonpregnant animals (Figure 4) showed a decrease ($P \leq 0.05$) in concentration of TNF-α from d 7 to d 21 in nonpregnant cows, which occurred similarly in P4 in this same experimental group. Previously, it has been reported by our laboratory that low concentrations of TNF-α are linked to low concentrations of P4 in nonpregnant cows [10]. The nonpregnant group additionally showed a greater ($P \leq 0.05$) concentration of TNF-α on d 7 compared to the pregnant group for reasons unable to be determined with these results. However, it is noteworthy that contrary to nonpregnant animals, pregnant cows maintained steadier concentrations of TNF-α through the entire experimental period. Interestingly, TNF-α has been reported having luteolytic properties. Some investigators [46–48] have suggested that TNF-α is deleterious to young embryos and promotes the process of luteolysis, thereby stimulating the release of PGF2α. On the other hand, other investigators [28] suggest that TNF-α may provide both luteolytic and luteotropic tendencies. Thus, the increased concenrations of P4 in pregnant animals may have played a role in inhibiting the luteolytic properties of TNF-α [49, 50]; nevertheless, the decreasing concentrations of TNF-α in the nonpregnant cows, seems to be associated with the luteolytic properties and consequently low concentrations of P4 as it has been reported in some other species and in cattle [28, 51].

3.3. Prostaglandin F2α. There were no significant differences in concentrations of PGFM ($P \geq 0.05$) between the treatment groups on d 14 (0.30 ± 0.48, 0.37 ± 0.84, 0.33 ± 0.46, 0.43 ± 0.99 pg/mL in control, CIDR, GnRH, and hCG groups, resp.) or d 21 (0.51 ± 0.11, 0.64 ± 0.69, 0.55 ± 0.14, 0.62 ± 0.85 pg/mL in control, CIDR, GnRH, and hCG groups, resp.) or between the pregnant and nonpregnant animals within treatment groups. Many studies have associated increased concentrations of PGF2α with the termination of pregnancy [26], as PGF2α is released from the uterus to essentially cause spontaneous luteolysis in cattle. However, in these current data, animals in the pregnant group actually had more steady concentrations of PGF2α on d 21, inferred from the measurement of PGFM, compared to the nonpregnant group on that same day (Table 3).

Prostaglandin F2α is released in pulses from the endometrium of the uterus and 80% of it is metabolized during one passage of the lungs, which helps create a short half-life for PGF2α as well as fluctuations in concentrations [52]. As expected, variation existed among the six samples collected over the 2 h period for each cow. These data are supported by fellow investigators [32, 53] who also reported variations within concentration of PGF2α between cyclic and noncyclic ewes. With the exception of pregnant cows on d 21, on both d 14 and d 21 there were consistently one or two samples within both the pregnant and nonpregnant animals that were different ($P \leq 0.05$) than the other samples collected on one of those days (Table 3). Furthermore, concentrations of PGFM in samples 5 and 6 within d 21 were significantly increased ($P \leq 0.05$) in the pregnant (0.69 ± 0.69; 0.57 ± 0.69) cows compared to the nonpregnant

TABLE 3: LSMeans and standard errors for concentrations of PGFM (ng/mL) for d 14 and 21 in nonpregnant and pregnant cows.

[1]Serum samples	Pregnant		Nonpregnant		All pregnant	All nonpregnant
	Day 14	Day 21	Day 14	Day 21		
1	0.38 ± 0.60^{ab}	0.68 ± 0.69^{a}	0.37 ± 0.32^{ab}	0.67 ± 0.49^{a}	0.49 ± 0.15	0.52 ± 0.15
2	0.36 ± 0.54^{ab}	0.68 ± 0.69^{a}	0.35 ± 0.32^{a}	0.66 ± 0.49^{a}	0.52 ± 0.16	0.51 ± 0.16
3	0.33 ± 0.60^{a}	0.71 ± 0.69^{a}	0.33 ± 0.32^{a}	0.67 ± 0.49^{a}	0.52 ± 0.19	0.50 ± 0.17
4	0.31 ± 0.54^{a}	0.77 ± 0.74^{a}	0.30 ± 0.32^{a}	0.68 ± 0.52^{a}	0.54 ± 0.23	0.49 ± 0.19
5	0.31 ± 0.54^{a}	0.69 ± 0.69^{a}	0.29 ± 0.32^{a}	0.45 ± 0.49^{b}	0.50 ± 0.19	0.37 ± 0.08
6	0.51 ± 0.54^{cb}	0.57 ± 0.69^{a}	0.46 ± 0.32^{b}	0.40 ± 0.49^{b}	0.54 ± 0.03	0.43 ± 0.03
Mean	0.36 ± 0.03^{x}	0.68 ± 0.03^{y}	0.35 ± 0.03^{x}	0.59 ± 0.05^{y}	0.52 ± 0.16^{x}	0.47 ± 0.12^{x}

[a,b,c]Means within the same column lacking a common superscript are significantly different.
[x,y]Means within row and within treatment group lacking a common superscript are significantly different ($P \leq 0.05$).
($P \leq 0.05$).
[1]Serum samples taken 15 minute apart on each day.

cows (0.45 ± 0.49; 0.40 ± 0.49), respectively. Nevertheless, concentrations of PGFM were not correlated on either d 14 or d 21 of the study with concentrations of P4. These findings are supported by other investigators [27, 54] who found that PGF2α actually increases during pregnancy. This suggests that the pattern of uterine secretion is altered during pregnancy and that this increased concentration of PGF2α now becomes luteo-protective rather than a luteolytic pattern of secretion [55]. One possible luteo-protective mechanism for the pregnant animal is to lower their sensitivity to the luteolytic effects of PGF2α [56]. Sensitivity may be lowered by the steady release of PGF2α in pregnant animals, where nonpregnant animals have more peaks and variations in their PGF2α release [57]. This steady release would allow the CL to become desensitized and have less PGF2α receptors, which would induce a more rapid metabolism of PGF2α to the inactive PGFM. Alternatively, along with the steady secretion of PGF2α, the uterus may receive signals by the conceptus via interferon tau to induce the release of PGF2α, which would consequently reduce the luteolytic effects of PGF2α [58].

4. Conclusion

These results indicate that the strategy of boosting endogenous P4 in cattle by injecting GnRH immediately at the transfer of embryos results in low pregnancy rates. Although treatment with hCG resulted in being the best treatment to boost systemic P4, this did not translate into a higher percent pregnancy compared to the other treatments in this study. Instead, similar concentrations of P4 between d 7 and d 21 are more suggestive of the survival of transferred embryos. Furthermore, with the exception of GnRH, pregnant animals in the other experimental groups had a significant increase in concentrations of P4 from d 0 to d 7. In addition, increased concentrations of P4 seem to be linked with TNF-α, perhaps by inhibiting the luteolytic effects of TNF-α as more of these cows maintained pregnancy. Concentrations of PGFM were steadier in pregnant animals.

Conflict of Interests

The authors declare that there is no conflict of interests regarding the publication of this paper.

References

[1] T. J. Parkinson and G. E. Lamming, "Interrelationships between progesterone, 13,14-dihydro-15-keto PGF-2α (PGFM) and LH in cyclic and early pregnant cows," *Journal of Reproduction and Fertility*, vol. 90, no. 1, pp. 221–233, 1990.

[2] K. L. Macmillan, V. K. Taufa, A. M. Day, and A. J. Peterson, "Effect of supplemental progesterone on pregnancy rates in cattle," *Journal of Reproduction and Fertility*, vol. 43, p. 304, 1991.

[3] Y.-P. Cheon, X. Xu, M. K. Bagchi, and I. C. Bagchi, "Immune-responsive gene 1 is a novel target of progesterone receptor and plays a critical role during implantation in the mouse," *Endocrinology*, vol. 144, no. 12, pp. 5623–5630, 2003.

[4] J. M. Burke, R. L. De La Sota, C. A. Risco, C. R. Staples, É. J.-P. Schmitt, and W. W. Thatcher, "Evaluation of timed insemination using a Gonadotropin-releasing hormone agonist in lactating dairy cows," *Journal of Dairy Science*, vol. 79, no. 8, pp. 1385–1393, 1996.

[5] S. H. Purcell, W. E. Beal, and K. R. Gray, "Effect of a CIDR insert and flunixin meglumine, administered at the time of embryo transfer, on pregnancy rate and resynchronization of estrus in beef cattle," *Theriogenology*, vol. 64, no. 4, pp. 867–878, 2005.

[6] T. van Werven, F. Waldeck, A. H. Souza, S. Floch, and M. Englebienne, "Comparison of two intravaginal progesterone releasing devices (PRID-Delta vs CIDR) in dairy cows: blood progesterone profile and field fertility," *Animal Reproduction Science*, vol. 138, no. 3-4, pp. 143–149, 2013.

[7] R. L. Butcher, J. E. Reber, A. W. Lishman et al., "Maintenance of pregnancy in postpartum beef cows that have short-lived corpora lutea," *Journal of animal science*, vol. 70, no. 12, pp. 3831–3837, 1992.

[8] J. D. Rhinehart, M. J. Starbuck-Clemmer, J. A. Flores et al., "Low peripheral progesterone and late embryonic/early fetal loss in suckled beef and lactating dairy cows," *Theriogenology*, vol. 71, no. 3, pp. 480–490, 2009.

[9] P. Lonergan, "Influence of progesterone on oocyte quality and embryo development in cows," *Theriogenology*, vol. 76, no. 9, pp. 1594–1601, 2011.

[10] M. Mason, E. J. Cuadra, T. H. Elsasser, J. Lopez, and J. Yoon-sung, "Evaluating the interaction between progesterone, tumor necrosis factor-alpha and cortisol on early loss of transferred embryo in beef cows," *Canadian Journal of Animal Science*, vol. 93, no. 2, pp. 217–225, 2013.

[11] R. G. Loy, R. G. Zimbelman, and L. E. Casida, "Effects of injected ovarian hormones on the corpus luteum of the estrual cycle in cattle," *Journal of Animal Science*, vol. 19, no. 1, pp. 175–182, 1960.

[12] R. G. Zimbelman, A. L. Pope, and L. E. Casida, "Effect of exogenous progesterone on the corpus luteum of the bred ewe," *Journal of Animal Science*, vol. 18, no. 4, pp. 1327–1332, 1959.

[13] D. C. Busch, J. A. Atkins, J. F. Bader et al., "Effect of ovulatory follicle size and expression of estrus on progesterone secretion in beef cows," *Journal of Animal Science*, vol. 86, no. 3, pp. 553–563, 2008.

[14] M. W. Peters and J. R. Pursley, "Timing of final GnRH of the Ovsynch protocol affects ovulatory follicle size, subsequent luteal function, and fertility in dairy cows," *Theriogenology*, vol. 60, no. 6, pp. 1197–1204, 2003.

[15] J. S. Stevenson, D. E. Tenhouse, M. A. Portaluppi, and A. Lloyd, "Post-AI intervention in lactating dairy cattle," *Journal of Animal Science*, vol. 84, p. 47, 2006.

[16] T. Nakao, S. Narita, K. Tanaka et al., "Improvement of first-service pregnancy rate in cows with gonadotropin-releasing hormone analog," *Theriogenology*, vol. 20, no. 1, pp. 111–119, 1983.

[17] H. F. Schels and D. Mostafawi, "The effect of Gn-RH on the pregnancy rate of artificially inseminated cows," *The Veterinary Record*, vol. 103, no. 2, pp. 31–32, 1978.

[18] J. S. Stevenson, E. P. Call, R. K. Scoby, and A. P. Phatak, "Double insemination and gonadotropin-releasing hormone treatment of repeat-breeding dairy cattle," *Journal of Dairy Science*, vol. 73, no. 7, pp. 1766–1772, 1990.

[19] N. Beindorff, A. Honnens, Y. Penno, V. Paul, and H. Bollwein, "Effects of human chorionic gonadotropin on luteal blood flow and progesterone secretion in cows and in vitro-microdialyzed corpora lutea," *Theriogenology*, vol. 72, no. 4, pp. 528–534, 2009.

[20] F. de Rensis, F. López-Gatius, I. García-Ispierto, and M. Techakumpu, "Clinical use of human chorionic gonadotropin in dairy cows: an update," *Theriogenology*, vol. 73, no. 8, pp. 1001–1008, 2010.

[21] J. S. Stevenson, M. A. Portaluppi, D. E. Tenhouse et al., "Interventions after artificial insemination: conception rates, pregnancy survival, and ovarian responses to gonadotropin-releasing hormone, human chorionic gonadotropin, and progesterone," *Journal of Dairy Science*, vol. 90, no. 1, pp. 331–340, 2007.

[22] R. Rajamahendran and P. C. Sianangama, "Effect of human chorionic gonadotrophin on dominant follicles in cows: formation of accessory corpora lutea, progesterone production and pregnancy rates," *Journal of Reproduction and Fertility*, vol. 95, no. 2, pp. 577–584, 1992.

[23] J. E. P. Santos, W. W. Thatcher, L. Pool, and M. W. Overton, "Effect of human chorionic gonadotropin on luteal function and reproductive performance of high-producing lactating Holstein dairy cows," *Journal of Animal Science*, vol. 79, no. 11, pp. 2881–2894, 2001.

[24] G. H. L. Marquezini, C. R. Dahlen, S. L. Bird, and G. C. Lamb, "Administration of human chorionic gonadotropin to suckled beef cows before ovulation synchronization and fixed-time insemination: replacement of gonadotropin-releasing hormone with human chorionic gonadotropin1," *Journal of Animal Science*, vol. 89, no. 10, pp. 3030–3039, 2011.

[25] N. Shams-Esfandabadi, A. Shirazi, P. Mirshokrai, and M. Bonyadian, "Influence of hCG administration after AI on conception rates and serum progesterone concentration in cattle," *Pakistan Journal of Biological Sciences*, vol. 10, no. 16, pp. 2709–2713, 2007.

[26] T. L. Watts and J. W. Fuquay, "Response and fertility of dairy heifers following injection with prostaglandin F2α during early, middle or late diestrus," *Theriogenology*, vol. 23, no. 4, pp. 655–661, 1985.

[27] G. S. Lewis, "Role of ovarian progesterone and potential role of prostaglandin F 2α and prostaglandin E2 in modulating the uterine response to infectious bacteria in postpartum ewes," *Journal of Animal Science*, vol. 81, no. 1, pp. 285–293, 2003.

[28] K. Okuda and R. Sakumoto, "Multiple roles of TNF super family members in corpus luteum function," *Reproductive Biology and Endocrinology*, vol. 1, article 95, 2003.

[29] L. Miller and J. S. Hunt, "Regulation of TNF-α production in activated mouse macrophages by progesterone," *Journal of Immunology*, vol. 160, no. 10, pp. 5098–5104, 1998.

[30] R. W. Whitman, *Weight change, body condition and beef cow reproduction [Ph.D. dissertation]*, Colorado State University, Fort Collins, Colo, USA, 1975.

[31] D. J. Putney, W. W. Thatcher, M. Drost, J. M. Wright, and M. A. DeLorenzo, "Influence of environmental temperature on reproductive performance of bovine embryo donors and recipients in the southwest region of the United States," *Theriogenology*, vol. 30, no. 5, pp. 905–922, 1988.

[32] J. E. Pexton, C. W. Weems, and E. K. Inskeep, "Prostaglandins F in uterine and ovarian venous plasma from nonpregnant and pregnant ewes collected by cannulation," *Prostaglandins*, vol. 9, no. 3, pp. 501–509, 1975.

[33] D. C. Kenison, T. H. Elsasser, and R. Fayer, "Radioimmunoassay for bovine tumor necrosis factor: concentrations and circulating molecular forms in bovine plasma," *Journal of Immunoassay*, vol. 11, no. 2, pp. 177–198, 1990.

[34] J. A. Vizcarra, R. P. Wettemann, J. C. Spitzer, and D. G. Morrison, "Body condition at parturition an dpostpartum weight gain influence luteal activity and concentrations of glucose, insulin, and noesterified faty acids in plasma of primiparous beef cows," *Journal of Animal Science*, vol. 76, no. 4, pp. 927–936, 1998.

[35] G. E. Selk, R. P. Wettemann, K. S. Lusby et al., "Relationship among weight change, body condition and reproductive performance of range beef cows," *Journal of Animal Science*, vol. 66, no. 12, pp. 3153–3159, 1988.

[36] R. W. Shephard, J. M. Morton, and S. T. Norman, "Effects of administration of gonadotropin-releasing hormone at artificial insemination on conception rates in dairy cows," *Animal Reproduction Science*, vol. 144, no. 1-2, pp. 14–21, 2014.

[37] A. P. Phatak, H. L. Whitmore, and M. D. Brown, "Effect of gonadotrophin releasing hormone on conception rate in repeat-breeder dairy cows," *Theriogenology*, vol. 26, no. 5, pp. 605–609, 1986.

[38] W. W. Thatcher, P. J. Hansen, T. S. Gross, S. D. Helmer, C. Plante, and F. W. Bazer, "Antiluteolytic effects of bovine trophoblast protein-1," *Journal of Reproduction and Fertility. Supplement*, vol. 37, pp. 91–99, 1989.

[39] T. Diaz, E. J.-P. Schmitt, R. L. De La Sota, M.-J. Thatcher, and W. W. Thatcher, "Human Chorionic Gonadotropin-induced alterations in ovarian follicular dynamics during the estrous cycle of heifers," *Journal of Animal Science*, vol. 76, no. 7, pp. 1929–1936, 1998.

[40] P. M. Fricke, L. P. Reynolds, and D. A. Redmer, "Effect of human chorionic gonadotropin administered early in the estrous cycle on ovulation and subsequent luteal function in cows.," *Journal of animal science*, vol. 71, no. 5, pp. 1242–1246, 1993.

[41] R. Harper, W. A. Bennett, E. J. Cuadra, C. F. Vaughn, and N. S. Whitworth, "Effects of GnRH in combination with PGF2α on the dynamics of follicular and luteal cells in post-pubertal Holstein heifers," *Journal of Livestock Science*, vol. 117, no. 1, pp. 88–92, 2008.

[42] M. Zerani, G. Catone, M. Maranesi, A. Gobbetti, C. Boiti, and F. Parillo, "Gonadotropin-releasing hormone 1 directly affects corpora lutea lifespan in mediterranean buffalo (*Bubalus bubalis*) during diestrus: presence and in vitro effects on enzymatic and hormonal activities," *Biology of Reproduction*, vol. 87, no. 2, article 45, 2012.

[43] E. E. Nilsson, J. Stanfield, and M. K. Skinner, "Interactions between progesterone and tumor necrosis factor-α in the regulation of primordial follicle assembly," *Reproduction*, vol. 132, no. 6, pp. 877–886, 2006.

[44] Y. Li, N. Matsuzaki, K. Masuhiro et al., "Trophoblast-derived tumor necrosis factor-α induces release of human chorionic gonadotropin using interleukin-6 (IL-6) and IL-6-receptor-dependent system in the normal human trophoblasts," *The Journal of Clinical Endocrinology and Metabolism*, vol. 74, no. 1, pp. 184–191, 1992.

[45] V. Montgomery Rice, S. D. Limback, K. F. Roby, and P. F. Terranova, "Changes in circulating and ovarian concentrations of bioactive tumour necrosis factor α during the first ovulation at puberty in rats and in gonadotrophin-treated immature rats," *Journal of Reproduction and Fertility*, vol. 113, no. 2, pp. 337–341, 1998.

[46] A. El-Sayed, M. Hoelker, F. Rings et al., "Large-scale transcriptional analysis of bovine embryo biopsies in relation to pregnancy success after transfer to recipients," *Physiological Genomics*, vol. 28, no. 1, pp. 84–96, 2006.

[47] P. J. Hansen and J. Block, "Towards an embryocentric world: The current and potential uses of embryo technologies in dairy production," *Reproduction, Fertility and Development*, vol. 16, no. 1-2, pp. 1–14, 2004.

[48] G. D. Niswender, J. L. Juengel, P. J. Silva, M. K. Rollyson, and E. W. McIntush, "Mechanisms controlling the function and life span of the corpus luteum," *Physiological Reviews*, vol. 80, no. 1, pp. 1–29, 2000.

[49] M. Candolfi, G. Jaita, V. Zaldivar et al., "Progesterone antagonizes the permissive action of estradiol on tumor necrosis factor-α-induced apoptosis of anterior pituitary cells," *Endocrinology*, vol. 146, no. 2, pp. 736–743, 2005.

[50] G. Luo, V. M. Abrahams, S. Tadesse et al., "Progesterone inhibits basal and tnf-α-induced apoptosis in fetal membranes: a novel mechanism to explain progesterone-mediated prevention of preterm birth," *Reproductive Sciences*, vol. 17, no. 6, pp. 532–539, 2010.

[51] S. Bilodeau-Goeseels and J. P. Kastelic, "Factors affecting embryo survival and strategies to reduce embryonic mortality in cattle," *Canadian Journal of Animal Science*, vol. 83, no. 4, pp. 659–671, 2003.

[52] T. M. Nett, R. B. Staigmiller, A. M. Akbar, M. A. Diekman, W. E. Ellinwood, and G. D. Niswender, "Secretion of prostaglandin F2alpha in cycling and pregnant ewes," *Journal of Animal Science*, vol. 42, no. 4, pp. 876–880, 1976.

[53] G. D. Thorburn, R. I. Cox, W. B. Currie, B. J. Restall, and W. Schneider, "Prostaglandin F and progesterone concentrations in the utero-ovarian venous plasma of the ewe during the oestrous cycle and early pregnancy," *Journal of Reproduction and Fertility*, vol. 18, pp. 151–158, 1973.

[54] K. M. Burgess, M. M. Ralph, G. Jenkin, and G. D. Thorburn, "Effect of oxytocin and estradiol on uterine prostaglandin release in nonpregnant and early-pregnant ewes," *Biology of Reproduction*, vol. 42, no. 5-6, pp. 822–833, 1990.

[55] E. Choudhary, B. A. Costine, M. E. Wilson, E. K. Inskeep, and J. A. Flores, "Prostaglandin F2α (PGF2α) independent and dependent regulation of the bovine luteal endothelin system," *Domestic Animal Endocrinology*, vol. 27, no. 1, pp. 63–79, 2004.

[56] W. J. Silvia and G. D. Niswender, "Maintenance of the corpus luteum of early pregnancy in the ewe. IV. Changes in luteal sensitivity to prostaglandin F2α throughout early pregnancy," *Journal of Animal Science*, vol. 63, no. 4, pp. 1201–1207, 1986.

[57] W. E. Ellinwood, T. M. Nett, and G. D. Niswender, "Maintenance of the corpus luteum of early pregnancy in the ewe. I. Luteotropic properties of embryonic homogenates," *Biology of Reproduction*, vol. 21, no. 2, pp. 281–288, 1979.

[58] G. D. Niswender, J. L. Juengel, W. J. McGuire, C. J. Belfiore, and M. C. Wiltbank, "Luteal function: the estrous cycle and early pregnancy," *Biology of Reproduction*, vol. 50, no. 2, pp. 239–247, 1994.

Preliminary Study of Pet Owner Adherence in Behaviour, Cardiology, Urology, and Oncology Fields

Zita Talamonti, Chiara Cassis, Paola G. Brambilla, Paola Scarpa, Damiano Stefanello, Simona Cannas, Michela Minero, and Clara Palestrini

Università degli Studi di Milano, Dipartimento di Scienze Veterinarie e Sanità Pubblica (DIVET), Via Celoria 10, 20133 Milan, Italy

Correspondence should be addressed to Zita Talamonti; zita.talamonti@gmail.com

Academic Editor: Remo Lobetti

Successful veterinary treatment of animals requires owner adherence with a prescribed treatment plan. The aim of our study was to evaluate and compare the level of adherence of the owners of patients presented for behavioural, cardiological, urological, and oncological problems. At the end of the first examination, each owner completed a questionnaire. Then, the owners were called four times to fill out another questionnaire over the phone. With regard to the first questionnaire, statistically significant data concern behavioral medicine and cardiology. In the first area the owner's worry decreases during the follow-up and the number of owners who would give away the animal increases. In cardiology, owners who think that the pathology harms their animal's quality of life decreased significantly over time. With regard to the 9 additional follow-up questions, in behavioural medicine and urology the owner's discomfort resulting from the animal's pathology significantly decreases over time. Assessment of adherence appears to be an optimal instrument in identifying the positive factors and the difficulties encountered by owners during the application of a treatment protocol.

1. Introduction

Owner compliance or adherence to treatment recommendations can determine the success of veterinary treatment [1]. The term compliance describes the observance of a medical recommendation, but it also includes how well laws, regulations, and guidelines are applied when administering prescribed treatments. The concept of compliance in veterinary medicine involves the consistency and accuracy with which a client follows the regime recommended by the veterinarian or other veterinary health care team members [2]. The term "compliance" (or "observance") suggests that a patient adapts to, submits to, or obeys the instructions of a doctor and implies a submissive role with a professional in a position of authority. The negative connotation of the term has caused the medical world to increasingly distance itself from the term compliance, replacing it with "adherence"; in other words, the tendency to adhere to the doctor's instructions, carrying them out quickly, respectfully, and accurately [3]. The World

Health Organization defines adherence as "the extent to which a person's behaviour, taking medication, following a diet, and/or executing lifestyle changes, corresponds with agreed recommendations given by a health care provider" [4]. For these reasons, the term adherence is preferred to compliance and will be used throughout the text in this paper.

In veterinary medicine, adherence is the centrepiece for fulfilling the veterinary profession's obligation to advocate on behalf of the pet's best interest. Adherence is based on effective communication of recommendations, resulting in informed client acceptance and efficient follow-through for patient care [2]. The successful outcome of a prescribed treatment depends on several factors, including a correct diagnosis, the prescription of the right treatment, and the adherence shown by the patient. The veterinarian plays a fundamental role in owner adherence to treatment of and the management of the patient, so it appears to be the result of cooperation between both persons. Since the application of any diagnostic and therapeutic option requires the owner's consent, it is of prime importance for the attending doctor to achieve their adherence to treatment, so as to achieve a successful therapeutic outcome and client satisfaction [1]. A high level of adherence in the veterinary field is dependent on two basic factors: the owner's view of his/her animal (and the resulting importance of the said animal to the owner) and the owner's understanding of the medical situation [5, 6]. The goal is to provide what the client wants, which happens to be congruent with the health care team's delivering the care the patient needs and deserves; by increasing the client's understanding of veterinary recommendations and through the health care team's reinforcement of clarifications, adherence ratios increase [2]. Adherence to treatment also appears to be influenced by the duration and frequency of the treatment, by the consultation time offered by the clinician and by the quality of interaction between the veterinarian, the pet, and the owner. With regard to the duration of the treatment, several studies have shown a negative correlation between the level of adherence and a long treatment period. In fact, if a long-term treatment is prescribed, nonadherence of the owner may occur over time which, in the case of prolonged administration of drugs, leads to reduced intake by the patient. However, with regard to the relationship between adherence and the frequency with which the treatment must be administered, it seems that a higher frequency of drug administration leads to reduced adherence to treatment; adherence is therefore inversely proportional to the increase of daily doses [7]. There is also a relationship between adherence and the time devoted by the veterinarian to the consultation: the level of adherence is generally higher in owners who believe that the veterinarian has devoted more time to the consultation [8]. In the same way, the therapist's ability to adequately explain the reasons underlying a given behaviour/symptom manifested by the animal may have a positive influence on the owner's adherence to the treatment [9]. One of the reasons that causes an owner not to adhere to the treatment is his/her belief that the treatment is not necessary, thus emphasising the need to provide a better explanation of the benefits that can be obtained through the treatment and its correct application [10]. In this way, the owners see themselves as an active part of the healing process or the maintenance of the animal's state of well-being, which has a clear positive effect on adherence to protocols that are often demanding in terms of time and economy. In line with the aim of enhancing adherence levels, the veterinarian should provide maximum clarity concerning the pathology and the necessary therapeutic protocols, so that the owner can really understand the problem and the importance of applying the correct treatments. The veterinarian should then try to empathise with the owner, through an understanding of the difficulties that the owner may encounter in the application of specific therapeutic protocols [10]. Studies performed on human psychotherapy have shown how a reliable, empathic, and flexible attitude from the therapist has a positive impact on the cooperation of the patient, while a professional with an attitude perceived as rigid, aloof, tense, distracted, and insecure has a negative influence on the adherence shown by the patient [11]. Excessive lifestyle changes can have a negative influence on adherence to treatment: asking a patient to

change their lifestyle in order to improve a treatment (e.g., combining proper physical exercise and diet) is more difficult than following the pharmacological treatment alone [1]. Good adherence to treatment can also be obtained by inviting the owner to regular, scheduled follow-up visits to ensure that the treatment is being implemented correctly by the owner, modifying certain aspects based on the animal's response and encouraging the owner to express any doubts about the correct application of the treatment [12]. Only a few studies on compliance in veterinary medicine have been published and, to the authors' knowledge, no study to date has compared the pet owners' adherence in different veterinary areas. This study assessed and compared the adherence levels of the owners of patients with behavioural, cardiological, urological, and oncological problems. We investigated how the owners perceive the disease of their animal and what they think about the feasibility of the treatment proposed. Finally, we have assessed the perception of the owner related to the usefulness of the treatment and the difficulties they have encountered in implementing it.

2. Materials and Methods

The study was conducted on dogs that attended the clinical visit at the Behavioural, Cardiology, Urology, and Oncology Services of the Veterinary Sciences and Public Health Department of the University of Milan from November 2012 to October 2013.

The observational prospective study was comprised of an initial enrolment phase and a second follow-up monitoring phase.

Phase 1. Cases were chosen among dog patients presented at the veterinary clinic for specialist consultation in the different fields considered in this study. We used a convenience sampling technique as subjects were selected because of their convenient accessibility and proximity to the researcher. Enrolment coincided with the first examination and implied a written consent of the owners. The consultations were conducted by veterinarians, specialists in the field, and were of variable duration from 45 to 120 minutes. The clinical visit was composed of medical history-taking, clinical examination, classification of the pathology, explanation of the prescribed treatment and scheduled follow-up (with health checks on varying dates depending on the pathology and the observed need), and definition of clinical outcome and prognosis.

At the end of the first examination, the veterinarian carried out an initial questionnaire with the owner, composed of 6 multiple-choice questions. Each question was worded as a statement to which the respondent assigned a score expressed by means of a Likert scale, where 1 = strongly disagree; 2 = disagree; 3 = neither; 4 = agree; 5 = strongly agree.

Phase 2. Then, the owners were called by phone 15 days, 1 month, 3 months, and 6 months after the examination. During the telephone calls, a questionnaire was carried out which included, in addition to the initial 6 questions, further 9 follow-up questions (Table 1).

TABLE 1: Questionnaire: 1 = strongly disagree; 2 = disagree; 3 = neither; 4 = agree; and 5 = strongly agree.

| | Questionnaire | Follow-up | | | | |
		1	2	3	4	5
First visit	(1) I am concerned about the disorder of my animal					
	(2) I could abandon my animal because of the disorder					
	(3) I could euthanize my animal because of the disorder					
	(4) My daily routine have changed because of the disorder of my animal					
	(5) It is challenging to apply the new management rules					
	(6) My animal quality of life is compromised by its disorder					
	(7) The disorder of my animal has been explained in detail					
	(8) The disorder of my animal bothers me					
	(9) The disorder of my animal bothers my neighbors or roommates					
	(10) The pharmacological treatment has been explained in detail					
	(11) It is simple to follow pharmacological recommendation					
	(12) I am consistent in administering drugs					
	(13) It is useful to administer prescribed drugs					
	(14) My animal refuses to take drugs					
	(15) The new management rules has been explained in detail					

3. Data Analysis

The answers to the questionnaire were classified with scores from 1 to 5 and entered into a database for later statistical analysis. The data analysis was performed by means of IBM SPSS Statistics 22 software [13]. The data was subject to a descriptive analysis and then a Chi Square test to compare the observed and expected frequencies in each response category.

4. Results

This study analysed a total of 48 cases (26 spayed females, 2 intact females, 3 neutered males, and 17 intact males, with different ages ranging from 8 months to 14 years old), including 20 in the behavioural medicine area, 14 in cardiology, 8 in urology, and 6 in oncology. Some owners decided to terminate their involvement in the study (8.6%), some animals died (8.5%), and others were given away (3%) or euthanized (0.8%) (Table 2).

Phase 1. The analysis of the questionnaires gathered during the first examination showed how most owners (60.6%) proved to be concerned by their animal's disease (agree 33.5% and strongly agree 27.1%). Nevertheless, 42.2% of owners believe that the disease does not harm the animal's quality of life (strongly disagree 32.8%, disagree 9.4%) and are not thinking of giving it away or euthanizing it as a result of the pathology (70.3% strongly disagree). Of those interviewed, 40.4% believe that their day-to-day habits have not changed (strongly disagree 37.7%, disagree 7.6%) as a result of the animal's pathology and 53.5% find it easy to apply the new management rules recommended by the veterinarian (50.8% strongly disagree, 2.7% disagree).

These percentages vary depending on the area analysed. Table 3, in which the "strongly agree" responses are aggregated with the "agree" responses and "disagree" is aggregated

with "strongly disagree," details the results obtained in the four areas. Owners of urological patients were the most worried about the disorder of their dogs; furthermore they did not consider abandonment or euthanasia as an option or a solution for their animals' problems.

Daily routine was more affected in owners in cardiological and behavioral areas. In addition, owners in the latter category found it more difficult than others to apply the new management rules and many of them were convinced that the disease could compromise the quality of life of their animal (Table 3).

Phase 2. The changes in the responses given by owners over time showed that, in relation to the behavioural medicine area, the concern caused by the animal's pathology significantly falls during the follow-up visits ($p < 0.05$) (Figure 1). On the contrary, the percentage of owners who consider giving their dog away as a result of the pathology increases significantly over time ($p < 0.05$). The responses to any changes in day-to-day habits and the commitment to the new management rules remain constant throughout the entire duration of the study, as is also the case with owner's responses in the cardiology and urology areas. In cardiology, the number of owners who think that the pathology harms their animal's quality of life falls significantly over time ($p < 0.05$) (Figure 2). In the oncology area, although there are a higher number of owners who, during the follow-up visits, consider the possibility of euthanizing the animal, this variation is not significant.

With regard to the 9 additional questions in the follow-up questionnaires, the only significant data relates to the behavioural medicine and urology areas, in which the owner's discomfort resulting from the animal's pathology significantly decreases over time ($p < 0.05$). In the behavioural medicine area, the discomfort caused to cohabitants and neighbours also significantly decreases ($p < 0.05$).

TABLE 2: Number of owners who abandoned the study and number of patients abandoned, euthanized, and dead (BM = behavioural medicine; C = cardiology; U = urology; and O = oncology).

	First visit				15 days				1 month				3 months				6 months				Total			
	BM	C	U	O	BM	C	U	O	BM	C	U	O	BM	C	U	O	BM	C	U	O	BM	C	U	O
Owners who abandoned the study	0	0	0	0	2	1	0	0	0	0	0	0	2	0	0	0	0	0	0	0	**4**	**1**	**0**	**0**
Patients abandoned	0	0	0	0	0	0	0	0	0	0	0	0	3	0	0	0	1	0	0	0	**4**	**0**	**0**	**0**
Patients euthanized	0	0	0	0	0	0	0	0	0	0	0	0	1	0	0	0	0	0	0	0	**1**	**0**	**0**	**0**
Patients dead	0	0	0	0	1	0	0	1	0	1	0	0	0	1	1	0	0	3	0	3	**1**	**5**	**1**	**4**

TABLE 3: Results obtained by the four fields during the first visit.

	Behavioural medicine		Cardiology		Urology		Oncology	
	Agree	Disagree	Agree	Disagree	Agree	Disagree	Agree	Disagree
I am concerned about the disorder of my animal	49%	26%	71,2%	9,1%	77,5%	15,5%	53,3%	21%
I could abandon my animal because of the disorder	9%	61%	4,5%	75,8%	2,5%	90%	0%	76,7%
I could euthanize my animal because of the disorder	1%	74%	6%	71,2%	2,5%	82,5%	23,3%	50%
My daily routine have changed because of the disorder of my animal	37%	36%	37,9%	42,4%	22,5%	67,5%	20%	53,3%
It is challenging to apply the new management rules	32,9%	36,7%	15,4%	62,5%	9,4%	75%	4,2%	62,5%
My animal quality of life is compromised by its disorder	41,4%	29,3%	36,5%	42,4%	17,5%	70%	16,6%	43,6%

5. Discussion

The aim of our study was to assess the adherence levels of owners of patients in the behavioural, cardiological, urological, and oncological sectors of veterinary medicine. Given the lack of published research on pet owners' adherence in different veterinary areas, this pilot study was planned as a first step to determine if and how it is possible to assess and compare adherence in each of the considered sectors of veterinary medicine. The main limitation of this study is the relatively small sample of animals included, and this means that caution should therefore be exercised so as not to generalize these results and more patients should be involved in order to transfer the results to the entire population.

Overall, the owners who participated in the study appeared to be concerned by their animal's disorder; this information could be very important in improving the owner's adherence, because the concern for the pathology could represent a concrete reason for the person to adhere to the prescribed treatment [1]. However, the owner's concern does not appear to go hand in hand with the harm to the animal's quality of life. In fact, most interviewees believe that the pathology does not affect the animal's quality of life. This could be linked to poor knowledge and an erroneous interpretation of the animal's body language by the owner, which can make it difficult to recognise signs of the animal's discomfort or pain. In fact, owners often have an anthropomorphic view of their animal's behaviour and, consequently, they expect human behaviours

and reactions from their animals, often creating misunderstandings in the communication and relationship with the dog [14]. Giving the animal away and putting it down are possibilities that are rarely considered by the owner. The man-animal bond of companionship changes considerably over the years and the new way of experiencing the relationship with the pet often translates into greater attention to its health and greater emotional involvement in living with its disease and its loss [15]. This greater involvement of the owner not only causes him/her not to feel the influence of the pathology on their own day-to-day habits or to encounter difficulties in adapting to the needs pertaining to their animal's pathology, but also represents an effective instrument that can be used to obtain greater adherence.

When comparing the four clinical areas investigated, the owners of patients with behavioural problems stated that they were less worried about the problem manifested by their animal and this concern tends to fall over time. This could be linked to the fact that, to date, behavioural medicine and behavioural problems are not well-known by owners and this may lead them to underestimate or not recognize the seriousness of their dog or cat's disorder or the necessary commitment to their treatment, thus reducing their adherence level. It would therefore be necessary for owners to receive more in depth information from the attending veterinarians related to the possibility of onset of behavioural pathologies [9]. Owners who, in the first visit, appeared to be most concerned were those of the urology area. In our study, patients in this

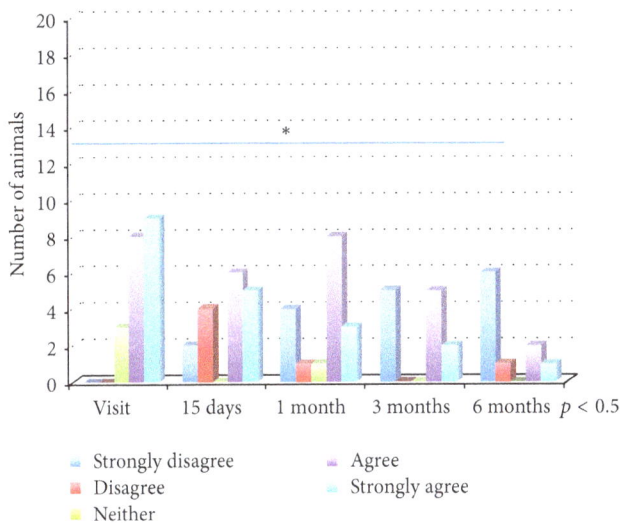

FIGURE 1: Behavioural medicine: "I am concerned about the disorder of my animal."

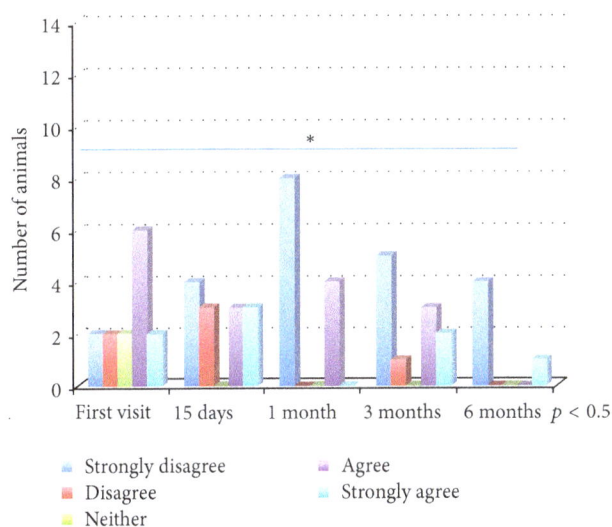

FIGURE 2: Cardiology: "My animal's quality of life is compromised by its disorder."

area were mainly cats and currently, as a result of veterinary information, the owners of these animals have a certain level of awareness of the possibility of elderly cats developing renal pathologies; their concern could therefore be based on knowledge of such serious pathologies. A simple explanation of the pathology may encourage the owner to follow the therapeutic protocol with a greater level of participation and attention. In fact, it seems that one of the reasons that causes an owner not to adhere to the treatment is his/her belief that the treatment is not necessary or useless, thus underlining the importance of providing a clear explanation of the benefits that can be obtained through the treatment and its correct application [10]. In this way, the owners see themselves as an active part of the healing process or the maintenance of the animal's state of well-being, which has a clear positive effect

on adherence to protocols that are often demanding in terms of time and money. In order to increase the adherence level, it seems important to ask owners to express their concerns about the health condition of the animal. This makes it possible to establish a dialogue with the owner, to make them feel free to express any concerns about the health of the animal and therefore add any important elements to the diagnostic process and the resulting treatment [16].

Among the four areas investigated, the owners who, upon the first visit, least consider the idea of putting down or giving the animal away as a result of the pathology are those in the urology area, followed by those of cardiology, oncology, and behavioural medicine. During the follow-up visits, the situation remains unchanged for the first three areas (in which no subject was given away or euthanized), while, in the behavioural area, four animals were given away and one was put down. For this purpose, it is important to consider the social aspect of behavioural pathology; behavioural problems often have a strong impact on the animal itself, the owner, and their cohabitants and neighbours, and this is why an owner could be more willing to give away or put down their animal [17]. Furthermore, owners often do not have sufficient information to manage the behavioural problem, they are not referred to specific, specialised professionals, and they attend specialist consultations when the problem has already been apparent for some time (thus compromising the prognosis [17, 18]). In addition to this, this factor could be influenced by the effect of time on the owner-dog relationship. In fact, in most cases, heart, urological, and oncological pathologies occur at an advanced age, that is to say, after years of close cohabitation between the person and the animal, with the resulting creation of a strong and deep-rooted bond; conversely, behavioural pathologies often arise in young animals or those recently adopted and, sometimes, this brief period is not sufficient to create a close and deep relationship. The increase in owners of patients in behavioural medicine who have given their animal away by the third follow-up can be traced back to the fact that, at this point in the treatment, the owner expects results that do not materialise because, in most cases, behavioural treatment requires time and commitment and results may not be visible after only one month from the start [18]. In this regard, it seems that the veterinarian can help to increase adherence levels by also inviting the owner to regular, scheduled follow-up visits: this would enable the veterinarian to ensure that the treatment is being implemented correctly by the owner and possibly change any aspects depending on the animal's response [1, 19].

When comparing the four areas investigated, the management rules laid down by the behavioural veterinary doctor as well as the day-to-day habits appear to be the most demanding. This may be derived from the fact that behavioural treatment, unlike that which is generally prescribed by specialists in the other three areas, is comprised of changes to the rules of management and interaction with the animal, in addition to administration of a pharmacological treatment where necessary [19]. Since the ease of applying the treatment has a positive effect on adherence levels, it is advisable to limit the amount of information provided, use clear and plain language, and speak slowly to enable the owner to absorb each indication given [2, 9, 20, 21]. Clear and simple explanations often give rise not only to greater adherence to the treatment, but also to an increase in the value attributed by the owner to the veterinary recommendations [10]. In fact, adherence to treatment appears to be significantly influenced by the importance and value given by the owner to the veterinary recommendations [10].

When comparing the four areas investigated, there are a greater number of owners in the behavioural medicine and cardiology groups who believe that the pathology harms the animal's quality of life. In the case of cardiology, there is a significant reduction of this value over time and this points to the effectiveness of the treatment enabling the owner to take into account the clinical improvements of their animal. This consideration is also reinforced by the fact that, in the same area, there is a significant decrease in the discomfort caused to the owner during the follow-up visits. The same information has also been obtained in the behavioural medicine area, in which there is also a reduction in the discomfort caused to the owner by the pathology [18].

6. Conclusions

In the veterinary field, the management of the patient is the result of cooperation between the veterinarian and the owner. The role of the veterinarian is therefore fundamental in enabling an increase in the levels of adherence to the therapeutic protocols by the owners of animals.

To achieve good adherence levels, constant contact between the doctor and owner is necessary. It is therefore essential that the owner be allowed to clarify any doubts with the veterinarian that may arise during treatment and to receive constant support in the administration of the treatment and coping with the animal's pathology. Assessment of adherence appears to be an optimal instrument in identifying the positive factors and the difficulties encountered by owners during the application of a treatment requiring the administration of specific drugs and the implementation of precise management rules. The results set out here should be considered as preliminary to research that we are conducting on a wider sample of animals for a longer follow-up period.

Conflict of Interests

The authors declare that there is no conflict of interests regarding the publication of this paper.

Acknowledgment

The authors acknowledge the assistance of Kirk T. Ford for the revision of the English paper.

References

[1] American Animal Hospital Association, *The Path to High-Quality Care. Practical Tips for improving Compliance*, American Animal Hospital Association, Lakewood, Colo, USA, 2003.

[2] C. J. Wayner and M. L. Heinke, "Compliance: crafting quality care," *Veterinary Clinics of North America: Small Animal Practice*, vol. 36, no. 2, pp. 419–436, 2006.

[3] T. Klauer and U. K. Zettl, "Compliance, adherence, and the treatment of multiple sclerosis," *Journal of Neurology*, vol. 255, no. 6, supplement, pp. 87–92, 2008.

[4] World Health Organization, *Adherence to Long-Term Therapies*, World Health Organization, Geneva, Switzerland, 2003.

[5] R. A. S. White, "The approach to the tumor patient," in *Manual of Small Animal Oncology*, R. A. S. White, Ed., pp. 13–16, British Small Animal Veterinary Association (BSAVA), 1991.

[6] P. A. Ciekot, "Consulenza al cliente per il cancro: considerazioni per una presentazione professionale ed intelligente delle opzioni, dei rischi e degli scopi terapeutici," in *Oncologia Chirurgica*, S. D. Gilson, Ed., vol. 9, no. 2, pp. 215–227, Medicina-Scienze, 1998.

[7] V. J. Adams, J. R. Campbell, C. L. Waldner, P. M. Dowling, and C. L. Shmon, "Evaluation of client compliance with short-term administration of antimicrobials to dogs," *Journal of the American Veterinary Medical Association*, vol. 226, no. 4, pp. 567–574, 2005.

[8] K. Grave and H. Tanem, "Compliance with short-term oral antibacterial drug treatment in dogs," *Journal of Small Animal Practice*, vol. 40, no. 4, pp. 158–162, 1999.

[9] B. A. Berger, "Assessing and interviewing patients for meaningful behavioral change: part 1," *The Case Manager*, vol. 15, no. 5, pp. 46–50, 2004.

[10] T. W. Lue, D. P. Pantenburg, and P. M. Crawford, "Impact of the owner-pet and client-veterinarian bond on the care that pets receive," *Journal of the American Veterinary Medical Association*, vol. 232, no. 4, pp. 531–540, 2008.

[11] S. J. Ackerman and M. J. Hilsenroth, "A review of therapist characteristics and techniques negatively impacting the therapeutic alliance," *Psychotherapy*, vol. 38, no. 2, pp. 171–185, 2001.

[12] L. Pagliaro, "Medicina basata sule evidenze," *Recenti Progressi in Medicina*, vol. 89, no. 3, 1998.

[13] IBM, *IBM SPSS Statistics 22 Command Syntax Reference*, IBM, Chicago, Ill, USA, 2013.

[14] J. W. S. Bradshaw and R. A. Casey, "Anthropomorphism and anthropocentrism as influences in the quality of life of companion animals," *Animal Welfare*, vol. 16, pp. 149–154, 2007.

[15] L. Lagoni, C. Butler, and S. J. Withrow, "Companion animal death and pet owner grief," in *Small Animal Clinical Oncology*, S. J. Withrow and E. G. MacEwen, Eds., pp. 547–559, WB Saunders, 2nd edition, 1996.

[16] J. R. Shaw, B. N. Bonnett, C. L. Adams, and D. L. Roter, "Veterinarian-client-patient communication patterns used during clinical appointments in companion animal practice," *Journal of the American Veterinary Medical Association*, vol. 228, no. 5, pp. 714–721, 2006.

[17] L. Notari and B. Gallicchio, "Owners' perceptions of behavior problems and behavior therapists in Italy: a preliminary study," *Journal of Veterinary Behavior: Clinical Applications and Research*, vol. 3, no. 2, pp. 52–58, 2008.

[18] K. L. Overall, *La clinica comportamentale del cane e del gatto*, C.G. Edizioni Medico Scientifiche, 2001.

[19] Y. Takeuchi, K. A. Houpt, and J. M. Scarlett, "Evaluation of treatments for separation anxiety in dogs," *Journal of the American Veterinary Medical Association*, vol. 217, no. 3, pp. 342–345, 2000.

[20] R. P. C. Kessels, "Patients' memory for medical information," *Journal of the Royal Society of Medicine*, vol. 96, no. 5, pp. 219–222, 2003.

[21] C. Bower, "Il ruolo della medicina comportamentale nella pratica veterinaria," in *Terapia comportamentale del cane e del gatto*, D. F. Horwitz, D. S. Mills, and S. Heath, Eds., UTET, 2004.

25

Kennel Disinfectants for *Microsporum canis* and *Trichophyton* sp.

Karen A. Moriello

Department of Medical Sciences, School of Veterinary Medicine, University of Wisconsin-Madison, 2015 Linden Drive West, Madison, WI 53706, USA

Correspondence should be addressed to Karen A. Moriello; moriellk@svm.vetmed.wisc.edu

Academic Editor: Douglas Morck

The antifungal efficacy of commonly used kennel disinfectants for large surfaces was tested using naturally infective material from untreated animals (*M. canis* and *Trichophyton* sp.) soaked and macerated but unfiltered leaving visible fluorescing hairs and/or scales in the test inoculum to create a robust challenge. Disinfectants included sodium hypochlorite (1 : 32 and 1 : 100), enilconazole (1 : 100), accelerated hydrogen peroxide (1 : 16), potassium peroxymonosulfate (1% and 2%), and calcium hypochlorite "dry bleach." Disinfectants were tested at a 1 : 10, 1 : 5, and 1 : 1 dilution of test inoculum to disinfectant with a 10 min contact time. Good efficacy was defined as a disinfectant resulting in no growth. Control plates grew >300 colonies of each pathogen per plate. Enilconazole, sodium hypochlorite (all dilutions), accelerated hydrogen peroxide, and 2% potassium peroxymonosulfate (but not 1%) inhibited all growth of both pathogens at 1 : 10, 1 : 5, and 1 : 1 dilutions. Calcium hypochlorite showed no antifungal efficacy (>300 colonies per plate). Enilconazole (1 : 100), sodium hypochlorite (1 : 32 or 1 : 100), accelerated hydrogen peroxide (1 : 16), and 2% potassium peroxymonosulfate are recommended for decontamination of kennels exposed to dermatophyte pathogens.

1. Introduction

Environmental disinfection is an important component of the prevention and control of dermatophytosis and is of particular importance in facilities housing large numbers of animals (e.g., animal shelters, boarding kennels, etc.). Many factors need to be considered when selecting a kennel disinfectant including, but not limited to, efficacy, lack of toxicity or irritancy to animals or workers, cost, ease of application, and lack of corrosiveness to surfaces, for example, cages.

Although sodium hypochlorite is a commonly used disinfectant in multianimal facilities, there is increasing interest in using compounds that are inexpensive, easier to use, and less corrosive to cages. One of these compounds is calcium hypochlorite, also referred to as "dry bleach" because it is supplied in pellets and packages. This compound is most commonly used to disinfect foods, swimming pools, and water supplies [1–3]. It is also used in over-the-counter bathroom cleaners and disinfectants and to kill moss and algae. It is an increasingly popular kennel disinfectant because it is automatically diluted and dispensed using a water house, is inexpensive, and is not very corrosive [4].

Although the commercial products do not claim antifungal efficacy, the lay literature on kennel disinfectants often claims it is effective in the control and treatment of dermatophytosis; however published studies to support this could not be found.

One laboratory method used to test the field efficacy of antifungal disinfectants is the isolated infected spore model [5]. In this methodology, infected hairs harvested from untreated animals are used to produce a test inoculum that contains naturally infective material. In this model, the test inoculum is filtered to remove organic debris. A valid criticism of the isolated infective spore test inoculum is that it may not be a robust enough test because it lacks organic material, specifically particulate infective hairs or scales. If the filtering step is omitted the test inoculum contains a marked amount of organic material, that is, small pieces of infective hairs, scales, and debris similar to what would be found on a kennel surface deemed "visibly clean" prior to application of

TABLE 1: Mean number of colony forming units after exposure to disinfectants.

	M. canis			Trichophyton sp.		
	1:10	1:5	1:1	1:10	1:5	1:1
Water	>100	>100	>100	>100	>100	>100
Sodium hypochlorite 1:10	0	0	0	0	0	0
Sodium hypochlorite 1:32	0	0	0	0	0	0
Sodium hypochlorite 1:100	0	0	0	0	0	0
AHP 1:16	0	0	0	0	0	0
Enilconazole 1:100	0	0	0	0	0	0
2% potassium peroxymonosulfate	0	0	0	0	0	0
1% potassium peroxymonosulfate	4 ± 5	15 ± 6	23 ± 3	0	2 ± 3	7 ± 4
Calcium hypochlorite	>100	>100	>100	>100	>100	>100

Mean of the agar plates ± standard deviation.
AHP: accelerated hydrogen peroxide (Accel).

a disinfectant. The objective of this study was to determine the antifungal efficacy of six kennel disinfectants against a robust challenge of naturally infective material.

2. Materials and Methods

2.1. Test Pathogens. *Microsporum canis* was obtained from kittens with untreated spontaneous infections. For testing of a *Trichophyton* sp. pathogen, infective crusts were obtained from juvenile hedgehogs with spontaneous untreated infections (i.e., *T. erinacei*).

2.2. Preparation of Infective Spore Suspensions. Infective spore suspensions were prepared using a modification of previously published method [5]. Briefly, naturally infective material was soaked in sterile water for 15 min and minced with a sterile scalpel blade three times. Using a tissue macerator the suspension was macerated until an opaque solution was obtained. For this study, the solution was not filtered and hair and scales were grossly visible. Wood's lamp examination of the *M. canis* spore suspension revealed large numbers of fluorescing particles and microscopic examination of the *Trichophyton* sp. suspension revealed intact crusts and identifiable scales.

2.3. Fungal Cultures. Mycosel Agar (Becton Dickinson, Cockeyville, MD, USA) was used for fungal cultures. Plates were incubated at 30°C and examined daily for growth for 14 days. Colony forming units (cfu) for each plate were determined as the maximum number of colonies at day 14 of culture. Potential pathogens were identified microscopically using established morphological criteria.

2.4. Kennel Disinfectants. Disinfectants tested included 5.5% sodium hypochlorite diluted 1:32 and 1:100, accelerated hydrogen peroxide at 1:16 (Accel Concentrate 4.25%, Virox Technologies, Oakville, Ontario, Canada), potassium peroxymonosulfate at 1% and 2% (Trifectant: Vetoquinol, Fort Worth, TX), and enilconazole at 1:100 (Clinafarm, Schering Plough Animal Health, Union, New Jersey) and calcium hypochlorite (Wysiwash, Wysiwash, South Daytona,

FL, USA). For calcium hypochlorite one liter of test solution was collected midstream after allowing the hose to run for 3 min. All test solutions were prepared fresh and used within 3 h. Sterile distilled water and 5.5% sodium hypochlorite (1:10 dilution) were used as untreated and treated controls, respectively.

2.5. Testing Protocol. Infective spore suspensions were tested at a 1:10, 1:5, and 1:1 dilution of spores to disinfectant with a contact time of 10 min. Testing solutions were vortexed four times (0 min, 5 min, 9 min, and 10 min) during the contact time to ensure adequate exposure of spores to disinfectant. Four 100 μL aliquots of each test suspension were inoculated on fungal culture plates by spreading the suspension evenly on the surface with a sterile loop. Stock suspensions were repeatedly vortexed before and between samplings to ensure fungal spores and hairs did not settle in the test tube. All testing was done in triplicate. Disinfectants lacking antifungal efficacy were retested using isolated infected spores, that is, filtered test inoculum.

2.6. Data Analysis. Descriptive data was collected. The number of colony forming units per plate was counted and presented as the mean ± standard deviation. For the purposes of this study, good efficacy was defined as a disinfectant that produced no growth.

3. Results and Discussion

A 100 μL inoculum of each pathogen grew too many to count colonies per plate. Serial dilutions estimated the 5×10^5 and 8×10^6 infective spores per mL for *M. canis* and *Trichophyton* sp., respectively. However this number likely underestimated the test inoculum since it cannot account for the spore challenge in particulate hair or scales. Pre-, mid-, and postexperiment 100 μL inoculums grew >300 cfu/plate for both pathogens. Enilconazole, AHP, 2% potassium peroxymonosulfate, and all dilutions of sodium hypochlorite were 100% fungicidal (Table 1) against both pathogens. Calcium hypochlorite lacked fungicidal activity (Table 1) in this test model and when retested using isolated infected spores (i.e., filtered test inoculum). 1% potassium peroxymonosulfate was not considered to have good efficacy compared to 2% potassium peroxymonosulfate.

In this study, calcium hypochlorite demonstrated no fungicidal activity against naturally infective material. This is most likely due to the fact that this product is primarily an algaecide.

Decontamination of surfaces exposed to dermatophytes requires a "hard clean." Specifically, all gross material should be mechanically removed and the area washed with a detergent until visibly clean, rinsed to remove residual detergents and excess water removed to prevent dilution of the disinfectant, and then finally sprayed with a disinfectant. Disinfectants are intended to kill any remaining spores not removed via mechanical cleaning. With respect to this, it is important to note two things. First, there was a strict 10 min contact time. Second, although the test suspensions contained visible hair and skin debris no other organic material was present (e.g., feces, serum, and food) that could prevent contact between the infective material and the disinfectant. Although these disinfectants were highly efficacious against a robust spore challenge, proper surface preparation is still a necessity for good sanitation.

One of the reasons this study was conducted was to answer anecdotal comments that original isolated infective spore model results were not representative of the "real world" because hair and debris were removed. The findings in this study are similar to those previously published using filtered isolated infective spores in either suspension tests or textile disinfectant testing [5–7]. This is supporting evidence that the original isolated infective spore model is a robust challenge and that data using that model is valid. The advantage of the isolated infective spore model over the procedure used in this study was that less naturally infective material is needed.

4. Conclusions and Clinical Relevance

In practice, these findings suggest that if obvious organic debris is removed and the surface is visibly clean, the use of sodium hypochlorite (1 : 32 and 1 : 100), enilconazole 1 : 16, 2% potassium peroxymonosulfate, or accelerated hydrogen peroxide 1 : 16 with a 10 min contact time is an efficacious disinfectant for any residual remaining infective material of dermatophytosis.

Conflict of Interests

The author declares that there is no conflict of interests regarding the publication of this paper.

Acknowledgments

This project was funded by the Companion Animal Fund School of Veterinary Medicine, University of Wisconsin-Madison, and the Winn Foundation for Feline Research. The author thanks Lauren Mullen and the staff at the San Francisco SPCA, San Francisco, California, USA, for providing resources for this study and Dr. Julie Levy, College of Veterinary Medicine, University of Florida, for donation of the calcium hypochlorite dispensing system.

References

[1] H. Ding, T.-J. Fu, and M. A. Smith, "Microbial contamination in sprouts: how effective is seed disinfection treatment?" *Journal of Food Science*, vol. 78, no. 4, pp. R495–R501, 2013.

[2] B. F. Arnold and J. M. Colford Jr., "Treating water with chlorine at point-of-use to improve water quality and reduce child diarrhea in developing countries: a systematic review and meta-analysis," *The American Journal of Tropical Medicine and Hygiene*, vol. 76, no. 2, pp. 354–364, 2007.

[3] J. A. Wojtowicz, "Water treatment of swimming pools, spas, and hot tubs," in *Kirk-Othmer Encyclopedia of Chemical Technology*, John Wiley & Sons, Hoboken, NJ, USA, 5th edition, 2004.

[4] M. Spindel, "Sanity Animal Sheltering," 2011, http://www.animalsheltering.org/, http://www.animalsheltering.org/resources/magazine/may_jun_2011/shelter_med_sanitation_sanity.pdf.

[5] K. A. Moriello, D. J. Deboer, L. M. Volk, A. Sparkes, and A. Robinson, "Development of an *in vitro*, isolated, infected spore testing model for disinfectant testing of *Microsporum canis* isolates," *Veterinary Dermatology*, vol. 15, no. 3, pp. 175–180, 2004.

[6] K. A. Moriello and H. Hondzo, "Efficacy of disinfectants containing accelerated hydrogen peroxide against conidial arthrospores and isolated infective spores of *Microsporum canis* and *Trichophyton* sp," *Veterinary Dermatology*, vol. 25, no. 3, p. 191-e48, 2014.

[7] K. A. Moriello, D. Kunder, and H. Hondzo, "Efficacy of eight commercial disinfectants against *Microsporum canis* and *Trichophyton* spp: infective spores on an experimentally contaminated textile surface," *Veterinary Dermatology*, vol. 24, no. 6, pp. 621–623, 2013.

26

Claw Lesions Causing Clinical Lameness in Lactating Holstein Frisian Crossbred Cows

Umar Nazir Zahid,[1] Swaran Singh Randhawa,[2] Syed Ashaq Hussain,[2]
Sarnarinder Singh Randhawa,[3] Vishal Mahajan,[4] and Kirti Dua[2]

[1] Department of Animal Husbandry, Jammu and Kashmir 190019, India
[2] Department of Veterinary Medicine, Guru Angad Dev Veterinary and Animal Sciences University, Ludhiana,
  Punjab 141004, India
[3] Guru Angad Dev Veterinary and Animal Sciences University, Ludhiana, Punjab 141004, India
[4] Animal Disease Research Centre, Guru Angad Dev Veterinary and Animal Sciences University, Ludhiana, Punjab 141004, India

Correspondence should be addressed to Syed Ashaq Hussain; draashiqhussain@gmail.com

Academic Editor: William Ravis

The objective of this study was to identify claw lesions causing clinical lameness in lactating Holstein Frisian (HF) crossbred cows in dairy cattle. Seventy dairy farmers were interviewed at the monthly meetings of Progressive Dairy Farmers Association of Ludhiana, Punjab, India. Ten dairy farms were randomly selected as per probability proportional to size and a total of 450 lactating HF crossbred cows were taken into the study. All the lactating cows were scored for locomotion and rear leg view index. Trimming was done in all the clinically lame animals (animals with locomotion scores 2 and 3) and equal number of animals selected randomly from those with locomotion scores 0 and 1. Various claw lesions were evaluated in both the groups. There was a significant relationship between locomotion score and rear leg view index to identify lameness. Sole ulcers and white line fissures were the lesions responsible for clinical lameness. Other lesions did not cause clinical lameness but increased the asymmetry in lactating HF crossbred cows. Both locomotion score and rear leg view index could be reliably used to identify clinical lameness in lactating cattle.

1. Introduction

Lameness is one of the greatest economic concerns of present day dairy industry. The major ill effects of lameness include pain, distress, loss in production, a negative impact on reproductive performance, and an increased risk of culling [1]. It is reported that 60% of herd may become lame at least once a year [2] and about 90–99% of lameness incidents occur due to claw lesions [3, 4]. Clinical lameness is comparatively more concerned because of high rate of culling [5] and marked reduction in milk yield [6].

The mere presence of a lesion is not associated with clinical lameness [7] but it also depends on severity of foot lesion. Only a few studies have investigated the relationship between locomotion score and the type of foot lesion present [8–10]. Sole ulcer, double sole, interdigital purulent inflammation,

and severe stages of digital dermatitis have been associated with clinical lameness [7, 11]. Keeping in view the increasing population of HF crossbred cows in Punjab, India, this study seemed to be necessary. The present study was designed to identify the foot lesions responsible for clinical lameness in lactating HF crossbred cattle. Another objective was to evaluate the reliability of locomotion score and rear leg view index for identifying clinical lameness.

2. Materials and Methods

2.1. Selection of Animals. Seventy farmers were interviewed at the monthly meetings of Progressive Dairy Farmers Association of Ludhiana, Punjab, India. The farmers were questioned about general management, housing system, claw trimming

TABLE 1: Association between locomotion scores (2 and 3) and various lesions.

Lesions	Coefficients	Standard error	P value	Lower 95%	Upper 95%
Intercept	2.107	0.116	0.00	1.876	2.339
HE	−0.0029	0.014	0.842	−0.031	0.026
SH	0.0027	0.027	0.921	−0.051	0.056
WLH	0.1100	0.11	0.322	−0.11	0.329
SA	0.0117	0.014	0.392	−0.015	0.039
US	−0.0047	0.049	0.925	−0.103	0.094
OS	0.0391	0.071	0.586	−0.104	0.182
OH	−0.0465	0.226	0.838	−0.499	0.406
WLF	0.0707*	0.034	0.044	0.002	0.14
IDH	0.0680	0.224	0.762	−0.38	0.516
SU	0.478*	0.147	0.002	0.184	0.773

*Significant at $P \leq 0.05$.
HE: heel erosion, SH: sole haemorrhage, WLH: white line haemorrhage, SA: sole avulsion, US: underrun sole, OS: overgrown sole, OH: overgrown hoof, WLF: white line fissure, IDH: interdigital hyperplasia, SU: sole ulcer.

TABLE 2: Association between locomotion scores (0 and 1) and various lesions.

Lesions	Coefficients	Standard error	P value	Lower 95%	Upper 95%
Intercept	0.71	0.088	0.000	0.537	0.890
HE	0.015	0.013	0.263	−0.012	0.042
SH	0.010	0.035	0.780	−0.060	0.080
WLH	0.006	0.093	0.948	−0.180	0.192
SA	0.003	0.026	0.894	−0.049	0.055
US	0.068	0.044	0.128	−0.020	0.157
OS	−0.146	0.086	0.095	−0.317	0.026
OH	−0.741	0.427	0.088	−1.597	0.115
WLF	0.039	0.143	0.784	−0.247	0.325
IDH	0.021	0.095	0.824	−0.169	0.211

HE: heel erosion, SH: sole haemorrhage, WLH: white line haemorrhage, SA: sole avulsion, US: underrun sole, OS: overgrown sole, OH: overgrown hoof, WLF: white line fissure, IDH: interdigital hyperplasia.

routines, milk production, nutrition, number of lame animals, presence of lameness chute, and knowledge about lameness and its ill effects. Among these seventy enrolled farmers, ten farms were selected randomly as per probability proportional to size sampling [12]. A total of 450 lactating HF cross bred cows were included in the study. All these animals were kept in loose housing system with provision of both soft and concrete flooring. The average milk yield of these animals was 3000–4000 litres/lactation. Majority of the animals were fed maize silage along with concentrate feed @ 400 gram for every kilogram of milk production.

2.2. Locomotion Score and Rear Leg View Index (RLVI). All the ten farms were visited after the morning milking. Locomotion score and rear leg view index of all the 450 animals were evaluated independently by two observers, working together. For locomotion score, the cows were allowed to walk on a flat surface for up to 30 meters. Locomotion score of each animal was assessed on a five-point scale as described by Wells et al. [13]. RLVI of each animal was recorded as normal/score 0 (when there was no inward knuckling of hocks and hocks were straight) and cow hock/score 1 (when

there was inward knuckling of hocks), when observed from rear side [14].

2.3. Hoof Examination. Hoof trimming was done as per standard procedure [14] and different foot lesions were observed in all the lame animals (locomotion scores 2 and 3) and equal number of animals selected randomly from those with locomotion scores 0 and 1 [12]. Each animal was properly restrained in trimming chute and then each foot was examined for any lesion before and after paring a layer of approximately 1 mm of horn from the weight bearing surface. Heel erosions, sole haemorrhages, sole avulsions, white line haemorrhages, and white line fissures were scored for severity on hoof maps, as per Randhawa et al. [15]. The rest of the foot lesions, namely, sole ulcers, underrun soles, double soles, overgrown hooves, overgrown soles, and interdigital hyperplasia, were categorized as 1 (when present) and 0 (when absent) [14].

2.4. Statistical Analysis. In order to identify the lesions responsible for lameness, regression analysis was carried out using statistical package for social sciences (SPSS for windows

TABLE 3: Correlation between lesions within cows having locomotion scores 2 and 3 (first row = correlation coefficient, second row = probability value).

Lesion	HE	SH	WLH	SA	US	OS	OH	WLF	IDH	SU
HE	1									
	.									
SH	0.1	1								
	0.201	.								
WLH	−0.019	−0.047	1							
	0.332	0.346	.							
SA	0.26*	0.008	−0.07	1						
	0.013	0.473	0.277	.						
US	0.224*	0.003	−0.025	−0.083	1					
	0.029	0.49	0.415	0.243	.					
OS	−0.051	−0.163	0.125	−0.083	0.299**	1				
	0.333	0.084	0.145	0.244	0.005	.				
OH	0.315**	0.025	−0.041	−0.011	0.096	−0.062	1			
	0.003	0.415	0.364	0.462	0.211	0.301	.			
WLF	−0.02	−0.076	0.082	0.123	0.029	0.134	−0.081	1		
	0.433	0.26	0.244	0.149	0.404	0.128	0.249	.		
IDH	−0.121	0.084	−0.084	−0.053	0.089	0.033	−0.028	−0.087	1	
	0.154	0.241	0.239	0.327	0.227	0.391	0.406	0.233	.	
SU	−0.059	−0.104	0.041	−0.181	−0.189	−0.028	−0.039	0.253**	−0.081	1
	0.31	0.191	0.364	0.062	0.055	0.406	0.37	0.015	0.249	.

*Significant at 0.05 level; **significant at 0.01 level.
HE: heel erosion, SH: sole haemorrhage, WLH: white line haemorrhage, SA: sole avulsion, US: underrun sole, OS: overgrown sole, OH: overgrown hoof, WLF: white line fissure, IDH: interdigital hyperplasia, SU: sole ulcer.

TABLE 4: Correlation between lesions within cows having locomotion scores 0 and 1 (first row = correlation coefficient, second row = probability value).

Lesion	HE	SH	WLH	SA	US	OS	OH	WLF	IDH
HE	1								
	.								
SH	0.151	1							
	0.225	.							
WLH	0.025	0.45**	1						
	0.842	0	.						
SA	0.093	0.241	0.17	1					
	0.456	0.051	0.173	.					
US	−0.062	−0.107	−0.141	−0.096	1				
	0.623	0.392	0.26	0.445	.				
OS	0.386**	−0.038	−0.081	−0.016	0.205	1			
	0.001	0.764	0.516	0.899	0.099	.			
OH	−0.053	0.08	0.162	−0.039	0.008	0.103	1		
	0.672	0.522	0.193	0.759	0.951	0.412	.		
WLF	0.109	0.011	−0.114	0.097	0.062	0.101	0.095	1	
	0.384	0.929	0.364	0.438	0.622	0.422	0.45	.	
IDH	0.034	0.014	−0.119	0.146	0.143	0.006	0.044	0.884**	1
	0.785	0.91	0.343	0.242	0.254	0.964	0.728	0	.

**Significant at 0.01 level.
HE: heel erosion, SH: sole haemorrhage, WLH: white line haemorrhage, SA: sole avulsion, US: underrun sole, OS: overgrown sole, OH: overgrown hoof, WLF: white line fissure, IDH: interdigital hyperplasia.

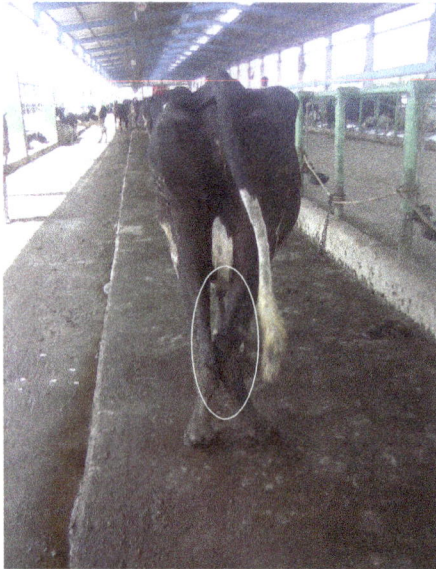

FIGURE 1: Cow hock: rear leg view index.

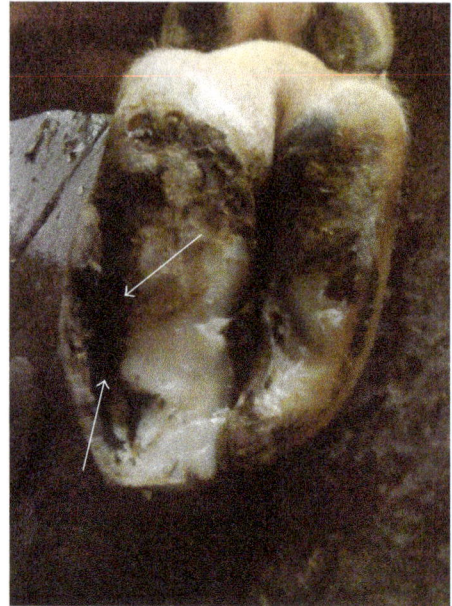

FIGURE 2: Heel erosion.

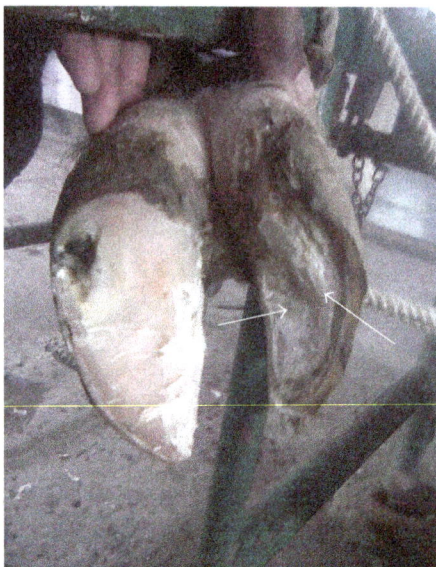

FIGURE 3: Sole avulsion.

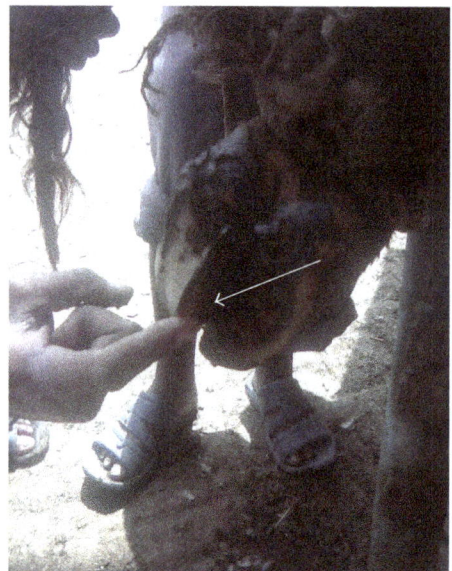

FIGURE 4: White line fissure.

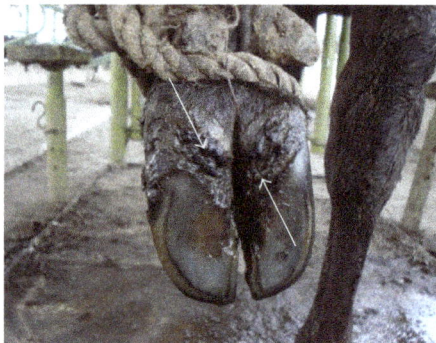

FIGURE 5: Underrun sole.

version 11-0-1; SPSS Inc, Chicago, Illinois). The correlation between different lesions within cow was investigated and correlated at $P \leq 0.05$ and $P \leq 0.01$. The relationship between locomotion score and rear leg view was analyzed by Chi square analysis. The reliability of locomotion scores assigned by two observers was analyzed by calculating Spearman's rank correlation coefficient.

3. Results

Out of 450 cows, 8.6% ($n = 39$), 73.7% ($n = 332$), 12.8% ($n = 58$), and 4.6% ($n = 21$) were having 0, 1, 2, and 3 locomotion score, respectively. The association between

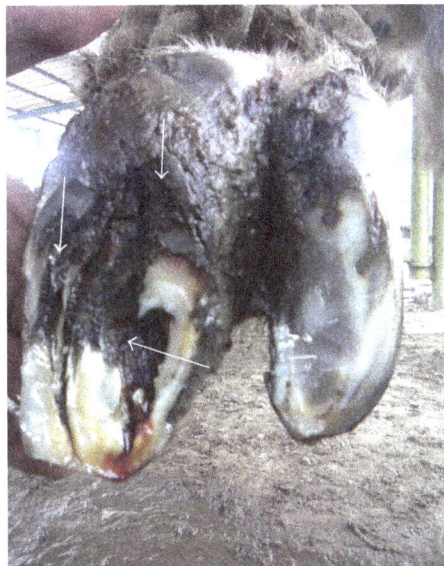

FIGURE 6: Heel erosion, white line fissure, and underrun sole.

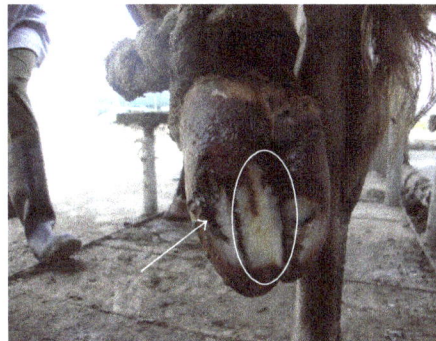

FIGURE 7: Overgrown sole.

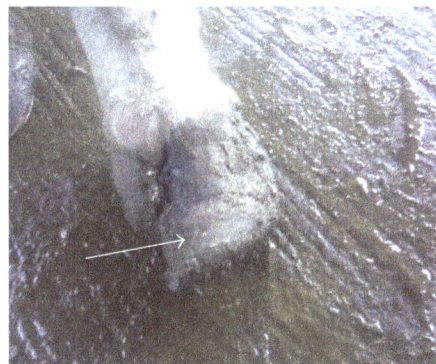

FIGURE 8: Overgrown sole and white line fissure.

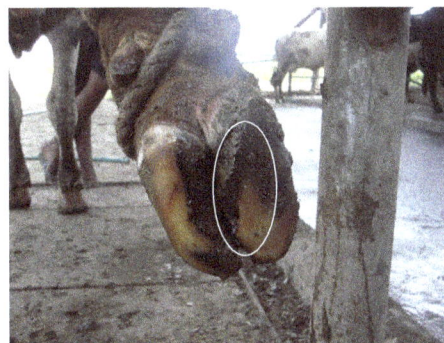

FIGURE 9: Overgrown hoof.

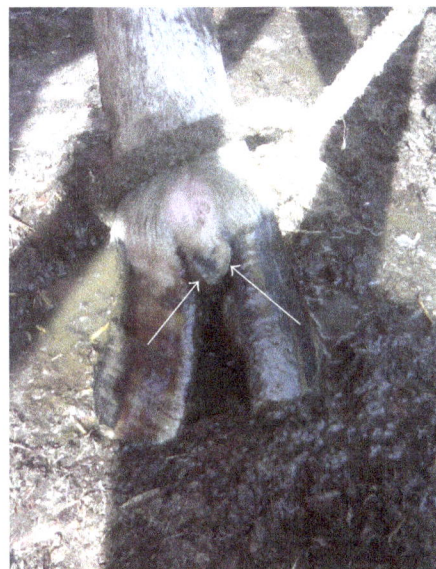

FIGURE 10: Interdigital hyperplasia.

locomotion score and various lesions is presented in Tables 1 and 2 and the photographs of various lesions and RLVI are depicted in Figures 1, 2, 3, 4, 5, 6, 7, 8, 9, and 10. Heel erosions were present in about 70% of the animals with locomotion score 2 and about 28% of the animals with locomotion score 3 (Figures 11(a) and 11(b)) but they failed to cause apparent lameness. In contrast, sole ulcers and white line fissures had a close association with poor locomotion, with figures of 11.11% and 88.89% for sole ulcer and 15.58% and 84.42% for white line fissures, for locomotion scores 2 and 3, respectively (Figure 11(b)). All the other lesions did not cause clinical lameness but tend to increase asymmetry (Table 1).

In case of normal animals (locomotion score 0) and asymmetric animals (locomotion score 1) the presence of lesions was associated with increased locomotion score. In other words the degree of asymmetry was more in animals with foot lesions (Figures 12(a) and 12(b)). However, despite the presence of lesions, these animals were not clinically lame.

In clinically lame cows (locomotion scores 2 and 3) there was a significant correlation between sole avulsions and heel erosions (0.26; $P \leq 0.05$), underrun soles and heel erosions (0.224; $P \leq 0.05$), overgrown hooves and heel erosions (0.315; $P \leq 0.01$), overgrown sole and underrun soles (0.299; $P \leq 0.01$), and sole ulcers and white line fissures (0.253; $P \leq 0.01$) (Table 3). In cows with locomotion scores 0 and 1 there was a significant correlation between overgrown soles and heel erosions (0.386; $P \leq 0.01$), white line haemorrhages and sole

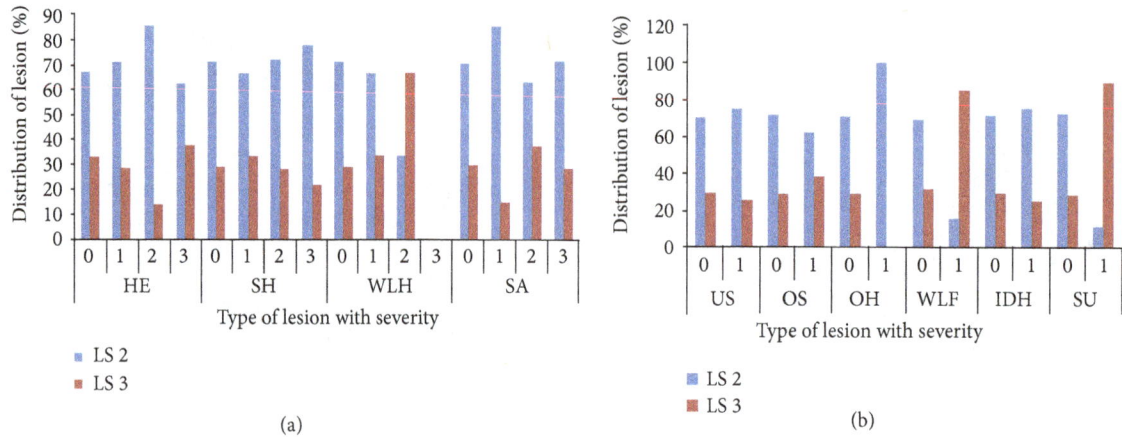

LS 2
LS 3
(a)

LS 2
LS 3
(b)

FIGURE 11: (a) Distribution of severities of lesions in cows with locomotion score 2 and 3, HE: heel erosion, SH: sole haemorrhage, WLH: white line haemorrhage, SA: sole avulsion, LS: locomotion score. (b) Distribution of severities of lesions in cows with locomotion score 2 and 3, US: under run sole, OS: overgrown sole, OH: overgrown hoof, WLF: white line fissure, IDH: interdigital hyperplasia, SU: Sole ulcer, LS: locomotion score.

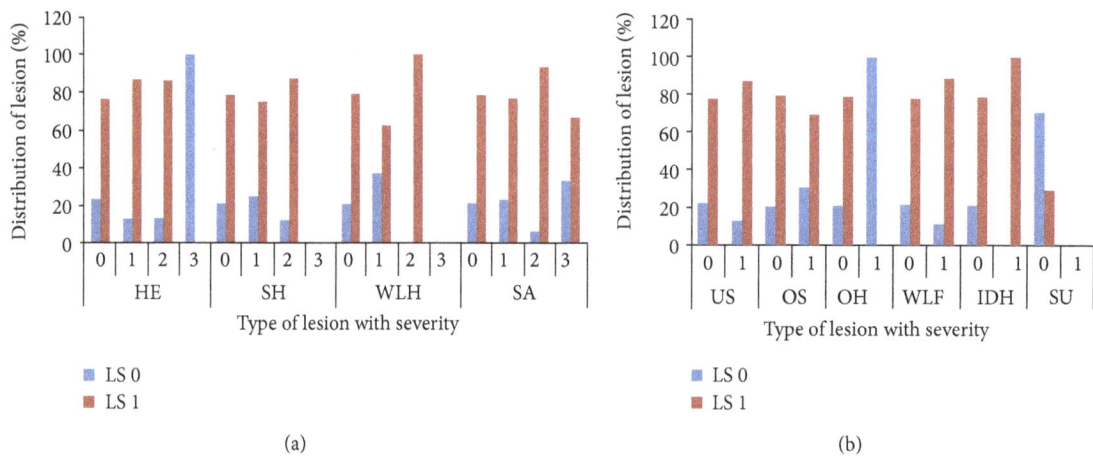

LS 0
LS 1
(a)

LS 0
LS 1
(b)

FIGURE 12: (a) Distribution of severities of lesions in cows with locomotion scores 0 and 1, HE: heel erosion, SH: sole haemorrhage, WLH: white line haemorrhage, SA: sole avulsion, LS: locomotion score. (b) Distribution of severities of lesions in cows with locomotion scores 0 and 1, US: underrun sole, OS: overgrown sole, OH: overgrown hoof, WLF: white line fissure, IDH: interdigital hyperplasia, SU: sole ulcer, LS: locomotion score.

haemorrhages (0.45; $P \leq 0.01$), and interdigital hyperplasia and white line fissures (0.884; $P \leq 0.01$) (Table 4).

There was a significant relationship between locomotion score and RLVI ($\chi^2 = 4.87$; $P \leq 0.05$ for locomotion scores 2 and 3; $\chi^2 = 12.95$; $P \leq 0.05$ for locomotion scores 0 and 1) to identify lameness. Spearman's rank correlation coefficient for locomotion score from two observers was 0.637 ($P \leq 0.01$) and that for RLVI was 0.753 ($P \leq 0.01$).

4. Discussion

In the present study, despite the presence of lesions in the animals with locomotion scores 0 and 1, these animals did not show clinical lameness. The reason for this might be that several claw and digital lesions do not seem to inflict sufficient pain to cause clinical lameness [16]. Also, the individual susceptibility to foot lesions, pain, and resulting lameness

vary from animal to animal [17]. Furthermore the potentially painful corium insult occurs several weeks before the lesions are visible in the sole [18]. So, ignoring these cows with lesions in the feet may reduce the probability of detecting risks for lesion development by misclassifying these cows as nonlame in spite of having lesions in feet.

From Table 3, it can be inferred that presence of sole avulsions, underrun soles, and overgrown hooves increased the chances of occurrence of heel erosions; presence of overgrown soles increased the chances of underrun soles; and presence of sole ulcers increased the chances of occurrence of white line fissures. The association between underrun sole and heel erosions may be attributed to their common aetiopathogenesis of subclinical laminitis [19]. A disturbance of microvasculature of the corium results in the escape of blood components into the tubules of the horn of the sole and bulb. As recovery occurs and sound horn is produced, the event is recorded as a blood strained stratum. As the new horn grows, the haemorrhagic stratum moves towards the surface, and during wear (or if horn is pared) it appears in the substance of the horn until it is worn away. A haemorrhagic stratum often terminated as a groove on the heel or under running of the sole. This underrunning until avulsed is observed as underrun soles. But if the sole horn quality is poor due to improper nutrition/mineralization the soles may get avulsed leading to sole avulsions [19].

The correlation between overgrown hooves and heel erosions may be attributed to altered balance of the claw with heel erosions leading to more weight bearing on the toes, leading to overgrowth of hooves. The association between underrun soles and overgrown soles could be due to possible damage to the axial solar part of the medial claw initiating the development of underrun sole [19], because most of the overgrown soles were present in the lateral hind claws. The association between sole ulcer and white line fissure may be due to the fact that both appear as a sequel to sole haemorrhages and white line haemorrhages, respectively, which are common lesions associated with subclinical laminitis. Subclinical laminitis causes damage either in lamina portion of white line or in the sole bulb area, the common site of sole ulcer. The significant correlation between sole ulcers and white line fissures and poor locomotion in the present study was in concurrence with that of Tadich et al. [7]. Clarkson et al. [20] also observed that sole ulcer and white line disease were the lesions responsible for lameness while another study [21] demonstrated that the skin lesions, namely, digital dermatitis and interdigital phlegmon, were the important cause of lameness. Similar to previous studies [10, 22] heel erosions and sole haemorrhages were not associated with locomotion score. Correlation between sole ulcer and double sole has been reported previously [7, 23] but no such correlation was observed in our study.

In normal (lameness score 0) and asymmetric animals (lameness score 1), the presence of overgrown soles increased the chances of heel erosions or vice versa and white line haemorrhages increased the chances of occurrence of sole haemorrhages or vice versa. The possible reason for these correlations could be similar to that for the clinically lame animals. White line fissures may have increased the proximity of hooves and interdigital space to the underfoot manure/slurry and may have led to interdigital dermatitis and in turn interdigital hyperplasia [19].

The significant correlation between locomotion score and RLVI indicated that the placement of claws gets disturbed due to pain of different lesions, leading to improper weight bearing. As more lesions were observed in hind lateral claws, the animals shift their weight to medial claws to relieve the pain in lateral claws resulting in inward knuckling of hocks (cow hock rear leg view). This change in the rear leg view conformation along with the type of lesion present may render the animal asymmetric or lame. Thus, a significant correlation between two indices indicates that both locomotion score and RLVI can be reliably used to identify clinical lameness on dairy farms, despite the subjective nature of clinical diagnosis.

5. Conclusions

It was concluded that sole ulcers and white line fissures were the lesions responsible for clinical lameness in lactating HF crossbred cows. Other lesions do not cause clinical lameness but tend to increase asymmetry in dairy cows. The presence of sole avulsions, underrun soles, and overgrown hooves increased the chances of occurrence of heel erosions; presence of overgrown soles and white line fissures increased the chances of occurrence of underrun soles and sole ulcers, respectively. Locomotion score can be reliably used to identify clinical lameness in dairy cattle.

Conflict of Interests

The authors declare that there is no conflict of interests regarding the publication of this paper.

Acknowledgment

The authors would like to thank Dr. A. S. Nanda, Director of Research, Guru Angad Dev Veterinary and Animal Sciences University, Ludhiana, India, for providing the research facilities.

References

[1] K. O'Callaghan, "Lameness and associated pain in cattle—challenging traditional perceptions," *In Practice*, vol. 24, no. 4, pp. 212–219, 2002.

[2] J. J. Vermunt, "Herd lameness—a review," in *Proceedings of the 13th International Symposium and 5th Conference on Lameness in Ruminants*, vol. 18, pp. 3–18, Maribor, Slovenija, 2004.

[3] J. Hernandez, J. K. Shearer, and D. W. Webb, "Effect of lameness on milk yield in dairy cows," *Journal of the American Veterinary Medical Association*, vol. 220, no. 5, pp. 640–644, 2002.

[4] S. R. Van Amstel and J. K. Shearer, "Review of pododermatitis circumscripta (ulceration of the sole) in dairy cows," *Journal of Veterinary Internal Medicine*, vol. 20, no. 4, pp. 805–811, 2006.

[5] P. J. Rajala-Schultz and Y. T. Gröhn, "Culling of dairy cows part I. Effects of diseases on culling in Finnish Ayrshire cows," *Preventive Veterinary Medicine*, vol. 41, no. 2-3, pp. 195–208, 1999.

[6] L. E. Green, V. J. Hedges, Y. H. Schukken, R. W. Blowey, and A. J. Packington, "The impact of clinical lameness on the milk yield of dairy cows," *Journal of Dairy Science*, vol. 85, no. 9, pp. 2250–2256, 2002.

[7] N. Tadich, E. Flor, and L. Green, "Associations between hoof lesions and locomotion score in 1098 unsound dairy cows," *Veterinary Journal*, vol. 184, no. 1, pp. 60–65, 2010.

[8] T. Manske, J. Hultgren, and C. Bergsten, "The effect of claw trimming on the hoof health of Swedish dairy cattle," *Preventive Veterinary Medicine*, vol. 54, no. 2, pp. 113–129, 2002.

[9] K. A. O'Callaghan, P. J. Cripps, D. Y. Downham, and R. D. Murray, "Subjective and objective assessment of pain and discomfort due to lameness in dairy cattle," *Animal Welfare*, vol. 12, no. 4, pp. 605–610, 2003.

[10] F. C. Flower and D. M. Weary, "Effect of hoof pathologies on subjective assessments of dairy cow gait," *Journal of Dairy Science*, vol. 89, no. 1, pp. 139–146, 2006.

[11] S. L. Berry, "Infectious diseases of the Bovine claw," in *Proceedings of the 14th International Symposium and 6th Conference on Lameness in Ruminants*, pp. 52–57, Colonia del Sacremento, Uruguay, 2006.

[12] M. Thrushfield, *Veterinary Epidemiology*, Blackwell, London, UK, 2007.

[13] S. J. Wells, A. M. Trent, W. E. Marsh, and R. A. Robinson, "Prevalence and severity of lameness in lactating dairy cows in a sample of Minnesota and Wisconsin herds," *Journal of the American Veterinary Medical Association*, vol. 202, no. 1, pp. 78–82, 1993.

[14] E. Toussaint Raven, *Cattle Foot Care and Claw Trimming*, Farming Press Limited, Ipswich, UK, 1989.

[15] S. S. Randhawa, K. Dua, C. S. Randhawa, S. S. Randhawa, and S. K. Munshi, "Effect of biotin supplementation on hoof health and ceramide composition in dairy cattle," *Veterinary Research Communications*, vol. 32, no. 8, pp. 599–608, 2008.

[16] T. Manske, J. Hultgren, and C. Bergsten, "Prevalence and interrelationships of hoof lesions and lameness in Swedish dairy cows," *Preventive Veterinary Medicine*, vol. 54, no. 3, pp. 247–263, 2002.

[17] J. J. Vermunt, "Risk factors of laminitis an overview," in *Proceedings of the 6th International Symposium on Disorders of Ruminant Digit and International Conference on Bovine Lameness*, pp. 34–45, Parma, Italy, 2000.

[18] K. A. Leach, D. N. Logue, S. A. Kempson, J. E. Offer, H. E. Ternent, and J. M. Randall, "Claw lesions in dairy cattle: development of sole and white line haemorrhages during the first lactation," *The Veterinary Journal*, vol. 154, no. 3, pp. 215–225, 1997.

[19] S. S. Randhawa, *Prevalence, biomechanics, pathogenesis and clinico-therapeutic studies on foot lameness in dairy animals [PhD Dissertation]*, Guru AngadDev Veterinary and Animal Sciences University, Ludhiana, India, 2006.

[20] M. J. Clarkson, D. Y. Downham, W. B. Faull et al., "Incidence and prevalence of lameness in dairy cattle," *Veterinary Record*, vol. 138, no. 23, pp. 563–567, 1996.

[21] J. E. Offer, D. McNulty, and D. N. Logue, "Observations of lameness, hoof conformation and development of lesions in dairy cattle over four lactations," *Veterinary Record*, vol. 147, no. 4, pp. 105–109, 2000.

[22] D. N. Logue, J. E. Offer, and J. J. Hyslop, "Relationship of diet, hoof type and locomotion score with lesions of the sole and white line in dairy cattle," *Animal Production*, vol. 59, pp. 173–181, 1994.

[23] N. Capion, S. M. Thamsborg, and C. Enevoldsen, "Prevalence and severity of foot lesions in Danish Holstein heifers through first lactation," *Veterinary Journal*, vol. 182, no. 1, pp. 50–58, 2009.

27

Pharmacological Overview of Galactogogues

Felipe Penagos Tabares, Juliana V. Bedoya Jaramillo, and Zulma Tatiana Ruiz-Cortés

Biogenesis Research Group, Agrarian Sciences Faculty, University of Antioquia, Medellin, Colombia

Correspondence should be addressed to Felipe Penagos Tabares; felipe.penagos@udea.edu.co
and Zulma Tatiana Ruiz-Cortés; biogenesis1995@gmail.com

Academic Editor: William Ravis

Galactogogues are substances used to induce, maintain, and increase milk production, both in human clinical conditions (like noninfectious agalactias and hypogalactias) and in massification of production in the animal dairy industry. This paper aims to report the state of the art on the possible mechanisms of action, effectiveness, and side effects of galactogogues, including potential uses in veterinary and human medicine. The knowledge gaps in veterinary clinical practice use of galactogogues, especially in the standardization of the lactogenic dose in some pure drugs and herbal preparations, are reviewed.

1. Introduction

Milk production is essential for optimal feeding of infants and has a direct impact on growth, development, and health in neonatal period [1]. Breastfeeding is influenced by nutritional and nonnutritional factors (associated with endocrinology, health, climate, and management) that affect milk synthesis and secretion. These factors modulate physiological actions that regulate situations such as noninfectious agalactias and hypogalactias, the latest being the main problem of breastfeeding women [2]. Galactogogues are synthetic or plants molecules used to induce, maintain, and increase milk production [3], which mediate complex processes involving interaction between physical and physiological factors. Among the most important factors are hormones such as prolactin (PRL). However, somatotropine, cortisol, insulin, leptin, estrogen, progesterone and medroxyprogesterone [2], oxytocin, recombinant bovine somatotropin (rBST), and thyrotropin releasing hormone (TRH) also play important role as galactogogues (Table 1).

Most common galactogogues for human use are metoclopramide, domperidone, chlorpromazine, and sulpiride (Table 1); their remarkable side effects in mothers are xerostomia (dry mouth syndrome or hyposalivation), gastrointestinal disorders, cardiac arrhythmia, lethargy, sedation, extrapyramidal symptoms such as hypertension, tremor, tic,

facial seborrhea, and hyperhidrosis, and even sudden death. In infants that ingested milk from treated mothers symptoms include intestinal discomfort, lethargy, and sedation [2]. The main galactogogue used in cattle is rBST which has reported adverse health effects that directly affect animal welfare [4, 5].

Plants with galactogogues components include fenugreek (*Trigonella graecum foecum*), fennel (*Foeniculum vulgare*), goat's rue (*Galega officinalis*), asparagus (*Asparagus racemosus*), anise (*Pimpinella anisum*), and milk thistle (*Silybum marianum*) [6, 7] (Table 2). Nowadays, herbal preparations are known to increase significantly milk production in women, goats, cows, and other species. This research area is very important for human breastfeeding medicine and in veterinary dairy industry [7–11].

There are numerous references about herbal medicine and breastfeeding. However, they are mainly based on empirical traditions and on human studies. This information could be deficient in systematization, is unstructured, heterogeneous, and thus has nonverifiable quality. From previously mentioned plants classified as galactogogues, there are currently available studies for efficacy and safety, but their mechanisms of action have not been elucidated yet [3, 12]. Publications generally focus on the effects with no emphasis on the mechanism by which milk production stimulation is achieved. The increased use of herbal medicine is also encouraged by a trend towards organic production, mainly

TABLE 1: Pharmacological overview of some galactogogues synthetic drugs.

Galactogogue drug	Proposed mechanism	Doses and dosage form	Adverse effects	Half-life
Metoclopramide	D2R antagonist, increase PRL secretion [2].	Human: 10 mg PO TID [31]. Canine/feline: 0.1–0.2 mg/kg, SC TID [32].	Humans: several gastrointestinal disorders, insomnia severe depression, and seizures and in infants that consume milk from treated mothers causing intestinal discomfort [2].	Humans: 156.7 minutes [29]. Dogs: 90 minutes [30].
Domperidone	D2R antagonist, increase PRL secretion [2].	Human: 10 mg PO TID [37]. Canine/feline: 2.2 mg/kg SC, every 12 hours for 4–6 days [36]. Equine: 1.1 mg/kg PO BID [38].	Humans: xerostomia, gastrointestinal disorders, cardiac arrhythmia, and sudden death [2].	Humans: 7.5 hours [36].
Chlorpromazine	D2R antagonist, increase PRL secretion [2].	Human: 25 mg PO TID [42]. Rat: 15 mg/kg [41].	Humans: extrapyramidal symptoms in mothers and lethargy in infants [2, 40]. Feline: in high doses tremors, shivering, rigidity, and loss of the righting, reflexes, lethargy, diarrhea, and loss of anal sphincter tone [30]. Equine: ataxic reactions, excitation, panic reactions and violent consequences, sedation [30], and phototoxic reactions [45, 46].	Humans: 16–30 hours [43].
Sulpiride	D2R antagonist, increase PRL secretion [2].	Human: 50 mg PO TID [49]. Equine: 1.1 mg/kg PO BID [54] or 0.5 BID IM [38].	Humans: headache, fatigue, extrapyramidal symptoms, acute dystonic reactions, and endocrine disruption [2, 50].	Dogs: 1.6–3.4 hours [51]. Humans: 7.15 hours [53].
Oxytocin	Induce milk ejection and this promotes milk synthesis by FIL decrease [28].	Canine and feline: 0.5–2.0 IU/kg dose SC EM [32]. Bovine: 20 IU SC EM [70]. Sheep and goat: 1–5 IU EM [71]. Swine: 0.025 and 0.05 IU IV EM [72]. Equine: 20 UI IM EM [73].	When used appropriately at reasonable dosages, oxytocin rarely causes significant adverse reactions [30]. Result of using the drug in inappropriate individuals (adequate physical exam and monitoring of patient are essential) or at too high doses [26]. In high doses they may cause discomfort, uterine cramping, hazardous of uterine rupture, and fetuses-placental compromise. [30].	Goat: 22 minutes [61]. Swine: 127 seconds [62]. Rat: 1.46 minutes [63]. Bovine: 7–9 minutes and 25 minutes [64, 65]. Equine: 6.8 minutes [66]. Humans: 272 seconds [67].
Recombinant bovine somatotropin (rBST)	Increase basal metabolic rate and nutrients bioavailability, in mammary gland Increase MEC proliferation, survival and milk synthesis [92].	Bovine: 500 mg SC every 14 days [5].	Bovine: low pregnancy rates, increased open days [94], increase incidences of retained placenta [95], clinical and subclinical, reduced food intake, allergic reactions, laminitis digestive disorders [5], decreased hemoglobin and hematocrit [98], and mastitis [96, 97].	Bovine: 54.8 minutes [93].
Thyrotropin releasing hormone (TRH)	Increase PRL blood levels [102].	Humans: 20 mg PO TID [105].	Humans: hyperthyroidism and brief episodes of sweating [106, 108].	Rat: 4.16 minutes [109].
Medroxyprogesterone	Not reported	Humans: 150 mg IM every 3 months [122].	Human: amenorrhea [121].	Human: 40–60 hrs [119].

Abbreviations: BID, twice daily; TID, three times daily; PO, oral administration; SC, subcutaneous; IM, intramuscular; EM, every milking.

TABLE 2: Pharmacological overview of some botanical galactogogues.

Herbal galactogogue	Proposed mechanism	Common doses and dosage form	Adverse Effects	Half-life
Fenugreek (*Trigonella graecum foenum*)	Estrogenic action?	Goat: dry plant 10 g SID [127]	Not reported.	Not reported.
Fennel (*Foeniculum vulgare*)	Estrogenic action?	Not reported	Not reported.	Not reported.
Anise (*Pimpinella anisum*)	Estrogenic action?	Rat: ethanolic and aqueous extract 1 g/kg IP [156]	Not reported.	Not reported.
Goat's rue (*Galega officinalis*)	Estrogenic action?	Sheep: Plant (dry), 2 g/kg body weight in diet daily [158].	Sheep: doses over 5 g/kg were toxic [161].	Not reported.
Asparagus (*Asparagus racemosus*)	Estrogenic action?	Human: concentrated root extract, 60 mg/kg PO SID [166]. Rat: Plant (dry), 2% of the diet [167].	Rat: methanol roots extract in dose of 100 mg/Kg/day for 60 days showed teratological disorders as increased resorption of fetuses, gross malformations as swelling in legs, and intrauterine growth retardation with a small placental size [171].	Not reported.
Milk thistle (*Silybum marianum*)	Estrogenic action?	Bovine: plant (dry), 10 g PO SID [176].	Human: gastrointestinal disturbances have been reported: nausea and diarrhea. Patients who have allergies to other members of the *Asteraceae/Compositae* plant family (including ragweed, marigolds, daisies, etc.) may exhibit allergic reactions to Milk Thistle derivatives [30].	Human: silymarin elimination half-life average 6 hours [30].

Abbreviations: SID, once daily; BID, twice daily; TID, three times daily; PO, oral administration; SC, subcutaneous; IM, intramuscular; IP, intraperitoneal.

in European markets, and the growing evidence on its safety and efficacy [13]. Several factors explain the tendency to use botanical galactogogues: adverse effects of synthetic drugs and a better understanding of chemistry, pharmacology and clinical use of botanical drugs and their derivatives, the development of analytical methods that facilitate quality control, and the development of new ways of preparation and administration [14, 15]. Many nutraceutical and phytopharmaceutical preparations are not approached in many countries; to develop and sale these preparations, it is necessary to have the basic knowledge of their chemical composition and of the mechanisms implicated on its galactogogue action. The following are also required: good agricultural practices (GAP), good laboratory practices (GLP), good manufacturing practices (GMP), and quality control standards to ensure the efficacy, safety, and composition of the products produced from these plants [16–18]. The use of herbal products in dairy industry relies on the new trend in dairy sector of organic dairy farming [19].

This paper reports and reviews potential uses of galactogogues in human and veterinary medicine, in both clinical uses and feeding practices of dairy animals, with emphasis on the possible mechanism of action relating drugs and plants knowledge, their efficacy and adverse effects. It also exposes gaps knowledge about galactogogues in veterinary clinical practice, especially in dose standardization of some pure drugs (with only one molecule in the pharmaceutical preparation) and herbal preparations.

2. Synthetic Galactogogues

Among synthetic molecules used to increase lactation, the dopamine antagonists, such as antiemetics metoclopramide and domperidone and such as antipsychotics sulpiride and chlorpromazine. Hormone synthetic analogs such as oxytocin, rBST, TRH, and medroxyprogesterone are also included in the synthetic galactogogues list [2]. Figure 1 depicts the basic structures of synthetic galactogogues mentioned in this review.

2.1. Dopamine Antagonists. These drugs block the dopamine 2 receptors (D2R) in the central nervous system which induces an increase of PRL synthesis in lactotrophic cells of the anterior pituitary [20–22]. Activation by an agonist of D2R, a G protein receptor, induces via subunit Gα0 the K^+ channels opening, increases intracellular concentration of this ion, and reduces Ca^{2+} entry and its intracellular concentration. This effect is also induced by another pathway: inhibition of phospholipase C (PLC) and protein kinase C (PKC); reducing the Ca^{2+} mobilization from endoplasmic reticulum (ER), the low Ca^{2+} inhibits vesicle formation and PRL secretion. The activation of D2R also turns active the subunit Gαi, which inhibits adenylyl cyclase (AC), and decreases the concentration of adenine monophosphate (cAMP) [23], suppressing cAMP dependent protein kinase (PKA). Finally, inhibition of both kinases, PKC and PKA, inactivates PRL gene expression [24, 25].

When an antagonist binds to the receptor, those pathways are blocked, and the synthesis and release of PRL are activated. This high blood level of PRL increases milk protein synthesis rate and mammary epithelial cells (MEC) proliferation (Figure 2) [26].

2.1.1. Metoclopramide. This drug was originally commercialized in Europe as an antipsychotic and later in the US as a gastrokinetic agent that increases gastrointestinal motility. Its first reported use as a galactogogue was in 1975 [27] and has been evaluated in many clinical trials [28]. In humans, adverse effects have been reported in mothers such as anxiety, and several gastrointestinal disorders, insomnia [2], severe depression, and seizures and in infants that consume milk from treated mothers cause intestinal discomfort [2]. Half-life reported in humans is 156.7 minutes [29] and its plasma half-life in dogs is about 90 minutes [30]. In humans, 10 mg administered by oral route (PO) three times a day during 10 days increases milk production [31]. It is used in small animal veterinary medicine to treat cases of secondary hypogalactia or agalactia at doses of 0.1-0.2 mg/kg subcutaneously (SC) every 6–8 hours for 4 to 6 days [32].

2.1.2. Domperidone. Its first use as a galactogogue was reported in 1983 [33]. It was used to increase milk production in mothers of premature infants [34], but it was not approved by the Food and Drug Administration (FDA) in the US and domperidone use in human clinical trials has not been associated with adverse effects in infants, but in mothers it was associated with xerostomia, gastrointestinal disorders, cardiac arrhythmia, and sudden death, and this should be taken into account in veterinary practice [2]. There are recent human data where no maternal or neonatal adverse effects were reported [35]. The half-life reported in human is 7.5 hours [36]. Women enhance lactation with 10 mg of domperidone PO 3 times daily [37]. In dogs and cats, the domperidone medical use in secondary agalactia or hypogalactia is recommended at doses of 2.2 mg/kg SC, every 12 hours for 4–6 days [32]. In equine domperidone administered dose is 1.1 mg/kg PO every 12 hours to increase PRL blood concentration and milk production [38]. Domperidone is effective in preventing the signs of tall fescue toxicosis (including hypogalactia or agalactia) in horses without neuroleptic side effects [39].

2.1.3. Chlorpromazine. Like in other neuroleptics, little is known about pharmacokinetics of chlorpromazine in mothers or infants during breastfeeding [40]. Chlorpromazine administered in doses of 15 mg/kg of body weight in rats during 5 days was effective in inducing lobuloalveolar growth and initiation of milk secretion initially primed with 10 μg estradiol daily for 10 days [41]. Also, this neuroleptic increases milk production and weight gain in women with hypogalactia at doses of 25 mg, 3 times a day for a week [42]. The half-life reported in humans is 16–30 hours [43]. Short and long term use cause adverse effects in the development of the central nervous system (CNS) as documented by extrapyramidal symptoms in mothers and lethargy in infants that consumed milk. This could induce changes in CNS development in

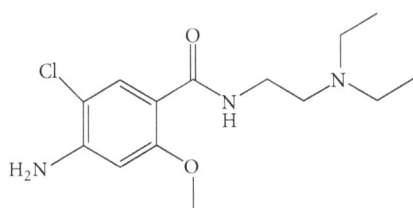

2.1.1. Metoclopramide

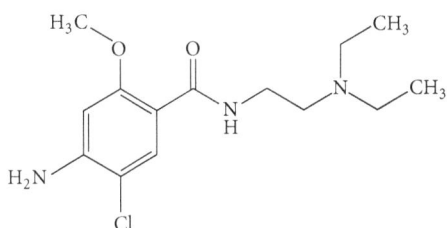

2.1.2. Domperidone

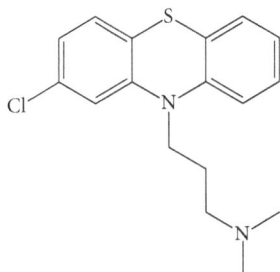

2.1.3. Chlorpromazine

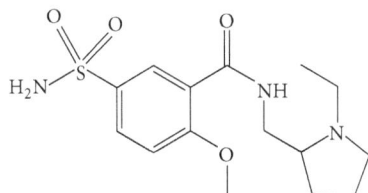

2.1.4. Sulpiride

2.2. Oxytocin

Phe-Pro-Thi-Ie-Pro-Leu-Ser-Arg-Leu-Phe-Asp-Asn-Ala-Mei-Leu-Arg-Ala-His-
Arg-Leu-His-Gln-Leu-Ala-Phe-Asp-Thi-Tyr-Gln-Glu-Phe-Glu-Glu-Ala-Tyr-IIe-
Pro-Lys-Glu-Gli-Lys-Tyr-Ser-Phe-Leu-Gln-Asn-Pro-Gln-Thi-Ser-Leu-Cys-Phe
-Ser-Glu-Ser-Ile-Pro-Thr-Pro-Ser-Asn-Arg-Glu-Glu-Thr-Gln-Gln-Lys-Ser-Asn-
Leu-Glu-Leu-Leu-Arg-Ie-Ser-Leu-Leu-Leu-Ie-Gli-Ser-Trp-Leu-Glu-Pro-Val-Gln
-Phe-Leu-Arg-Ser-Val-Phe-Ala-Asn-Ser-Leu-Val-Tyr-Gly-Ale-Ser-Asp-Ser-Asn
-Val-Tyr-Asp-Leu-Leu-Lys-Asp-Leu-Glu-Glu-Gly-Ile-Gln-Thr-Leu-Mei-Gly-Arg-
Leu-Glu-Asp-Gly-Ser-Pro-Arg-Thi-Gly-Gln-Ile-Phe-Lys-Gln-Thi-Tyi-Ser-Lys-
Phe-Asp-Thr-Asn-Ser-His-Asn-Asp-Asp-Ala-Leu-Leu-Lys-Asn-Tyr-Gly-Leu-
Leu-Tyr-Cys-Phe-Arg-Lys-Asp-Met-Asp-Lys-Val-Glu-Thr-Phe-Leu-Arg-Ie-
Val-Gln-Cys-Arg-Ser-Val-Glu-Gly-Cye-Gly-Phe

2.3. Recombinant bovine somatotropin (rBST)

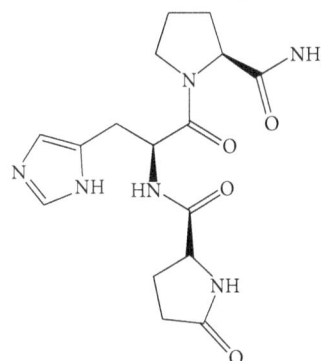

2.4. Thyrotropin releasing hormone (TRH)

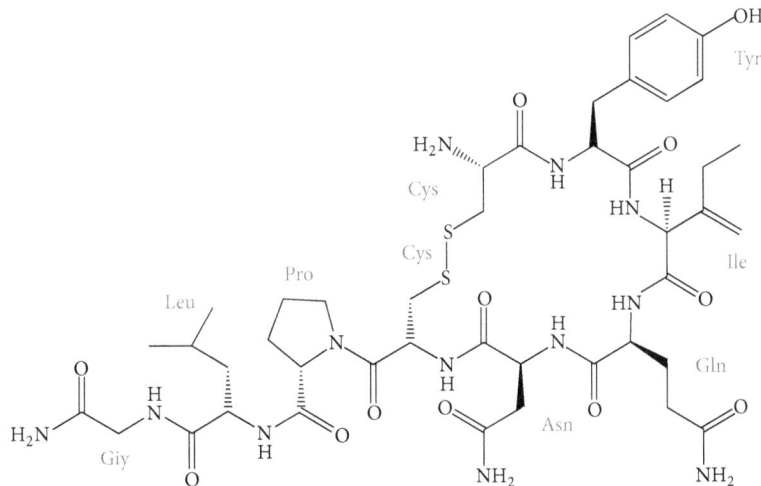

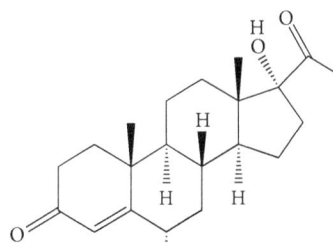

2.5. Medroxyprogesterone

FIGURE 1: Synthetics galactogogue drugs structure.

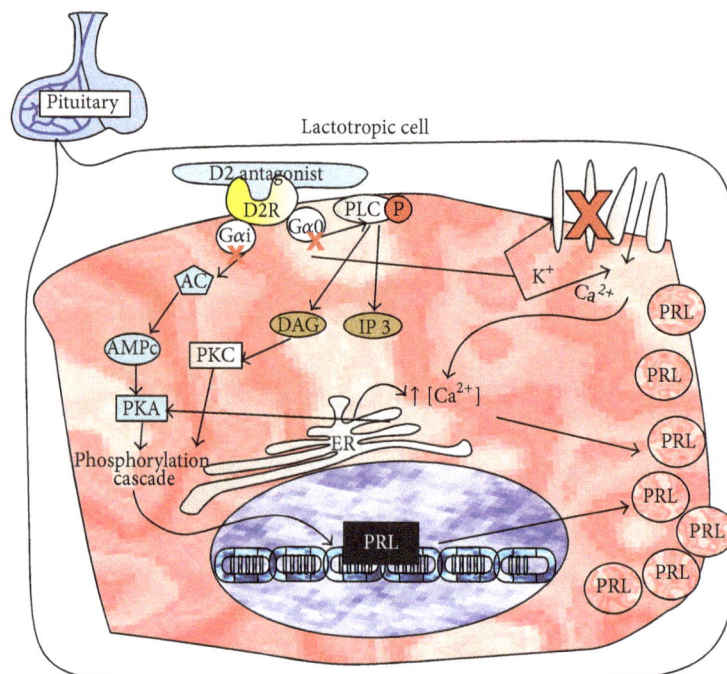

FIGURE 2: Proposed mechanism of action of dopamine 2 antagonists. In the pituitary gland, antagonists bind to the receptor (D2R) dopamine 2 and induce PRL gene expression, blood level of PRL increases, milk protein synthesis rate increases, and mammary epithelial cells (MEC) proliferation is stimulated.

neonate because of alterations in the undeveloped brain [44]. The possible effects listed for the acepromazine use in animals are hypotension and contradictory effects such as CNS stimulation and bradycardia [30]. In felines chlorpromazine may cause extrapyramidal signs when used at high dosages. These can include tremors, shivering, rigidity, and loss of the righting reflexes. Lethargy, diarrhea, and loss of anal sphincter tone may also be seen [30]. In horses ataxic reactions with resultant excitation, panic reactions, and violent consequences may develop. These ataxic periods may cycle with periods of sedation. Because of this effect, chlorpromazine is rarely used in equine medicine today [30]. Animals in treatment with chlorpromazine should not be exposed to sun because it may induce phototoxic reactions [45, 46].

2.1.4. Sulpiride. It was shown as a drug with galactogogue potential effect when increased serum PRL was observed in women [47]. Several clinical studies support its efficacy; one of these included 130 primiparous women: 66 treated with doses of 50 mg of oral sulpiride, every 12 hours during 7 days, and 64 as placebo group. The treatment resulted in an increase in PRL serum levels as in milk secretion [48]. A previous study reported an effective oral sulpiride dose of 50 mg every 8 hours for 4 weeks in women with hypogalactia; in this investigation serum PRL concentrations increased during the first 2 weeks, while the control group decreased and infants of treated mothers showed higher weight gain than those of the placebo group after 28 days of sulpiride treatment [49]. These results were confirmed by other studies [48, 50]. Plasma half-life of sulpiride in dogs was 1.6–3.4 hours [51, 52]

and in humans was 7.15 hours [53]. Adverse effects reported in women were headache, fatigue, extrapyramidal symptoms, acute dystonic reactions, and endocrine disruption [2, 50]. In equine, sulpiride used at dose of 1.1 mg/kg PO twice a day [54] and 0.5 mg/kg intramuscularly (IM) twice a day increased PRL blood concentration and milk production [38].

2.2. Oxytocin (OT). The major sites of expression of this peptide hormone are located in the magnocellular neuron region in the supraoptic and paraventricular hypothalamic nuclei [55]. It has been used to induce milk ejection in cases where dysfunction has been associated with this reflex [56]. This hormone induces contraction of myoepithelial cells via G protein receptor, and PLC is activated and induces the formation of diacylglycerol (DAG) and inositol 1,4,5-triphosphate (IP3), by hydrolysis of membrane lipid phosphatidylinositol 4, 5-bisphosphate (IPI2). The IP3 induces intracellular Ca^{2+} release, and this active Ca^{2+}-calmodulin system triggers the activation of myosin light-chain kinase (MLCK) which initiates smooth muscle contraction in mammary myoepithelial cells [55] (Figure 3). In rabbit, OT not only stimulates milk ejection by the contraction of mammary myoepithelial cells, but also induces exocytosis of milk synthesis in the MEC [57]. With effects in myoepithelial and MEC, OT induces milk ejection and this milk removal also removes feedback inhibitor of lactation (FIL), a milk glycoprotein that induces reversible block of protein synthesis of the MEC. Thus, reduction of FIL induces milk synthesis [58] (Figure 3). OT can increase milk production and is indicated in agalactia or hypogalactia for dysfunction of

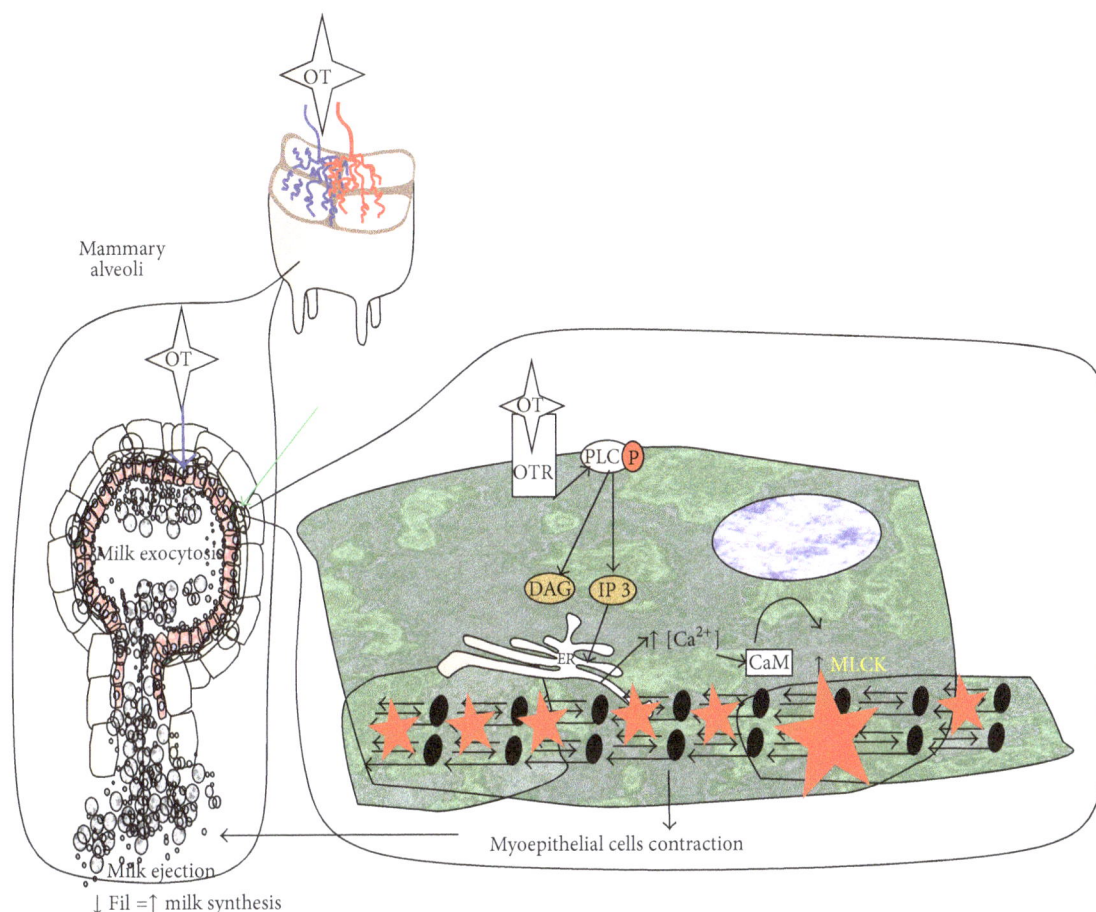

FIGURE 3: Proposed mechanism of action of oxytocin (OT). This hormone induces contraction of the myoepithelial cells (green arrow), via a G protein receptor. OT also induces exocytosis of milk in MEC (blue arrow) by intracellular Ca^{2+} increased pathways. Myoepithelial cells contraction and MEC exocytosis induce milk ejection; the continued milk ejection results in a decrease of a protein milk synthesis reversible blocker: feedback inhibitor of lactation (FIL), and this milk and FIL removal of mammary gland will promote then the milk synthesis.

milk ejection reflex in stress or premature birth cases [56]; it is also used in mastitis treatment [59, 60]. The half-life reported in goats is 22 minutes [61]; in pigs, 127 seconds [62]; in rats, 1.46 minutes [63]; in cows, two half-life data were reported: 7–9 minutes and 25 minutes [64, 65]; in equines it was determined to be 6.8 minutes [66]; in humans, 272 seconds [67]. There are no reports about OT adverse effects in women or infants [2, 68]. When used appropriately at reasonable dosages, oxytocin rarely causes significant adverse reactions [30]. Most adverse effects are a result of using the drug in inappropriate individuals (adequate physical exam and monitoring of patient are essential) or at too high doses [30]. Most of the older dosage recommendations for dogs or cats are obsolete as minidoses have been found to improve the frequency of uterine contractility and are less hazardous to the bitch (uterine rupture) and to the fetuses (placental compromise) [30]. Repeated bolus injections of oxytocin may cause uterine cramping and discomfort [30]. The use of oxytocin in dairy animal as galactogogue is banned in India and other countries because its continuous use in each milking affects the animal welfare [69]. In dogs and cats reported medicated doses are 0.5–2.0 IU/kg dose SC every

two hours [32]. In bovine SC injection dose of 20 IU per animal at each milking throughout lactation increased milk production [70]. The doses mostly used in goat and sheep are 1–5 IU SC every milking [71]. In swine reported doses are between 0.025 and 0.05 IU in intravenously (IV) rapid injection every milking [72]. Equine reported IM dose 20 IU per animal every milking [73].

2.3. Recombinant Bovine Somatotropin (rBST). The rBST approved in dairy cows is the 190-amino-acid variant with leucine at position 127, and it has an extra methionine at the NH2 terminus [5, 74] (Figure 1). In 1979, rBST was developed in bioreactors (an *E. coli* strain); three years later its *in vivo* galactagogue action was published [75]. Its use was approved in US in 1993 and commercialized one year later. The rBST increases milk production approximately 2.25 to 6.6 liters/cow/day and increases lactancy in 30 to 100 days [5, 76]. In 1998 more than 100 million doses of rBST were sold around the world and it is estimated that in 1999 about 30% of 9 million dairy cows in the US were treated with this drug. Cows were treated with 500 mg SC every 14 days throughout the lactation period and maximum increase in production is achieved after third or fourth injection [5].

This hormone has direct effects on breast parenchyma and basal metabolic rate. This promotes increases in milk synthesis, blood flow, and viability of MEC, along with increases in insulin-like growth factor 1 (IGF-1) protein in liver and mammary tissues [77, 78]. Other effects were observed on lipolysis, gluconeogenesis, and production of 1,25 dihydroxycholecalciferol and Ca^{2+} absorption [73, 78]. The effects on mammary epithelium are mediated by stimulation of somatotropine receptor (ST-R), which in synergy with the PRL pathway stimulates the Janus kinase/signal transducer and activator of transcription 5 (STAT5), the main lactogenic mediator of MEC proliferation, survival, and milk gene expression signaling [79–81]. Activation of the IGF-IR occurs following IGF-I binding to the α-subunit of the IGF-IR on epithelial cells, leading to autophosphorylation of the β-subunit by an intrinsic tyrosine kinase. These events can lead to the activation of a number of downstream [82, 83] pathways including the insulin receptor substrate (IRS) phosphorylation, which are involved in the upregulation phosphorylation of the phosphatidylinositol 4,5-bisphosphate (PIP_2) to phosphatidylinositol (3,4,5)-triphosphate (PIP_3) by phosphatidylinositol 3-kinase (PI3K); the PIP_3 increment is followed by phosphoinositide dependent kinase-1 (PDK1) [84], serine/threonine kinasealso known as protein kinase B (Akt/PKB), and mammalian target of rapamycin (mTOR) activation that induces MEC proliferation, survival (anti-apoptotic), and milk synthesis gene expression [83, 85–87]. Another IGF-1 activated pathway is the rat sarcoma protein [88]/rapidly accelerated Fibrosarcoma kinase (Raf)/mitogen activated protein kinase (MAPK) (also known as Ras-Raf-mitogen-activated protein kinase kinase (MEK)-ERK pathway), which, after the binding of IGF-1 to its receptor, induces phosphorylation of tyrosine residues, docking protein such as growth factor receptor-bound protein 2 (GRB2). This factor contains an Src homology 2 domain (Shc) that binds to the phosphotyrosine residues of the activated receptor GRB2 and binds to Son of Sevenless (SOS) to produce GRB2-SOS complex and docks to phosphorylated IGFR, SOS becomes activated and then induces Ras activation, Ras activates Raf, and this induces a phosphorylation cascade that activates MEK and mitogen-activated protein kinase also known as extracellular signal-reduced kinases MAPK/ERK [89–91]. Both IRS/PI3K/AKT(PKB)/mTOR pathway and Ras/Raf/(MAPK/ERK) pathway activated by IGF-1 and the JAK/STAT5 pathway activated by rBST/ST-R induce MEC proliferation and survival and increase milk protein synthesis, finally explaining the galactogogue actions of rBST [92] (Figure 4). Its half-life in Holstein cows is 54.8 minutes [93]. Somatotropin is the main galactogogue used in cattle. However, its use not only results in gain in productive efficiency and profitability but has also generated ethical dilemmas, in terms of animal welfare and health and potential risks for consumers. Contraindications in cattle include low pregnancy rates, increased open days [94], increased incidences of retained placenta [95], clinical and subclinical mastitis [96, 97], laminitis, digestive disorders, reduced feed

intake, allergic reactions [4], and decreased hemoglobin and hematocrit [98]. The FDA reports that between 1994 and 2005 they received about 2408 cases of adverse reactions to this treatment [4]. These facts triggered the decision of the European Union members, Canada, and other countries to prohibit its administration [4, 5].

2.4. Thyrotropin Releasing Hormone (TRH). This peptide hormone is synthesized in the hypothalamus, stimulating the secretion of thyroid stimulating hormone (TSH) and PRL by the anterior pituitary [99–101]. TRH is the principal physiological factor stimulating the fast release of PRL [99, 102]. Synthetic TRH applied IV can significantly increase serum PRL in proestrous female and in normal and estrogen-primed male rats, 10 min after injection [103]. Subcutaneous administration of TRH was also effective to increase plasma PRL levels in lactating cows [104]. Women treated with synthetic TRH 20 mg PO three times a day had high blood concentrations of PRL [105]. In another study, TRH administration for one month, at doses of 5 mg twice a day PO, did not change PRL blood concentration in human [106]. TRH has been effective in the induction of lactation in mothers with agalactia 10–150 days after birth [107], but its galactogogue effect is variable [108]. Its half-life in rats was found to be 4.16 minutes [109]. The TRH molecule binds to its receptor in the lactotrophic cells triggering the activation of PLC and increasing the formation of diacylglycerol (DAG) and inositol 1,4,5-triphosphate (IP3). DAG activates protein kinase C (PKC) and PKC promotes phosphorylation pathways that culminate in PRL gene expression; IP3 induces release of Ca^{2+} from endoplasmic reticulum, forming the complex Ca^{2+}-calmodulin (CaM) [110], and this complex induces the PRL gene expression [111, 112]. Furthermore, the increase of intracellular CA^{2+} and CaM stimulates the release of the PRL stored in vesicles [112, 113] (Figure 5).

About its elimination in milk, no data are available [2]. TRH administration increases maternal plasma levels of thyroxine T4 and triiodothyronine T3; however, both hormones appear in low concentrations in milk [99]. No side effects have been found in infants [105]. Some cases of iatrogenic hyperthyroidism and brief episodes of sweating have been reported in mothers [106, 108]. There are no clinical studies about its use in veterinary medicine, and more research is needed.

2.5. Medroxyprogesterone. It is a steroidal synthetic progesterone (a progestin). This drug causes hyperplasia of mammary secretory epithelium in macaques [114] and mice, with its activity being associated with epidermal growth factor (EGF) [115]. However, there are limited clinical studies in women suggesting that this drug is effective in increasing serum PRL and milk production [116–118]. Medroxyprogesterone acetate biological half-life in human is 40–60 hrs [119]. In human, medroxyprogesterone was found in plasma and in milk at a 1 : 1 ratio [120]. No adverse effects were reported in infants and in mothers amenorrhea was described [121]. Reported effective dose in humans is 150 mg IM every 3 months, beginning at week 2 postpartum and repeating at

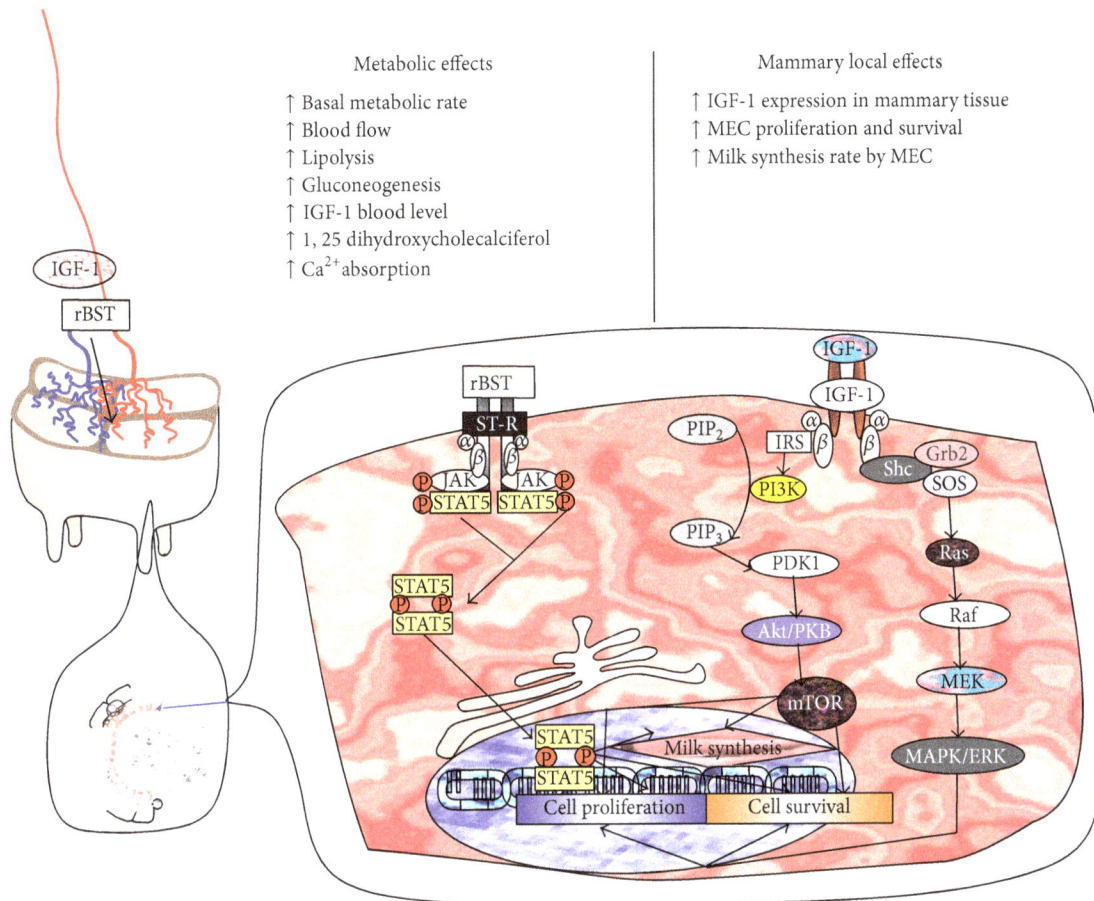

FIGURE 4: Proposed mechanism of action of recombinant bovine somatotropin (rBST). This hormone has direct effects on basal metabolic rate and breast parenchyma; the effects on the MEC (blue arrow) are mediated by rBST/ST-R complex, which stimulates JAK2/STAT5 pathway and by IGF-1R/IGF-1 which promotes and upregulates IRS/PI3K/(AKT/PKB)/mTOR and Ras/Raf/(MAPK/ERK) pathways. This will induce cell proliferation and survival and increase milk protein synthesis in MEC.

week 14 [122]. It is considered compatible with breastfeeding [121] and its mechanism of action is not well known [2].

3. Herbal Galactogogues

Some plants have been used in many cultures to stimulate milk production in women and in dairy animals [123]. Galactogogue effect of various plants has been studied and there is evidence that milk synthesis can be increased and that most of them are safe in humans [40], cows [7, 88, 124, 125], goats [126–129], and buffaloes [130–132]. Several herbal galactogogues have been reported as safe substances that in appropriate and economic doses can be used therapeutically in domestic animals [67] and in food supplements of dairy herds [7, 126]. The herbal derivative products use in dairy industry relies on the new trend in dairy sector of organic dairy farming [19, 133]. Some herbs demonstrate efficacy in increasing milk production in women with mammary hypoplasia [134].

However, pharmacokinetics and pharmacodynamics of active ingredients present in galactogogues plants are not

well characterized and further research is compulsory to determine their mechanisms of action and to establish therapeutic ranges, dosage, and possible side effects in different domestic species and humans [123]. Some clinical trial results have shown several limitations including small sample size, insufficient randomization methods, poorly defined eligibility criteria, use of poly-herbal interventions, and variable breastfeeding practices among enrolled subjects [3]. Plant drugs, also known as herbal drugs, phytopharmaceuticals, or phytomedicines are plant-derived medicines that contain a chemical compound or more usually mixtures of chemical compounds that act individually or in combination on the animal body to prevent disorders and to restore or maintain health [16] or to improve the animal production [135].

Crude plants, herbal teas, decoction, and alcoholic extracts are also traditional ways of using medicinal plants. Very often these plant materials are used in a nonstandardized manner [16]. However, nowadays more and more emphasis is being put on the use of standardized materials and preparations to ensure the efficacy, safety, and composition; this is called as pharmaceutical quality [16–18]. To develop and sale these preparations studies of phytochemical

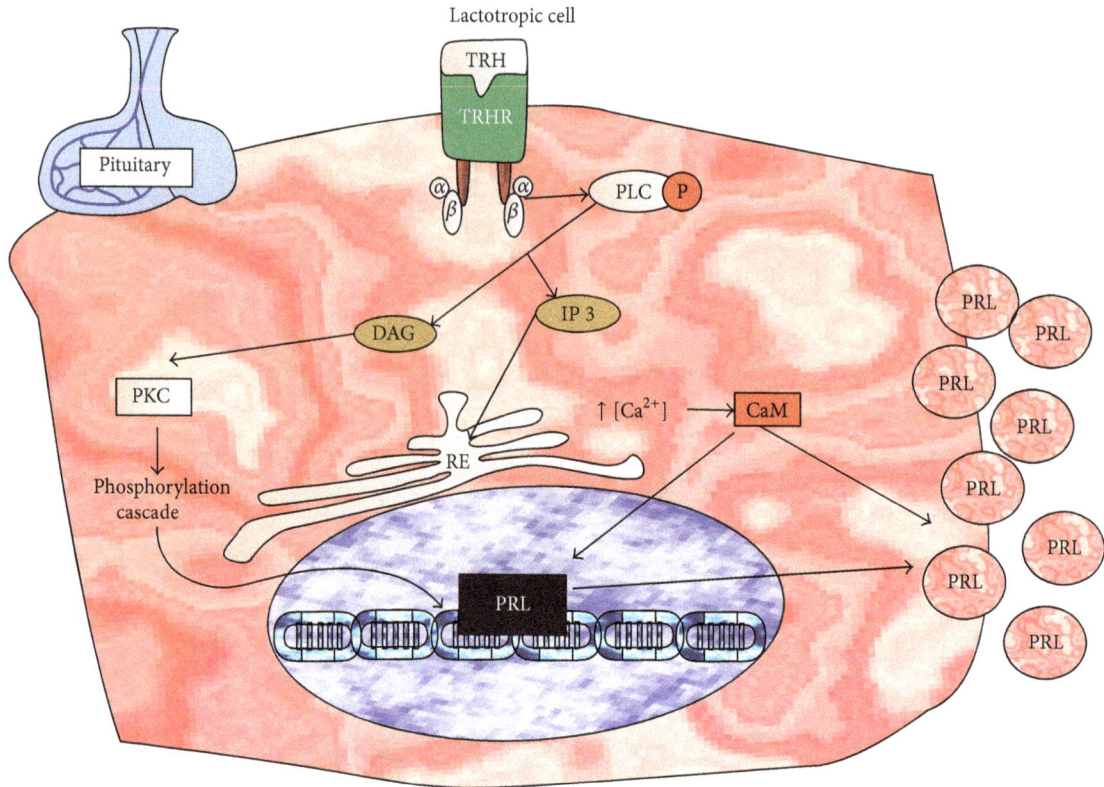

FIGURE 5: Proposed mechanism of action of thyrotropin releasing hormone (TRH). The TRH molecule binds to its receptor in lactotrophic cells of the pituitary gland and stimulates Ca^{2+}/CaM release, which induces the PRL gene expression. Furthermore, the increase in intracellular CA^{2+}/CaM stimulates the release of PRL stored in vesicles. This will increase PRL blood levels and promotes more milk synthesis.

composition, pharmacodynamic and pharmacokinetic are necessary, but also good agricultural practices (GAP), good laboratory practices (GLP), good manufacturing practices (GMP), and quality control standards are required [16–18]. The complementarity of analytical methods like high performance liquid chromatography (HPLC) and gas chromatography (GC) is of paramount importance for analyzing both the lead and the minor compounds [16]. For the pharmaceutical quality level also it is important to make assessment of microbial contamination, raw materials adulteration, and side-effects (toxicity) of plant extracts [16, 136].

It is necessary to develop well-designed and well-conducted clinical trials that address the above limitations to generate strong evidence of the efficacy and safety, as a basis for producing herbal galactogogues preparations [3, 137]. The pharmacological research of botanical galactogogues should study nutritional values (macro- and micronutrients) as wells as therapeutic potentials (secondary metabolites and their activities) [138]. Turkyilmaz et al. suggested that the herbal galactogogues effect could be mediated by phytoestrogenic action [139] and that some molecules may have effects similar to 17β-estradiol (E2), an endogenous estrogen that promotes the proliferation of MEC [140]. The supply of genistein (isoflavone phytoestrogen) induces mammary gland hyperplasia in sows [141]. Figure 6 depicts the chemical structures of phytoestrogens that are mentioned in this review. We

hypothesize that if the phytoestrogen molecules have E2-like action, these molecules could induce the expression of PRL receptor (PRLR) [142] and EGF receptor (EGFR) [143] and could upregulate casein production and lactose synthetase activity in MEC [144]. E2 triggers PRL gene expression through at least two independent and undetermined pathways in pituitary lactotropic cells. A first route is characterized to act through the intracellular receptor E2 (E2R) that finally increases levels of PRL [145, 146] and increases secretion of milk. These effects are mediated by the pathway triggered by α isoform of the membrane-associated estrogen receptor (mE2R) (Figure 7). The second route inhibits the pathway activated by D2R dopamine receptor, stimulating PRL production and proliferation of lactotrophic cells by increasing cAMP ending in PKA phosphorylation pathways that trigger PRL gene expression [107] (Figure 7). The following sections will review information about commonly used galactogogues plants.

3.1. Trigonella foenum graecum (Fenugreek/fenugreek). It is the most used commonly herbal galactogogue [3, 147]. It is a member of the Leguminosaefamily that is cultivated in many parts of the world, particularly in India, Mediterranean countries, north Africa, and southern Europe [123]. Reports indicate that seeds have mastogenic effect, stimulating growth of mammary gland [138]. This plant is used around the world as galactagogue in women due to its

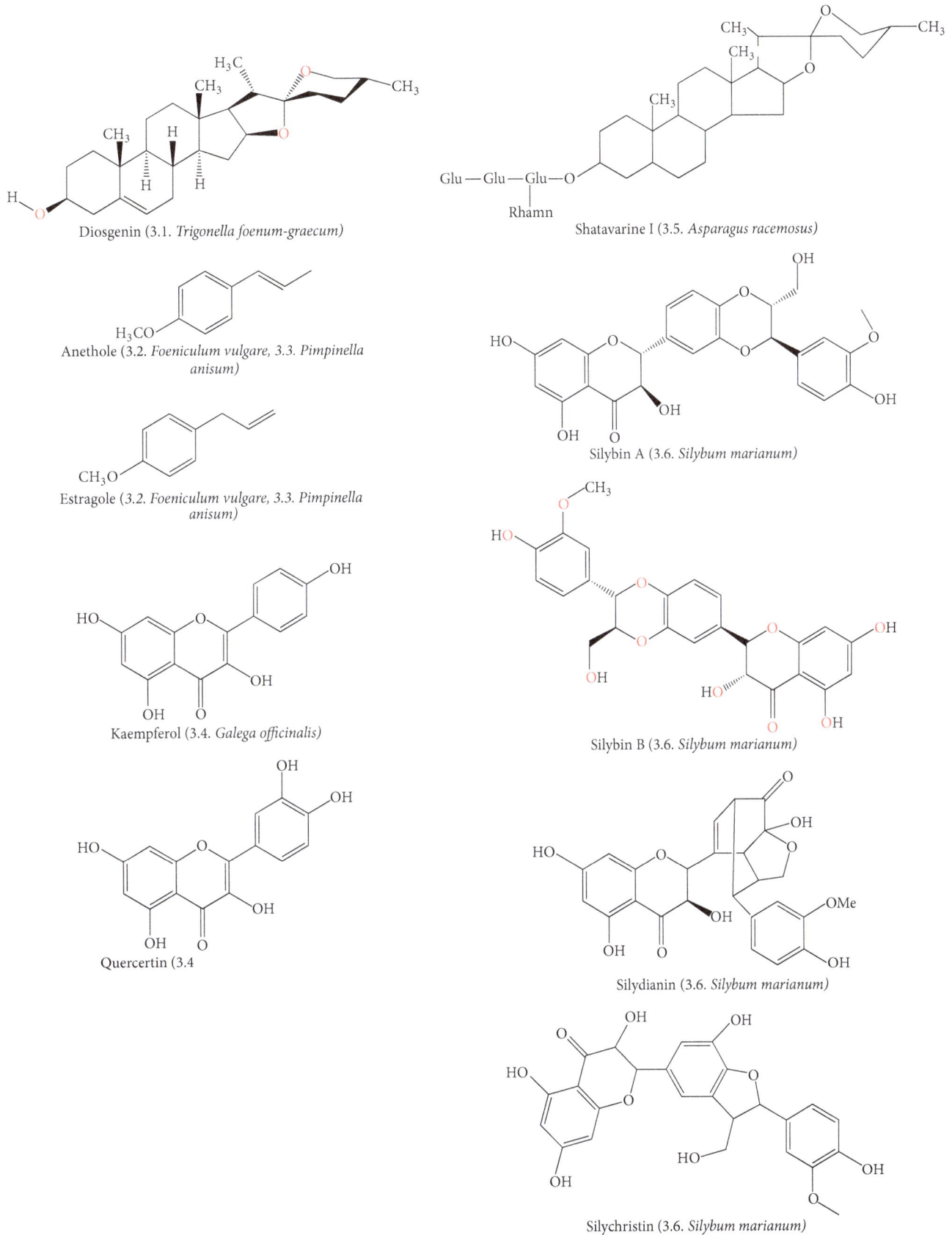

FIGURE 6: Phytoestrogenic molecules present in some botanical galactogogues.

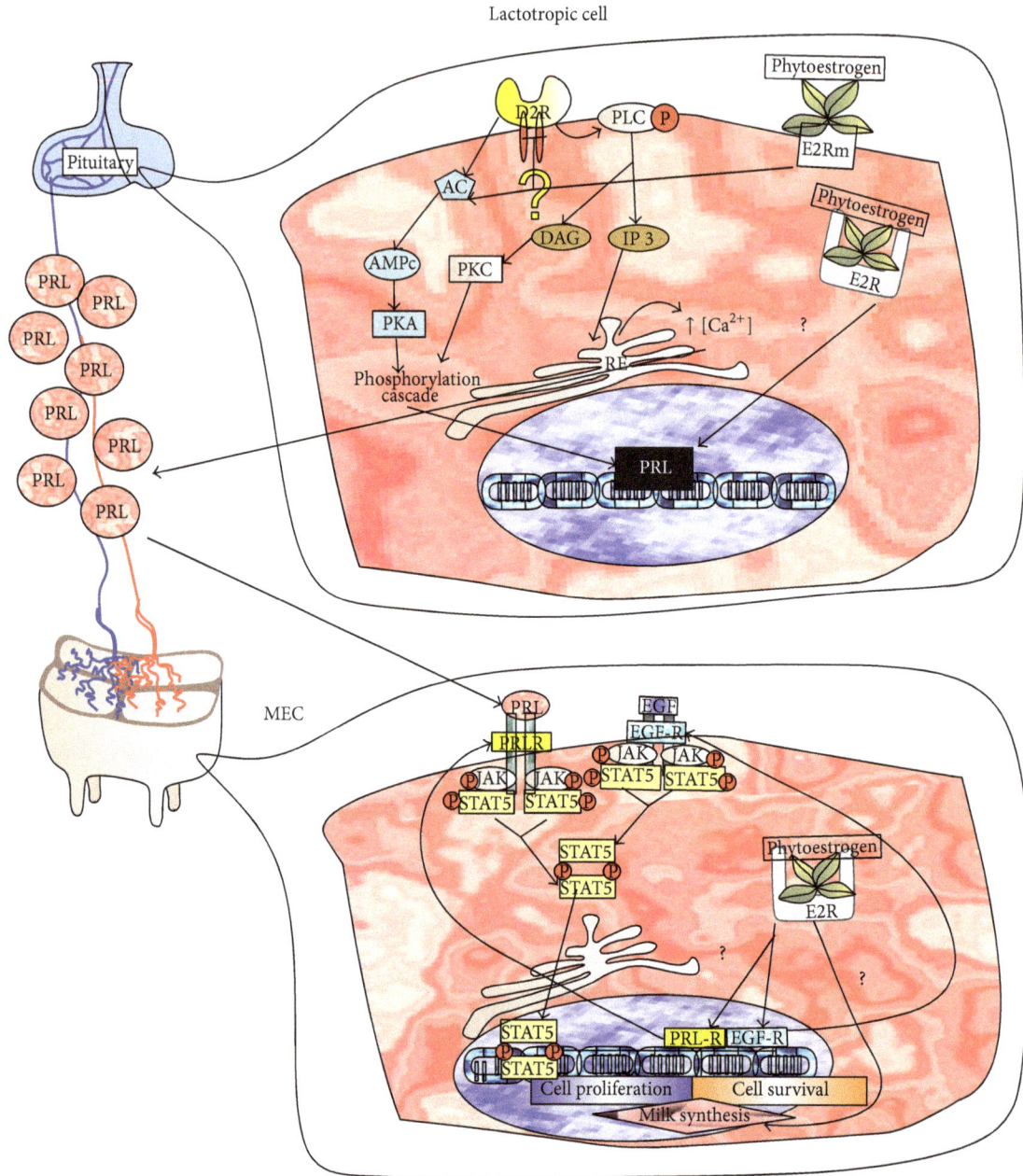

FIGURE 7: Proposed galactogogue mechanism of action of phytoestrogen molecules in anterior pituitary and mammary gland. The E2-like action may induce PRL expression in anterior pituitary lactotrophic cells and milk production in MEC by indeterminate pathways (?). In lactotrophic cells, upregulation of PRL gene expression and secretion occurs directly by E2R and indirectly by mE2R inducing D2R inhibition. In MEC, PRL-R and EGF-R expressions are induced and milk synthesis, cell proliferation, and survival gene expression are suggested.

phytoestrogens' significant levels [148]. One study using *in vitro* assays found that fenugreek seeds contain estrogen-like compounds and that they stimulate pS2 (estrogen-induced protein) expression in a breast cancer cell line Michigan Cancer Foundation-7 (MCF-7); pS2 is frequently used as a marker for assessing the estrogenicity of a compound [148]. Phytoestrogens as diosgenin, a type of steroidal sapogenin, could explain the observed milk flow increase [3].

Recently, it was found that fenugreek induces a significant increase in milk production in women and decrease the time of neonates recovery weight [139]. Despite its widespread use, there is little research conducted on its pharmacodynamic and pharmacokinetics properties to determine the extent to which its components are excreted in milk.

Moreover, this plant has been shown to influence the maintenance of lactation in ruminants; buffaloes fed with seeds increase milk production, but it has not been clearly demonstrated whether its composition is altered [130]. In goats, it has been reported that feeding with 10 g daily of fenugreek seed increases milk production [127]. Attempting to elucidate the mechanism by which this plant increases milk production, it is proposed that the galactogenic effect could be mediated through increased feed intake in buffaloes [131].

Other studies suggest that stimulation of endogenous hormones secretion may be the way by which fenugreek exerts its action on increasing milk production. In goats feeding with fenugreek increased milk production and this effect might be mediated via PRL stimulation, because PRL concentrations were found to be significantly higher in the fenugreek fed goats compared to control group [149]. Similarly, in a recent study performed in goats, an increase of 13% in milk production was paralleled to an increase of serum somatotropine [128]. It is suggested also that plasma growth hormone in buffaloes could be candidate in mediating fenugreek action [131].

3.2. Foeniculum vulgare (Fennel).

It is the only species in the genus *Foeniculum*, found in temperate zones around the world, and it is a perennial and aromatic plant native of southern Europe, especially the Mediterranean coast, where it is considered as a wild herb [150]. The first report of its galactagogue properties was by a Greek botanist Pedanius Dioscorides (40–90 A.D). This plant may increase milk production and milk fat content in goats [151]. It has been used as a galactogogue in humans and no adverse effects have been reported yet [6, 123], in mice [152] or goats [136]. *F. vulgare* has been used as an estrogenic agent for centuries. It has been reported to increase milk secretion, improve the reproductive cyclicity, facilitate birth, and increase libido [150]. It contains E2-like molecules, such as anethole and estragole [153, 154] (Figure 6).

3.3. Pimpinella anisum (Anise).

This herbal galactogogue is part of the Apiaceae family, a plant found in West Asia, Eastern Mediterranean, Mexico, and Spain. The main oil constituents, obtained from dried fruits, are trans-anethole (93,9%) and estragole (2,4%), which are pharmaceutical compounds that possess strong estrogenic activity which justifies its use as a galactagogue [7, 123, 155]. Aqueous and ethanolic extracts of *P. anisum* seeds can increase milk production in rats [156]. The aqueous (1 g/kg) and ethanolic extracts (1 g/kg) increased rats milk production significantly in about 68.1% and 81%, respectively, compared to the control group [156].

3.4. Galega officinalis (Goat's Rue).

It is an herbaceous plant from central and southern Europe. Its lactogenic value has to be considered according to reported increase in milk yield and lactation persistency when included in a daily diet in cows [88, 124, 129, 157] and sheep [158]. However, several members of the genus *Galega* have been listed as poisonous to livestock in New Zealand and USA [158, 159]. Genus *Galega* is considered to be of low palatability and high toxicity [159]; this latter due to high concentrations of guanidine derived molecules hidroxigalegin and galegin [160]. The toxic effects

of *G. officinalis* in sheep may vary among individuals, but in all cases, doses over 5 g/kg are toxic [161]. In contrast with these reports of toxicity, lactogenic properties of *G. officinalis* were confirmed in sheep at daily doses of 2 g of dry matter/kg body weight from the first month after lambing and during 60 days; the result was a 16.9% increase in total milk yield, without any signs of toxicity [158]. In cows any adverse effects were reported in a diet of 25% concentrate feeds and 75% *G. officinalis*, with *ad libitum* intake [132]. In this regard, the administration of phytoestrogens in low doses or foods containing them could promote activation of some estrogen receptors in the animal and increase milk production. Several phytoestrogens have been isolated from methanol extracts of Goat's rue such as flavonol triglycosides, kaempferol, and quercetin [158, 162].

3.5. Asparagus racemosus (Shatavari).

This plant belongs to the Asparagaceaefamily and has its origins in India; its role as a milk production enhancing substance has been mentioned in several ancient Ayurvedic text books such as *Charaka Samhita* and *Susruta Samhita* [163]. It has phytoestrogenic properties [163] and it has been observed to increase milk secretion following administration of *A. racemosus* as Ricalex tablets in women suffering from hypogalactia [164]; the gradual decrease in milk secretion, on withdrawal of the drug, suggested that the increase in milk secretion was due to drug therapy only and not to any psychological effect [165]. In 2011, the root powder oral administration in women in a double-blind randomized clinical trial has demonstrated a threefold increase in PRL level in subjects of the research group compared to the control group [166]. However, in previous works authors did not observe any increase in PRL levels in *A. racemosus* treated females suffering from a secondary lactational failure [163]. In rats supplemented with the plant (2% of their diet), a lactogenic effect was reported [167]. Systemic administration of alcohol extract of *A. racemosus* in weaning rats increased weight of mammary glands, inhibited involution of lobuloalveolar tissue, and maintained milk secretion [168]. Other studies with alcohol extract of Shatavari demonstrated estrogenic effects in genital organs and in mammary glands in rats with hyperplasia in alveolar tissues and acini and with increased milk production [163]. A significant increase in milk yield has also been observed in pigs and goats after feeding with lactare (commercial herbal galactogogues with *A. racemosus* in its formulation) which also increased growth of the mammary glands, alveolar tissues, and acini [169]. Roots of *A. racemosus* also have shown galactogogue effect in buffaloes [170]. In rats, its methanolic roots extract in a dose of 100 mg/Kg/day for 60 days showed teratological disorders in terms of increased fetuses resorption, malformations as legs swelling, and intrauterine growth retardation with a small placental size [171]. Chemical analysis of Shatavari roots reveals the presence of steroidal saponins (as Shatavarins I-IV). Shatavarin I is the most glycosided molecule with 3 glucose and a rhamnose moieties attached to sarsasapogenin [172]; one hypothesis states that the estrogenic activity results from the hormone-like actions of these steroidal saponins

[163, 166]. Another hypothesis declares that the growth of mammary tissue is caused by the action of released corticoids or PRL [163, 165, 166]. Although estrogens have a stimulating effect on the ductal epithelial cells, causing them to lengthen, their primary role seems to be the potentiation of PRL production [3].

3.6. Silybum marianum (Milk Thistle). This medicinal plant has been used from ancient times by Theophrastus (4th century BC) who was probably the first to describe it under the name of "Pternix," and later it was mentioned by Dioskurides in his "Materia medica" and by Plinius (1st century AD) [173]. Silymarin is a mixture of flavonoids extracted from seeds of this plant, which contains silybin, silydianin, and silychristin; molecules that show estrogenic effect in ovariectomized rats [174] and its major component, silibinin, bind to cytosolic estrogen receptors [175]. Human and animal studies suggest that milk thistle has promising lactogenic properties. In a study, after treatment with 10 g silymarin/cow/days PO in the peripartum (from 10 day sbefore calving to 15 days after calving), an increase in milk production of 5-6 L/day per cow was observed [176]. It is thought that the administration of silymarin after calf delivery improves physiological status of the cow, which leads to faster recovery, increased feed intake, and increased milk production. This finding was supported by the observation of reduction of blood β-hydroxybutyric acid and decreased outcomes of ketonuria in cows treated with silymarin [164, 176]. Silymarin elimination half-life in humans averages 6 hours [30]. Silymarin is apparently well tolerated when administered orally. In humans, GI disturbances have been reported on occasion (nausea to diarrhea). Patients who have allergies to other members of the *Asteraceae/Compositae* plant family (includes ragweed, marigolds, daisies, etc.) may exhibit allergic reactions to Milk Thistle derivatives [30]. In women orally treated for 63 days with 420 mg/day of silymarin a clear galactogogue effect was evident with an increase of 85.94% of daily milk production compared to 32.09% of the placebo group [154]. Female rats treated for 14 days with 25–200 mg/kg orally increased, in a dose dependent manner, the serum PRL levels [177]. It is known that silymarin elicited partial ER activation and silybin B were probably responsible for a majority of the weak ER-mediated activities of silymarin, whereas, its diastereomer, silybin A, was found to be inactive [173].

4. General Conclusions and Research Needs

Galactogogues, both synthetics and herbal, have been poorly studied in veterinary medicine. Most of the information about the effectiveness and safety of these substances as galactogogues was obtained by research in human; these studies were included in the review as a relevant comparative element, which are the basis for developing applications in veterinary and livestock practice, especially in massive dairy production. Nowadays, limited pharmacological knowledge exists about botanical galactogogues. The mechanisms of action and relevant pharmacological data were reviewed

and hypotheses about its mechanism of action are postulated. *In vitro* studies in mammary secretory epithelial and lactotrophic cells are considered as reference models for pharmacological essays and determination of galactogogues action mechanisms and pathways; its limitations in terms of pharmacokinetic processes and systemic metabolic effects study in *in vitro* models are, however, recognized. Because of limited literature on this topic in veterinary practices, it is of interest to characterize the doses, characterization of phytochemical composition (molecules), formulations, and mechanisms of action, side effects, and drug interactions of galactogogues, mainly the herbals ones. This is an innovative research area that could be projected as sustainable strategies for massification and optimization of milk production in the dairy and swine industry (e.g., increasing weaning weight). These plants could be given as feed rations or its concentrated extracts (essential oils, alcohol extracts, lyophilized extract, among others) as supplements. Apparently, they are compatible with animal welfare but further basic and applied research about this issue is proposed.

Conflict of Interests

The authors did not receive financial compensation for the investigation and declare that there is no conflict of interests with respect to the research, authorship, and publication of this paper.

Acknowledgments

This research is supported by the Estrategia de Sostenibilidad, University of Antioquia, to Biogenesis Group 2013-2014 and by the Programática-Ciencias Biomédicas y de la Salud 2012-2013.

References

[1] S. Sjolin, Y. Hofvander, and C. Hillervik, "Factors related to early termination of breast feeding: a retrospective study in Sweden," *Acta Paediatrica Scandinavica*, vol. 66, no. 4, pp. 505–511, 1977.

[2] A. A. Zuppa, P. Sindico, C. Orchi et al., "Safety and efficacy of galactogogues: substances that induce, maintain and increase breast milk production," *Journal of Pharmacy and Pharmaceutical Sciences*, vol. 13, no. 2, pp. 162–174, 2010.

[3] M. Mortel and S. D. Mehta, "Systematic review of the efficacy of herbal galactogogues," *Journal of Human Lactation*, vol. 29, no. 2, pp. 154–162, 2013.

[4] M. Melnyk, *Recombinant bovine somatotropin: challenging Canada's science-based regulatory system and the emergence of post-normal science [Doctoral, thesis]*, Department of Sociology, University of Saskatchewan, Saskatoon, Canada, 2005.

[5] Scientific Committee on Animal Health and Animal Welfare, "Report on the animal welfare aspects of the use of bovine somatotrophin," 1999, http://ec.europa.eu/food/fs/sc/scah/out21.

[6] I. P. Agrawala, M. V. Achar, R. V. Boradkar, and N. Roy, "Galactagogue action of *Cuminum cyminum* and *Nigella staiva*," *Indian Journal of Medical Research*, vol. 56, no. 6, pp. 841–844, 1968.

[7] R. E. Westfall, "Galactagogue herbs: a qualitative study and review," *Canadian Journal of Midwifery Research and Practice*, vol. 2, no. 2, pp. 22–27, 2003.

[8] S. N. Bharti, N. K. Sharma, A. K. Gupta, K. Murari, and A. Kumar, "Pharmacological actions and potential uses of diverse Galactogogues in Cattle," *International Journal of Clinical Pharmacology and Therapeutics*, vol. 2, no. 1, pp. 24–28, 2012.

[9] M. A. Underwood, "Human milk for the premature infant," *Pediatric Clinics of North America*, vol. 60, no. 1, pp. 189–207, 2013.

[10] A. Zapantis, J. G. Steinberg, and L. Schilit, "Use of herbals as galactagogues," *Journal of Pharmacy Practice*, vol. 25, no. 2, pp. 222–231, 2012.

[11] M. I. Baig and V. G. Bhagwat, "Study the efficacy of Galactin Vet Bolus on milk yield in dairy cows," *Veterinary World*, vol. 2, no. 4, pp. 140–142, 2009.

[12] E. Romano-Santos, B. Fernández-González, L. Díez-Soro, and S. Martínez-Bonafont, "¿Qué sabemos de los galactogogos?" *Matronas Profesión*, vol. 10, no. 4, pp. 27–30, 2009.

[13] T. Frankič, M. Voljč, J. Salobir, and V. Rezar, "Use of herbs and spices and their extracts in animal nutrition," *Acta Agriculturae Slovenica*, vol. 94, no. 2, pp. 95–102, 2009.

[14] C. Vanaclocha and S. Cañigueral, *Fitoterapia: Vademécum de Prescripción*, Masson, Barcelona, 4th edition, 2003.

[15] F. J. Haya, *Uso práctico de la fitoterapia en ginecología*, Médica Panamericana, Madrid, Spain, 2007.

[16] A. Gurib-Fakim, "Medicinal plants: traditions of yesterday and drugs of tomorrow," *Molecular Aspects of Medicine*, vol. 27, no. 1, pp. 1–93, 2006.

[17] K. Chan, "Some aspects of toxic contaminants in herbal medicines," *Chemosphere*, vol. 52, no. 9, pp. 1361–1371, 2003.

[18] S. Verma and S. P. Singh, "Current and future status of herbal medicines," *Veterinary World*, vol. 1, no. 11, pp. 347–350, 2008.

[19] M. Oruganti, "Organic dairy farming: a new trend in dairy sector," *Veterinary World*, vol. 4, no. 3, pp. 128–130, 2011.

[20] A. Kauppila, S. Kivinen, and O. Ylikorkala, "A dose response relation between improved lactation and metoclopramide," *The Lancet*, vol. 317, no. 8231, pp. 175–177, 2001.

[21] R. A. Ehrenkranz and B. A. Ackerman, "Metoclopramide effect on faltering milk production by mothers of premature infants," *Pediatrics*, vol. 78, no. 4, pp. 614–620, 1986.

[22] A. P. Gupta and P. K. Gupta, "Metoclopramide as a lactogue," *Clinical Pediatrics*, vol. 24, no. 5, pp. 269–272, 2005.

[23] P. de Camilli, D. Macconi, and A. Spada, "Dopamine inhibits adenylate cyclase in human prolactin-secreting pituitary adenomas," *Nature*, vol. 278, no. 5701, pp. 252–254, 1979.

[24] R. C. Rogers, M. J. Barnes, and G. E. Hermann, "Leptin 'gates' thermogenic action of thyrotropin-releasing hormone in the hindbrain," *Brain Research*, vol. 1295, pp. 135–141, 2009.

[25] N. Ben-Jonathan and R. Hnasko, "Dopamine as a prolactin (PRL) inhibitor," *Endocrine Reviews*, vol. 22, no. 6, pp. 724–763, 2001.

[26] R. M. Akers, D. E. Bauman, A. V. Capuco, G. T. Goodman, and H. A. Tucker, "Prolactin regulation of milk secretion and biochemical differentiation of mammary epithelial cells in periparturient cows," *Endocrinology*, vol. 109, no. 1, pp. 23–30, 1981.

[27] V. Guzman, G. Toscano, E. S. Canales, and A. Zarate, "Improvement of defective lactation by using oral metoclopramide," *Acta Obstetricia et Gynecologica Scandinavica*, vol. 58, no. 1, pp. 53–55, 1979.

[28] P. O. Anderson and V. Valdés, "A critical review of pharmaceutical galactagogues," *Breastfeeding Medicine*, vol. 2, no. 4, pp. 229–242, 2007.

[29] D. N. Bateman, C. Kahn, and D. S. Davies, "The pharmacokinetics of metoclopramide in man with observations in the dog," *British Journal of Clinical Pharmacology*, vol. 9, no. 4, pp. 371–377, 1980.

[30] C. Plumb, *Veterinary Drug Handbook*, PharmaVet, Stockholm, Wis, USA, 6th edition, 2008.

[31] J. Ingram, H. Taylor, C. Churchill, A. Pike, and R. Greenwood, "Metoclopramide or domperidone for increasing maternal breast milk output: a randomised controlled trial," *Archives of Disease in Childhood: Fetal and Neonatal Edition*, vol. 97, no. 4, pp. F241–F245, 2012.

[32] M. Kahn, *Manual Merck de Veterinaria*, Grupo Editorial Océano, Barcelona, España, 2007.

[33] J. A. Barone, "Domperidone: a peripherally acting dopamine2-receptor antagonist," *Annals of Pharmacotherapy*, vol. 33, no. 4, pp. 429–440, 1999.

[34] E. W. Wan, K. Davey, M. Page-Sharp, P. E. Hartmann, K. Simmer, and K. F. Ilett, "Dose-effect study of domperidone as a galactagogue in preterm mothers with insufficient milk supply, and its transfer into milk," *The British Journal of Clinical Pharmacology*, vol. 66, no. 2, pp. 283–289, 2008.

[35] A. Osadchy, M. E. Moretti, and G. Koren, "Effect of domperidone on insufficient lactation in puerperal women: a systematic review and meta-analysis of randomized controlled trials," *Obstetrics and Gynecology International*, vol. 2012, Article ID 642893, 7 pages, 2012.

[36] J. Heykants, R. Hendriks, W. Meuldermans, M. Michiels, H. Scheygrond, and H. Reyntjens, "On the pharmacokinetics of domperidone in animals and man. IV. The pharmacokinetics of intravenous domperidone and its bioavailability in man following intramuscular, oral and rectal administration," *European Journal of Drug Metabolism and Pharmacokinetics*, vol. 6, no. 1, pp. 61–70, 1981.

[37] O. P. Da Silva and D. C. Knoppert, "Domperidone for lactating women," *Canadian Medical Association Journal*, vol. 171, no. 7, pp. 725–726, 2004.

[38] D. Guillaume, P. Chavatte-Palmer, Y. Combarnous et al., "Induced lactation with a dopamine antagonist in mares: different responses between ovariectomized and intact mares," *Reproduction in Domestic Animals*, vol. 38, no. 5, pp. 394–400, 2003.

[39] D. L. Cross, L. M. Redmond, and J. R. Strickland, "Equine fescue toxicosis: signs and solutions," *Journal of Animal Science*, vol. 73, no. 3, pp. 899–908, 1995.

[40] K. Yoshida, B. Smith, M. Craggs, and R. Kumar, "Neuroleptic drugs in breast-milk: a study of pharmacokinetics and of possible adverse effects in breast-fed infants," *Psychological Medicine*, vol. 28, no. 1, pp. 81–91, 1998.

[41] P. K. Talwalker, J. Meites, C. S. Nicoll, and T. F. Hopkins, "Effects of chlorpromazine on mammary glands of rats," *The American Journal of Physiology*, vol. 199, pp. 1073–1076, 1960.

[42] C. E. Weichert, "Lactational reflex recovery in breast-feeding failure," *Pediatrics*, vol. 63, no. 5, pp. 799–803, 1979.

[43] G. Wampler, "The pharmacology and clinical effectiveness of phenothiazines and related drugs for managing chemotherapy-induced emesis," *Drugs*, vol. 25, no. 1, pp. 35–51, 1983.

[44] M. P. Gabay, "Galactogogues: medications that induce lactation," *Journal of Human Lactation*, vol. 18, no. 3, pp. 274–279, 2002.

[45] M. Jeanmougin, M. Sigal-Nahum, J. R. Manciet, A. Petit, B. Flageul, and L. Dubertret, "Photosensibilisation rémanente induite par la chlorproéthazine," *Annales de Dermatologie et de Vénéréologie*, vol. 120, no. 11, pp. 840–843, 1993.

[46] A. S. Zelickson and H. C. Zeller, "A new and unusual reaction to chlorpromazine," *The Journal of the American Medical Association*, vol. 188, no. 4, pp. 394–396, 1964.

[47] A. M. Mancini, A. Guitelman, C. A. Vargas, L. Debeljuk, and N. J. Aparicio, "Effect of sulpiride on serum prolactin levels in humans," *Journal of Clinical Endocrinology and Metabolism*, vol. 42, no. 1, pp. 181–184, 1976.

[48] T. Aono, T. Aki, K. Koike, and K. Kurachi, "Effect of sulpiride on poor puerperal lactation," *The American Journal of Obstetrics and Gynecology*, vol. 143, no. 8, pp. 927–932, 1982.

[49] F. Polatti, "Sulpiride isomers and milk secretion in puerperium," *Clinical and Experimental Obstetrics and Gynecology*, vol. 9, no. 3, pp. 144–147, 1982.

[50] O. Ylikorkala, A. Kauppila, S. Kivinen, and L. Viinikka, "Sulpiride improves inadequate lactation," *British Medical Journal*, vol. 285, no. 6337, pp. 249–251, 1982.

[51] A. S. Alam, A. R. Imondi, J. Udinsky, and L. M. Hagerman, "Bioavailability of 14C-sulpiride in dogs," *Archives Internationales de Pharmacodynamie et de Therapie*, vol. 242, no. 1, pp. 4–13, 1979.

[52] J. Segura, L. Borja, and O. M. Bakke, "Pharmacokinetics of sulpiride after oral and intravenous administration in the rat and dog," *Archives Internationales de Pharmacodynamie et de Therapie*, vol. 223, no. 1, pp. 88–95, 1976.

[53] F. A. Wiesel, G. Alfredsson, M. Ehrnebo, and G. Sedvall, "The pharmacokinetics of intravenous and oral sulpiride in healthy human subjects," *European Journal of Clinical Pharmacology*, vol. 17, no. 5, pp. 385–391, 1980.

[54] P. Chavatte-Palmer, G. Arnaud, C. Duvaux-Ponter et al., "Quantitative and qualitative assessment of milk production after pharmaceutical induction of lactation in the mare," *Journal of Veterinary Internal Medicine*, vol. 16, no. 4, pp. 472–477, 2002.

[55] G. Gimpl and F. Fahrenholz, "The oxytocin receptor system: structure, function, and regulation," *Physiological Reviews*, vol. 81, no. 2, pp. 629–683, 2001.

[56] M. J. Renfrew, S. Lang, and M. Woolridge, "Oxytocin for promoting successful lactation," *Cochrane Database of Systematic Reviews*, no. 2, 2000.

[57] V. Lollivier, P. Marnet, S. Delpal et al., "Oxytocin stimulates secretory processes in lactating rabbit mammary epithelial cells," *Journal of Physiology*, vol. 570, no. 1, pp. 125–140, 2006.

[58] M. Peaker and C. J. Wilde, "Feedback control of milk secretion from milk," *Journal of Mammary Gland Biology and Neoplasia*, vol. 1, no. 3, pp. 307–315, 1996.

[59] J. E. Hillerton and K. E. Kliem, "Effective treatment of *Streptococcus uberis* clinical mastitis to minimize the use of antibiotics," *Journal of Dairy Science*, vol. 85, no. 4, pp. 1009–1014, 2002.

[60] S. Jonsson and M. O. Pulkkinen, "Mastitis today: incidence, prevention and treatment," *Annales Chirurgiae et Gynaecologiae*, vol. 208, pp. 84–87, 1994.

[61] A. M. Homeida and R. G. Cooke, "Biological half-life of oxytocin in the goat," *Research in Veterinary Science*, vol. 37, no. 3, pp. 364–365, 1984.

[62] J. D. Cleverley and S. J. Folley, "The blood levels of oxytocin during machine milking in cows with some observations on its half-life in the circulation," *Journal of Endocrinology*, vol. 46, no. 3, pp. 347–361, 1970.

[63] T. Higuchi, K. Honda, T. Fukuoka, H. Negoro, and K. Wakabayashi, "Release of oxytocin during suckling and parturition in the rat," *Journal of Endocrinology*, vol. 105, no. 3, pp. 339–346, 1985.

[64] D. Schams, B. Schmidt-Polex, and V. Kruse, "Oxytocin determination by radioimmunoassay in cattle. I. Method and preliminary physiological data," *Acta Endocrinologica*, vol. 92, no. 2, pp. 258–270, 1979.

[65] E. A. Wachs, R. C. Gorewit, and W. B. Currie, "Half-life, clearance and production rate for oxytocin in cattle during lactation and mammary involution I," *Domestic Animal Endocrinology*, vol. 1, no. 2, pp. 121–140, 1984.

[66] D. L. Paccamonti, J. F. Pycock, M. A. M. Taverne et al., "PGFM response to exogenous oxytocin and determination of the half-life of oxytocin in nonpregnant mares," *Equine Veterinary Journal*, vol. 31, no. 4, pp. 285–288, 1999.

[67] G. Rydén and I. Sjöholm, "Half-life of oxytocin in blood of pregnant and non-pregnant women." *Acta Endocrinologica*, vol. 61, no. 3, pp. 425–431, 1969.

[68] R. Rani, S. Medhe, K. R. Raj, and M. Srivastava, "Standardization of HPTLC method for the estimation of oxytocin in edibles," *Journal of Food Science and Technology*, vol. 50, no. 6, pp. 1222–1227, 2013.

[69] M. S. Fewtrell, K. L. Loh, A. Blake, D. A. Ridout, and J. Hawdon, "Randomised, double blind trial of oxytocin nasal spray in mothers expressing breast milk for preterm infants," *Archives of Disease in Childhood*, vol. 91, no. 3, pp. F169–F174, 2006.

[70] H. Ruis, R. Rolland, W. Doesburg, G. Broeders, and R. Corbey, "Oxytocin enhances onset of lactation among mothers delivering prematurely," *The British Medical Journal*, vol. 283, no. 6287, pp. 340–342, 1981.

[71] J. L. Linzell and M. Peaker, "The effects of oxytocin and milk removal on milk secretion in the goat," *The Journal of Physiology*, vol. 216, no. 3, pp. 717–734, 1971.

[72] F. Ellendorff, M. L. Forsling, and D. A. Poulain, "The milk ejection reflex in the pig," *The Journal of Physiology*, vol. 333, no. 1, pp. 577–594, 1982.

[73] H. F. Schryver, O. T. Oftedal, J. Williams, L. V. Soderholm, and H. F. Hintz, "Lactation in the horse: the mineral composition of mare milk," *Journal of Nutrition*, vol. 116, no. 11, pp. 2142–2147, 1986.

[74] T. D. Etherton and D. E. Bauman, "Biology of somatotropin in growth and lactation of domestic animals," *Physiological Reviews*, vol. 78, no. 3, pp. 745–761, 1998.

[75] I. R. Dohoo, L. DesCôteaux, K. Leslie et al., "A meta-analysis review of the effects of recombinant bovine somatotropin 2. Effects on animal health, reproductive performance, and culling," *Canadian Journal of Veterinary Research*, vol. 67, no. 4, pp. 252–264, 2003.

[76] D. E. Bauman, M. J. de Geeter, C. J. Peel, G. M. Lanza, R. C. Gorewit, and R. W. Hammond, "Effect of recombinantly derived bovine growth hormone (bGH) on lactational performance of high yielding dairy cows," *Journal of Dairy Science*, vol. 65, no. 1, p. 121, 1982.

[77] R. J. Collier, M. A. Miller, C. L. McLaughlin, H. D. Johnson, and C. A. Baile, "Effects of recombinant bovine somatotropin (rbST) and season on plasma and milk insulin-like growth factors I (IGF-I) and II (IGF-II) in lactating dairy cows," *Domestic Animal Endocrinology*, vol. 35, no. 1, pp. 16–23, 2008.

[78] C. F. M. Molento, E. Block, R. I. Cue, and D. Petitclerc, "Effects of insulin, recombinant bovine somatotropin, and their

interaction on insulin-like growth factor-1 secretion and milk protein production in dairy cows," *Journal of Dairy Science*, vol. 85, no. 4, pp. 738–747, 2002.

[79] D. E. Bauman, "Bovine somatotropin and lactation: from basic science to commercial application," *Domestic Animal Endocrinology*, vol. 17, no. 1–3, pp. 101–116, 1999.

[80] M. I. Gallego, N. Binart, G. W. Robinson et al., "Prolactin, growth hormone, and epidermal growth factor activate Stat5 in different compartments of mammary tissue and exert different and overlapping developmental effects," *Developmental Biology*, vol. 229, no. 1, pp. 163–175, 2001.

[81] Y. Cui, G. Riedlinger, K. Miyoshi et al., "Inactivation of stat5 in mouse mammary epithelium during pregnancy reveals distinct functions in cell proliferation, survival, and differentiation," *Molecular and Cellular Biology*, vol. 24, no. 18, pp. 8037–8047, 2004.

[82] X. Liu, G. W. Robinson, K. Wagner, L. Garrett, A. Wynshaw-Boris, and L. Hennighausen, "Stat5a is mandatory for adult mammary gland development and lactogenesis," *Genes and Development*, vol. 11, no. 2, pp. 179–186, 1997.

[83] S. A. Burgos and J. P. Cant, "IGF-1 stimulates protein synthesis by enhanced signaling through mTORC1 in bovine mammary epithelial cells," *Domestic Animal Endocrinology*, vol. 38, no. 4, pp. 211–221, 2010.

[84] A. Wickenden and C. J. Watson, "Key signalling nodes in mammary gland development and cancer. Signalling downstream of PI3 kinase in mammary epithelium: a play in 3 Akts," *Breast Cancer Research*, vol. 12, article 202, 2010.

[85] S. A. Burgos, M. Dai, and J. P. Cant, "Nutrient availability and lactogenic hormones regulate mammary protein synthesis through the mammalian target of rapamycin signaling pathway," *Journal of Dairy Science*, vol. 93, no. 1, pp. 153–161, 2010.

[86] L. Wang, Y. Lin, Y. Bian et al., "Leucyl-tRNA synthetase regulates lactation and cell proliferation via mTOR signaling in dairy cow mammary epithelial cells," *International Journal of Molecular Sciences*, vol. 15, no. 4, pp. 5952–5969, 2014.

[87] X. Cui, P. Zhang, W. Deng et al., "Insulin-like growth factor-I inhibits progesterone receptor expression in breast cancer cells via the phosphatidylinositol 3-kinase/Akt/mammalian target of rapamycin pathway: progesterone receptor as a potential indicator of growth factor activity in breast cancer," *Molecular Endocrinology*, vol. 17, no. 4, pp. 575–588, 2003.

[88] G. Sharif yanov, R. M. Kharrasov, and F. S. Khaziakhmetov, "Goat's rue (Galega officinalis) in rations for cows," *Zootekhniya*, vol. 5, pp. 15–16, 1996.

[89] J. A. McCubrey, L. S. Steelman, W. H. Chappell et al., "Roles of the Raf/MEK/ERK pathway in cell growth, malignant transformation and drug resistance," *Biochimica et Biophysica Acta*, vol. 1773, no. 8, pp. 1263–1284, 2007.

[90] A. Shukla, J. Grisouard, V. Ehemann, A. Hermani, H. Enzmann, and D. Mayer, "Analysis of signaling pathways related to cell proliferation stimulated by insulin analogs in human mammary epithelial cell lines," *Endocrine-Related Cancer*, vol. 16, no. 2, pp. 429–441, 2009.

[91] E. Marshman and C. H. Streuli, "Insulin-like growth factors and insulin-like growth factor binding proteins in mammary gland function," *Breast Cancer Research*, vol. 4, no. 6, pp. 231–239, 2002.

[92] R. M. Akers, "Major advances associated with hormone and growth factor regulation of mammary growth and lactation in dairy cows," *Journal of Dairy Science*, vol. 89, no. 4, pp. 1222–1234, 2006.

[93] P. L. Toutain, D. Schams, M. P. Laurentie, and T. D. Thomson, "Pharmacokinetics of a recombinant bovine growth hormone and pituitary bovine growth hormone in lactating dairy cows," *Journal of Animal Science*, vol. 71, no. 5, pp. 1219–1225, 1993.

[94] A. Azza, A. S. Khalil, H. T. El-Hamamsy, and O. H. Ezzo, "The effect of recombinant bovine somatotropin administration on milk production, some hemato-biochemical parameters and reproductive performance of lactating cows," *Global Veterinaria*, vol. 4, pp. 366–373, 2010.

[95] J. K. Oldenbroek, G. J. Garssen, L. J. Jonker, and J. I. Wilkinson, "Effects of treatment of dairy cows with recombinant bovine somatotropin over three or four lactations," *Journal of Dairy Science*, vol. 76, no. 2, pp. 453–467, 1993.

[96] L. J. Judge, R. J. Erskine, and P. C. Bartlett, "Recombinant bovine somatotropin and clinical mastitis: incidence, discarded milk following therapy, and culling," *Journal of Dairy Science*, vol. 80, no. 12, pp. 3212–3218, 1997.

[97] P. Willeberg, "Bovine somatotropin and clinical mastitis: epidemiological assessment of the welfare risk," *Livestock Production Science*, vol. 36, no. 1, pp. 55–66, 1993.

[98] J. L. Burton, B. W. McBride, B. W. Kennedy, J. H. Burton, T. H. Elsasser, and B. Woodward, "Hematological profiles in dairy cows treated with recombinant bovine somatotropin.," *Journal of Animal Science*, vol. 70, no. 5, pp. 1488–1495, 1992.

[99] G. Briggs, R. K. Freeman, and S. J. Yaffe, *Drugs in Pregnancy and Lactation: A Reference Guide to Fetal and Neonatal Risk with Access Code*, Lippincott Williams and Wilkins, New York, NY, USA, 2002.

[100] O. Ylikorkala, S. Kivinen, and A. Kauppila, "Oral administration of TRH in puerperal women: effect on insufficient lactation, thyroid hormones and on the responses of TSH and prolactin to intravenous TRH," *Acta Endocrinologica*, vol. 93, no. 4, pp. 413–418, 1980.

[101] A. H. Tashjian Jr., N. J. Barowsky, and D. K. Jensen, "Thyrotropin releasing hormone: direct evidence for stimulation of prolactin production by pituitary cells in culture," *Biochemical and Biophysical Research Communications*, vol. 43, no. 3, pp. 516–523, 1971.

[102] M. E. Freeman, B. Kanyicska, A. Lerant, and G. Nagy, "Prolactin: structure, function, and regulation of secretion," *Physiological Reviews*, vol. 80, no. 4, pp. 1523–1631, 2000.

[103] G. P. Mueller, H. J. Chen, and J. Meites, "In vivo stimulation of prolactin release in the rat by synthetic TRH," *Experimental Biology and Medicine*, vol. 144, no. 2, pp. 613–615, 1973.

[104] T. Johke, "Effects of TRH on circulating growth hormone, prolactin and triiodothyronine levels in the bovine," *Endocrinologia Japonica*, vol. 25, no. 1, pp. 19–26, 1978.

[105] S. Zárate, G. Jaita, J. Ferraris et al., "Estrogens induce expression of membrane-associated estrogen receptor α isoforms in lactotropes," *PLoS ONE*, vol. 7, no. 7, Article ID e41299, 2012.

[106] J. E. Tyson, A. Perez, and J. Zanartu, "Human lactational response to oral thyrotropin releasing hormone," *Journal of Clinical Endocrinology and Metabolism*, vol. 43, no. 4, pp. 760–768, 1976.

[107] A. Sengupta and D. K. Sarkar, "Estrogen inhibits D2S receptor-regulated Gi3 and Gs protein interactions to stimulate prolactin production and cell proliferation in lactotropic cells," *Journal of Endocrinology*, vol. 214, no. 1, pp. 67–78, 2012.

[108] F. Peters, J. Schulze-Tollert, and W. Schuth, "Thyrotrophin-releasing hormone—a lactation-promoting agent?" *British Journal of Obstetrics and Gynaecology*, vol. 98, no. 9, pp. 880–885, 1991.

[109] T. W. Redding and A. V. Schally, "On the half life of thyrotropin-releasing hormone in rats," *Neuroendocrinology*, vol. 9, no. 4, pp. 250–256, 1972.

[110] Z. J. Cui, F. S. Gorelick, and P. S. Dannies, "Calcium/calmodulin-dependent protein kinase-II activation in rat pituitary cells in the presence of thyrotropin-releasing hormone and dopamine," *Endocrinology*, vol. 134, no. 5, pp. 2245–2250, 1994.

[111] B. A. White and C. Bancroft, "Ca²⁺/Calmodulin regulation of prolactin gene expression," *Methods in Enzymology*, vol. 139, pp. 655–667, 1987.

[112] A. Lachowicz, F. van Goor, A. C. Katzur, G. Bonhomme, and S. S. Stojilkovic, "Uncoupling of calcium mobilization and entry pathways in endothelin-stimulated pituitary lactotrophs," *The Journal of Biological Chemistry*, vol. 272, no. 45, pp. 28308–28314, 1997.

[113] B. Muller, L. Caccavelli, I. Manfroid et al., "Régulation tran-scriptionnelle du gène de la prolactine humaine," *Medicine Sciences*, vol. 14, no. 5, pp. 580–587, 1998.

[114] J. M. Cline, G. Soderqvist, E. Von Schoultz, L. Skoog, and B. Von Schoultz, "Effects of conjugated estrogens, medroxypro-gesterone acetate, and tamoxifen on the mammary glands of macaques," *Breast Cancer Research and Treatment*, vol. 48, no. 3, pp. 221–229, 1998.

[115] M. Molinolo, S. Simian, S. Vanzulli et al., "Involvement of EGF in medroxyprogesterone acetate [154]-induced mammary gland hyperplasia and its role in MPA-induced mammary tumors in BALB/c mice," *Cancer Letters*, vol. 126, no. 1, pp. 49–57, 1998.

[116] E. Guiloff, A. Ibarra Polo, C. Toscanini, T. W. Mischler, and C. Gómez-Rogers, "Effect of contraception on lactation," *The American Journal of Obstetrics and Gynecology*, vol. 118, no. 1, pp. 42–45, 1974.

[117] P. R. Hannon, A. K. Duggan, J. R. Serwint, J. W. Vogelhut, F. Witter, and C. DeAngelis, "The influence of medroxyproges-terone on the duration of breast-feeding in mothers in an urban community," *Archives of Pediatrics and Adolescent Medicine*, vol. 151, no. 1, pp. 490–496, 1997.

[118] M. Karim, R. Ammar, S. el-Mahgoub, B. el-Ganzoury, F. Fikri, and I. Abdou, "Injected progestogen and lactation," *The British Medical Journal*, vol. 1, no. 742, pp. 200–203, 1971.

[119] E. D. B. Johansson, P. B. Johansen, and S. N. Rasmussen, "Medroxyprogesterone acetate pharmacokinetics following oral high-dose administration in humans: a bioavailability evalua-tion of a new MPA tablet formulation," *Acta Pharmacologica et Toxicologica*, vol. 58, no. 5, pp. 311–317, 1986.

[120] B. N. Saxena, K. Shrimanker, and J. G. Grudzinskas, "Levels of contraceptive steroids in breast milk and plasma of lactating women," *Contraception*, vol. 16, no. 6, pp. 605–613, 1977.

[121] J. J. Kelsey, "Hormonal contraception and lactation," *Journal of Human Lactation*, vol. 12, no. 4, pp. 315–318, 1996.

[122] R. R. Chaudhury, S. Chompootaweep, N. Dusitsin, H. Friesen, and M. Tankeyoon, "The release of prolactin by medroxy progesterone acetate in human subjects," *British Journal of Pharmacology*, vol. 59, no. 3, pp. 433–434, 1977.

[123] K. Abascal and E. Yarnell, "Botanical galactagogues," *Alternative and Complementary Therapies*, vol. 14, no. 6, pp. 288–294, 2008.

[124] J. Latvietis, J. Drikis, V. Auzins, A. Trupa, and H. Kaldmae, "Some types of grass silage used in feeding cows," in *Proceedings of the Animal Nutritions Conference*, pp. 7–15, Tartu, Estonia, 2002.

[125] V. I. Brikman, M. I. Lopatko, Z. M. Arkhipova, and N. I. Roi, "Intake of some plants by cow," *Zootekhniya*, vol. 5-6, pp. 14–15, 1992.

[126] M. Alamer, "Effect of feeding fennel straw (*Foeniculum vulgare* Mill) on performance of lactating goats," *Journal of Applied Animal Research*, vol. 36, no. 1, pp. 61–64, 2009.

[127] M. Kholif and M. A. M. Abd El-Gawad, "Medical plant seeds supplementation of lactating goats diets and its effects on milk and cheese quantity and quality," *Egyptian Journal of Dairy Science*, vol. 29, pp. 139–150, 2001.

[128] M. A. Alamer and G. Basiouni, "Feeding effects of fenugreek seeds (*Trigonella foenum-graecum* L) on lactation performance, some plasma constituents and growth hormone level in goats," *Pakistan Journal of Biological Science*, vol. 25, no. 11, pp. 28–46, 2005.

[129] Z. G. Bikbulatov, F. A. Zainutdinov, and B. G. Sharifyanov, " Feeds from goats rue in diets for cows," *Kormoporizvodstvo*, vol. 7, pp. 28–31, 1997.

[130] A. El-Alamy, H. M. Khattab, S. A. El-Nor, F. A. F. Salam, and M. M. A. Abdou, "Milk production response to supplementing rations with some medical herbs of lactating buffaloes," in *Proceedings of the 8th Egyptian Conference for Dairy Science and Technology*, pp. 675–686, Cairo, Egypt, November 2001.

[131] K. S. Tomar, V. P. Singh, and R. S. Yadav, "Effect of feeding maithy (*Trigonella foenum-graecum*) and chandrasoor (*Lepid-ium sativum* L.) seeds on milk and blood constituents of Murrah buffaloes," *Indian Journal of Animal Sciences*, vol. 66, no. 11, pp. 1192–1193, 1996.

[132] S. A. H. Abo El-Nor, "Influence of fenugreek seeds as a galactagogue on milk yield, milk composition and different blood biochemical of lactating buffaloes during mid-lactation," *Egyptian Journal of Dairy Science*, vol. 27, no. 1, pp. 231–238, 1999.

[133] K. A. E. Mullen, K. L. Anderson, and S. P. Washburn, "Affil-iations, Effect of 2 herbal intramammary products on milk quantity and quality compared with conventional and no dry cow therapy," *Journal of Dairy Science*, vol. 97, no. 6, pp. 3509–3522, 2014.

[134] M. W. Arbour and J. L. Kessler, "Mammary hypoplasia: not every breast can produce sufficient milk," *Journal of Midwifery and Women's Health*, vol. 58, no. 4, pp. 457–461, 2013.

[135] H. Greathead, "Plants and plant extracts for improving animal productivity," *Proceedings of the Nutrition Society*, vol. 62, no. 2, pp. 279–290, 2003.

[136] B. T. Schaneberg and I. A. Khan, "Analysis of products sus-pected of containing *Aristolochia* or *Asarum* species," *Journal of Ethnopharmacology*, vol. 94, no. 2-3, pp. 245–249, 2004.

[137] A. B. Forinash, A. M. Yancey, K. N. Barnes, and T. D. Myles, "The use of galactogogues in the breastfeeding mother," *Annals of Pharmacotherapy*, vol. 46, no. 10, pp. 1392–1404, 2012.

[138] T. Gbadamosi and O. Okolosi, "Botanical galactogogues: nutri-tional values and therapeutic potentials," *Journal of Applied Biosciences*, vol. 61, no. 1, pp. 4460–4469, 2013.

[139] C. Turkyilmaz, E. Onal, I. M. Hirfanoglu et al., "The effect of galactagogue herbal tea on breast milk production and short-term catch-up of birth weight in the first week of life," *The Journal of Alternative and Complementary Medicine*, vol. 17, no. 2, pp. 139–142, 2011.

[140] M. Foidart, C. Colin, X. Denoo et al., "Estradiol and pro-gesterone regulate the proliferation of human breast epithelial cells," *Fertility and Sterility*, vol. 69, no. 5, pp. 963–970, 1998.

[141] C. Farmer, M. F. Palin, G. S. Gilani et al., "Dietary genistein stimulates mammary hyperplasia in gilts," *Animal*, vol. 4, no. 3, pp. 454–465, 2010.

[142] J. Dong, C. H. Tsai-Morris, and M. L. Dufau, "A novel estradiol/estrogen receptor α-dependent transcriptional mechanism controls expression of the human prolactin receptor," *The Journal of Biological Chemistry*, vol. 281, no. 27, pp. 18825–18836, 2006.

[143] R. J. Vanderboom and L. G. Sheffield, "Estrogen enhances epidermal growth factor-induced DNA synthesis in mammary epithelial cells," *Journal of Cellular Physiology*, vol. 156, no. 2, pp. 367–372, 1993.

[144] F. Borellini and T. Oka, "Growth control and differentiation in mammary epithelial cells," *Environmental Health Perspectives*, vol. 80, no. 1, pp. 85–99, 1989.

[145] R. A. Maurer, "Estradiol regulates the transcription of the prolactin gene," *The Journal of Biological Chemistry*, vol. 257, no. 5, pp. 2133–2136, 1982.

[146] G. Benker, C. Jaspers, G. Häusler, and D. Reinwein, "Control of prolactin secretion," *Wiener klinische Wochenschrift*, vol. 68, no. 23, pp. 1157–1167, 1990.

[147] U. C. Yadav and N. Z. Baquer, "Pharmacological effects of *Trigonella foenum-graecum* L. in health and disease," *Pharmaceutical Biology*, vol. 52, no. 2, pp. 243–254, 2013.

[148] S. Sreeja and V. S. Anju, "*In vitro* estrogenic activities of fenugreek *Trigonella foenum graecum* seeds," *Indian Journal of Medical Research*, vol. 131, no. 1, pp. 814–819, 2010.

[149] A. K. Janabi, "Feeding effects of fenugreek seeds (*Tringonella foenum-graceum*) on lactation performance, some serum constituents and prolactin hormone level in damascus crossbred goats," *Diyala Agricultural Sciences Journal*, vol. 4, no. 1, pp. 1–8, 2012.

[150] M. A. Rather, B. A. Dar, S. N. Sofi, B. A. Bhat, and M. A. Qurishi, "*Foeniculum vulgare*: a comprehensive review of its traditional use, phytochemistry, pharmacology, and safety," *Arabian Journal of Chemistry*, 2012.

[151] S. Mills and K. Bone, *Principles and Practice of Phytotherapy: Modern Herbal Medicine*, Churchill Livingstone, Edinburgh, UK, 2000.

[152] A. H. Shah, S. Qureshi, and A. M. Ageel, "Toxicity studies in mice of ethanol extracts of *Foeniculum vulgare* fruit and *Ruta chalepensis* aerial parts," *Journal of Ethnopharmacology*, vol. 34, no. 2-3, pp. 167–172, 1991.

[153] M. Albert-Puleo, "Fennel and anise as estrogenic agents," *Journal of Ethnopharmacology*, vol. 2, no. 4, pp. 337–344, 1980.

[154] L. Gori, E. Gallo, V. Mascherini, A. Mugelli, A. Vannacci, and F. Firenzuoli, "Can estragole in fennel seed decoctions really be considered a danger for human health? A fennel safety update," *Evidence-based Complementary and Alternative Medicine*, vol. 2012, Article ID 860542, 10 pages, 2012.

[155] M. M. Özcan and J. C. Chalchat, "Chemical composition and antifungal effect of anise (*Pimpinella anisum* L.) fruit oil at ripening stage," *Annals of Microbiology*, vol. 56, no. 4, pp. 353–358, 2006.

[156] H. Hosseinzadeh, M. Tafaghodi, S. Abedzadeh, and E. Taghiabadi, "Effect of aqueous and ethanolic extracts of *Pimpinella anisum* L. seeds on milk production in rats," *Journal of Acupuncture and Meridian Studies*, vol. 6, no. 1, pp. 18–23, 2013.

[157] V. Kudrna, J. Rendla, and E. Markalous, "Stimulation of milk production by feeding with *Galega officinalis*," *Fytotechnicka Rada*, vol. 9, no. 1, article 254, 1992.

[158] F. González-Andrés, P. A. Redondo, R. Pescador, and B. Urbano, "Management of *Galega officinalis* L. and preliminary results on its potential for milk production improvement in sheep," *New Zealand Journal of Agricultural Research*, vol. 47, no. 2, pp. 233–245, 2004.

[159] K. Parton and A. N. Bruere, "Plant poisoning of livestock in New Zealand," *New Zealand Veterinary Journal*, vol. 50, no. 3, pp. 22–27, 2002.

[160] M. H. Benn, G. Shustov, L. Shustova, W. Majak, Y. Bai, and N. A. Fairey, "Isolation and characterization of two guanidines from *Galega orientis* Lam. Cv. Gale (Fodder Galega)," *Journal of Agricultural and Food Chemistry*, vol. 44, no. 9, pp. 2779–2781, 1996.

[161] R. F. Keeler, D. C. Baker, and J. O. Evans, "Individual animal susceptibility and its relationship to induced adaptation or tolerance in sheep to *Galega officinalis* L," *Veterinary and Human Toxicology*, vol. 30, no. 5, pp. 420–423, 1988.

[162] Y. Champavier, D. P. Allais, A. J. Chulia, and M. Kaouadji, "Acetylated and non-acetylated flavonol triglycosides from *Galega officinalis*," *Chemical and Pharmaceutical Bulletin*, vol. 48, no. 2, pp. 281–282, 2000.

[163] K. Sharma and M. Bhatnagar, "*Asparagus racemosus* (Shatavari): a versatile female tonic," *International Journal of Pharmaceutical and Biological Archive*, vol. 2, no. 3, pp. 855–863, 2011.

[164] F. di Pierro, A. Callegari, D. Carotenuto, and M. M. Tapia, "Clinical efficacy, safety and tolerability of BIO-C (micronized Silymarin) as a galactagogue," *Acta Biomedica de l'Ateneo Parmense*, vol. 79, no. 3, pp. 205–210, 2008.

[165] R. K. Goyal, J. Singh, and H. Lal, "*Asparagus racemosus*—an update," *Indian Journal of Medical Sciences*, vol. 57, no. 9, pp. 408–414, 2003.

[166] M. Gupta and B. Shaw, "A double-blind randomized clinical trial for evaluation of galactogogue activity of asparagus racemosus willd," *Iranian Journal of Pharmaceutical Research*, vol. 10, no. 1, pp. 167–172, 2011.

[167] S. K. Pandey, A. Sahay, R. S. Pandey, and Y. B. Tripathi, "Effect of *Asparagus racemosus* rhizome (Shatavari) on mammary gland and genital organs of pregnant rat," *Phytotherapy Research*, vol. 19, no. 8, pp. 721–724, 2005.

[168] P. B. Sabnis, B. B. Gaitonde, and M. Jetmalani, "Effects of alcoholic extracts of *Asparagus racemosus* on mammary glands of rats," *Indian Journal of Experimental Biology*, vol. 6, no. 1, pp. 55–57, 1968.

[169] K. A. Narendranath, S. Anuradha, and I. S. Rao, "Effect of herbal galactogogue (lactare). A pharmacological and clinical observation," *Medicine and Surgery*, vol. 26, no. 4, pp. 19–22, 1986.

[170] A. B. Patel and U. K. Kanitkar, "*Asparagus racemosus* willd—form bordi, as a galactogogue, in buffaloes," *Indian Veterinary Journal*, vol. 46, no. 8, pp. 718–721, 1969.

[171] R. K. Goel, T. Prabha, M. Mohan Kumar, M. Dorababu, and G. Singh, "Teratogenicity of *Asparagus racemosus* willd. root, a herbal medicine," *Indian Journal of Experimental Biology*, vol. 44, no. 7, pp. 570–573, 2006.

[172] G. Saxena, M. Singh, and M. Bhatnagar, "Phytoestrogens of *Asparagus racemosus* wild," *Journal of Herbal Medicine and Toxicology*, vol. 4, no. 1, pp. 15–20, 2010.

[173] V. Kren and D. Walterová, "Silybin and silymarin: new effects and applications," *Biomedical Papers*, vol. 149, no. 1, pp. 29–41, 2005.

[174] V. Kummer, J. Mašková, J. Čanderle, Z. Zralý, J. Neča, and M. Machala, "Estrogenic effects of silymarin in ovariectomized rats," *Veterinarni Medicina*, vol. 46, no. 1, pp. 17–23, 2001.

[175] D. Seidlová-Wuttke, T. Becker, V. Christoffel, H. Jarry, and W. Wuttke, "Silymarin is a selective estrogen receptor β (ERβ) agonist and has estrogenic effects in the metaphysis of the femur but no or antiestrogenic effects in the uterus of ovariectomized (ovx) rats," *The Journal of Steroid Biochemistry and Molecular Biology*, vol. 86, no. 2, pp. 179–188, 2003.

[176] D. Tedesco, A. Tava, S. Galletti et al., "Effects of silymarin, a natural hepatoprotector, in periparturient dairy cows," *Journal of Dairy Science*, vol. 87, no. 7, pp. 2239–2247, 2004.

[177] R. Capasso, G. Aviello, F. Capasso et al., "Silymarin BIO-C, an extract from *Silybum marianum* fruits, induces hyperprolactinemia in intact female rats," *Phytomedicine*, vol. 16, no. 9, pp. 839–844, 2009.

28

Prevalence and Risk Factors Associated with Faecal Shedding of *Cryptosporidium* Oocysts in Dogs in the Federal Capital Territory, Abuja, Nigeria

Gbemisola Magaret Olabanji, Beatty Viv Maikai, and Gbeminiyi Richard Otolorin

Department of Veterinary Public Health and Preventive Medicine, Faculty of Veterinary Medicine, Ahmadu Bello University, Zaria, Kaduna State, Nigeria

Correspondence should be addressed to Gbemisola Magaret Olabanji; golabanji@yahoo.com

Academic Editor: Cynthia C. Powell

Cryptosporidium is one of the causes of diarrhoeal illness in man and animals worldwide. The aim of the study was to determine the prevalence and risk factors associated with faecal shedding of *Cryptosporidium* oocysts in dogs in FCT Abuja, Nigeria. A total of 276 dog faecal samples were examined using Modified Acid Fast (MAF) technique and Enzyme Linked Immunosorbent Assay (ELISA). Fifteen (5.4%) and 51 (18.5%) out of the 276 dog faecal samples examined were positive for *Cryptosporidium* oocysts and coproantigens, respectively. There was a fair agreement (0.371) between the two tests used in this study. The prevalence of *Cryptosporidium* infection was highest in 4 dogs (21.0%) between 3 and 9 months of age. Ten diarrhoeic dogs (30.3%) and 31 dogs from rural settlements were more infected (22.46%) with *Cryptosporidium* oocysts. There was statistical association between prevalence of *Cryptosporidium* and confinement of dogs (OR = 0.41; 95% CI on OR: 0.21 < OR < 0.80). However, there was no statistical association ($P > 0.05$) between prevalence of *Cryptosporidium* and age, diarrhoeic status of the dogs, sex, breed, and location. A total of 62.7% respondents did not have prior knowledge about dogs harbouring organisms that can infect humans. The finding of this research is of public health significance.

1. Introduction

Cryptosporidium is an obligate intracellular, protozoan parasite of great public health significance that causes cryptosporidiosis in animals and humans [1]. Due to unrestricted movement of dogs across major cities across the nations, dogs are exposed to both the endemic and nonendemic intestinal protozoan infections in Nigeria [2]. It has been suggested for some time that dogs can be a significant source of human cryptosporidiosis [3]. *Cryptosporidium parvum* and *Cryptosporidium hominis* are the two most common species found in humans and account for more than 90% of humans cases in the world. Other species and genotypes of *Cryptosporidium* have occasionally been recorded in humans including *Cryptosporidium canis* [4, 5]. It is speculated that humans may acquire infection from naturally infected dogs [6]. Zoonotic transmission from a dog was suspected in one case when a veterinary student working in a ward where an infected dog was being cared for developed acute self-limiting diarrhoea and *Cryptosporidium* oocysts were identified in her feces [6].

Dogs can be naturally infected with *Cryptosporidium canis*, *Cryptosporidium parvum*, and *Cryptosporidium meleagridis* [7, 8]. *Cryptosporidium canis* is reported to be the most frequently identified species of *Cryptosporidium* in dogs. In addition, small numbers of zoonotic *C. parvum*, *C. muris*, and *C. meleagridis* have also been detected in dogs. *Cryptosporidium canis* infections in dogs are usually asymptomatic but may cause severe diarrhoea, malabsorption, and weight loss [9]. Recent molecular study indicates that dogs may transmit the cattle genotype, which is known to be pathogenic to humans [10]. Dogs are the most commonly domesticated pet animals primarily used for security purposes in Nigeria, making their population density high in major cities including Abuja; however there is no readily available data on canine cryptosporidiosis as an emerging zoonoses in Abuja, on the potential hazard these oocysts from dogs poses to public health in Abuja, Nigeria, and in general, therefore making it necessary to investigate the prevalence of canine cryptosporidiosis and also understand the risk factors that lead to the transmission and possible spread of infection in animals in Abuja, Nigeria.

2. Materials and Methods

2.1. Study Area and Study Design. The Federal Capital Territory is the home of Abuja, the capital of Nigeria. A cross-sectional study was used. Three (3) area councils in Abuja were selected using convenience sampling method. One area council, namely, Abuja municipal, was selected as a representative of major urban settlement with the highest population of dogs in the territory, while the remaining two were Abaji and Kwali, both representing the rural setting in the territory.

2.2. Sample Collection. A total of 276 faecal samples were collected. 138 faecal samples were collected from Abuja municipal area council (23 samples each from Central area, Garki, Wuse, Maitama, Asokoro, and Gwarimpa districts) while 69 faecal samples each were collected from Abaji (23 samples each from Abaji, Toto, Nasarawa, and Kotokarfe) and Kwali (23 samples each from Kwali, Lambata, and Kwaita towns) area councils, respectively. Convenience sampling technique was used to select houses in districts and wards of each area council for the selection of individual dog-owning households in the study areas. Sampling was done between July and September 2014. Faecal sample was collected from the rectum of each animal by means of a disposable plastic bag and emptied into a wide-mouthed disposable plastic container [11]. Faecal samples collected were stored in 10% formalin prior to transportation to the Parasitic Zoonoses Laboratory of the Department of Veterinary Public Health and Preventive Medicine, Ahmadu Bello University, Zaria, for processing.

2.3. Administration of Questionnaires. Prior to sample collection, structured questionnaires were used to obtain information for each dog from which faecal sample was collected and also to obtain information that may help identify risk factors for the faecal shedding of *Cryptosporidium* in dogs. The questionnaire consisted of two sections: *Section A* contained biodata of respondents and questions relating to transmission of the disease; *Section B* contained questions on age, sex, breed, confinement of dogs, source of drinking water, and presence of diarrhoea or loose faeces.

2.4. Sample Processing and Laboratory Procedure Using Modified Acid Fast Technique and ELISA. The faecal samples were treated using formol-ether concentration method and stained using Modified Acid Fast (MAF) [12]. Each faecal sample collected was correspondingly examined for the presence of *Cryptosporidium* spp. antigens by ELISA using a commercial kit (*Copro*ELISA for detection of *Cryptosporidium* antigen in faeces, Savyon Diagnostics Limited, Israel). Samples with optical density (OD) higher than 0.5 were reported as positive

TABLE 1: Level of agreement between MAF and ELISA using Kappa's Statistic.

Type of test	Number positive	Specific rate (%)	κ-value
Modified Acid Fast[Ref]	15	5.4	
ELISA	51	18.5	0.371

Note: κ-value means Kappa value.
Kappa value within the range 0.21–0.40 indicates a fair agreement between the outcome of the two tests.
Note: Ref refers to reference category.

while those with OD less than 0.5 were reported as negative for *Cryptosporidium* coproantigens.

2.5. Data Analysis. The results obtained were presented using tables and charts (descriptive statistics). Using the Statistical Package for Social Science (SPSS) version 17.0 (SPSS Inc., Chicago, IL, USA), Chi-square and Fisher's exact tests were used to check for association between *Cryptosporidium* and factors studied. Odds ratio (OR) and 95% confidence intervals were calculated for dichotomous variables using EP1 INFO version 3.1. OR values greater than unity denote association and less than unity denote that the factor may have a protective effect. Values of $P < 0.05$ were considered statistically significant.

3. Results and Discussion

Out of the 276 dog faecal samples examined using Modified Acid Fast (MAF) staining, 15 (5.4%) samples were positive for *Cryptosporidium* oocysts, while 51 (18.5%) dog faecal samples were positive for *Cryptosporidium* coproantigens using Enzyme Linked Immunosorbent Assay (ELISA). The infection rates from this study were higher than that reported by Adejimi and Osayomi [2]. From this study it was observed that ELISA test was more sensitive than MAF. There was a fair agreement (κ-value: 0.371) between the two tests used in this research (Table 1), indicating a fair outcome between both tests because of the varied number of positives obtained between the two tests.

The presence of *Cryptosporidium* in household dogs may cause cryptosporidiosis in humans due to zoonotic transmission of the infection through close contact with dogs and other domestic animals [13–15]. Abuja is an urban area where dogs are freely kept by most households, usually for security purposes and as pets. Humans have close interactions with companion animals, sharing their living space, and consequently are exposed to microorganisms/parasites that may cause diseases [16]. *Cryptosporidium* spp. isolated in dogs have been found to infect healthy children and adults [4, 17]; hence its control in dogs and other domestic animals is very important.

Infection rates in dogs sampled were higher in dogs between 3 and 9 months of age (Table 2). This result is in contrast to other works where *Cryptosporidium* infection was highest in younger dogs [16, 18, 19]. The high proportion of *Cryptosporidium* infection in older dogs was probably due to the use of older dogs for security purposes thereby increasing

TABLE 2: Effect of age on the prevalence of *Cryptosporidium* infection in dogs using ELISA and MAF techniques in the FCT, Abuja.

Age group (months)	Number of dogs examined	Number positive (%)		Chi-square χ^2	P value & df
		*MAF	**ELISA		
<3	77	2 (2.60)	13 (16.88)	*2.010	0.366; 2
>3–9	100	9 (9.00)	21 (21.00)		
>9	99	4 (4.04)	17 (17.17)	**0.664	0.717; 2

*Chi-square χ^2 in reference to MAF.
**Chi-square χ^2 in reference to ELISA.

TABLE 3: Odds ratio and 95% confidence interval on effect of diarrhoea on the prevalence of *Cryptosporidium* infection in dogs using MAF and ELISA in the FCT, Abuja.

Diarrhoea	Number examined	Number positive	Specific rate (%)	Odds ratio (OR)	95% confidence interval on OR
MAF					
Present[Ref]	33	8	24.24	1.00	
Absent	243	7	2.88	10.79	3.21–36.74
ELISA					
Present[Ref]	33	10	30.30	1.00	
Absent	243	41	16.87	2.14	0.88–5.16

Note: Ref refers to reference category.

TABLE 4: Odds ratio and 95% confidence interval on effect of sex on the prevalence of *Cryptosporidium* infection in dogs using MAF and ELISA in the FCT, Abuja.

Sex	Number examined	Number positive	Specific rate (%)	Odds ratio (OR)	95% confidence interval on OR
MAF					
Male[Ref]	181	12	6.63	1.00	
Female	95	3	3.16	2.18	0.55–9.99
ELISA					
Male[Ref]	181	32	17.68	1.00	
Female	95	19	20.00	0.86	0.44–1.69

Note: Ref refers to reference category.

their tendency to move around more often and possibly getting infected with the *Cryptosporidium* oocysts.

Prevalence of *Cryptosporidium* infection was highest in 8 (24.24%) and 10 (30.30%) dogs with diarrhoea with the use of MAF and ELISA, respectively, as compared to 7 (2.88%) and 41 (16.87%) in the corresponding dogs without diarrhoea. There was statistical significance ($P < 0.05$) between prevalence of *Cryptosporidium* in the MAF (OR = 10.79; 95% CI on OR: 3.21 < OR < 36.74) (Table 3). The higher rate of infection in diarrhoeic dogs may probably be because some of the dogs tested were already manifesting the disease undetected as one of the clinical signs of cryptosporidiosis is diarrhoea [20]; various authors have reported higher rates of infection in dogs, humans, and other domestic animals with diarrhoea [13, 14, 21].

Prevalence of *Cryptosporidium* infection was more in females (20.0%) than males (17.68%) in samples examined using ELISA. There was no statistical significance between prevalence of *Cryptosporidium* in both the MAF (OR = 2.18; 95% CI on OR: 0.55 < OR < 9.99) and ELISA (OR = 0.86; 95% CI on OR: 0.44 < OR < 1.69) (Table 4). The higher rate of infection in females than in male dogs, examined with the use of ELISA, may be probably due to a reduced immunity at

certain periods in females physiologic cycle. A similar study conducted in China and Brazil reported similar findings [22].

Prevalence of *Cryptosporidium* infection was more in crossbreed of dogs (19.23%) compared to exotic and local breed of dogs in samples examined using ELISA. There was no statistical significant association between prevalence of *Cryptosporidium* in both the MAF (χ^2 = 0.379, df = 2, and P value = 0.827) and ELISA (χ^2 = 0.052, df = 2, and P value = 0.974) with the breed of the dog sampled (Table 5). This is in contrast with results gotten by Adejimi and Osayomi [2] who reported a higher prevalence of *Cryptosporidium* infection in local breed of dogs. Prevalence of *Cryptosporidium* infection was highest in 10 (7.25%) and 31 (22.46%) dogs in the rural area councils with the use of MAF and ELISA, respectively, as compared to 5 (3.62%) and 20 (14.49%) in the corresponding dogs in the urban area council. The high prevalence in household dogs from rural part of the study area is in agreement with work done by Adriana et al. [23]. This high prevalence can be correlated with the dogs living close to other domestic animals as cattle and sheep that may be infected and shedding the *Cryptosporidium* oocyst and also dogs in this area are prone to roam about and may easily be infected.

TABLE 5: Effect of breed and location on the prevalence of *Cryptosporidium* infection in dogs using ELISA and MAF in the FCT, Abuja.

Variable	Number of dogs examined: $n = 276$	Number positive (%)		Chi-square χ^2	P value & df
		*MAF	**ELISA		
Breed					
Exotic	150	9 (6.00)	27 (18.00)	*0.379	0.827; 2
Local	74	3 (4.05)	14 (18.92)		
Cross	52	3 (5.77)	10 (19.23)	**0.052	0.974; 2
Location					
Urban	138	5 (3.62)	20 (14.49)	*1.762	0.144; 1
Rural	138	10 (7.25)	31 (22.46)	**2.910	0.060; 1

*Chi-square χ^2 in reference to MAF.
**Chi-square χ^2 in reference to ELISA.

TABLE 6: Odds ratio and 95% confidence interval on effect of confinement on the prevalence of *Cryptosporidium* infection in dogs using MAF and ELISA in the FCT, Abuja.

Confinement	Number examined	Number positive	Specific rate (%)	Odds ratio (OR)	95% confidence interval on OR
MAF					
Yes[Ref]	201	8	3.98	1.00	
No	75	7	9.33	0.40	0.13–1.29
ELISA					
Yes[Ref]	201	29	14.42	1.00	
No	75	22	29.33	0.41	0.21–0.80

Note: Ref refers to reference category.

TABLE 7: Factors associated with the prevalence of *Cryptosporidium* infection in dogs within sampled households in the FCT, Abuja.

Variable	Frequency (%)	Number of ELISA positive samples (%)	Chi-square χ^2	P value & df
Close contact to dogs				
Yes	162 (58.7)	23		
No	114 (41.3)	28	4.771	0.029; 1
Knowledge about dogs harbouring organisms that can infect humans				
Yes	103 (37.3)	15		
No	173 (62.7)	36	1.672	0.196; 1
Housing of dogs within premises				
Specially constructed house/cage	181 (65.6)	32		
In-house passage way	48 (17.4)	7		
Anywhere in the premises	47 (17.0)	12	2.112	0.348; 2
Total	276			

Prevalence of *Cryptosporidium* infection was highest in 7 (9.33%) and 22 (29.33%) dogs that were not confined with the use of MAF and ELISA, respectively, as compared to 8 (3.98%) and 29 (14.42%) in the corresponding dogs that were confined. There was statistically significant association between the prevalence of *Cryptosporidium* in both the MAF (OR = 0.40; 95% CI on OR: 0.13 < OR < 1.29) and ELISA (OR = 0.41; 95% CI on OR: 0.21 < OR < 0.08) with dog confinement (Table 6). Dogs that were allowed to roam the neighbourhood by their owners had the highest rate of infection, as they are prone to exposure to *Cryptosporidium* oocysts as they move within the neighbourhood interacting with other animals and

infectious material. Free-roaming dogs in urban areas constitute nuisance and promote indiscriminate shedding of parasitic organism in the environment and are an important public health issue; studies performed worldwide have demonstrated the presence of parasitic elements within samples of canine faecal material collected from public urban areas [24].

About 58.7% of the respondents said that they and other members of their households have close contact with the dogs in their premises. There was statistically significant association between prevalence of *Cryptosporidium* (χ^2 = 4.771, df = 1, and P value = 0.029) and humans contact with dogs (Table 7). A total of 62.7% respondents did not have knowledge about dogs harbouring organisms that can infect humans and there was no statistically significant association between prevalence of *Cryptosporidium* ($\chi^2 = 1.672$, df = 1, and *P* value = 0.196) and humans knowledge about dogs harbouring potentially harmful organisms to them. About 65.6% of the dogs were housed in specially constructed houses/cages while 17.4% and 17% of dogs in these households were housed on households' passage way and anywhere in the households, respectively. Individuals having close contact with pet animals have been shown to be a source of transmission of zoonotic infection between humans and animals, especially when humans are exposed to discharges and faeces of these animals [15]. Also most of the respondents did not have knowledge about dogs harbouring organisms that can infect humans and this poor knowledge recorded by the respondents may increase their exposure and interfere with the control of *Cryptosporidium* infection in the dogs in the study area.

4. Conclusion

This research was able to establish a higher sensitivity and specificity rate for ELISA in routine diagnosis of *Cryptosporidium* in dogs in comparison to MAF. The presence of *Cryptosporidium* infection in household dogs in the study area is of public health concern as infected dogs can serve as vehicle of transmission of the infection to humans. There was a fair agreement between the two tests used in this study. There was no statistical association between the prevalence of *Cryptosporidium* infection and age, sex, and breed in dogs sampled within the study area. Rate of infection was higher in diarrhoeic dogs and free-roaming dogs. A significant number of respondents in the households surveyed were unaware that dogs can shed organisms in their faeces that can be harmful to their health. Hence it is important that adequate public health programme is organized to educate dog owners about adequate protective measures to take to protect themselves. However the study has shown that associated risk factors such as dog confinement and their contact with man are of great significance.

Conflict of Interests

The authors declare that there is no conflict of interests regarding the publication of this paper.

References

[1] M. Mirzaei, "Epidemiological survey of *Cryptosporidium* spp. in companion and stray dogs in Kerman, Iran," *Veterinaria Italiana*, vol. 48, no. 3, pp. 291–296, 2012.

[2] J. O. Adejimi and J. O. Osayomi, "Prevalence of intestinal protozoan parasites of dogs in Ibadan, south western Nigeria," *Journal of Animal & Plant Sciences*, vol. 7, no. 2, pp. 783–788, 2010.

[3] L. Xiao and Y. Feng, "Zoonotic cryptosporidiosis," *FEMS Immunology & Medical Microbiology*, vol. 52, no. 3, pp. 309–323, 2008.

[4] L. Xiao, C. Bern, J. Limor et al., "Identification of 5 types of *Cryptosporidium* parasites in children in Lima, Peru," *Journal of Infectious Diseases*, vol. 183, no. 3, pp. 492–497, 2001.

[5] V. A. Cama, C. Bern, I. M. Sulaiman et al., "*Cryptosporidium* species andgenotypes in HIV-positive patients in Lima Peru," *Journal of Eukaryotic Microbiology*, vol. 50, pp. 531–533, 2003.

[6] C. E. Greene, G. J. Jacobs, and D. Prickett, "Intestinal malabsorption and cryptosporidiosis in an adult dog," *Journal of the American Veterinary Medical Association*, vol. 197, no. 3, pp. 365–367, 1990.

[7] R. Fayer, J. M. Trout, L. Xiao, U. M. Morgant, A. A. Lal, and J. P. Dubey, "*Cryptosporidium canis* n. sp. from domestic dogs," *Journal of Parasitology*, vol. 87, no. 6, pp. 1415–1422, 2001.

[8] O. Hajdušek, O. Ditrich, and J. Šlapeta, "Molecular identification of *Cryptosporidium* spp. in animal and human hosts from the Czech Republic," *Veterinary Parasitology*, vol. 122, no. 3, pp. 183–192, 2004.

[9] P. J. Irwin, "Companion animal parasitology: a clinical perspective," *International Journal for Parasitology*, vol. 32, no. 5, pp. 581–593, 2002.

[10] N. Abe, I. Kimata, and M. Iseki, "Identification of genotypes of *Cryptosporidium parvum* isolates from a patient and a dog in Japan," *Journal of Veterinary Medical Science*, vol. 64, no. 2, pp. 165–168, 2002.

[11] S. Jongwutiwes, R. Tiangtip, S. Yentakarm, and N. Chantachum, "Simple method for long-term copro-preservation of *Cryptosporidium oocysts* for morphometric and molecular analysis," *Tropical Medicine and International Health*, vol. 7, no. 3, pp. 257–264, 2002.

[12] WHO, *Basic Laboratory Methods in Medical Parasitology*, World Health Organization, Geneva, Switzerland, 1991.

[13] H. O. Tariuwa, I. Ajogi, C. L. Ejembi et al., "Incidence of *Cryptosporidium* infection in port-harcourt rivers state Nigeria based on regular contact with domestic animals," *Nigerian Veterinary Journal*, vol. 28, no. 3, 2007.

[14] B. V. Makai, J. U. Umoh, J. K. P. Kwaga, V. Maikai, and S. C. Egege, "Prevalence and risk factors associated with faecal sheding of *Cryptosporidium oocysts* in piglets, Kaduna state, Nigeria," *Journal of Parasitology and Vector Biology*, vol. 1, no. 1, pp. 001–004, 2009.

[15] F. Jian, M. Qi, X. He et al., "Occurrence and molecular characterization of *Cryptosporidium* in dogs in Henan Province, China," *BMC Veterinary Research*, vol. 10, article 26, 2014.

[16] N. E. Ramirez, L. A. Ward, and S. Sreevatsan, "A review of the biology and epidemiology of cryptosporidiosis in humans and animals," *Microbes and Infection*, vol. 6, no. 8, pp. 773–785, 2004.

[17] S. Pedraza-Diaz, C. Amar, A. M. Iversen, P. J. Stanley, and J. McLauchlin, "Unusual *Cryptosporidium* species recovered from human faeces: first description of *Cryptosporidium felis* and *Cryptosporidium* 'dog type' from patients in England," *Journal of Medical Microbiology*, vol. 50, no. 3, pp. 293–296, 2001.

[18] I. S. Hamnes, B. K. Gjerde, and L. J. Robertson, "A longitudinal study on the occurrence of *Cryptosporidium* and *Giardia* in dogs during their first year of life," *Acta Veterinaria Scandinavica*, vol. 49, no. 1, article 22, 2007.

[19] A. Titilincu, V. Mircean, D. Achelariei, and V. Cozma, "Prevalence of *Cryptosporidium* spp. in asymptomatic dogs by ELISA and risk factors associated with infection," *Lucrări Stiinţifice Medicină Veterinară*, vol. 43, no. 1, 2010.

[20] R. C. Thompson, A. Armson, and U. M. Ryan, *Cryptosporidium: From Molecules to Disease*, Elsevier, 2003.

[21] A. O. Akinkuotu, B. O. Fagbemi, E. B. Otesile, M. A. Dipeolu, and A. B. Ayinmode, "*Cryptosporidium* infection in cattle in Ogun state, Nigeria," *Sokoto Journal of Veterinary Sciences*, vol. 12, article 2, 2014.

[22] J. Wang, P. Li, X. Xue et al., "Investigation on the infection situation of *Cryptosporidium* in dogs in hefei city," *Chinese Journal of Veterinary Parasitology*, vol. 16, no. 5, pp. 20–23, 2008 (Chinese).

[23] T. Adriana, M. Viorica, D. Achelaritei, and V. Cozma, "Prevalence of *Cryptosporidium* spp. Inasymptomatic dogs by elisa and risk factors associated with infection," *Lucrări Stiinţifice Medicină Veterinară*, vol. 13, no. 1, 2010.

[24] L. Rinaldi, M. P. Maurelli, V. Musella et al., "Giardia and *Cryptosporidium* in canine faecal samples contaminating an urban area," *Research in Veterinary Science*, vol. 84, no. 3, pp. 413–415, 2008.

29

Comparison of the Effect of Two Purification Methods on the Immunogenicity of Recombinant Outer Membrane Protein H of *Pasteurella multocida* Serovar A:1

Arunee Thanasarasakulpong,[1] **Pichayanut Poolperm,**[2] **Weerapongse Tangjitjaroen,**[1] **Thanya Varinrak,**[1] **Takuo Sawada,**[2] **Dirk Pfeiffer,**[1,3] **and Nattawooti Sthitmatee**[1]

[1]*Faculty of Veterinary Medicine, Chiang Mai University, Chiang Mai 50100, Thailand*
[2]*Laboratory of Veterinary Microbiology, Nippon Veterinary and Life Science University, Tokyo 180-8602, Japan*
[3]*Veterinary Epidemiology, Economics and Public Health Group, Royal Veterinary College, London AL9 7TA, UK*

Correspondence should be addressed to Nattawooti Sthitmatee; drneaw@gmail.com

Academic Editor: Francesca Mancianti

Recombinant outer membrane protein H (rOmpH) of *Pasteurella multocida* strain X-73 can be purified using affinity chromatography but this adversely affects its immunogenicity. The current study presents the results from an intervention study comparing the immunogenicity of rOmpH purified using electroelution with rOmpH purified using affinity chromatography and native OmpH purified using electroelution and a nonimmunized control group. Chickens immunized with rOmpH purified using electroelution produced the highest ELISA antibody levels against *P. multocida* strains. Chickens in each of the 5 treatment groups were split into two subgroups for challenge with two different *P. multocida* strains. The average number of adhesions to CEF cells was statistically significantly lower in sera from chickens immunized with rOmpH or native OmpH purified using electroelution than in those of the three other treatment groups. The survival amongst chickens immunized with rOmpH or native OmpH purified using electroelution indicated high levels of protection. In contrast, survival probability was zero or low in the groups immunized with rOmpH purified using affinity chromatography and in the nonimmunized group. These findings show that the rOmpH purified using electroelution retains its immunogenicity and stimulates high levels of protection in chickens against *P. multocida* infection.

1. Introduction

Recombinant proteins with 6×His-tagged protein are routinely purified by a Ni-NTA affinity chromatography as recommended by their manufacturers. However, Luo et al. [1] and Rimler [2] suggested that this process resulted in a change in the structure of the recombinant outer membrane protein H (rOmpH) of avian *Pasteurella multocida* strain X-73 affecting its immunogenicity. The OmpH, a porin protein, is stable in the homotrimer form at room temperature and was fully dissociated into monomers which correlated with the unfolded or denatured form of protein after purification of the protein using a denatured condition of affinity chromatography. In contrast, Sthitmatee et al. [3] successfully improved the immunogenicity of rOmpH using a hybrid condition of affinity chromatography to purify rOmpH. But this method is unstable, is of low reproducibility, and results in a high loss of protein yield [3]. This suggests that affinity chromatography may be unsuitable for purification of this recombinant protein. The electroelution method is widely used for analytic purposes [4–6]. The method employs polyacrylamide gel electrophoresis (PAGE) which is easy to perform and has high resolution and good reproducibility. This system also has advantages in terms of having high loading capacity of sample protein and allowing easy monitoring of the elution process. Previous studies using electroelution to purify target proteins showed that the method provides an effective purification method for protection of immunogenicity of the target proteins [7–10]. Interestingly, the method has been used for purification of a native form of OmpH

TABLE 1: Experimental design and results of *P. multocida* challenge of immunized and nonimmunized chickens.

Treatment groups	Type of immunogen	*P. multocida* strain challenge subgroup Number of survivors/total (% protection)	
		X-73	P-1059
1	rOmpH purified using electroelution	9/10 (90)*	8/10 (80)*
2	rOmpH purified using a denatured condition of affinity chromatography	2/10 (20)	3/10 (30)
3	Native OmpH purified using electroelution	10/10 (100)*	10/10 (100)*
4	Incomplete Freund's adjuvant	0/5 (0)	0/5 (0)
5	No immunization	0/5 (0)	0/5 (0)

*Significantly difference ($p < 0.05$).

while completely protecting its immunogenicity [8]. This suggests that the electroelution method could also be applied for purification of rOmpH. The present intervention study aimed at comparing the performance of the electroelution and affinity chromatography methods for purification of the rOmpH in terms of their effect on the immunogenicity of the recombinant protein.

2. Materials and Methods

2.1. Experimental Design. An intervention study was used with five treatment groups; there were four immunized groups and one nonimmunized group (Table 1). The treatments included group 1, immunized with rOmpH purified using electroelution, group 2, immunized with rOmpH purified using a denatured condition of affinity chromatography [1], group 3, immunized with native OmpH purified using electroelution [8], group 4, immunized with incomplete Freund's adjuvant, and group 5, a nonimmunized group, respectively. Each of the five treatment groups was divided into two subgroups, one challenged with *P. multocida* serovar A:1 and the other with serovar A:3. There were therefore in total 10 treatment-challenge subgroups. Hisex brown chickens at the age of 21 weeks sourced from RPM Farm & Feed Co. Ltd., Chiang Mai, Thailand, were used in this study. The outcome variables which were compared between the treatment groups were immunological and clinical parameters. The former consisted of serum antibody and cell adhesion levels in response to infection challenge, both measured after vaccination, and the latter of survival of chickens. The chickens were randomly allocated to the 10 treatment-challenge subgroups, with 10 chickens in each of the six subgroups immunized with rOmpH or OmpH purified using electroelution and 5 chickens in each of the four other subgroups. The group size of 10 was sufficient to detect a reduction in mortality in a pairwise comparison from 100 to 40% at 95% confidence level and with 80% power. A group size of 10 in each of the OmpH or rOmpH immunized and 5 in each of the two comparison groups allowed for detection of a reduction in mortality from 100 to 30% at 95% confidence level and with 80% statistical power. Chickens in groups 1–3 were intramuscularly immunized two times at a 2-week interval with a total volume of 1 mL of 100 μg rOmpH or OmpH emulsified with an equal volume of incomplete Freund's adjuvant (Sigma-Aldrich), specifically

group 1 with rOmpH purified using electroelution, group 2 with a denatured condition of affinity chromatography, and group 3 with native OmpH purified using electroelution. Chickens in group 4 were intramuscularly immunized with incomplete Freund's adjuvant in PBS buffer and group 5 was not immunized (Table 1). Chickens in the 4 immunized groups were immunized twice, once on day 0 and again on day 14. All groups were intramuscularly challenged with either approximately 2×10^6 cfu/mL or 4.3×10^6 cfu/mL of live *P. multocida* strains X-73 or P-1059 [3], respectively, at 2 weeks after the second immunization.

Blood samples from each chicken were collected from the wing veins on days 0, 7, 14, 21, and 28 after immunization. Sera were assayed using western blot, indirect ELISA, and the adhesion inhibition assay. All chickens were observed every day for clinical signs and behavioral changes during the experiments. Once chickens showed clinical signs of the disease, they were euthanised according to the protocol in the AVMA guideline for the euthanasia of animals, version 2013 [11]. The experimental use of animals in this study was approved by the animal welfare and laboratory animal ethics committee of the Faculty of Veterinary Medicine, Chiang Mai University, Chiang Mai, Thailand (approval number R15/2555).

2.2. Bacterial Strains, Gene, and Plasmid. The challenge experiments were conducted using *P. multocida* strains X-73 (serovar A:1, ATCC15742) and P-1059 (serovar A:3, ATCC11039), which as major etiologic strains of fowl cholera are widely considered to be appropriate for assessing the protection of chickens against infection with all *P. multocida* strains. They were grown in brain heart infusion broth (BHI; Merck, Darmstadt, Germany) for 6 h at 37°C. Then the bacteria were subcultured onto a blood agar and incubated at 37°C for 18 h. *E. coli* strain PQE-ompH, which carried the 6×Histidine tag fused *ompH* gene of the *P. multocida* strain X-73 plasmid in the *E. coli* strain M15 from our previous study [3], was grown in Luria-Bertani (LB) broth or on LB agar containing 100 μg/mL ampicillin and 25 μg/mL kanamycin (Sigma-Aldrich, St. Louis, MO, USA) at 37°C.

2.3. Purification of Native OmpH. Native OmpH was prepared using the electroelution method as described elsewhere [8]. Briefly, crude capsular extract (CCE) was prepared using the saline extraction method as described previously [8].

Then, target 39 kDa protein of native OmpH was purified by electroelution (electroelution electrophoresis apparatus, ATTO) in 20 mM Tris base, 150 mM glycine, and 0.01% SDS buffer at 100 V for 1 h in an icebox. The conditions for protein collection were 200 min for delay time, 2 min for EP time, 100 s for filling time, 120 s for collecting time, and 15 mA for electrical current. The eluted native OmpH was passed through the detergent removing minicolumn (Ampure DT, Amersham, Japan). Then, the total protein in the supernatant was quantified using the BCA protein assay kit (Pierce, Rockford, IL, USA) and the eluted protein was kept at $-20°C$ until use.

2.4. Preparation and Purification of rOmpH.

The rOmpH was expressed via *E. coli* strain PQE-ompH as described in our previous study [3]. Then, the expression of the recombinant protein was induced by the addition of isopropyl-β-D-thiogalactopyranoside (IPTG; Amresco, Solon, OH, USA) to a final concentration of 1 mM and continually incubated under the same conditions for a further 5 h. Finally, the bacterial cells were harvested by centrifugation at 4,000 ×g at 4°C for 20 min. The supernatant was discarded and the cell pellets were stored in $-20°C$ for further utilization.

E. coli cell pellets were lysed and purified using the electroelution method or a denatured condition of affinity chromatography [1]. Purification of the recombinant protein using the electroelution method was explained as follows. The 5 g wet weight of cell pellets was lysed in 10 mL of a native lysis buffer (50 mM NaH_2PO_4, 300 mM NaCl, and 10 mM imidazole, pH 8.0). The solution was gently mixed, at 4°C, and then the homogenate was centrifuged at 10,000 ×g at 4°C. The supernatant containing 1,500 μg of total protein was run on a preparative 12.5% sodium dodecyl sulfate polyacrylamide gel column (10 mm stacking gel and 30 mm separating gel) in a sample buffer (4% SDS, 50 mM, Tris, 20% of glycerol, and 0.005% of bromophenol blue) using the electroelution apparatus (Nativen, ATTO, Tokyo, Japan). The conditions for protein collection were 200 min for delay time, 2 min for EP time, 100 s for filling time, 120 s for collecting time, and 15 mA for electrical current. Protein fractions were collected in buffer (371 mM Tris, 5% sucrose, pH 8.8) and the total protein was quantified using the BCA protein assay kit (Pierce) before being kept at $-20°C$.

2.5. Protein Fraction Analyses.

Each 10 μg protein fraction was identified on the basis of presence of the target protein by 12.5% SDS-PAGE according to the Laemmli method [12] and then subjected to western blotting. Protein fractions were transferred onto nitrocellulose membrane and immunostained with an anti-HisG-HRP antibody (Invitrogen, Carlsbad, CA, USA). After incubation with antibodies, the membranes were washed thoroughly with PBST. The protein bands were visualized following incubation with 3,3'-diaminobenzidine (DAB; Invitrogen) as a chromogenic substrate.

2.6. Determination of Antibody Responses.

Specific antibody responses of the chicken sera were determined through measuring the Immunoglobulin Y (IgY) titers using a commercial indirect ELISA test kit for fowl cholera (ProFLOK, Synbiotics, Kansas City, MO, USA). The plates were evaluated using an ELISA plate reader (Immuno Mini NJ 2300, Intermed, Japan) and the average sample per positive (S/P) ratio of each group was calculated according to the manufacturer's recommendation. The S/P ratios were calculated according to the following equation: S/P ratio (%) = [corrected optical density of a sample/corrected optical density of a positive reference serum]. There is no quantitative test sensitivity and specificity information available for this test.

2.7. Chicken Embryo Fibroblast (CEF) Cell Culture.

The CEF cells were obtained from 10-day-embryonated chicken eggs (The Upper Northern Veterinary Research and Development Center, Hang Chat, Lam Pang, Thailand). Approximately 48 h before the experiment, a total of 2.5×10^5 cells/mL in 2 mL Dulbecco's Modified Eagle Medium (DMEM; Invitrogen) supplemented with 5% fetal bovine serum (Invitrogen), 1% L-glutamine (Invitrogen), and 100 U/mL of penicillin and streptomycin (Invitrogen) were seeded into 35 mm Corning culture dishes containing 22×22 mm cover slips in the bottom of the well. The dishes were incubated at 37°C with 5% CO_2. After the incubation, the dishes were washed three times with 2 mL of sterile PBS pH 7.4 and used for the adhesion inhibition assay.

2.8. Adhesion Inhibition Assay.

The adhesion inhibition assay was modified based on a previous study [8]. Briefly, *P. multocida* strains were grown separately on blood agar at 37°C for 18 h and were resuspended in sterile PBS and suspension turbidity was adjusted to 0.5 of McFarland Standard (approximately 2.8×10^8 cfu/mL) at the wavelength of 600 nm. The day after vaccination with the highest average S/P value in the indirect ELISA across all serum samples was identified, and samples from that day were pooled within each of the 10 treatment-challenge groups and used for this assay. To represent the bacterial challenge *in vitro*, for each of the 10 treatment-challenge groups 2 mL of the bacterial suspension was added to 3 mL of pooled chicken serum and incubated at 37°C for 1 h. After the incubation, the resulting suspension was inoculated onto the monolayer of CEF cells and incubated at 37°C with 5% CO_2 for 1 h. Nonadherent bacteria were removed by washing with 2 mL of sterile PBS. The washing step was repeated for 4 times. After washing the cover slips were fixed with 4% formaldehyde and stained with Wright Giemsa solution (Sigma-Aldrich). The cover slips were examined under a light microscope with 1000x power of magnification. For each of the treatment-challenge subgroups, 100 CEF cells with intact structure were selected and the number of adhering bacteria was counted. The selection of CEF cells occurred randomly by scanning a magnification field from the left to the right and from the top to the bottom of the cover slips. The counts for each selected CEF cell were performed twice and the mean was used in the analysis.

2.9. Experimental Infection in Chickens.

After allowing two weeks following the second immunization for chickens to

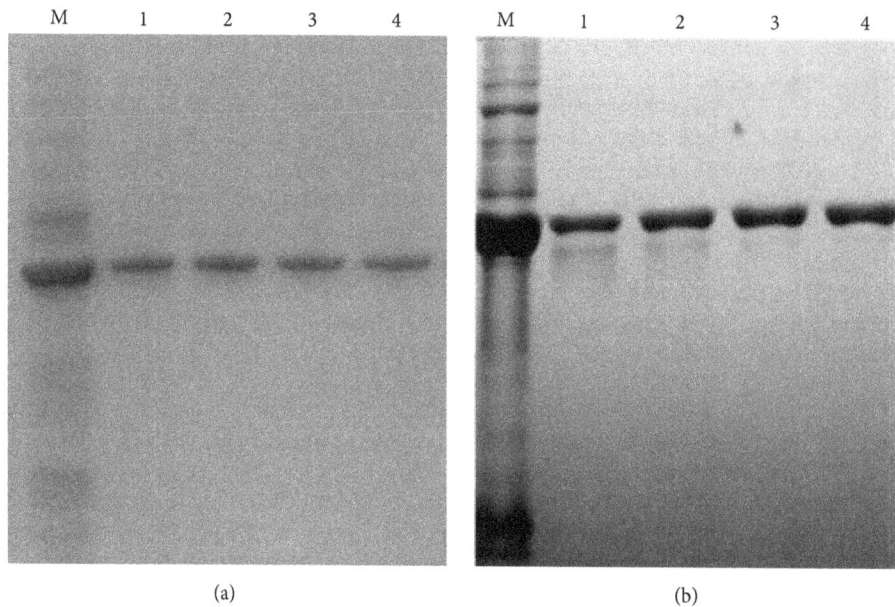

FIGURE 1: The fractions of rOmpH purified by electroelution were analyzed using SDS-PAGE (a) and probed with anti-HisG-HRP antibody (b). Lane M: cell lysates of the *E. coli* host. Lanes 1–4: rOmpH fractions purified using electroelution.

develop an immune response, chickens in all groups were challenged with the bacteria by intramuscular injection of 1 mL of bacterial suspension containing 2×10^6 cfu/mL of strain X-73 or 4.3×10^6 cfu/mL of P-1059 [3], respectively. The birds were examined for clinical signs over a 7-day postchallenge period, and mortality was recorded.

2.10. Statistical Analysis. The results were analyzed using Stata SE 13.1 software (StataCorp LP, College station, TX, USA) and IBM SPSS Statistics version 22. No statistical analysis was performed for the antibody response data as only summary statistics were available. A general linear model analysis was used to compare the average adhesion inhibition of bacteria to CEF cells counts between treatment groups and *in vitro* infection challenge groups, as well as their interaction. The means between different groups were compared using simple contrasts. The survival of chickens was compared between different treatment and *in vivo* infection challenge groups using binary logistic regression. Exact estimation was used given the small sample sizes in this study.

3. Results

3.1. Expression and Purification of rOmpH. *E. coli* cell whole cell lysates showed an overexpressed band at approximately 39 kDa on sodium dodecyl sulfate polyacrylamide gel electrophoresis (SDS-PAGE; Figure 1). The rOmpH fractions from the electroelution apparatus, which was employed in order to check whether the eluted fractions had been extracted, showed a single protein band with the same target molecular mass, as shown in Figure 1. The western blotting, probed with anti-6×Histidine tagged-antibody, also confirmed the overexpressed band of rOmpH which was tagged with the 6×Histidine, as shown in Figure 1. Additionally, all

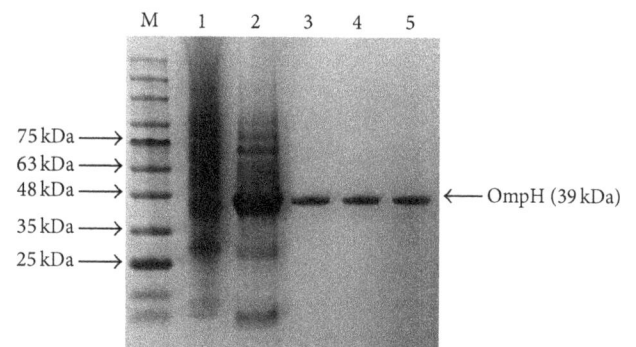

FIGURE 2: SDS-PAGE of proteins used in this study. Lanes: M: molecular mass standards; 1: whole cell lysate of strain X-73; 2: prepurified rOmpH; 3: rOmpH purified by electroelution; 4: rOmpH purified by a hybrid condition of affinity chromatography; and 5: native OmpH of strain X-73 purified by electroelution.

the proteins used in this study were analyzed using SDS-PAGE (Figure 2). The molecular mass of those 3 proteins, native OmpH, and the two types of rOmpH produced using different purification methods were identical with approximately 39 kDa.

3.2. Antibody Responses after Vaccination. It is to be noted that the findings in relation to antibody data are based on visual analysis of the data, since only summary statistics were available. The levels of serum antibody in the chickens immunized with native OmpH or rOmpH, both purified using the electroelution method, increased following the first and second immunizations (Figure 3). Immune responses to native OmpH reached a maximal point 7 days after first dose and began to plateau after 14 days but responses were also

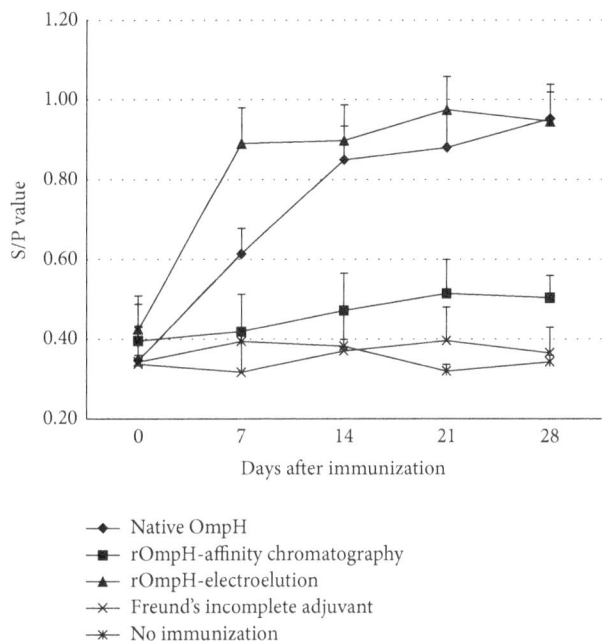

FIGURE 3: The temporal pattern of the average S/P value of chicken sera (including standard error) based on indirect ELISA (ProFLOK) for each of the five treatment groups (first vaccination on day 0 and the second on day 14).

slightly increased at days 21 and 28. In contrast, rOmpH reached a maximal point after 7 days and began to plateau at day 7 after first dose. Moreover, responses were also slightly increased at day 21 (rOmpH) but do not appear to be significantly different to the responses at day 14 and therefore were considered to have reached a maximum at day 14. In contrast, low antibody levels were observed in the chickens immunized with the rOmpH purified using affinity chromatography, those receiving incomplete Freund's adjuvant, and the nonimmunized groups.

3.3. Bacterial Adhesion following In Vitro Challenge with P. multocida Strains. The general linear model analysis indicates that the mean number of adherent bacteria differs amongst treatment groups ($p < 0.001$) and between the two challenge strains ($p < 0.001$). There was no statistically significant interaction between treatment group and challenge strain ($p = 0.07$). Compared with the counts for the nonvaccinated group, the samples from chickens immunized with Freund's incomplete adjuvant had average bacterial adhesion counts per CEF which were lower by 8.9 (95% CI 5.9–11.9), those immunized with rOmpH purified using affinity chromatography were lower by 15.0 (95% CI 12–18), those immunized with rOmpH purified using electroelution were lower by 35 (95% CI 32.4–38.5), and those immunized with OmpH purified using electroelution were lower by 45 (95% CI 42.6–48.2). The pooled sera challenged *in vitro* with *P. multocida* strain P-1059 had on average 4.1 (95% CI 2.3–5.9) more adherent bacteria per CEF cell than those challenged with X-73. The distributions of counts of bacteria adherent to CEF cells for each of the 10 treatment-challenge groups are shown in Figure 4.

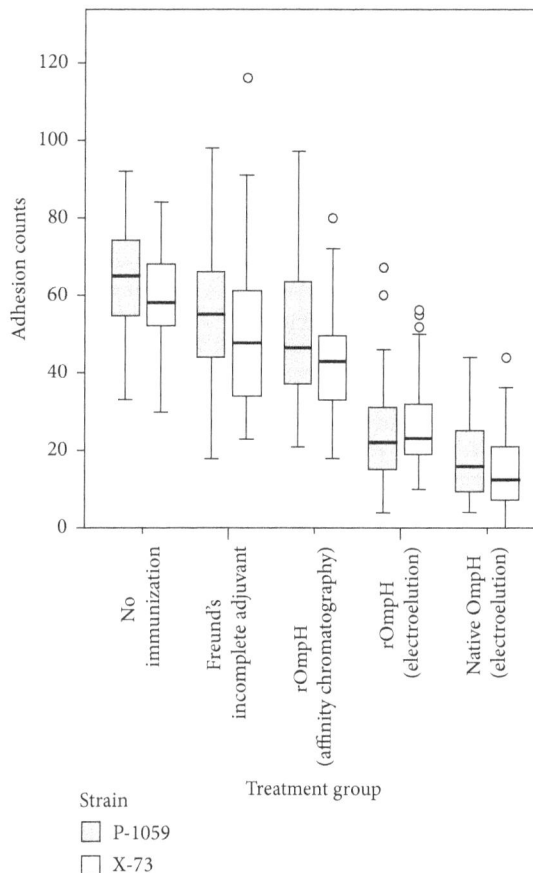

FIGURE 4: Box-and-whisker plot of counts of adhesions to CEF cells by treatment group and *P. multocida* challenge strains.

3.4. Survival following In Vivo Infection Challenge with P. multocida Strains. Amongst chickens developing clinical disease, clinical signs were observed from 12 hours following bacterial challenge. There was no statistically significant difference in survival between the two challenge strain groups, and this effect did not vary between treatment groups (median unbiased estimate of odds ratio = 1, exact 95% CI 0.19–5.1). There was a statistically significant difference in survival between treatment groups. Using nonvaccinated chickens as the reference group, there was a higher survival proportion in chickens immunized with either OmpH (median unbiased estimate of odds ratio = 238, exact 95% CI 33–infinity) or rOmpH purified using electroelution against challenge with one of the two *P. multocida* strains (median unbiased estimate of odds ratio = 55, exact 95% CI 9–infinity). The other two groups did not differ in their survival from the reference group. Table 1 shows the proportions of surviving chickens for each treatment and *P. multocida* strain challenge group.

4. Discussion

The structural integrity of the expressed protein is one of the main concerns in recombinant protein production. This is due partly to the original protein structure having an important role in inducing specific antibodies. The antigenic epitope and structure of the recombinant protein must also be conserved during the purification process. Electroelution is used to extract a particular protein of interest from an electrophoresis gel by applying an electric current [6, 13]. The method is considered to be an effective purification method for separating a small target band of proteins from a crude whole protein sample [7–10]. Other chromatography methods are less able to uniquely separate the target protein band [6]. The electroelution method uses polyacrylamide gel electrophoresis (PAGE) which allows effective separation of the target protein band from a crude original protein [6, 13]. Indeed, PAGE is routinely used to determine protein or nucleotide purity. Amongst its advantages is also the absence of sodium dodecyl sulfate (SDS) and urea in the gel composition. In the current study, electroelution was applied to purify the rOmpH from cell lysate in order to protect the immunogenicity of the protein.

Outer membrane protein H (OmpH) is a porin protein which is considered to be highly conserved among Gram-negative bacteria including *P. multocida* strains [14]. A native form of OmpH is a homotrimer of approximately 110 kDa while a monomeric form of this protein can be obtain by induced denaturation and ranges from 34 to 42 kDa. The variation in the size of the monomer depends on the serotype and the electrophoretic system used for the analysis [1, 15, 16]. Chevalier et al. [15] demonstrated the use of size exclusion chromatography to purify the native form of OmpH and successfully protected the immunogenicity of the protein. Subsequently, Luo et al. [1] employed the same method and used the protein as an immunogen in chickens. The native form of OmpH produced effective protection in chickens against homologous challenge-exposure. Recombinant OmpH of *P. multocida* strain X-73 has been cloned and expressed by Luo et al. [1]. The rOmpH was purified by a denatured condition of affinity chromatography and characterized the immunogenicity. The protection in chickens conferred by immunization with rOmpH in that study was low when compared with a native form of OmpH. Luo et al. [1] suggested that the structure of the recombinant outer membrane protein H (rOmpH) of avian *P. multocida* strain X-73 had changed and affected its immunogenicity following purification by a denatured condition of affinity chromatography. According to previous reports on immunization with bacterial porins in animal models, the trimeric or native conformation of porin is considered essential for induction of protective immunity [1, 2]. Until now, there has been only one application of the electroelution method for purification of a native form of OmpH (Borrathybay et al., 2003); however, the application for purification of rOmpH has not been demonstrated yet. Borrathybay et al. [8] attempted to purify a native form of OmpH of *P. multocida* strain P-1059 from crude capsular extract. The purified OmpH provided effective protection in chicken against challenge with different *P. multocida* strains. This suggested that the electroelution method used in that study had no adverse effect on the immunogenicity of OmpH after purification. According to the results from the current study, the protection conferred by immunization with OmpH or rOmpH purified using the electroelution method resulted in a higher level of protection amongst chickens compared with other purification methods. This indicates that the electroelution method can be used for purification of rOmpH

without adversely affecting its immunogenicity. Furthermore, given that there was no statistically significant difference in the performance of native OmpH and rOmpH both purified using electroelution, it can be concluded that the recombinant OmpH of *P. multocida* can be used as effectively as the native one.

The ability to induce cross-immunity among *P. multocida* serovars is important in the development of poultry vaccines. Similar to this study, Sthitmatee et al. [3] and Borrathybay et al. [8] also demonstrated that OmpH and rOmpH of *P. multocida* strains are cross-protective immunogens against avian *P. multocida* strains. The method used for purification of the protein influences its immunogenicity, including its cross-protection potential. This is important since a natural fowl cholera outbreak can be caused by strains that are different from the vaccination strain or may involve multiple strains. A previous study suggested that the natural expression of the antigen responsible for cross-protection is limited under the *in vitro* growth conditions during the proliferation process [17].

The current study demonstrates that both native OmpH and rOmpH purified using electroelution induce effective *in vitro* antibody protection that inhibits the adhesion of two common avian *P. multocida* strains to CEF cells. In contrast, the antibodies induced by rOmpH purified by a denatured condition of affinity chromatography resulted in a high number of adhesions of bacteria to CEF cells. This result provides strong evidence that the electroelution was successful at refolding the protein conformation. In accordance with the previous study [8], the native form of OmpH induced an efficient antibody which inhibited the bacterium from adhering to CEF cells. Moreover, low amounts of OmpH in bacterial capsule affected the cross-protectivity [18]. However, the method requires further basic biochemistry coupled with bioinformatics tools to verify the protein structure. The result was confirmed in the *in vivo* challenge experiment where survival in the groups immunized with rOmpH purified using electroelution was 85% compared with 25% in the groups immunized with rOmpH purified using affinity chromatography. These *in vitro* and *in vivo* results demonstrate the potential of rOmpH purified using electroelution for protection of chickens against *P. multocida* infection.

5. Conclusion

The rOmpH purified using the electroelution method retains its immunogenicity as demonstrated by being able to induce specific antibodies against avian *P. multocida* strains. It successfully protected against homologous strain challenge as measured by *in vitro* and *in vivo* challenge with two different avian *P. multocida* strains. The rOmpH purified using the affinity chromatography method achieved poor protection in the challenge experiment.

Conflict of Interests

The authors declare that there is no conflict of interests regarding the publication of this paper.

Acknowledgment

This research (Grant no. P-10-11170) was financially supported by the National Science and Technology Development Agency (NSTDA), Ministry of Science and Technology, Thailand.

References

[1] Y. Luo, J. R. Glisson, M. W. Jackwood et al., "Cloning and characterization of the major outer membrane protein gene (ompH) of Pasteurella multocida X-73," *Journal of Bacteriology*, vol. 179, no. 24, pp. 7856–7864, 1997.

[2] R. B. Rimler, "Purification of a cross-protective antigen from *Pasteurella multocida* grown *in vitro* and *in vivo*," *Avian Diseases*, vol. 45, no. 3, pp. 572–580, 2001.

[3] N. Sthitmatee, S. Numee, E. Kawamoto et al., "Protection of chickens from fowl cholera by vaccination with recombinant adhesive protein of *Pasteurella multocida*," *Vaccine*, vol. 26, no. 19, pp. 2398–2407, 2008.

[4] B. Chellan, P. S. Appukuttan, and N. N. Jayakumari, "Electroelution of lipoprotein(a) [Lp(a)] from native polyacrylamide gels: a new, simple method to purify Lp(a)," *Journal of Biochemical and Biophysical Methods*, vol. 68, no. 1, pp. 43–53, 2008.

[5] P. Sá-Pereira, J. Duarte, and M. Costa-Ferreira, "Electroelution as a simple and fast protein purification method: isolation of an extracellular xylanase from *Bacillus* sp. CCMI 966," *Enzyme and Microbial Technology*, vol. 27, no. 1-2, pp. 95–99, 2000.

[6] M. Shoji, M. Kato, and H. Shuichi, "Electrophoretic recovery of proteins from polyacrylamide gel," *Journal of Chromatography A*, vol. 698, no. 1-2, pp. 145–162, 1995.

[7] P. J. Barrell, O. W. Liew, and A. J. Conner, "Expressing an antibacterial protein in bacteria for raising antibodies," *Protein Expression and Purification*, vol. 33, no. 1, pp. 153–159, 2004.

[8] E. Borrathybay, T. Sawada, Y. Kataoka et al., "A 39 kDa protein mediates adhesion of avian *Pasteurella multocida* to chicken embryo fibroblast cells," *Veterinary Microbiology*, vol. 97, no. 3-4, pp. 229–243, 2003.

[9] U. Kaur, S. Khurana, U. N. Saikia, and M. L. Dubey, "Immunogenicity and protective efficacy of heparan sulphate binding proteins of *Entamoeba histolytica* in a guinea pig model of intestinal amoebiasis," *Experimental Parasitology*, vol. 135, no. 3, pp. 486–496, 2013.

[10] A. R. Pinto, C. G. P. Beyrodt, R. A. M. Lopes, and C. L. Barbiéri, "Identification of a 30 kDa antigen from *Leishmania* (L.) *chagasi* amastigotes implicated in protective cellular reponses in a murine model," *International Journal for Parasitology*, vol. 30, no. 5, pp. 599–607, 2000.

[11] American Veterinary Medical Association, *AVMA Guidelines for the Euthanasia of Animals*, American Veterinary Medical Association Press, Schaumburg, Ill, USA, 2013.

[12] U. K. Laemmli, "Cleavage of structural proteins during the assembly of the head of bacteriophage T4," *Nature*, vol. 227, no. 5259, pp. 680–685, 1970.

[13] M. G. Harrington, "Purification procedures: electrophoretic methods elution of protein from gels," in *Guide to Protein Purification, Methods in Enzymology*, M. P. Deutscher, Ed., pp. 488–498, Academic Press, San Diego, Calif, USA, 1990.

[14] T. Hatfaludi, K. Al-Hasani, J. D. Boyce, and B. Adler, "Outer membrane proteins of *Pasteurella multocida*," *Veterinary Microbiology*, vol. 144, no. 1-2, pp. 1–17, 2010.

[15] G. Chevalier, H. Duclohier, D. Thomas, E. Shechter, and H. Wroblewski, "Purification and characterization of protein H, the major porin of *Pasteurella multocida*," *Journal of Bacteriology*, vol. 175, no. 1, pp. 266–276, 1993.

[16] A. Lübke, L. Hartmann, W. Schröder, and E. Hellmann, "Isolation and partial characterization of the major protein of the outer membrane of *Pasteurella haemolytica* and *Pasteurella multocida*," *Zentralblatt für Bakteriologie*, vol. 281, no. 1, pp. 45–54, 1994.

[17] P. A. Rebers and K. L. Heddleston, "Fowl cholera: induction of cross-protection in turkeys with bacterins prepared from host-passaged *Pasteurella multocida*," *Avian Diseases*, vol. 21, no. 1, pp. 50–56, 1977.

[18] N. Sthitmatee, T. Yano, K. N. Lampang, C. Suphavilai, Y. Kataoka, and T. Sawada, "A 39-kDa capsular protein is a major cross-protection factor as demonstrated by protection of chickens with a live attenuated *Pasteurella multocida* strain of P-1059," *Journal of Veterinary Medical Science*, vol. 75, no. 7, pp. 923–928, 2013.

30

Brazilian Spotted Fever with an Approach in Veterinary Medicine and One Health Perspective

Sabrina Destri Emmerick Campos,[1] **Nathalie Costa da Cunha,**[2] **and Nádia Regina Pereira Almosny**[1]

[1]*Departamento de Patologia e Clínica Veterinária, Universidade Federal Fluminense, 24230-340 Niterói, RJ, Brazil*
[2]*Departamento de Saúde Coletiva Veterinária e Saúde Pública, Universidade Federal Fluminense, 24230-340 Niterói, RJ, Brazil*

Correspondence should be addressed to Sabrina Destri Emmerick Campos; s.destri@gmail.com

Academic Editor: Francesca Mancianti

There is increasing interaction between man and pathogens transmitted by arthropods, especially by ticks. It is on this background that a holistic approach stands out, for the sake of Public Health. Brazilian Spotted Fever is an endemic disease at the country's southeast, with *Amblyomma sculptum* as its major contributor, followed by *A. aureolatum* and potentially *Rhipicephalus sanguineus*. Dogs have been considered sentinels, and in some areas the disease in dogs can precede human disease. Considering the importance of this disease for human health, the serological evidence in dogs, and the transmission of ticks between dogs and their owners, this review aimed to elucidate the importance of the epidemiological investigation, the diagnosis in dogs, and the role of veterinarians in Public Health to control vector-borne zoonotic diseases. We encourage veterinarians to include this rickettsial infection in the diagnosis of febrile diseases of common occurrence in dogs.

1. Introduction

Vector-borne diseases are globally important to human and animal health, since pathogens, vectors, and animal hosts reveal interactions through pathologies and their epidemiology, which differ among geographic zones, and may change over time [1]. Ticks and wildlife are among the main reservoirs of pathogens transmitted by arthropods of veterinary importance [2].

Human beings are causing important changes in the ecosystem, such as habitat fragmentation, global warming, and exploitation of natural resources, which have allowed interaction between man and pathogens potentially transmitted by arthropods [3, 4]. The global Strategic Framework for health has been created to decrease the risk and minimize the impact of emerging infectious diseases at the animal-human-ecosystem and socioeconomic interface [3]. Shaffer [5] suggested the use of surveillance policies for animals as part of an approach in One Health Perspective, in order to contribute to more coordinated actions towards human health.

It is against this background that stands out a holistic approach for the sake of Public Health, applying the concept of One Health, which recognizes that human welfare is linked to animals and the environment and so it seeks a combined action between physicians, ecologists, and veterinarians in the control of threats to Public Health.

Rickettsia rickettsii is the major bacterium responsible for the Brazilian Spotted Fever (BSF), a highly fatal disease with challenging diagnosis due to its nonspecific signs [6, 7]. To assist the epidemiological surveillance, studies have been searching for sentinel animals, such as horses and dogs, with positive serological reaction in endemic areas [8, 9].

Based on the importance of BSF to human health, the evidence of clinical illness in dogs from areas with laboratory-confirmed BSF in humans, and the potential transmission of ticks between dogs and their owners, this review aimed to discuss the importance of epidemiological surveys and laboratory diagnosis of BSF in dogs for Public Health, inspired by the principles of One World, One Health, a Strategic Framework that has been raised jointly by specialized agencies, such as World Health Organization (WHO), United Nations (UN) Food and Agriculture Organization (FAO), International Organization for Animal Health (OIE), and UN Children's Fund (UNICEF).

2. The One Health Idea

The idea that humans, animals, and the ecosystems are closely related has been under discussion since the late nineteenth century, when the first movements to integrate activities and research in human and animal health were raised [3, 10].

It is believed that emerging infectious diseases are related to socioeconomic conditions and ecological features, which allow identifying potential hotspots of injuries of animal origin, particularly at low latitudes, at areas where the notifications are substantially weak [11], a pattern that fits the epidemiological situation of BSF.

The Strategic Framework establishes a more interdisciplinary approach with international cooperation, in order to ensure health for humans, animals, and ecosystems [3, 10, 12]. However, people are reservoir of only a small number of zoonotic pathogens, so it is understood that an effective monitoring system requires the integration of physicians, who can identify human outbreaks, and veterinarians, that can identify animal reservoirs and sentinels [5, 13].

Veterinarians can contribute to the promotion of health through their knowledge on environmental conservation, the use of domestic animals as sentinels for the circulation of pathogens in the domestic and/or wildlife arenas, and occupational risk (due to the exposure to ticks) [12, 14, 15]. A study with veterinary students revealed that animal treatment with acaricides, avoiding contact with ticks, keeping vegetation cut down, and inspecting the body every three hours for the presence of ticks were the main prevention methods cited in control of BSF [15].

We believe that interdisciplinary participation in epidemiological investigation research and dissemination of articles and reports to scientific and health care assistance communities could be a mechanism to integrate information and improve strategies to control this disease.

3. Brazilian Spotted Fever

3.1. History. A disease caused by *Rickettsia rickettsii* was first described in the USA, and since then it has been confirmed in several countries, including Canada, Mexico, Panama, Costa Rica, Colombia, Brazil, Argentina, and possibly Guatemala [16–21]. In Brazil, this disease has been called Brazilian Spotted Fever (BSF) and it was first discovered in the state of São Paulo in 1928, where it was originally treated as "Exanthematic Typhus" [22]. The return of BSF reports in the 80s has shown that the disease has never ceased to occur; however it became detected as an acute disease affecting people from the same household or labor, albeit isolated cases have been described [23, 24]. Since 2001, BSF is a nationally notifiable disease, considered endemic in southeastern Brazil [23, 25].

According to the Center of Disease Control, the gold standard serologic test for diagnosis of the disease is the indirect immunofluorescence assay (IFA) with *R. rickettsii* antigen, performed on two paired serum samples to demonstrate a significant (fourfold) rise in IgG antibody titers, since molecular diagnosis is not always routinely available to confirm cases (http://www.cdc.gov/rmsf/symptoms). In Brazil, 1141 human cases confirmed by IFA were notified between 2007 and 2015, being 61.26% (699/1141) in the southeast, especially in the states of São Paulo (43.21%, 493/1141), Minas Gerais (8.15%, 93/1141), and Rio de Janeiro (7.19%, 82/1141). The state of Santa Catarina is highlighted with 23.05% of human cases (263/1141). Amapá, Rondônia, and Amazonas contributed with a single confirmed human case each, in 2007, 2008, and 2011 (http://www.saude.gov.br/sinan).

3.2. Vectors, Reservoir, and Amplifying Hosts. Due to their capability to transmit a variety of zoonotic pathogens, ticks stand out on the concept of One Health. Brazil contains many biomes, rich and abundant fauna, and several species of arthropods, such as ticks of the *Amblyomma* genus, widely distributed in the Neotropical region [21].

Based on recent reassessment of the taxonomic and morphological status of *Amblyomma cajennense* (Fabricius, 1787), currently, the name *A. cajennense sensu lato* (*s.l.*) refers to a group of six species. According to geographical distributions, and host associations, *A. cajennense sensu stricto* (*s.s.*) applies to the tick found in the Amazonian region of South America, while *A. sculptum* applies to the tick found in the coastal states, and degraded areas of the Atlantic Forest, including all states in the southeast [26, 27].

Interestingly, the low host specificity of *A. cajennense s.l.* allows for their detection in many mammals including cattle, deer, and wild and domestic canids, besides man [7, 28, 29]. *Amblyomma cajennense s.l.* is implicated as the major species responsible for BSF, followed by *A. aureolatum* [29, 30]. In addition, the potential disease-transmission role of *Rhipicephalus sanguineus* is also increasingly studied [9, 31–35].

In the tick, transstadial and transovarian systems maintain the bacteria, which are transmitted to the vertebrate host during blood feeding, making arthropods simultaneously vector and reservoir [36–39]. However, infection rates by *R. rickettsii* in ticks under natural conditions tend to be low (<1%), evidencing that *R. rickettsii* is pathogenic to ticks, and reinforcing the need of an amplifying host to ensure the maintenance of bacteria, such as capybaras, especially in endemic areas of São Paulo [40–44].

3.3. Amblyomma sculptum. In southeastern Brazil, the area with the highest concentration of BSF reports, the ecological setting in which the disease occurs is well described, including a voluminous population of *Amblyomma* ticks [21]. Horses and capybaras are among the most important primary hosts for all parasitic stages of *A. cajennense s.l.* [38, 45]. The capybara population has greatly increased in the state of São Paulo, and at this point it raises suspicions of its relationship to the emergence of BSF [44].

Although massive infestations with adult ticks occur in horses and capybaras in southeastern Brazil, nymphs of *A. cajennense s.l.* have shown better competence as vectors of

R. rickettsii experimentally [46, 47], which is important, since these stages have less requirements regarding their hosts including dogs and people [28, 29]. In fact, most human cases of BSF seem to occur during the nymphs season of *A. cajennense s.l.*, from July to November, possibly related to the aggressive behavior of nymphs, their effective spreading through the environment, and their small size, making their removal quite difficult [48].

3.4. Amblyomma aureolatum. *Amblyomma aureolatum* is yet another vector involved in BSF, with its ecological peculiarities. The "yellow dog tick" is found mainly in subtropical areas, with high humidity and mild temperatures throughout the year [49]. The population of *A. aureolatum* tends to be low and in southeastern Brazil, its distribution is restricted to Atlantic Forest, typically occurring in dogs with free access to rainforest [30, 49].

There are few reports of adults of *A. aureolatum* biting humans [50, 51]. Thus, human cases transmitted by *A. aureolatum* seem to occur when dogs get infected by adults of this tick during incursions into the rainforest and go on to carry *A. aureolatum* to their households [21]. However, experimentally, this tick was more susceptible to *R. rickettsii* infection and more efficient to maintain the pathogen by transstadial and transovarian transmission than *A. sculptum* [52]. Another study with experimental infection of *A. aureolatum* demonstrated that *R. rickettsii* was preserved between transstadial and transovarial stages in 100% of the *A. aureolatum* ticks for several consecutive generations, and larvae, nymphs, and adults transmitted *R. rickettsii* to susceptible guinea pigs [53]. Recently it was suggested that the adult *A. aureolatum* needs only approximately 10 minutes attached to the body of a vertebrate host to transmit *R. rickettsii* [35].

Note that in some areas of southeastern Brazil, particularly in areas of the state of São Paulo, *A. aureolatum* can replace *A. sculptum* as the main vector of *R. rickettsii* to humans, being even more effective in transmitting the pathogen [30, 31, 53].

3.5. Amblyomma ovale. In the past years, *A. ovale* has been implicated as a possible vector of new rickettsiosis in Brazil, since a human case of febrile disease with eschar (*tache noire*) was observed after tick biting in an Atlantic (ATL) Rainforest region of the state of São Paulo. Phylogenetic analysis revealed a new human rickettsiosis of the Spotted Fever Group (SFG), named ATL Rainforest Rickettsiosis, distinct from that caused by *R. rickettsia* [54]. Due to its phylogenetic similarity to *R. parkeri*, this new strain was called *R. parkeri* strain ATL Rainforest, which has been detected naturally infecting *A. ovale* ticks [55, 56]. So far *A. triste* was the vector associated with infection by *R. parkeri* in South America, including Brazil [57, 58].

Experimentally, 100% of transstadial and transovarian transmission of *R. parkeri* to *A. ovale* was confirmed by PCR. Larvae and nymphs demonstrated high competence in transmission of the bacteria because all animals infested by these ticks' stages presented seroconversion when tested by IFA using *R. parkeri* antigens, but only half of the animals presented seroconversion after being infested by infected-adult

ticks. Reproductive parameters of infected *A. ovale* females were low when compared to uninfected females, indicating deleterious effect of *R. parkeri* on this tick [56].

Amplifier hosts and reservoir in the ATL Rainforest Rickettsiosis have not been determined so far, but small rodents were shown to be important for *A. ovale* immature stages and high seroconversion prevalence [59]. Krawczak [56] suggested that *A. ovale* is an important vector on the epidemiology of *R. parkeri* strain ATL Rainforest, since this tick is often found in the ATL Rainforest ecosystem. Moreover, human bites by adult *A. ovale* tick are common [50]. Thus, humans can become infected if bitten by ticks detached from the dogs, suggesting the importance of dogs from the forests of endemic areas, mainly infested with *A. ovale* ticks [21, 59].

Serology studies have reported that dogs seroconvert, attaining very high titers against *R. parkeri* antigens [55, 59, 60]. Furthermore, Medeiros et al. [60] reported identical sequences to *R. parkeri* strain ATL Rainforest in dogs coinfested with *A. ovale* ticks. So far, it can be supposed that some febrile human cases diagnosed as mild BSF were in fact ATL Rainforest Rickettsiosis [59].

3.6. Rhipicephalus sanguineus. The "brown dog tick" is possibly the tick with greater distribution, inhabiting urban and rural environments where dogs and humans live [18]. It is a three-host tick that feeds primarily on dogs and occasionally on other hosts [61]. Participation of *Rh. sanguineus* in the transmission of BSF is still a source of speculation, although this tick is already an important vector and reservoir of *R. conorii* responsible for the Mediterranean Spotted Fever in Europe, Africa, and Asia [21].

In Brazil, human parasitism by *Rh. sanguineus* has been reported [61] but is still considered a rare event, particularly considering the close proximity of these ticks with man [51, 61]. Natural infection of *Rh. sanguineus* by *R. rickettsii* in Brazil has been observed in endemic areas for BSF [30, 33, 62]. And even if the transmission to humans has not been proven yet, there is a favorable outlook in urban areas where *Rh. sanguineus* is often found in pet or stray dogs [21]. Furthermore, these dogs can often move between urban and rural farming areas, being parasitized by ticks from both environments [30].

It is noteworthy that *Rh. sanguineus* tends to be less aggressive to man, making the transmission occasional, particularly for those dealing with dogs most of the time [21].

The traditional mechanism by which the tick gets infected by *R. rickettsia* is during blood feeding of the vertebrate host or by transstadial and transovarian transmission [36, 37]. However, under natural conditions, low infection rates among tick populations suggest that these mechanisms are not enough to maintain the pathogen in the ecosystem [40, 41]. It is important to consider that *R. rickettsii* is pathogenic to the tick, causing decreased fertility and death [41]. Cofeeding transmission of *R. rickettsii* is not fully elucidated but may have an important role in the transmission of bacteria among ticks that feed in close proximity at the same host [39].

Considering that dogs can become infected by *A. aureolatum* during incursions into the rainforest and that bacteria-infected *A. aureolatum* can remain on the dog for several weeks, it is possible that tick-infested dogs carry infected ticks back to human households. The ticks may then drop off from the dog, contaminate the household environment, and accidentally bite humans. In a different scenario, *Rh. sanguineus* ticks can become infected by cofeeding on the same dog with infected *A. aureolatum* ticks [21, 49, 59].

4. *Rickettsia rickettsii* Infection in Dogs and the Role of Sentinels in Brazil

Clinical disease caused by *R. rickettsii* in dogs is not easy to diagnose and has not been well described in South America, with few cases reported in the state of São Paulo, Brazil [7, 63].

Experimentally, dogs developed clinical illness characterized by fever, lethargy, anorexia, bilateral ocular discharge, scleral congestion, conjunctival edema, thrombocytopenia, and anemia [64]. *Rickettsia rickettsii*-reactive antibodies were shown in serum samples, and rickettsial DNA was detectable in blood 3 to 13 days after infection, indicating that a Brazilian strain of *R. rickettsii* is pathogenic for dogs [64].

Dogs, which remain close to both humans and naturally infected areas, can play a role as sentinels in an epidemiological approach [34, 65]. The use of serological methods for the detection of anti-*Rickettsia* spp. antibodies in dogs has been reported in several Brazilian states, especially in the southeast [9, 32, 34, 62, 66].

According to Cunha et al. [34], the dog's habit of entering rainforest regions and living in rural environments indicated a risk factor to the presence of anti-SFG rickettsiae antibodies.

Although SFG species share antigens that might cause group reactive serological responses, IFA is a highly sensitive and specific technique, used as the method of choice in serosurvey and screening tests in Brazil [67, 68]. In addition, if serology to several SFG antigens demonstrates titers to one antigen at least fourfold higher than the others, we can assume which pathogen stimulated the immune response [9]. High titers to *R. rickettsii* in endemic areas for BSF, up to 1 : 4096, or more, reinforce this hypothesis [34].

Clinical signs in dogs and humans may be similar, in such a way that the disease in dogs can precede the disease in humans, reinforcing the role of dogs as sentinels of BSF, a hypothesis that becomes stronger in USA, where cases of *R. rickettsii* in dogs and their owners have been found [8, 69, 70].

In Brazil, canine monocytic ehrlichiosis (CME), caused by *Ehrlichia canis*, is the most common tick-transmitted canine disease [71]. As many clinical and laboratorial findings described in CME, fever, depression, petechial hemorrhage, and thrombocytopenia, are also described in dogs infected by *R. rickettsii* [72], and given that doxycycline is the treatment of choice for both diseases, it is possible that rickettsial infection in dogs is being misdiagnosed as CME [7, 9, 72].

Differential diagnosis is a great challenge, because dogs may present with subclinical infections or nonspecific clinical signs, often misdiagnosed as other diseases transmitted by arthropods like CME, Lyme's disease, babesiosis, leishmaniasis, anaplasmosis, and any febrile disease of unspecified etiology [73].

According to Labruna et al. [7], definitive diagnosis of naturally infected dogs is based on (1) serological analysis of paired samples; (2) anti-*R. rickettsii* titers fourfold higher than other spotted-fever group antigens occurring in Brazil; (3) rickettsial DNA detection in blood; (4) both clinical and laboratorial findings compatible with the disease; (5) doxycycline responsive treatment; and (6) epidemiological history with tick infestation and exposure to endemic areas.

Besides the dog, authors have attempted to elucidate the role of other domestic animals as sentinels of the BSF. Horses, considered primary hosts of *A. cajennense s.l.*, are also an important object of study in the epidemiology of the disease.

Participation of horses as sentinels of infections caused by SFG has also been reported. One study suggested the ecological importance of cart horses as sentinels for BSF, since these horses are extensively used for transporting humans and heavy loads in urban and rural areas, being heavily infested with ticks [74]. Vianna et al. [75] believed that horses could be better sentinels to *R. rickettsii* than dogs, due to the presence of antibodies anti-*R. rickettsii* in 100% of the equine sera tested by IFA. However, Cunha et al. [34] after serosurvey in human foci of BSF observed that if the vector is not *A. sculptum*, horses present low serological reaction rate, which rules out these animals as good sentinels, while dogs can perform the role of sentinel for different vectors, since they can be parasitized by *A. sculptum*, *A. aureolatum*, *A. ovale*, and *Rh. sanguineus*. This was reinforced by other studies in the state of São Paulo, which observed a higher frequency of horses with positive serology in areas with strong evidence that the main vector was *A. cajennense s.l.* [66].

5. Conclusion and Perspectives

Ticks of domestic animals may be involved in the epidemiology of several vector-borne diseases, which also affect humans. Even though the dogs are not the main host for *R. rickettsii*, they may carry infected ticks into the human dwellings. One of the most effective ways to assess the evidence of SFG pathogens circulation in sentinel animals is through serological tests, among which the IFA has been widely employed in dogs, particularly because of the easy access to samples, their intimate relationship with man, and parasitism by the same ticks.

Due to this challenging outlook it is possible that BSF in dogs is underestimated, since the nonspecific clinical signs may get confused with EMC, which is the most prevalent tick-borne disease in dogs. As doxycycline is an effective treatment for patients with BSF or EMC, it is possible that dogs with acute febrile illness are not being routinely molecularly tested for BSF, since its cost is a limiting factor. Veterinarians should include rickettsial infections in the differential diagnosis of CME and other febrile diseases of nonspecific signs transmitted by common ticks, facilitating monitoring of BSF, since it is an important zoonosis with human fatalities when the diagnosis is delayed and treatment cannot be implemented in time.

Serology of these dogs could indicate prior exposure to rickettsial agents by the presence of IgG antibodies even before the reporting of human cases of BSF, warning about circulation of the bacteria, which added to the knowledge of the presence of ticks could help to improve BSF monitoring.

When physicians, veterinarians, and other health professionals face every challenge the same way, they will understand that the traditional mechanisms for the study of diseases are full of unresolved gaps that can be addressed with interdisciplinary actions.

Conflict of Interests

The authors declare that there is no conflict of interests regarding the publication of this paper.

Acknowledgments

The authors are thankful to CNPq, Capes, and Faperj for the financial support.

References

[1] S. Harrus and G. Baneth, "Drivers for the emergence and re-emergence of vector-borne protozoal and bacterial diseases," *International Journal for Parasitology*, vol. 35, no. 11-12, pp. 1309–1318, 2005.

[2] D. D. Colwell, F. Dantas-Torres, and D. Otranto, "Vector-borne parasitic zoonoses: emerging scenarios and new perspectives," *Veterinary Parasitology*, vol. 182, no. 1, pp. 14–21, 2011.

[3] World Organisation for Animal Health (OIE), *Contributing to One World, One Health. A Strategic Framework for Reducing Risks of Infectious Diseases at the Animal-Human-Ecosystems Interface*, World Organisation for Animal Health (OIE), Paris, France, 2008.

[4] A. K. Silveira and A. H. Fonseca, *Caracterização de Ambientes com Potencial para Ocorrência de Carrapatos Transmissores de Agentes Patogênicos para Humanos*, vol. 13 of *Boletim do Parque Nacional Do Itatiaia*, Ministério do Meio Ambiente, Instituto Chico Mendes de Conservação da Biodiversidade, ICMBio, 2011.

[5] L. E. Shaffer, "Role of surveillance in disease prevention and control: crossspecies surveillance contribution to one medicine," in *Proceedings of the 145th AVMA Annual Convention*, Schaumburg, Ill, USA, July 2008.

[6] D. H. Walker, "*Rickettsia rickettsii*: as virulent as ever," *The American Journal of Tropical Medicine and Hygiene*, vol. 66, no. 5, pp. 448–449, 2002.

[7] M. B. Labruna, O. Kamakura, J. Moraes-Filho, M. C. Horta, and R. C. Pacheco, "Rocky mountain spotted fever in dogs, Brazil," *Emerging Infectious Diseases*, vol. 15, no. 3, pp. 458–460, 2009.

[8] C. D. Paddock, O. Brenner, C. Vaid et al., "Short report: concurrent Rocky Mountain spotted fever in a dog and its owner," *The American Journal of Tropical Medicine and Hygiene*, vol. 66, no. 2, pp. 197–199, 2002.

[9] A. Pinter, M. C. Horta, R. C. Pacheco, J. Moraes-Filho, and M. B. Labruna, "Serosurvey of *Rickettsia* spp. in dogs and humans from an endemic area for Brazilian spotted fever in the State of São Paulo, Brazil," *Cadernos de Saúde Pública*, vol. 24, no. 2, pp. 247–252, 2008.

[10] P. D. Van Helden, L. S. Van Helden, and E. G. Hoal, "One world, one health: humans, animals and the environment are inextricably linked—a fact that needs to be remembered and exploited in our modern approach to health," *EMBO Reports*, vol. 14, no. 6, pp. 497–501, 2013.

[11] K. E. Jones, N. G. Patel, M. A. Levy et al., "Global trends in emerging infectious diseases," *Nature*, vol. 451, no. 7181, pp. 990–993, 2008.

[12] D. Frank, "One world, one health, one medicine," *Canadian Veterinary Journal*, vol. 49, no. 11, pp. 1063–1065, 2008.

[13] J. Childs, R. E. Shope, D. Fish et al., "Emerging zoonoses," *Emerging Infectious Diseases*, vol. 4, no. 3, pp. 453–454, 1998.

[14] D. A. Jessup, M. A. Miller, C. Kreuder-Johnson et al., "Sea otters in a dirty ocean," *Journal of the American Veterinary Medical Association*, vol. 231, no. 11, pp. 1648–1652, 2007.

[15] P. M. R. Barros-Silva, L. X. Fonseca, M. E. Carneiro, K. M. A. Vilges, S. V. Oliveira, and R. Gurgel-Gonçalves, "Occupational risk of spotted fever: an evaluation of knowledge, attitudes and prevention practices among veterinary medicine students," *Revista de Patologia Tropical*, vol. 43, no. 4, pp. 389–397, 2014.

[16] A. S. Chapman, S. M. Murphy, L. J. Demma et al., "Rocky Mountain spotted fever in the United States, 1997–2002," *Vector-Borne and Zoonotic Diseases*, vol. 6, no. 2, pp. 170–178, 2006.

[17] D. Estripeaut, M. G. Aramburú, X. Sáez-Llorens et al., "Rocky Mountain spotted fever, Panama," *Emerging Infectious Diseases*, vol. 13, no. 11, pp. 1763–1765, 2007.

[18] D. Raoult and P. Parola, *Rickettsial Diseases (Infectious Disease and Therapy)*, CRC Press, New York, NY, USA, 2007.

[19] L. Hun, X. Cortés, and L. Taylor, "Molecular characterization of Rickettsia rickettsii isolated from human clinical samples and from the rabbit tick *Haemaphysalis leporispalustris* collected at different geographic zones in Costa Rica," *American Journal of Tropical Medicine and Hygiene*, vol. 79, no. 6, pp. 899–902, 2008.

[20] M. E. Eremeeva, E. Berganza, G. Suarez et al., "Investigation of an outbreak of rickettsial febrile illness in Guatemala, 2007," *International Journal of Infectious Diseases*, vol. 17, no. 5, pp. e304–e311, 2013.

[21] M. P. J. Szabó, A. Pinter, and M. B. Labruna, "Ecology, biology and distribution of spotted-fever tick vectors in Brazil," *Frontiers in Cellular and Infection Microbiology*, vol. 3, no. 27, pp. 1–9, 2013.

[22] E. Dias and A. V. Martins, "Spotted fever in Brazil," *American Journal of Tropical Medicine*, no. 19, pp. 103–108, 1939.

[23] E. R. S. De Lemos, F. B. F. Alvarenga, M. L. Cintra et al., "Spotted fever in Brazil: a seroepidemiological study and description of clinical cases in an endemic area in the state of São Paulo," *The American Journal of Tropical Medicine and Hygiene*, vol. 65, no. 4, pp. 329–334, 2001.

[24] M. A. M. Galvão, "Diagnósticos e inquéritos sorológicos para riquetsioses do gênero rickettsia no Brasil," *Revista Brasileira de Parasitologia Veterinária*, vol. 13, no. 1, pp. 188–189, 2004.

[25] J. Brites-Neto, F. A. Nieri-Bastos, J. Brasil et al., "Environmental infestation and rickettsial infection in ticks in an area endemic for Brazilian spotted fever," *Revista Brasileira de Parasitologia Veterinaria*, vol. 22, no. 3, pp. 367–372, 2013.

[26] T. F. Martins, A. R. M. Barbieri, F. B. Costa et al., "Estudo do complexo *Amblyomma cajennense* (Acari: Ixodidae) no Brasil," *BEPA, Boletim Epidemiológico Paulista*, vol. 10, no. 117, pp. 8–13, 2013.

[27] S. Nava, L. Beati, M. B. Labruna, A. G. Cáceres, A. J. Mangold, and A. A. Guglielmone, "Reassessment of the taxonomic status of *Amblyomma cajennense* (Fabricius, 1787) with the description of three new species, *Amblyomma tonelliae* n. sp., *Amblyomma interandinum* n. sp. and *Amblyomma patinoi* n. sp., and reinstatement of *Amblyomma mixtum* Koch, 1844, and *Amblyomma sculptum* Berlese, 1888 (Ixodida: Ixodidae)," *Ticks and Tick-Borne Diseases*, vol. 5, no. 3, pp. 252–276, 2014.

[28] M. B. Labruna, C. E. Kerber, F. Ferreira, J. L. Faccini, D. T. De Waal, and S. M. Gennari, "Risk factors to tick infestations and their occurrence on horses in the state of São Paulo, Brazil," *Veterinary Parasitology*, vol. 97, no. 1, pp. 1–14, 2001.

[29] M. B. Labruna, "Ecology of *Rickettsia* in South America," *Annals of the New York Academy of Sciences*, vol. 1166, pp. 156–166, 2009.

[30] M. Ogrzewalska, D. G. Saraiva, J. Moraes-Filho et al., "Epidemiology of Brazilian spotted fever in the Atlantic Forest, state of Sao Paulo, Brazil," *Parasitology*, vol. 139, no. 10, pp. 1283–1300, 2012.

[31] A. Pinter and M. B. Labruna, "Isolation of *Rickettsia rickettsii* and *Rickettsia bellii* in cell culture from the tick *Amblyomma aureolatum* in Brazil," *Annals of the New York Academy of Sciences*, vol. 1078, pp. 523–529, 2006.

[32] J. Moraes-Filho, A. Pinter, R. C. Pacheco et al., "New epidemiological data on Brazilian spotted fever in an endemic area of the state of São Paulo, Brazil," *Vector-Borne and Zoonotic Diseases*, vol. 9, no. 1, pp. 73–78, 2009.

[33] N. C. Cunha, A. H. Fonseca, J. Rezende et al., "First identification of natural infection of *Rickettsia rickettsii* in the *Rhipicephalus sanguineus* tick, in the State of Rio de Janeiro," *Pesquisa Veterinaria Brasileira*, vol. 29, no. 2, pp. 105–108, 2009.

[34] N. C. Cunha, E. R. S. Lemos, T. Rozental et al., "Rickettsiae of the Spotted Fever group in dogs, horses and ticks: an epidemiological study in an endemic region of the State of Rio de Janeiro, Brazil," *Revista Brasileira de Medicina Veterinária*, vol. 36, no. 3, pp. 294–300, 2014.

[35] D. G. Saraiva, H. S. Soares, J. F. Soares, and M. B. Labruna, "Feeding period required by *Amblyomma aureolatum* ticks for transmission of *Rickettsia rickettsii* to vertebrate hosts," *Emerging Infectious Diseases*, vol. 20, no. 9, pp. 1504–1510, 2014.

[36] D. Raoult and V. Roux, "Rickettsioses as paradigms of new or emerging infectious diseases," *Clinical Microbiology Reviews*, vol. 10, no. 4, pp. 694–719, 1997.

[37] M. A. M. Galvão, L. J. da Silva, E. M. Mendes Nascimento, S. B. Calic, R. de Sousa, and F. Bacellar, "Riquetsioses no Brasil e Portugal: ocorrência, distribuição e diagnóstico," *Revista de Saude Publica*, vol. 39, no. 5, pp. 850–856, 2005.

[38] E. Guedes, R. C. Leite, M. C. A. Prata, R. C. Pacheco, D. H. Walker, and M. B. Labruna, "Detection of *Rickettsia rickettsii* in the tick *Amblyomma cajennense* in a new Brazilian spotted fever-endemic area in the state of Minas Gerais," *Memórias do Instituto Oswaldo Cruz*, vol. 100, no. 8, pp. 841–845, 2005.

[39] P. Parola, C. D. Paddock, and D. Raoult, "Tick-borne rickettsioses around the world: emerging diseases challenging old concepts," *Clinical Microbiology Reviews*, vol. 18, no. 4, pp. 719–756, 2005.

[40] J. E. McDade and V. F. Newhouse, "Natural history of *Rickettsia rickettsii*," *Annual Review of Microbiology*, vol. 40, pp. 287–309, 1986.

[41] M. L. Niebylski, M. G. Peacock, and T. G. Schwan, "Lethal effect of *Rickettsia rickettsii* on its tick vector (*Dermacentor andersoni*)," *Applied and Environmental Microbiology*, vol. 65, no. 2, pp. 773–778, 1999.

[42] M. B. Labruna, T. Whitworth, M. C. Horta et al., "Rickettsia species infecting *Amblyomma cooperi* ticks from an area in the state of São Paulo, Brazil, where Brazilian Spotted Fever is endemic," *Journal of Clinical Microbiology*, vol. 42, no. 1, pp. 90–98, 2004.

[43] R. C. Pacheco, M. C. Horta, J. Moraes-Filho, A. C. Ataliba, A. Pinter, and M. B. Labruna, "Rickettsial infection in capybaras (*Hydrochoerus hydrochaeris*) from São Paulo, Brazil: serological evidence for infection by *Rickettsia bellii* and *Rickettsia parkeri*," *Biomédica*, vol. 27, no. 3, pp. 364–371, 2007.

[44] C. E. Souza, J. Moraes-Filho, M. Ogrzewalska et al., "Experimental infection of capybaras *Hydrochoerus hydrochaeris* by *Rickettsia rickettsii* and evaluation of the transmission of the infection to ticks *Amblyomma cajennense*," *Veterinary Parasitology*, vol. 161, no. 1-2, pp. 116–121, 2009.

[45] A. M. L. Vieira, C. E. Souza, M. B. Labruna, R. C. Mayo, S. S. L. Souza, and V. L. F. Camargo-Neves, *Manual de Vigilância Acarológica, Estado de São Paulo*, Secretaria de Saúde, Estado da São Paulo, São Paulo, Brazil, 2004.

[46] D. M. Barros-Battesti, M. Arzua, and G. H. Bechara, *Carrapatos de Importancia Médico-Veterinaria da Regiao Neotropical: Um Guia Ilustrado Para Identificação de Espécies*, Vox/ICTTD-3/Butantan, São Paulo, Brazil, 2006.

[47] J. F. Soares, H. S. Soares, A. M. Barbieri, and M. B. Labruna, "Experimental infection of the tick *Amblyomma cajennense*, cayenne tick, with *Rickettsia rickettsii*, the agent of Rocky Mountain spotted fever," *Medical and Veterinary Entomology*, vol. 26, no. 2, pp. 139–151, 2012.

[48] A. Pinter, A. C. França, C. E. Souza et al., "Febre Maculosa Brasileira," *BEPA Suplemento*, vol. 8, no. 1, pp. 3–31, 2011.

[49] A. Pinter, R. A. Dias, S. M. Gennari, and M. B. Labruna, "Study of the seasonal dynamics, life cycle, and host specificity of *Amblyomma aureolatum* (Acari: Ixodidae)," *Journal of Medical Entomology*, vol. 41, no. 3, pp. 324–332, 2004.

[50] A. A. Guglielmone, L. Beati, D. M. Barros-Battesti et al., "Ticks (Ixodidae) on humans in South America," *Experimental and Applied Acarology*, vol. 40, no. 2, pp. 83–100, 2006.

[51] N. M. Serra-Freire, "Occurrence of ticks (Acari: Ixodidae) on human hosts, in three municipalities in the State of Pará, Brazil," *Revista Brasileira de Parasitologia Veterinaria*, vol. 19, no. 3, pp. 141–147, 2010.

[52] M. B. Labruna, M. Ogrzewalska, T. F. Martins, A. Pinter, and M. C. Horta, "Comparative susceptibility of larval stages of *Amblyomma aureolatum*, *Amblyomma cajennense*, and *Rhipicephalus sanguineus* to infection by *Rickettsia rickettsii*," *Journal of Medical Entomology*, vol. 45, no. 6, pp. 1156–1159, 2008.

[53] M. B. Labruna, M. Ogrzewalska, J. F. Soares et al., "Experimental infection of *Amblyomma aureolatum* ticks with *Rickettsia rickettsii*," *Emerging Infectious Diseases*, vol. 17, no. 5, pp. 829–834, 2011.

[54] M. G. Spolidorio, M. B. Labruna, E. Mantovani, P. E. Brandão, L. J. Richtzenhain, and N. H. Yoshinari, "Novel spotted fever group rickettsiosis, Brazil," *Emerging Infectious Diseases*, vol. 16, no. 3, pp. 521–523, 2010.

[55] G. S. Sabatini, A. Pinter, F. A. Nieri-Bastos, A. Marcili, and M. B. Labruna, "Survey of ticks (Acari: Ixodidae) and their rickettsia in an Atlantic rain forest reserve in the state of São Paulo, Brazil," *Journal of Medical Entomology*, vol. 47, no. 5, pp. 913–916, 2010.

[56] F. S. Krawczak, *Avaliação da dinâmica da infecção por Rickettsia parkeri cepa Mata Atlântica, agente etiológico de uma nova riquetsiose brasileira, em carrapatos Amblyomma ovale Koch, 1844 naturalmente infectados [M.S. dissertation]*, Universidade de São Paulo, São Paulo, Brazil, 2012, http://www.teses.usp.br/teses/disponiveis/10/10134/tde-11062013-155536/pt-br.php.

[57] Y. Romer, A. C. Seijo, F. Crudo et al., "*Rickettsia parkeri* rickettsiosis, Argentina," *Emerging Infectious Diseases*, vol. 17, no. 7, pp. 1169–1173, 2011.

[58] I. Silveira, R. C. Pacheco, M. P. J. Szabó, H. G. C. Ramos, and M. B. Labruna, "*Rickettsia parkeri* in Brazil," *Emerging Infectious Diseases*, vol. 13, no. 7, pp. 1111–1113, 2007.

[59] M. P. J. Szabó, F. A. Nieri-Bastos, M. G. Spolidorio, T. F. Martins, A. M. Barbieri, and M. B. Labruna, "*In vitro* isolation from *Amblyomma ovale* (Acari: Ixodidae) and ecological aspects of the Atlantic rainforest *Rickettsia*, the causative agent of a novel spotted fever rickettsiosis in Brazil," *Parasitology*, vol. 140, no. 6, pp. 719–728, 2013.

[60] A. P. Medeiros, A. P. de Souza, A. B. de Moura et al., "Spotted fever group *Rickettsia* infecting ticks (Acari: Ixodidae) in the state of Santa Catarina, Brazil," *Memórias do Instituto Oswaldo Cruz*, vol. 106, no. 8, pp. 926–930, 2011.

[61] F. Dantas-Torres, L. A. Figueredo, and S. P. Brandão-Filho, "*Rhipicephalus sanguineus* (Acari: Ixodidae), o carrapato vermelho do cão, parasitando humanos no Brasil," *Revista da Sociedade Brasileira de Medicina Tropical*, vol. 39, pp. 64–67, 2006.

[62] R. C. Pacheco, J. Moraes-Filho, E. Guedes et al., "Rickettsial infections of dogs, horses and ticks in Juiz de Fora, southeastern Brazil, and isolation of *Rickettsia rickettsii* from *Rhipicephalus sanguineus* ticks," *Medical and Veterinary Entomology*, vol. 25, no. 2, pp. 148–155, 2011.

[63] P. Parola, C. D. Paddock, C. Socolovschi et al., "Update on tick-borne rickettsioses around the world: a geographic approach," *Clinical Microbiology Reviews*, vol. 26, no. 4, pp. 657–702, 2013.

[64] E. M. Piranda, J. L. H. Faccini, A. Pinter et al., "Experimental infection of dogs with a Brazilian strain of *Rickettsia rickettsii*: clinical and laboratory findings," *Memorias do Instituto Oswaldo Cruz*, vol. 103, no. 7, pp. 696–701, 2008.

[65] L. D. Cardoso, R. N. Freitas, C. L. Mafra et al., "Caracterização de *Rickettsia* spp. circulante em foco silencioso de febre maculosa brasileira no município de Caratinga, Minas Gerais, Brasil," *Cadernos de Saúde Pública*, vol. 22, no. 3, pp. 495–501, 2006.

[66] M. C. Horta, M. B. Labruna, A. Pinter, P. M. Linardi, and T. T. S. Schumaker, "*Rickettsia* infection in five areas of the state of São Paulo, Brazil," *Memórias do Instituto Oswaldo Cruz*, vol. 102, no. 7, pp. 793–801, 2007.

[67] V. M. F. Del Guercio, M. M. M. Rocha, H. H. B. Melles, V. C. L. Lima, and M. G. Pignatti, "Febre maculosa no município de Pedreira, SP, Brasil. Inquérito sorológico," *Revista da Sociedade Brasileira de Medicina Tropical*, vol. 30, no. 1, pp. 47–52, 1997.

[68] H. H. Melles, S. Colombo, and E. R. S. Lemos, "Isolamento de rickettsia em cultura de célula vero," *Revista da Sociedade Brasileira de Medicina Tropical*, vol. 32, no. 5, pp. 469–473, 1999.

[69] L. Kidd, B. Hegarty, D. Sexton, and E. Breitschwerdt, "Molecular characterization of *Rickettsia rickettsii* infecting dogs and people in North Carolina," *Annals of the New York Academy of Sciences*, vol. 1078, pp. 400–409, 2006.

[70] B. N. Elchos and J. Goddard, "Implications of presumptive fatal Rocky Mountain spotted fever in two dogs and their owner," *Journal of the American Veterinary Medical Association*, vol. 223, no. 10, pp. 1450–1452, 2003.

[71] D. M. Aguiar, G. T. Cavalcante, A. Pinter, S. M. Gennari, L. M. A. Camargo, and M. B. Labruna, "Prevalence of *Ehrlichia canis* (Rickettsiales: Anaplasmataceae) in dogs and *Rhipicephalus sanguineus* (Acari: Ixodidae) ticks from Brazil," *Journal of Medical Entomology*, vol. 44, no. 1, pp. 126–132, 2007.

[72] C. B. Grindem, E. B. Breitschwerdt, P. C. Perkins, L. D. Cullins, T. J. Thomas, and B. C. Hegarty, "Platelet-associated immunoglobulin (antiplatelet antibody) in canine rocky mountain spotted fever and ehrlichiosis," *Journal of the American Animal Hospital Association*, vol. 35, no. 1, pp. 56–61, 1999.

[73] F. Dantas-Torres, "Canine vector-borne diseases in Brazil," *Parasites and Vectors*, vol. 1, no. 1, article 25, 2008.

[74] B. S. Milagres, A. F. Padilha, R. M. Barcelos et al., "*Rickettsia* in synanthropic and domestic animals and their hosts from two areas of low endemicity for Brazilian spotted fever in the Eastern Region of Minas Gerais, Brazil," *The American Journal of Tropical Medicine and Hygiene*, vol. 83, no. 6, pp. 1305–1307, 2010.

[75] M. C. B. Vianna, M. C. Horta, L. A. Sangioni et al., "Rickettsial spotted fever in Capoeirão village, Itabira, Minas Gerais, Brazil," *Revista do Instituto de Medicina Tropical de Sao Paulo*, vol. 50, no. 5, pp. 297–301, 2008.

Permissions

The contributors of this book come from diverse backgrounds, making this book a truly international effort. This book will bring forth new frontiers with its revolutionizing research information and detailed analysis of the nascent developments around the world.

We would like to thank all the contributing authors for lending their expertise to make the book truly unique. They have played a crucial role in the development of this book. Without their invaluable contributions this book wouldn't have been possible. They have made vital efforts to compile up to date information on the varied aspects of this subject to make this book a valuable addition to the collection of many professionals and students.

This book was conceptualized with the vision of imparting up-to-date information and advanced data in this field. To ensure the same, a matchless editorial board was set up. Every individual on the board went through rigorous rounds of assessment to prove their worth. After which they invested a large part of their time researching and compiling the most relevant data for our readers.

The editorial board has been involved in producing this book since its inception. They have spent rigorous hours researching and exploring the diverse topics which have resulted in the successful publishing of this book. They have passed on their knowledge of decades through this book. To expedite this challenging task, the publisher supported the team at every step. A small team of assistant editors was also appointed to further simplify the editing procedure and attain best results for the readers.

Apart from the editorial board, the designing team has also invested a significant amount of their time in understanding the subject and creating the most relevant covers. They scrutinized every image to scout for the most suitable representation of the subject and create an appropriate cover for the book.

The publishing team has been an ardent support to the editorial, designing and production team. Their endless efforts to recruit the best for this project, has resulted in the accomplishment of this book. They are a veteran in the field of academics and their pool of knowledge is as vast as their experience in printing. Their expertise and guidance has proved useful at every step. Their uncompromising quality standards have made this book an exceptional effort. Their encouragement from time to time has been an inspiration for everyone.

The publisher and the editorial board hope that this book will prove to be a valuable piece of knowledge for researchers, students, practitioners and scholars across the globe.

List of Contributors

Linda G. Shell, Belle M. Nibblett and Patrick Kelly
Department of Clinical Sciences, Ross University School of Veterinary Medicine (RUSVM), P.O. Box 334, Basseterre, Saint Kitts and Nevis

John Berezowski
Department of Biomedical Sciences, Ross University School of Veterinary Medicine (RUSVM), P.O. Box 334, Basseterre, Saint Kitts and Nevis
Veterinary Public Health Institute, Swiss Veterinary Faculty, University of Bern, Hochschulstrasse 4, 3012 Bern, Switzerland

Mark Rishniw
Department of Clinical Studies, Cornell University, 602 Tower Road, Ithaca, NY 14853, USA

T. K. W. Sikombe
Department of Disease Control, School of Veterinary Medicine, University of Zambia, P.O. Box 32379, Lusaka, Zambia
Central Veterinary Research Institute, P.O. Box 33980, Lusaka, Zambia

A. S. Mweene, John Muma and M. Simuunza
Department of Disease Control, School of Veterinary Medicine, University of Zambia, P.O. Box 32379, Lusaka, Zambia

C. Kasanga
Faculty of Veterinary Medicine, Sokoine University of Agriculture, P.O. Box 3021, Morogoro, Tanzania

Y. Sinkala
Department of Disease Control, School of Veterinary Medicine, University of Zambia, P.O. Box 32379, Lusaka, Zambia
National Livestock Epidemiology and Information Centre, P.O. Box 30041, Lusaka, Zambia

F. Banda
Central Veterinary Research Institute, P.O. Box 33980, Lusaka, Zambia

M. Mulumba
Southern African Development Community Secretariat, SADC House, Plot No. 54385, Central Business District, Private Bag 0095, Gaborone, Botswana

E. M. Fana
Botswana Vaccine Institute, Private Bag 0031, Gaborone, Botswana

C. Mundia
Department of Veterinary Services, Southern African Development Community, Trans-Boundary Animal Disease Section, Ministry of Agriculture and Livestock, P.O. Box 50060, Lusaka, Zambia

Diana L. Ríos, Catalina López and Jorge U. Carmona
Grupo de Investigación Terapia Regenerativa, Departamento de Salud Animal, Universidad de Caldas, Calle 65 No. 26-10, Manizales, Colombia

Amin Tamadon
Transgenic Technology Research Center, Shiraz University of Medical Sciences, Shiraz, Iran

Alireza Raayat Jahromi and Mohammad Ayaseh
Department of Clinical Sciences, School of Veterinary Medicine, Shiraz University, P.O. Box 1731-71345, Shiraz, Iran

Omid Koohi-Hosseinabadi
Laboratory Animal Center, Shiraz University of Medical Sciences, Shiraz, Iran

Reza Moghiminasr
Department of Stem Cells and Developmental Biology, Cell Science Research Center, Royan Institute for Stem Cell Biology and Technology, ACECR, Tehran, Iran

Farhad Rahmanifar
Department of Basic Sciences, School of Veterinary Medicine, Shiraz University, P.O. Box 1731-71345, Shiraz, Iran

Arvind Kumar Sharma, Amit Kumar and Shara Kumar Yadav
Department of Veterinary Microbiology, College of Veterinary Sciences and Animal Husbandry, Uttar Pradesh Pandit Deen Dayal Upadhyaya Pashu Chikitsa Vigyan Vishwavidyalaya Evam Go Anusandhan Sansthan (DUVASU), Mathura 281001, India

Anu Rahal
Department of Veterinary Pharmacology and Toxicology, College of Veterinary Sciences and Animal Husbandry, Uttar Pradesh Pandit Deen Dayal Upadhyaya Pashu Chikitsa Vigyan Vishwavidyalaya Evam Go Anusandhan Sansthan (DUVASU), Mathura 281001, India

Ashraf M. Abu-Seida
Department of Surgery, Anesthesiology & Radiology, Faculty of Veterinary Medicine, Cairo University, Giza 12211, Egypt

Supot Noopataya
Department of Veterinary Public Health, Faculty of Veterinary Medicine, Kasetsart University, Kamphaeng Saen Campus, Nakhon Pathom 73140, Thailand
Department of Livestock Development, Ministry of Agriculture and Cooperatives, Bangkok 10400, Thailand

Sukanya Thongratsakul and Chaithep Poolkhet
Department of Veterinary Public Health, Faculty of Veterinary Medicine, Kasetsart University, Kamphaeng Saen Campus, Nakhon Pathom 73140, Thailand

Ayman Atiba and Alaa Ghazy,
Department of Surgery, Anesthesiology and Radiology, Faculty of Veterinary Medicine, Kafrelsheikh University, Kafrelsheikh 33516, Egypt

Naglaa Gomaa
Department of Animal Medicine, Faculty of Veterinary Medicine, Kafrelsheikh University, Kafrelsheikh 33516, Egypt

Tarek Kamal
Department of Biochemistry, Faculty of Veterinary Medicine, Kafrelsheikh University, Kafrelsheikh 33516, Egypt

Mustafa Shukry
Department of Physiology, Faculty of Veterinary Medicine, Kafrelsheikh University, Kafrelsheikh 33516, Egypt

Faruku Bande
Department of Veterinary Pathology and Microbiology, Faculty of Veterinary Medicine, Universiti Putra Malaysia, 43400 UPM Serdang, Selangor, Malaysia
Department of Veterinary Services, Ministry of Animal Health and Fisheries Development, PMB 2109, Usman Faruk Secretariat, 840221 Sokoto, Sokoto State, Nigeria

Siti Suri Arshad and Zunita Zakaria
Department of Veterinary Pathology and Microbiology, Faculty of Veterinary Medicine, Universiti Putra Malaysia, 43400 UPM Serdang, Selangor, Malaysia

Latiffah Hassan
Department of Veterinary Laboratory Diagnostics, Faculty of Veterinary Medicine, Universiti Putra Malaysia, 43400 UPM Serdang, Selangor, Malaysia

Deniece R. Williams and John Champagne
Veterinary Medicine Teaching and Research Center, School of Veterinary Medicine, University of California, Davis, 18830 Road 112, Tulare, CA 93274, USA

Patrick Pithua
Department of Veterinary Medicine & Surgery, Veterinary Medicine Teaching Hospital, College of Veterinary Medicine, University of Missouri, 900 E. Campus Drive, Columbia, MO 65211, USA

Angel Garcia
Departamento de Producción y Sanidad Animal, Facultad de Veterinaria, Universidad CEU Cardenal Herrera, Moncada, 46113 Valencia, Spain

Deborah M. Haines
Department of Veterinary Microbiology, Western College of Veterinary Medicine, University of Saskatchewan, Saskatoon, SK, Canada S7N 5B4
The Saskatoon Colostrum Co. Ltd., 30Molaro Pl, Saskatoon, SK, Canada S7K 6A2

Sharif S. Aly
Veterinary Medicine Teaching and Research Center, School of Veterinary Medicine, University of California, Davis, 18830 Road 112, Tulare, CA 93274, USA
Department of Population Health and Reproduction, School of Veterinary Medicine, University of California, One Shields Avenue, Davis, CA 95616, USA

Mukhtar Taha Abu-Samra
Department of Veterinary Medicine and Surgery, College of Veterinary Medicine (CVM), Sudan University of Science and Technology (SUST), P.O. Box 204, Hilat Kuku, Khartoum North, Sudan

Yassir Adam Shuaib
Department of Preventive Veterinary Medicine, College of Veterinary Medicine (CVM), Sudan University of Science and Technology (SUST), P.O. Box 204, Hilat Kuku, Khartoum North, Sudan
Research Center Borstel, Parkallee 18, 23845 Borstel, Germany

Justin Shmalberg
Small Animal Clinical Sciences, College of Veterinary Medicine, University of Florida, Gainesville, FL 32608, USA

Mushtaq A. Memon
Department of Veterinary Clinical Sciences, College of Veterinary Medicine, Washington State University, Pullman, WA 99164, USA

Luca Lacitignola, Pasquale De Luca, Alessandro Guarracino and Antonio Crovace
Sezione di Cliniche Veterinarie e P.A., Dipartimento delle Emergenze e Trapianti di Organo, Università degli Studi di Bari "AldoMoro", s.p. per Casamassima km 3, Valenzano, 70010 Bari, Italy

Barbara Padalino
Department of Veterinary Medicine, University of Bari, Str. prov. Per Casamassima, km 3, 70010 Valenzano (Bari), Italy

Paola Zaccagnino
Dipartimento di Scienze delle Produzioni Animali, Università degli Studi della Basilicata, Via dell'Ateneo Lucano 10, 85100 Potenza, Italy

Pietro Celi
Faculty of Veterinary Science, University of Sydney, P.M.B. 4003, Narellan, NSW 2567, Australia
Melbourne School of Land and Environment, The University of Melbourne, Parkville, VIC 3010, Australia

J. J. Vargas-Duarte
Genetic Institute, National University of Colombia, Carrera 30 No. 45-03, Edificio 426, Bogotá D.C., Colombia
Unit of Integrated Veterinary Research, Department of Veterinary Medicine, University of Namur, rue de Bruxelles 61, 5000 Namur, Belgium

H. Lozano-Márquez
Unit of Integrated Veterinary Research, Department of Veterinary Medicine, University of Namur, rue de Bruxelles 61, 5000 Namur, Belgium
Faculty of Veterinary Medicine and Animal Science, National University of Colombia, Carrera 30 No. 45-03, Edificio 481, Bogotá D.C., Colombia

H. A. Grajales-Lombana and C. Manrique-Perdomo
Faculty of Veterinary Medicine and Animal Science, National University of Colombia, Carrera 30 No. 45-03, Edificio 481, Bogotá D.C., Colombia

D. A. Martínez-Bello
Faculty of Veterinary Medicine, Cooperative University of Colombia, Calle 30 No. 33-51, Bucaramanga, Colombia

C. Saegerman
Research Unit of Epidemiology and Risk Analysis Applied to Veterinary Sciences (UREAR), Fundamental and Applied Research for Animal and Health (FARAH), University of Liège, boulevard de Colonster 20, 4000 Liège, Belgium

M. Raes and N. Kirschvink
Unit of Integrated Veterinary Research, Department of Veterinary Medicine, University of Namur, rue de Bruxelles 61, 5000 Namur, Belgium

María Fernanda Posada-Guzmán
Maestría en Enfermedades Tropicales, Posgrado Regional en Ciencias Veterinarias Tropicales, Universidad Nacional, Campus Presb´ıtero Benjam´ın Nuñez, P.O. Box 86, 3000 Heredia, Costa Rica

Gaby Dolz
Maestría en Enfermedades Tropicales, Posgrado Regional en Ciencias Veterinarias Tropicales, Universidad Nacional, Campus Presbítero Benjamín Nuñez, P.O. Box 86, 3000 Heredia, Costa Rica
Programa de Investigación en Medicina Poblacional, Escuela de Medicina Veterinaria, Universidad Nacional, Campus Presbítero Benjamín Nuñez, P.O. Box 86, 3000 Heredia, Costa Rica

Juan José Romero-Zúñiga
Programa de Investigación en Medicina Poblacional, Escuela de Medicina Veterinaria, Universidad Nacional, Campus Presbítero Benjamín Nuñez, P.O. Box 86, 3000 Heredia, Costa Rica

Ana Eugenia Jiménez-Rocha
Laboratorio de Parasitología, Escuela de Medicina Veterinaria, Universidad Nacional, Campus Presbítero Benjamín Nuñez, P.O. Box 86, 3000 Heredia, Costa Rica

Y. Abba
Department of Veterinary Pathology, Faculty of Veterinary Medicine, University of Maiduguri, PMB 1069, Maiduguri 600233, Borno State, Nigeria
Department of Veterinary Pathology and Microbiology, Faculty of Veterinary Medicine, Universiti Putra Malaysia, 43400 Serdang, Selangor, Malaysia

I. O. Igbokwe
Department of Veterinary Pathology, Faculty of Veterinary Medicine, University of Maiduguri, PMB 1069, Maiduguri 600233, Borno State, Nigeria

Yu'e Wu, Fangui Min, Jinchun Pan, Jing Wang, Wen Yuan, Yu Zhang and Ren Huang
Guangdong Laboratory Animals Monitoring Institute, Guangdong Provincial Key Laboratory of Laboratory Animals, Guangzhou 510663, China

Lixin Zhang
Institute of Microbiology, Chinese Academy of Sciences, Beijing 100080, China

David Miller
P.O. Box 2786, Loveland, CO 80539-2786, USA

Bradford Jackson
University of Alabama at Birmingham, Birmingham, AL, USA

Heidi S. Riddle
Riddle's Elephant and Wildlife Sanctuary, AR, USA

Christopher Stremme
Elephant Health Care Program (EHCP) of the Veterinary Society for Sumatran Wildlife Conservation (Vesswic), Sumatra, Indonesia

Dennis Schmitt
WilliamH. Darr School of Agriculture, Missouri State University, Springfield, MO, USA
Ringling Bros. Center for Elephant Conservation, Polk City, FL, USA

Thaddeus Miller
University of North Texas Health Science Center, Fort Worth, TX, USA

Magda Patricia Carrillo, Nhora María Martinez, María del Pilar Patiño and Carlos Arturo Iregui
Pathobiology Group, Laboratory of Veterinary Pathology, Faculty of Veterinary Medicine and Zootechnics, National University of Colombia, Bogotá D.C., Colombia

Anu Rahal, Atul Prakash and Rajesh Mandil
Department of Veterinary Pharmacology and Toxicology, Uttar Pradesh Pandit Deen Dayal Upadhyaya Pashu Chikitsa Vigyan Vishwavidyalaya Evam Go-Anusandhan Sansthan (DUVASU), Mathura 281001, India

Abul Hasan Ahmad
Department of Veterinary Pharmacology and Toxicology, Govind Ballabh Pant University of Agriculture & Technology, Pantnagar 263145, India

Aruna T. Kumar
Directorate of Information and Publications of Agriculture, KAB-I, New Delhi 110012, India

Nektarios D. Giadinis, Vasiliki Papanikolopoulou, Evi Ioannidou and Harilaos Karatzias
Clinic of Farm Animals, Faculty of Veterinary Medicine, Aristotle University, 546 27Thessaloniki, Greece

Elias Papadopoulos, Sofia Karanikola and Anastasia Diakou
Laboratory of Parasitology and Parasitic Diseases, Faculty of Veterinary Medicine, Aristotle University, 541 24 Thessaloniki, Greece

Shawkat Q. Lafi
Department of Pathology and Animal Health, Faculty of Veterinary Medicine, Jordan University of Science and Technology, P.O. Box 3030, Irbid, Jordan

Vergos Vergidis
National Veterinary Laboratory, 69100 Komotini, Greece

Lihua Xiao
Division of Foodborne, Waterborne and Environmental Diseases, Centers for Disease Control and Prevention, Atlanta, GA, USA

M. C. Mason, J. Copeland and E. J. Cuadra
Department of Agriculture, Alcorn State University, 1000 ASU Drive No. 750, Alcorn State, Lorman, MS 39096, USA

T. H. Elsasser
Bovine Functional Genomics Laboratory Beltsville Agricultural Center, USDA ARS, Beltsville, MD 20705, USA

Y. Jung
Cooperative Agricultural Research Center, Prairie View A&M University, P.O. Box 519, AGRL No. 112, Prairie View, TX, USA

J. Larson
Department of Animal and Dairy Sciences, Mississippi State University, Mississippi State, MS 39762, USA

Zita Talamonti, Chiara Cassis, Paola G. Brambilla, Paola Scarpa, Damiano Stefanello, Simona Cannas, Michela Minero and Clara Palestrini
Università degli Studi di Milano, Dipartimento di Scienze Veterinarie e Sanitá Pubblica (DIVET), Via Celoria 10, 20133Milan, Italy

Karen A.Moriello
Department of Medical Sciences, School of Veterinary Medicine, University of Wisconsin-Madison, 2015 Linden Drive West, Madison, WI 53706, USA

Umar Nazir Zahid
Department of Animal Husbandry, Jammu and Kashmir 190019, India

Swaran Singh Randhawa, Syed Ashaq Hussain and Kirti Dua
Department of Veterinary Medicine, Guru Angad Dev Veterinary and Animal Sciences University, Ludhiana, Punjab 141004, India

Sarnarinder Singh Randhawa
Guru Angad Dev Veterinary and Animal Sciences University, Ludhiana, Punjab 141004, India

Vishal Mahajan
Animal Disease Research Centre, Guru Angad Dev Veterinary and Animal Sciences University, Ludhiana, Punjab 141004, India

Felipe Penagos Tabares, Juliana V. Bedoya Jaramillo and Zulma Tatiana Ruiz-Cortés
Biogenesis Research Group, Agrarian Sciences Faculty, University of Antioquia, Medellin, Colombia

Gbemisola Magaret Olabanji, Beatty Viv Maikai, and Gbeminiyi Richard Otolorin
Department of Veterinary Public Health and Preventive Medicine, Faculty of Veterinary Medicine, Ahmadu Bello University, Zaria, Kaduna State, Nigeria

Arunee Thanasarasakulpong, Weerapongse Tangjitjaroen, Thanya Varinrak and Nattawooti Sthitmatee
Faculty of Veterinary Medicine, Chiang Mai University, Chiang Mai 50100, Thailand

Pichayanut Poolperm and Takuo Sawada
Laboratory of Veterinary Microbiology, Nippon Veterinary and Life Science University, Tokyo 180-8602, Japan

Dirk Pfeiffer
Faculty of Veterinary Medicine, Chiang Mai University, Chiang Mai 50100, Thailand
Veterinary Epidemiology, Economics and Public Health Group, Royal Veterinary College, London AL9 7TA, UK

Sabrina Destri Emmerick Campos and Nádia Regina Pereira Almosny
Departamento de Patologia e Clínica Veterinária, Universidade Federal Fluminense, 24230-340 Niterói, RJ, Brazil

Nathalie Costa da Cunha
Departamento de Saúde Coletiva Veterinária e Saúde Pública, Universidade Federal Fluminense, 24230-340 Niterói, RJ, Brazil

www.ingramcontent.com/pod-product-compliance
Lightning Source LLC
Chambersburg PA
CBHW080507200326
41458CB00012B/4119